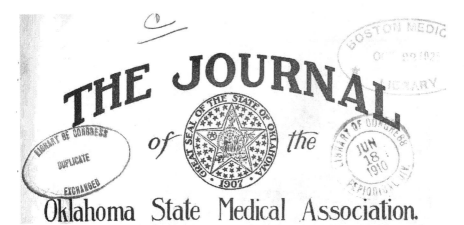

THE JOURNAL of the Oklahoma State Medical Association.

VOL. III NO. 1.   JUNE, 1910.   ANNUAL SUBSCRIPTION $1.00

PUBLISHED MONTHLY AT MUSKOGEE, OKLAHOMA, UNDER DIRECTION OF THE COUNCIL.

INDEX:

Address of the President, Dr. W. C. Bradford, Shawnee, Okla. 1

Surgical Section, Chairman's Address, Dr. Charles Blickensderfer, Shawnee, Okla. 5

Section on Pediatrics, Chairman's Address, Dr. H. M. Williams, Wellston, Okla. 8

Section on Pathology, Chairman's Address, Dr. Elizabeth Melvin, Guthrie, Okla. 11

The Need of Simplicity and Conciseness in the Practice of Medicine, Chairman's Address, Section on General Medicine, R. H. Harper, M. D., Afton Okla. 13

Supra-Pubic Prostatectomy, By F. W. Noble, M. D., Guthrie, Okla. 16

Some New Orleans Clinics, By V. Berry, M. D., Okmulgee, Okla. 22

The Eighteenth Annual Meeting of the Oklahoma State Medical Association, Tulsa, Okla., May 10, 11 and 12, 1910 24

Personal 29

Editorial 29

County Societies 30

Officers of the Association, Councillors, and Delegates to American Medical Association, 1911-1912... 31

Roster of Membership 31

Officers of County Societies 42

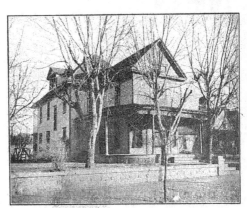

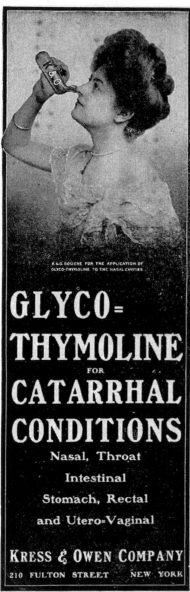
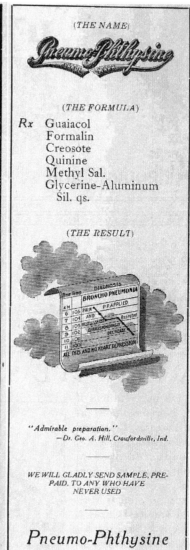

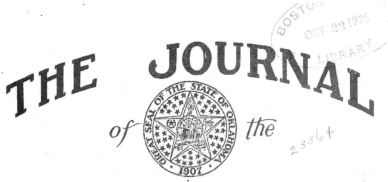

Oklahoma State Medical Association.

VOL. III.   MUSKOGEE, OKLAHOMA, JUNE, 1910.   NO. 1

DR. CLAUDE A. THOMPSON, Editor-in-Chief.

ASSOCIATE EDITORS AND COUNCILLORS.

DR. J. A. WALKER, Shawnee.   DR. JOHN W. DUKE, Guthrie.
DR. CHARLES R. HUME, Anadarko.   DR. A. B. FAIR, Frederick.
DR. F. R. SUTTON, Bartlesville.   DR. W. G. BLAKE, Tahlequah.
DR. I. W. ROBERTSON, Dustin.   DR. H. P. WILSON, Wynnewood.
DR. J. S. FULTON, Atoka.   DR. J. H. BARNES, Enid.

Entered at the Postoffice at Muskogee, Oklahoma, as second class mail matter, June, 1909.

This is the Official Journal of the Oklahoma State Medical Association. All communications should be addressed to the Journal of the Oklahoma State Medical Association, English Block, Muskogee, Oklahoma.

ADDRESS OF THE PRESIDENT

DR. W. C. BRADFORD, SHAWNEE, OKLAHOMA

As it is in accordance with precedent, and the authority vested in the office which you have chosen me to fill, it is my privilege to say a few words of greeting and I take this opportunity of expressing my appreciation of the great honor accorded me by your selection as president of the Oklahoma State Association for the past year. We are again assembled in annual meeting in this wonderful city and have received a most cordial welcome. Another year has passed and it finds the Oklahoma State Medical Association advancing, keeping pace with the wonderful improvement and development of the great New State of Oklahoma. But the present organization is but a beginning. We must further the interests of this association, leaving in the background petty politics and sectional differences and harmoniously pursue our labors in the perfecting of this useful organization, for a lack of unity will prevent us from gaining and maintaining the pre-eminent position to which we are entitled and upholding the dignity of a noble calling. The aim and end of the true physician's life is to bring health, happiness and comfort to the individual, the community, the world. To do this there is no avocation that demands a closer unity.

Heretofore we have failed to secure the support of the masses to the much needed sanitary reforms, because we have had to appeal to them as one individual to another without the weight of organization. They appreciate the saving of a human life which is near to death's door, by the skilful physician, but fail to appreciate the priceless jewels of preventive medicine and sanitary science.

The first great aim of the physician should be to take care of the sick, the next great work to teach the people how to live and prevent disease.

The great American Medical Association, of which we are a component part, having as its unit the county society, has done much to assist us, especially through the zeal of Dr. J. N. McCormack, who will be with us again this year and we hail his coming. For through his plan of public meeting and public instruction on preventive medicine and general sanitary matters, especially through the latter, great good has come. It is indeed time for the public to be taken into our confidence, for if we expect better results, we must enlighten the people. General sanitary matters of great importance are becoming understood through medical influence. The public is being educated in regard to the Great White Plague. Much good has been accomplished along this line by the Oklahoma Medical Association. Dr. H. H. Williams, appointed chairman of the Committee on Tuberculosis at our last annual meeting, has succeeded in organizing an Oklahoma Society for the Study and Prevention of Tuberculosis. Also throughout the state similar county societies have been organized and great good has been accomplished. The Exhibit No. 2, of the National Society for the Study and Prevention of Tuberculosis has exhibited in several cities of our State, and in each place it has received the support of the county society in which it was held, assisting in the public lectures and demonstrations. At each place the attendance and interest was beyond expectation. At Shawnee over eight thousand were in attendance during the ten days of the exhibition. I hope to see as much more accomplished during the coming year and commend the zeal of Doctor Williams for the past good service. The statistics of the State I am sure will show the effects of the diffusion of this knowledge.

Typhoid fever, another preventable disease is becoming better understood through medical influences, but there is room for improvement, and I hope the time will come when one who has been infected with typhoid fever from a city's neglect will have the same cause for damages as he who has fallen through a defective sidewalk and sustained a personal injury.

We must also teach the people of the great good which has resulted from the study of the habits of the mosquito, the short distance they fly from breeding places, and the short distance they fly without shelter, also the necessity of quarantining of malaria and yellow fever which they carry.

Thousands of deaths per annum, almost the sacrifice of an army daily, are caused by polluted water, impure and adulterated food and drugs, epidemics, and various preventable diseases, unclean cities and bad sanitation, which attest to the fact that the lessons have not been learned. Our Republican form of government affords individual freedom which many times interferes with and delays much needed legislation, with the result that many times that by the time the law can be passed, the immediate object to be attained has disappeared, the delays and changes caused by the ignorant through prejudice. This must be overcome.

In Germany vaccination has practically caused small-pox to disappear from the nation. But during the epidemic of small-pox through some of our Oklahoma cities this winter, a vociferous band of anti-vaccination agitators made life miserable for our health officers, consequently numerous cases and deaths from a preventable disease.

The building of the Panama canal will do much to educate our people along sanitary lines, for much publicity has been given to that portion of the work, the value of which is proven. The doctor made possible the building of the Panama canal—made the canal zone the most sanitary place in Latin America and the public realizes it. Medical science has also reduced the death rates from disease in the late wars, especially the Japanese-Russian war, to such an enormous extent that it also demanded public attention, and for the first time in history did bullets kill more men than disease, which was true in the Japanese army.

The discovery of the transmission of malaria and yellow fever by the mosquito, and of bubonic plague by the rat and ground squirrel has been a great boon to humanity, made possible by organization, regulation and education. Organized medicine has indeed done well, yet it is not hard to see a brighter future and the stamping out of all infectious and contagious diseases.

Another matter to consider is medical education. There is no place in the world where so many different systems of healing are practiced as in the United States. No place in the world has so many medical schools. We need a higher standard of requirement, and more and better supervision of medical schools. We need less schools and better ones, where less doctors are made and better ones. The Council on Medical Education of the American Medical Association, in which we have one representative, is working hard and has shown good results and we hope in the near future will show better ones.

I hope that organization will obliterate those imaginary state lines with regard to medical licensing and give us the individual freedom we should enjoy. We all live under the same constitution and belong to the same great Medical Association. Why not the examining boards adopt a more uniform examination and reciprocity. There is just one reason and that is, State laws. But we must look to this and not drop back a notch, as we did in Oklahoma.

We must not forget our relations to insurance companies, corporations and lodges. There is still an occasional insurance company asking members of the Pottawatomie County Medical Society to reduce their fees for examinations, as I suppose they do in other counties. Most of them, however, are paying a fair fee, and less should not be accepted. If this is done by all counties they will soon mend their ways. Lodge practice is a growing menace. Various lodges collect dues to give medical services at a low figure below the possible point for a professional man to live and continue his education. They will continue and grow unless condemned by the medical profession as they should be. The people are badly served, as competent physicians cannot be secured to do the work. Occasionally a lodge of this kind is organized in Pottawatomie County, but there are no lodge physicians in our county. There should not be one in Oklahoma, and I hope there is not. This brings to my mind the financial side of a doctor's life—the adjustment of which is a mighty problem, for it is a notorious fact that the doctor is a poor collector, a bad investor and a rainbow chaser. Yet his finances should be managed well. He owes it first to his family, second to the profession, and last, but not least, to the community at large. He must do so if he expects to pursue his studies and care for his patrons as he should. He does not need to be rich, for money interferes with the highest aims of a physician, and few of wealth have reached distinction. Money should not be the standard of success, but he should have a fair competence, and be free to pursue his labors. I know of none who have been burdened with wealth from the practice of medicine alone. Perhaps 'tis better so, but a due reward for our labor and skill is both right and desirable.

Beside money we must acquire knowledge, not only in college and in the medical school, but all through life. Here let me urge you to lay broad and deep foundations.

"Drink deep of the Pyerian spring,
   Or touch not at all,
For shallow drafts intoxicate the brain
   While drinking deeper sobers us again."

The superstructure can never be imposing unless the foundation be solid, yet the foundation is but the beginning of the structure, so graduation from a college is but the commencement of a life study of medicine. Graduation from a medical school is but a part of the foundation. In the practice of our profession the student days are never over. There are new and fundamental truths which follow each other so rapidly that we have scarcely been able to digest them, while before there was so much to be learned that a long and industrious life leaves us but a beginner, therefore we should have the reading habit, and the medical society habit. Lucky, indeed, is he who lives within easy access to a well organized medical society. If he ever does he will not live where there is not one. If there is not one where he is, he will organize one. The County Medical Society organized under the A. M. A. plan, as a unit of that organization and has done much, not only in stimulating scientific research through their post graduate courses, but in elevating the standard of medical ethics, assisting the health officers in enforcing the laws, and teaching the public the value of preventive medicine and sanitary science, and the application of the same. It is becoming a great organization and is becoming better every year.

Another important matter is your postgraduate work. Make frequent trips to the medical centers for the purpose of observation and studying with men who have gained reputation in special lines of work. In no other way can we avoid getting into a rut which limits our usefulness.

It has been customary for the retiring president to recommend to the association some lines of action which he deems of importance. I have given the matter careful study, and find that I have but very little to suggest at this time. However, I suggest that the Oklahoma State Association use every effort in assisting the Secretaries and councillors' societies. The county secretary is the life of his county society. The organization and the success of its scientific program depend upon him. The councillors hold practically the same position with regard to their district. The councillors and secretaries are the organizers of the State Association. I believe that the importance of this society, cannot be overestimated, and believe if well organized, will make the Oklahoma State Medical Association one of the greatest Medical associations of the United States. I therefore recommend that we assume the expenses of said society.

I also suggest that the Association investigate the physician's liability insurance. In several State Associations and county societies insurance has been furnished the members at a rate far below the cost of such protection were bought from corporations, in such business. I believe this idea is a good one.

Many Eastern cities are prohibiting the sale of fireworks and the Fourth of July casualties have been greatly reduced. I believe we should insist on the enactment of prohibitive regulations in this state.

Many socities are raising funds to alleviate the suffering of any of the profession who are unfortunate. I believe that we should do likewise.

With these few suggestions I will close my remarks, asking you at all times to strive for the honor and dignity of our profession, remembering that organization is the spirit of the times, and in this Association, we must have harmonious organization.

SURGICAL SECTION, CHAIRMAN'S ADDRESS

DR. CHARLES BLICKENSDERFER, SHAWNEE, OKLAHOMA

The stability of all government, national, state or municipal is dependent upon the following conditions:

First. The topography and geographical situation of its territory.

Second. Physical and mental vigor, and ample facilities for the proper education of its people.

Third. The maintenance of the health and integrity of its population unit.

The first of these influence to a great extent the remainder, since the topography governs, greatly, both the products of a country and transportation facilities for same, and the general commercial intercourse of contiguous nations. The topographical outlines, as well as the geographical location of a country, govern to a great extent, the physical development of the inhabitant and the cost of raising an individual from infancy to manhood. The first proposition is one over which we have no control, except in a minor degree, exemplified by the changes wrought by the construction of railroad, tunnels and canals, facilitating transportation and bringing into closer communication contiguous territories widely removed by natural barriers; the building of irrigation canals and dams increasing natural products, lowering the cost of maintenance and reducing to a minimum, so far as that feature is concerned the cost of raising a healthy human being from infancy to manhood, or, to a point where it will be self-sustaining. By way of comparison, it has been estimated that to raise an individual from infancy to adult age along the Nile during the early history of Egypt, cost approximately $14.00. The occupation of such a fertile country, places its people in possession of the most important requisite for becoming a great and enduring nation, provided that proper heed is given to the other requisites representing national stability.

Our racial types must be moulded to the highest physical development consistent with their possibilities. The physique and individual ideas of national and personal independence are in exact conformity with the natural surroundings of the individual concerned, being modified only by the mental emanations of tradition and the impress of racial or international intercourse. This feature was forcibly brought to the attention of Caesar during his conquest of Gaul. However, the physical development of members of communities can be largely controlled by proper attention to physiological requirements and should go hand in hand with the mental growth of each, for it cannot be expected to maintain mental entities of great functional capacity whose only support is a poorly developed and insufficiently nourished body.

The means of educating its young should be ample and along lines calculated to make the recipient a self reliant, self sustaining, productive member of society. This feature of his education appeals with great force to the State. But the knowledge of physical, physiological, natural and other scientific phenomena are more essential to national and personal welfare than if the "self-sustaining, self-reliant, productive social unit," the "human automaton," guided and controlled by influences and conditions wholly beyond his sphere of knowledge and power of reasoning, and whose only objective in life is animal comfort and competency. That this is true there can be no question, for whether an individual engages in manual labor with the object of an actual production of the material commodities, or confines his efforts along lines of professional activity, a scientific knowledge of the right sort is equally essential.

Knowledge.

Educational features, in order to be of the greatest benefit to the race, must be common property, widely disseminated, and bestowed with the object of securing for all life, physical and intellectual progression, proportionately commensurate with the progression of our planetary existence.

The maintenance of the health integrity of the population unit naturally occupies the third place in this discussion, not because of its relative unimportance, for all are equally important,—but because without the necessary knowledge of matter and its forces, referred to in the hypothesis, the maintenance of the health of a community would be a matter of instinctive results, whose variations would be subject to the wide fluctuations incident to the lives of the ignorant in densely or sparsely populated districts.

Nations and individuals, whether they will or no, must soon suffer extinction, or engage with the greatest energy of purpose in the struggle for the survival of the fittest, natural evidence of which are shown by the vast sums of money expended annually in the building of navies and fortifications. In a large sense of the word, we are all creatures of circumstances, in that according to our geographical location we are compelled to adapt ourselves to the conditions, climatic and otherwise, resulting from topographical inequalities, latitude and other physical phenomena, of our planetary location. The ability to thus accommodate oneself to prevailing conditions is instinctive in all animals and is also in conformity with the natural evolutional progression of all species from the simplest to the most complex forms of organic life.

From the evolutional point of view, this feature of life is exemplified in the development of the ovum—a cell, which of necessity is similar in structure and physiological functions to itself—but which, during its growth and development into the human body gives the phenomenon known as "cell differentiation," the final resultant being, cells endowed with the ability to perform specific functions. Therefore, if man or other animal, from the moment of his conception, has developed along lines influenced by conditions compelling anotomical and physiological necessities to the performance of certain functions, the instinctive performance of somewhat similar functions of the organism as a whole is not so difficult of comprehension.

As an example of the adaptability of organized life to surrounding conditions, may be mentioned the whale, illustrating to a high degree animal adaptability to local or general conditions. During the earlier stages of his life history, the whale was a land animal, but the inroads of the seas upon the land areas, cutting off his food supplies from that quarter, and the never ceasing relentless attacks of his natural enemies, compelled him to take to the seas, both as a matter of bodily protection and a means of obtaining an adequate food supply. In support of this view, we find the whale today a mammal, not a fish, the young being born and suckled as are other mammals, having lungs similar in structure and function as other land animals and like them also, compelled to breathe air.

Illustrating cell differentiation, we may mention the flattened horny cells of the outer skin and those of the cornea, whose chief function is protection; the ciliated epithelial cells of the thachea, whose chief function is the continuous removal of small foreign bodies, and the various active or secreting cells of the different glandular structures, whose functions are the production of the varied secretions of the body, and many others.

A sober consideration of this phase of our existence suggests not only a possibility but also a probability, that our lives have been, and are yet influenced and moulded more by these instinctive and extraneous circumstances than by a proper reference to those forces, such as reason and other mental faculties, the products of cerebral activity.

There can be no question but that knowledge and its proper application comprehends the worldly salvation of all living things. Booker T. Washington recognized that in education lay the salvation of the negro, and for this alone he deserved the everlasting gratitude of all his people, for what bondage can be more hateful than that of ignorance? These things being true, it is but natural to infer that our intellectual development is but scarcely begun. What vast possibilities must there not be for our future mental development if we but see to it, instead of catering to the more sordid desires of minds weakened by the insufficient support of diseased bodies, poorly nourished and wrecked by dissipation.

There must be foundations of force representing the greatest potentiality lying unexplored and dormant in our brains to-day, that are only awaiting development. When we consider the extent to which our lives and body functions are controlled by hereditary instinctive influences, the possibilities offered by the proper attention to intellectual requirements appeal illimitable.

Nature has been kind, generous, profligate, even wasteful in her labors that man might exist. The stupendous energies of her forces exercised in the aggregation of the mass and the setting in motion of the planetary bodies of our solar system, as resulted in but one, the earth, and perhaps Mars also, being so situated as to support life. A comparison of mass between Earth and the others, with man as the crowning point of her labors, establishes an equation which can only be satisfied by adding to the small organic representation an intellectuality of the highest conceivable order. To say that we are totally uneducated, or that our mental faculties are altogether untrained is manifestly untrue. But the trouble is, that our intellectual training is in the main based upon false premises. This becomes evident at once when we but consider the object of our education. Apparently they are for the sole purpose and object of increasing the wealth, social or political preferment of the recipient. The ultimate result is attained in the satisfaction enjoyed by a knowledge of the personal possession of these. It has been a characteristic of humanity to reach the goal, scientific or otherwise, by the most circuitous and indirect routes. As an example may be mentioned the telegraph and wireless telegraphy. Hundreds of examples corroborative of this statement, relative to this phase of our intellectual divergence may be cited. Paradoxical as it may seem, this only serves to show the inherent ability of the mind of man to ably work out the problems representing the results of cause and effect.

Our mental development has not yet reached such proportions enabling it to compete with animal instinct, for comparisons show that the latter at various times in the history of man has served to save him from total destruction, in that the compelling forces of nature impelled him to the most agreeable acceptances of her turn under distressing conditions which to recover from no doubt cost him many years or even cycles of time to effect, only to again accept equally discouraging terms because of a lack of intellectual development sufficient to enable him to take advantage of the situation. We therefore, do not wish to disparage the many virtues of instinct since it represents the natural, ever-present and ever ready escape from natural consequences.

But we do agree the cultivation of those higher psycological entities which when developed will enable man to scientifically cope with the natural and ever-changing problem with which he is daily confronted without a blind reference to his inherited animal instincts.

Through the channels of "public economy" we are caring for an ever-increasing number of insane, imbeciles and other types of incapacitated individuals the ultimate effect of which is to detract from the moral, physical and mental standards of the supporting class and to impoverish the producing supporters of such institutions both by example and by the divergence of funds that should be applied to racial and intellectual progression.

Under existing conditions these burdens will finally become unbearable and no adequate result will obtain.

Our highest examples of Art today are copies of those reproductions of the high types of physical man and womanhood brought about by the rigid and scarce selection of species during the early history of Sparta and Greece. The larger share of expense in the legal administration of all forms of government are directed to the suppression or holding in subjection the unnatural or harmful propensities of the race.

A generous proportion of this expense in time and treasure with a view of enlightening man along lines leading to his perpetuity as an unimpaired physical human unit will no doubt suffice to accomplish the desired end,—Health, long life and happiness.

SECTION ON PEDIATRICS, CHAIRMAN'S ADDRESS

DR. H. M. WILLIAMS, WELLSTON, OKLAHOMA

In discussing the subject of pediatrics, we are compelled, to a very large extent, to deal with the popular ignorance of the masses, as to hygiene and preventive medicine, and the care of those who are sick. And many cases of wide spread evils are placed beyond the power of the medical profession because of this existing condition.

The hygienic surroundings, the poorly nourished, these conditions together with the low resisting powers of the average child, make them the popular field for the invasion of numerous, bacteriological germs and parasitical organisms.

If the edict could but go forth that would compel all, who are responsible for the welfare, of those depending upon them, to require those responsible to not only acquire a practical knowledge of the above subject matter, but were made responsible for their proper application; it would be but a short time until the death rate would be reduced to the minimum among children. As a rule, the branch of medicine confined to the study of diseases of children, does not find the popularity among our profession, as do many other branches in our line of work; yet as to the actual results we offer no apology, when we say it ranks second to no other branch in importance. The competent physician, will make a more accurate diagnosis because he is required to make a careful examination, in order to arrive at his conclusion, and not rely upon the statements of the patient, who may have formed an erroneous idea as to his ailments, and thus give many imaginary symptoms to his physician, with a possibility of misguiding him.

It is not an uncommon occurrence in reviewing the recent advances made in our profession, to overlook the subject. There is no field, in which advances in both surgery and medicine are being more practically applied, than that of the diseases of children, within recent years rapid strides have been made in diagnosis; hygiene and preventive medicine, though not attained the highest standard in prefection are, to-day receiving more consideration, and given more prominence than at any previous period, therapeutic agents have revolutionized. Recent bacteriological developments have aided much in the line of diagnosis and prognosis, also added to our line of treatment in the infectious diseases.

The progress in infant feeding; the sterilization of food, prevention of sale of impure milk, laws prohibiting the sale of impure milk; have in a large measure done more for the prevention of spreading of disease than any other advancement made in recent years.

The hygienic condition of public buildings, schools, streets and alleys. The water supply, when carefully looked after, the sewerage disposals, the careful and thorough methods now employed in disinfecting houses, that have been occupied by those who have been suffering with contagious or infectious diseases; the enforcement of more strict quarantine laws; compulsory vaccination, when threatened with an epidemic of small-pox; public bath houses; all have had a marked benefit over that of former years, and many complaints

among children, that were at one time commonly seen, are now rarely met with; rickets, that were once so common, are scarcely seen; cretinism, that until recent years was considered hopeless, is now successfully treated. A comparison of the method of the treatment of diptheria by the use of the anti-toxin, of today; with the vague method of twenty years ago, has largely reduced the death rate.

Tuberculosis is now diagnosed early, and if the glands or extremeties are affected, the affected parts are promptly removed. If the skin or some of the vital organs are affected, the child is promptly placed on the proper road to recovery; when but a few years ago, the case was consigned to those of the hopelessly incurable, without, in many instances, as much as making an effort to give the child a chance for his life.

The indefinite and radiating pains that children frequently have, at one time were called growing pains, for the lack of the proper knowledge as to their cause; are now carefully studied, and in most cases a proper diagnosis is made, and we are able in the majority of cases to give effective relief and the term growing pains is now rarely found in the Doctor's vocabulary.

The medical inspection of the public schools is a means of cutting short an inestimable number of diseases, as well as prolonging the life of scores of children. Permitting them to develop into men and women with stronger minds and bodies, and thus building up a race of people who will be of greater use to our nation. The dull pupil instead of being punished by his teacher, as was once the custom, is now referred to a medical authority who carefully seeks out the cause, if found to be physical defect, this condition is corrected; not unfrequently it is the case in the larger cities, that the dullness is due to the lack of sufficient nourishment. By the above process children are found to be suffering with complaints of which the parents are wholly ignorant, and if not corrected early in life would be a permanent infliction.

Enlarged tonsils, polypus, and adenoid growths, which furnish rich fields for both infectious and contagious disease, are early removed; diseases of the middle ear are successfully treated; deficient eye sight is corrected; the teeth, when found to be in bad condition, are treated, as from this source, gastro-intestinal troubles are frequently set up.

Surgery is doing much for children; congentel-hip joint disease is now taken to the orthopedist and the bloodless operation done, and we are saved the sight of being confronted with the neglected hip-joint disease; at an unestimable benefit to the patient. Club footed children are now successfully treated at an early age and we now seldom see such deformities.

Much has been done along the line of reforms in child labor problem. We are able to study physical development by means of the X-Ray. The labor the child is placed at can be judged better from his development than from his age, as often children of the same age have a vast difference in development. This growth can be observed by this means.

The field of therapeutics has, in a very large measure, been improved practically as well as palitably. For the administration of remedies, vehicles have been found, and we can now eliminate the nausea and bitterness of drugs of former years, thus insuring a more prompt compliance with the doctor's orders, and better results in the end. In no line of medicine has serum therapy a more extensive and practicable use than in that of treating the diseases of children.

We endeavor to point out some of the more important advances that have been made during recent years to aid the better-

ment of the condition of children, yet there remains much to be done in our line in order to place this section of medicine upon that high plane, which should be accorded such an important branch.

By a careful study of the table of mortality of infancy and childhood, we find the death rate exceedingly high. A comparison of the death rate of our larger cities, since the rigid enforcement of pure food laws and stricter hygienic measures, has, in a large measure, reduced the per cent. of deaths among children. While these laws have done much for the cities; the towns, villages and rural districts have been neglected, and much work remains to be done by the advocates of pure milk, and hygienic laws.

We are told by Dr. Holt, "The physical development of the child is essentially the product of three factors—inheritance, surroundings, and food. The first of these is beyond the physicians power to alter; the second largely, and the third entirely within his control, at least in the more intelligent society." He concludes with the statement that, "Infant hygiene and infant feeding are the most important departments of Pediatrics." While in one sense it is true that the problem of inheritance is beyond the control of the physician, especially is it true of this present generation, but the physician, could in a large measure be of considerable service to those yet unborn.

The people should be educated to the consequence of married life, those who have contracted disease that would be injurious to their offspring, should be frankly informed and advised against marrriage, until absolutely cured of such physical ailments. It certainly would be the means of reducing the death rate to a great extent preventing much suffering and poverty, if all applicants for marriage license were required to present a certificate of good health before such license were issued.

The law of inheritance is an old law, and was evidently known to the ancient, as to who had sinned, the child or parent, for in the time of Christ, we find reference in case of one who was born blind.

If we expect to have strong and healthy children, we must see to it that the parents are strong and healthy; free from all diseases; for as certain as night follows day, that certain will an undeveloped and physically defected child be the result of a diseased parentage.

More advice should be given to one who is to be a mother. During this period of the expected mothers life, for lack of proper knowledge and care, the indulgence in intemperate habits, is often the cause of physical defects.

As to surroundings and food, the physician can aid much in the enforcement of our sanitary laws, by being a constant advocate of better hygienic conditions, and rigid enforcement of pure food laws. And in case that the law is not sufficient, he will be a strong factor in securing better laws if he will only lend his assistance.

In conclusion it is the opinion that no field of medicine offers a greater opportunity of reducing the mortality, than that of pediatrics. Let us by our work and earnest efforts, try and eliminate that erroneous idea held by many of the laity, that the doctor can not do much for the infants and children when sick; instead let us demonstrate that nowhere are results more satisfactorily accomplished.

It will require earnest and conscientious efforts on our part to advance the subject of children in the next twenty years, as it has in the past, let us give our best efforts and we shall be crowned with success.

SECTION ON PATHOLOGY, CHAIRMAN'S ADDRESS

DR. ELIZABETH MELVIN, GUTHRIE, OKLAHOMA

It is indeed a pleasure to be permitted to address this section in the capacity of chairman and I trust that there may be a bond of sympathy among all members and affilliates of this section throughout the meeting. I am sure you all realize the enormous difficulties which have confronted us, but I dare say the pioneer members of any similar section could tell the same story. No one recognizes more keenly than I, the shortcomings of the work this year,—how could it be otherwise when "dux femina facti?" However, we may flatter ourselves, that if we have not gained, at least we have not lost ground.

It is hard, sometimes, to realize that a small and seemingly unimportant section like ours is potentially the strongest in the Association and that its weakness or strength will serve as an indicator to the outside world of the importance of our state organization. As an observer is apt to measure the strength of a community by the number of its factories, its public buildings, its schools and the general progressiveness of its people, so the outside medical fraternity is apt to gauge the standing of the science and art of medicine in a city or state by the number of equipment of its laboratories. The recent graduate can remember enough of his laboratory training to do very creditable work for a while, and if there are several such in a town, each will doubtless fit up a tiny working place called by courtesy a laboratory; but as the practice and responsibilities of each increase, they find that such work absorbs too much time so they may concentrate on one man who shows a fondness or aptitude for such work, or they import someone from the outside. When a number of such persons are established in the work round about the state, they come together and form themselves into a section where they may exchange ideas for mutual benefit. The process is thus seen to be evolutionary. The sections on medicine and surgery were founded first, as they should be, for, in the primitive community, when a patient is found to have a chill, the all-important thing is to give him quinine and hope for results—not wait to import a pathologist from a neighboring state to find out if the malarial parasite is present.

The farther we go from empiricism and crudeness, the more important the pathologist comes to be.

In the present state of our development, it really seems, sometimes, as if a pathologist is looked upon as an expensive luxury and is called upon only when every available clinician has failed to make a diagnosis. Obviously, this is unfair. The physician and surgeon should regard the pathologist as his best friend, and as an invaluable adjunct to his diagnostic resources. The criterion of a clinician's knowledge is his ability rightly to interpret laboratory findings; while the ideal pathologist does not lose sight of the clinical side, but knows a reason for everything that comes to light in his test tube, or in the field of his microscope. The two working hand in hand, have almost occult powers, utterly incomprehensible to the one or the other working alone.

When the surgeon realizes that the pathologist is no less necessary to him than his anesthetist; when the internist learns to rely on the laboratory man equally with his favorite fever nurse, then we shall see a broader and a more profound awakening in scientific medicine.

If Edison's definition of genius, the infinite capacity for taking pains, could be taken literally, every conscientious laboratory worker would by virtue of his calling, measure up to the requirement; for pathological and bacteriological work is detail work from its very nature. The smaller and more obscure the object in view, the greater the liability for error the more thorough the safeguards which must be thrown about the process.

The foundation of a laboratory worker's equipment is, of course, knowledge of his subject. On this, volumes might be written but it may be passed with a word; and that, that knowledge depends first of all upon opportunity and comes with interest in the subject. The superstructure on which he builds is technique. Here the opportunities are almost unlimited and far from being mechanical and void of interest, technique in the laboratory is fascinating and always offers infinite range for originality. Even in imitative work there is satisfaction in the attaining of a certain standard better than someone's else, which is comparable to the feeling which a musician experiences when he feels that he has surpassed his rivals. In fact, the scientific man who loves his work is an artist, no less than the man who paints a landscape or one who excels in Shakesperean repertoire. I have seen the same absorbed, reverent expression on the face of a man working with solutions and pipettes, as may come on the face of a man working on canvass or the violin; and when he sees light ahead, saying, "I really think we have something good here" the exaltation is the same. Even, again in imitative work, the finding of an elusive bacterium or the diagnosing of a puzzling section, brings with it a sensation decidedly pleasurable.

The temptations are here, also, to run into fads, not to speak of ruts, to become infatuated with following one man's methods. One can guard against this by giving close attention to many methods, selecting those most suitable to his needs and being always open to conviction and on the look-out for better ways of doing things.

The coming year should see greater improvement along this line in this state. The general practitioner can no longer give as an excuse that there are no laboratory facilities available and the day is coming when the man who neither knows enough to employ a pathologist, nor cares to give his patient the benefit of such diagnostic aid will be left behind in the onward rush.

I think it would be an excellent plan for the members of this section to keep in touch with each other during the year, and give each other the benefit of such experience as may be useful. Hitherto we have all remained in heathen darkness as to what the others are doing. Do you not agree with me that this would be an incentive to better work and of far-reaching benefit? For my own part, when I find something interesting, I am anxious to tell someone who can understand and rejoice with me. If we had a small, modest bureau of exchange, the element of friendly competition would enter into our work, interest would be stimulated, and, who knows, some one among us might discover something of importance to us all.

In conclusion I wish to thank all who have been kind enough to help me with this program, particularly those who have contributed papers. I urge you to give my successor your united support in the coming year and to will and to do all in your power to make this a worthy section with real force in the Association.

THE NEED OF SIMPLICITY AND CONCISENESS IN THE PRACTICE OF MEDICINE, CHAIRMAN'S ADDRESS, SECTION ON GENERAL MEDICINE

R. H. HARPER, M. D., AFTON, OKLAHOMA

The great problems of life, with its infinite variety of phenomena, present themselves to the physician for a practical application to the conditions of health and disease, and the physical welfare of those who consult him. What constitutes Life, whether it is a concatenation of biological processes that are essentially chemical, or whether there is a methaphysical, suprapysical element, a vital principle involved in those structures that we call living, is a problem whose solution we must leave for those who follow us in the distant future, and whose senses will be more acute, who will possess methods and means of investigation that are unknown to us; for at present we lack both the fineness of sense and the evidence necessary to solve it.

It is but a superficial method to classify matter as living and not living, to say that one possesses life, the other does not; for those properties of matter known to us as gravitation, atomic and molecular force, chemical affinity, electricity, magnetism, heat, light, cohesion, elasticity, are as far beyond the comprehension of the human intelect as are any of the phenomena of that other group which we say are living; and the more we discover of the properties and reactions of living bodies, the more do they seem to be a part of the same molecular and atomic force that is common to all forms of matter.

As an illustration, the process of digestion and assimilation, a vital process, surely, with the disintegration of the food by the gastric and intestinal fluids, the selection and rejection of its component parts by the cells of the mucosa, its transference to distant parts, and its integration as a part of the body, differs, perhaps in no respect from the processes involved in the solution of a number of salts in a liquid, and their re-crystallization, each salt selecting its own molecules and rejecting all others. Even our language or our knowledge or both, are so limited that we use terms implying a degree of consciousness and intelligent action to both the vital and the chemical process, while admitting that the limited amount of knowledge of these phenomena that we possess would lead us to the opposite conclusion. We use, alike in describing a molecular or a vital process such terms as selection and rejection, attraction and repulsion, affinity and incompatibility, imparting to the process that we are attempting to describe, a part of that consciousness of intelligent action that we proudly believe ourselves to possess as a specially favored part of living beings.

But unfortunately, there is no other method within our reach by which the methods of investigation and the conclusions to be deduced therefrom can be expressed. It is to be hoped that in the vast period of time to come, mankind will develop a still higher form of cerebral cells than any that we now possess, enabling the man of the future to perceive structures and processes that we cannot, and to express his thoughts in language as much superior to ours as ours is to the chattering of the denizens of an African jungle. Such a hope is justified by the sublime and awe-inspiring processes of evolution, which, in the course of millions of years has raised us from the primitive forms of the paleozoic period to the infinitely varied and highly organized structures of the present time. and holds forth a promise of reaching ever higher and higher; and then as an anti-climax, to be gradually annihilated by the inevitable end of all life on our earth due to the physical limitations of the solar system and the infinity of time.

But amid these bewildering generalizations there has been established in the course of the ages and by infinite toil, failure, and success, and by the survival of the fittest, a normal and definite arrangement of phenomena common to all bodies, both in the molecular forces of inorganic bodies and in the vital processes of living organisms. This normal condition of equilibrium, of delicate adjustment of internal and external relations of organic structures constitutes the condition of normal life, or health; the action of a foreign or antagonistic factor, with its resulting disturbance of the normal adjustment and the consequent disorder in the mechanism and processes of the organism, we term disease. In different terms, one is a normal, physiological process, the other an abnormal, pathological series of events.

Here appears the chief difference between living and not living bodies; the living body has to a limited extent the faculty of molecular intussusception that we see as growth and repair. The piece of iron reduced to an oxide, is permanently disintegrated, and cannot restore or repair itself, but the organic or living have the innate ability, a seemingly purposeful process, of increasing its bulk as growth, or reconstructing lost parts as repair, and when the normal adjustment of itself to its surroundings is disturbed, to make an effort to return to an equilibrium. This apparently purposeful effort of the living organism to overcome abberrations and to return to a condition of adjustment to its environment, if not a complete adjustment, one in which its functions are performed in a manner approaching the normal, is the central fact to which this paper is devoted. In the human organism, as in all others, this return to the best possible adjustment is often not complete, but may be such as to make life endurable or useful; for it is a common observation that the most useful members of a community are not always those possessed of the highest physical perfections; and it is reiterated that this seeming purpose, this effort, of the organism to regain its normal condition as nearly as possible, and to perform its functions in the manner most suited to its continued existence, is the foundation upon which we base a hopeful prognosis in any case of sickness; if the disturbing factor is not insuperable or overpowering, the readjustment is made without assistance; if it is, we can often help by a judicious course of action.

We shall now consider that we have a human body whose structure we know moderately well, whose physiologic processes are slightly known and but dimly understood, and when perverted by pathologic aberrations, are absolutely bewildering in their infinite variety and complexity, but permeating them all, an endeavor on the part of the organism to return to the normal when disturbed by foreign or external factors. An attempt, more or less intelligent, to assist the body in this effort constitutes the practice of medicine, and a large part of this practice, has been devoted to the introduction of various substances of endless variety and complexity and with properties either unknown or but partially understood, into this human body, with results that are indifferent, often harmful, sometimes beneficial to a very limited extent. The properties and actions of most of our medicines can be studied in the chemical and physiological laboratory; the physiologic processes of the human body can be studied in such a manner only to a very limited extent, and it is attributed to Oliver Wendell Holmes to have said that therapeutics is the art of administering drugs, of which we know little, to a human being, of which we know less, and in the main this aphorism expresses the truth. A few fearless thinkers have proclaimed the futility of giving medicines with the intent to cure disease, but the majority of physicians seems to believe that it can be done, while to the laity the practice of medicine consists in finding the drug that will cure

the disease that is being treated, as attested by the innumerable patent cure-alls on the market, and a large part of the proprietaries offered to the profession are not much better; but the fact remains that with a few possible exceptions drugs have little or no influence on the processes of disease and often hinder the organism in its effort to recover its normal state. The variety of remedies that a physician uses in the treatment of a disease is often in inverse ratio to his knowledge of the causative pathologic processes involved; why are quinine and the antipyretics given to the extent they are in typhoid and pneumonia? Why are three-fourths of the medicines given that are used in any particular illness? Is it not often a failure to comprehend what we may of the processes going on in the sick body, and a concession to the patient, the family, and custom, to be doing something? What more interference does the average case of sickness need than cleaning outside and inside, rest in bed, limited diet, quiet and cheerful surroundings?

Do not think that I am making a plea for therapeutic nihilism; far from it; but I do advocate a deeper study of the fundamental principles of life in general, an intimate conception of physiologic and pathologic processes, a knowledge of the actions and uses of a few of the medicines that have stood the test of trial in the laboratory and at the bedside. The method of the past, and a part of that of the present may be compared to the blunderbuss, flintlock, shotgun, muzzle-loading, noisy, smoky, black powder age of fire arms; that of the scientific physician of the present and the future must be that of the modern high power, effective, smokeless and comparatively noiseless rifle; for a few drugs and the active principles of our best known medicines may be depended upon to give results that are fairly definite, in assisting the organism in its contest with the disturbing factor. These we, may use when a definite end is in view to be attained by their actions.

A summary of the ideas that has been the intent of this paper to express are, to know our patients and their diseases as well as we can; to know our remedies with their good and bad effects, and when we give one, to do so with a clear cut idea as to why and for what it is given, and its effect on the average patient, and not what we *hope* it *may* do for this one; that the effort of the organism is toward recovery, if the disturbing factor is not too great or sudden in its impact.

However, it must remain a fact that as our knowledge of our patients and our time are both limited, we cannot adhere very closely to this line of conduct; but it can be made an ideal toward which we should strive and the methods of attaining a degree of success will depend upon the personality of the physician. Nor should we conceal from our patient but very little if any, of the nature of the disease, its probable course, and the line of treatment, why we do this, or administer that; most people are intelligent enough to assist very materially in the line of action laid down by the doctor if they understand the reasons, they will attach less importance to the medicines, and more to common sense; and in conclusion, straightforward dealing, frankness, honesty, a reasonable explanation of the conditions to the patient and the family, conciseness in our knowledge and simplicity in treatment, is perhaps the ideal conduct in the practice of medicine.

SUPRA-PUBIC PROSTATECTOMY

BY F. W. NOBLE, M. D., GUTHRIE, OKLA., SURGEON TO OKLAHOMA METHODIST HOSPITAL AND FORT SMITH AND WESTERN RAILWAY

(Read before the Central Medical Society, April 12, 1910, at El Reno.)

Prostatectomy has been in the lime-light now for a few years as a proper field for helpful surgery. Yet it is only 10 or 12 years ago that the average surgeon did nothing of this work. His main reliance, in very bad cases where the common catheter or a Mercier catheter could not be used was upon perineal cystotmy with drainage. It will still be some years before the practitioners throughout this country recommend these cases to the surgeon, with the sense of duty performed and conscience satisfied, as is now the case when such practitioners meet with early cases of appendicitis.

Old men, who have successfully lengthened out their lives and eased their sufferings by the use of a catheter, are still pointed out as an example and an excuse for temporizing with these cases, that almost cry out for proper surgical treatment. For the catheter signifies as a rule the end or the beginning of the end. The early surgical treatment of enlarged prostate is a prophylactic as well curative measure; but most men and even doctors still regard prostatectomy as a most desperate remedy. To be used only as the last resort. Whereas it should be considered a prophylactic measure and the earlier it is advised and performed the safer it is for the patient.

Enucleation of adenomatous growths is readily performed if done early. But if the patient or the patient's medical adviser waits until changes occur which make the operation difficult or dangerous, it becomes an emergency operation and has a death rate equal to the major emergency operations. We see this well illustrated in hernia and appendicitis. Just as it is true that the operation for hernia, being left until strangulation occurs or the operation for appendicitis being left until peritonitis occurs, both these result in a vast increase in the dangers of these two operations, so to, when prostatectomy is left until cystitis, pyelitis, nephritis or cancerous changes occur, this latter operation becomes fraught with great danger. I firmly believe that supra-public prostatectomy, done before these changes occur, is no more dangerous than the interval operation for appendicitis.

For practical purposes aside from inflammatory conditions we know of two types of prostate:

1.—The large juicy gland, known as the epithelial type.

2.—The small hard gland, known as the connective tissue type.

Referring to the large juicy variety, Cahn states that the microscopic examination of the prostate, after its removal by Israel in forty cases, invariably revealed new growth starting from the epithelial tissue of the gland (microscopically papillary adenoma) and that in one of these cases the benign growth was in a state of transition to carcinomo.

Moscou reports the results of histologic study of the parts in a man of sixty-eight, who had been operated upon by the Fuller-Fryer technique, who died twenty-four hours afterwards. The anatomic findings showed that the enucleation of the adeno-myomatous growths of the prostate leaves a cavity the walls of which are formed by true prostatic tissue, which is the original prostate compressed and pushed back by the encroaching growth without loosing its integrity. I shall refer to this fact again. These findings suggest that hypertrophy of the prostate must be regarded as a true epithelial growth, with nothing in common with inflammatory changes.

The second or connective tissue type is much less common than the epithelial and is supposed to be the result of acute inflam-mation. In the old or middle aged the interstitial hyper plaisia does not cease and athrophy take place, as it does in the young; but, on account of the increased fibrosis of the aged and consequent thickening of the walls of the veins and lymphatics together with chronic congestion of the organ, this condition is prolonged with oedema and inflammatory exudate, and as a result of this overgrowth of connective tissue the muscle cells atrophy.

The history of hypertrophied prostate as given by the patient is usually dated from the time he first was forced to do something for the relief of pain or retention. The three symptoms complained of most are: frequent desire to make water, difficulty in making water and dribbling of the water. On inquiry we find that the first of these to bother was the increased frequency of micturition and that this increase in frequency is most marked during the night or early morning. Gradually the getting up at night becomes annoying and although the patient may sleep during the first part of the night toward morning the desire to urinate is so frequent as to make sleep impossible. Sometimes an early symptom is increased sexual desire with frequent and annoying morning erections: although in some cases, as in one of mine, the patient had been impotent for over a year.

Difficulty in making water is always early in making its appearance, the stream is hard to start, the patient standing for some minutes before being able to start the stream, meanwhile straining and manipulating the parts. The force of the stream is much lessened, as is the size. This causes it to strike the ground near his feet. The patient takes a much longer time to urinate and the stream does not shut off promptly at the end of the act; but decreases to a few spurts and ends by dribbling. As the case progresses the patient is unable to make even a stream of urine; but it flows by drops, and finally, owing to chilling or over indulgence in alcoholic or sexual excitement, he becomes unable to pass water at all and the doctor is called in to relieve him. After this is repeated several times, the patient may seek surgical aid.

The diagnosis of prostatic hypertrophy is usually easy. First the age and next from a carefully taken history. A rectal examination or a combined rectal and abdominal, together with an examination of the prostate between a sound in the bladder and the rectal finger will quite tell us that the gland is enlarged also which lobe and the consistency. We next ask the patient to make water while standing and observe the stream. In hypertrophy the stream is small, feeble and delayed, while if retention is present, micturition is impossible and the bladder will be distended. I have seen one case of this kind, where the doctor in charge called a surgeon to remove a tumor from the abdomen and another where the doctor in charge called a surgeon to operate for appendicitis.

After urination the patient is catheterized to find out the size of the bag of the bladder existing behind the prostate and also to determine the presence of cystitis from the characteristics of the urine. I believe the cystoscope is usually unnecessary and often a harmful instrument and can be dispensed with in doing a supra-pubic prostatectomy.

From stone we distinguish it by the history of gravel or renal stone, by the amount of blood in the urine, by the pain after micturition, by pain on riding, jumping, or going down stairs, by the improvement at night and the finding of the metallic click to the searcher.

From stricture by the youth of the patient, the history of gonorrhoea, the finding of the stricture by bougie and the use of the endoscope.

From cysto-spasm by the age, by the desire for frequent micturition occurring during the waking hours which is not accompanied by pain, the finding of phosphaturia, oxaluria and indicanuria and the fact that this occures in hysteria and neurasthenic persons.

Supra-pubic prostatectomy can be done successfully in progressive cases of prostatic hypertrophy, from fifty-five to sixty-five years of age, in which the bladder and kidneys are sound or not severely diseased. These patients may have such serious bladder or kidney disease co-existing as to make the question of operation very problematical; yet one of my patients was seventy-three years old and had chronic interstitial Brights disease.

Cases in patients above sixty-five who have already begun the use of the catheter and in whom the bladder is not septic may be operated upon. Cases, where serious heart trouble exists or where the kidneys are seriously damaged, must often be treat by palliative measures. In the past the operations which I believe will ultimately be adopted generally in all cases, except the small fibrous prostate, is the supra-pubic prostatectomy as done by Fryer, Deaver, Bevan, Stillman, Cahn, Weiner, and others.

It consists in shaving both pubes and perineum and preparing the parts by the usual antiseptic measures. The patient is catheterized with a soft rubber catheter and the bladder rinsed several times with boric acid solution after which a rubber bag, holding six to eight ounces, is inserted into the rectum and inflated with one half per cent. lysol solution or air, and clamped. Next the bladder is partly filled with six to eight ounces of boric acid solution and the rubber catheter clamped. The operation table is put in Trendelenburg position at an angle of about thirty degrees and the incision is made in the median line or slightly to the right of it from two inches above the symphysis to the symphysis in thin patients, and from five to six inches above the symphysis to the symphysis in fat patients. It goes through the skin, fascia and fat to the rectus muscle which is then separated by blunt dissection down to the peritoneum and prevesical fat. All bleeding is controlled by forceps and the peritoncum sought as it crosses the upper one third or half of the wound it is then pushed upward with gauze, and with the scissors we cut downward through the prevesical fat to the anterior walls of the bladder carefully stopping all hemorrhage. Two guy sutures of stout silk are stitched through the bladder walls about one-half inch apart and we open the bladder between these. We now lengthen the incision in the bladder. With the index finger we first seek the end of the rubber catheter in the urethra then we outline the prostate and feel for calculi which may be present. If such are found, we remove them with scoop or forceps. This being accomplished, we place from two to three retractors into the wound and dry out the bladder with sponge. Remove the rectal bag, then the assistant inserts a finger into the rectum and presses the prostate well up in view. At this point we scan the prostate for enlarged median lobe or a collar like ring around the uretha and note the size of the lateral lobe. If the trouble is caused by an enlarged median lobe will make an incision through the bladder wall to the prostate and shell it out with the finger. After this we can snip it off with the scissors or snare it off with a wire snare. If the obstruction is being caused by one or both lateral lobes, we make an incision parallel to the urethra over the summit of that lobe and inserting the index finger, follow the line of cleavage between the adenoma and its surroundings, passing first to the outer side of the lateral then working down and under the growth and next loosen it on its posterior aspects and finally when the growth is

quite well freed we separate the lateral and inferior surface of the apex from the triangular ligament. After one lobe has been loosened the other may be in like manner or we may dissect out the other lobe through the same incision. When this has been accomplished the growth is loose except when the urethra binds it to the triangular ligament and, as Deaver says, "At this stage one of two things happens, either the urethra slips from the center of the prostate remaining attached to the triangular ligament or the urethra tears off at the triangular ligament." The growth is now delivered into the bladder and taken out by the finger or forceps the cavity, where it was shrinks, in size and bleeding is stopped by irrigation with hot normal saline solution or by packing with gauze or by pad of gauze transfixed by a strong silk suture on a straight needle which is passed through the wound to the perineum and tied over a rubber tube; the operation is completed by stopping hemorrhage and placing a rubber drainage tube with two eyelets cut in the side and not too long into the bladder. We take a few stitches with number two iodized catgut in the fascia of the upper part of the wound so as to close this over the peritoneum. The guide sutures are removed and the upper part of the skin wound is closed with horse hair suture, while the lower part is left open. The rubber tube is fixed to the skin by silk worm gut suture and it is connected by long sterile tube with a urinal partly filled with a known quantity of a one to five hundred solution of bichloride of mercury. The wound is dressed with aseptic gauze and cotton and strapped with adhesive. If there a erno contra-indications we remove the drainage tube in two to three days. No sounds are passed and we do not irrigate unless there is a cystitis. When it is necessary to irrigate we use no catheter but irrigate directly through the urethra. Urine is usually passed by the natural channels in a few days and the wound closes very quickly.

This operation has been shown by Moscou to remove the Adenoma from the compressed and pushed back gland leaving the ejaculatory ducts unimpaired and apparently permeable which is the natural result of the preservation of the prostatic tissue. Moscou has also shown by the findings in his case that repair of the parts proceeds with a remarkably rapidity. While the retention of the ducts favors retention of the genital functions.

There is very little danger to the rectum, in supra-pubic prostatectomy, and urine passes naturally earlier and this has a very good effect on the patient's mind, for in no operation is the patient so apt to get downhearted, if early progress is not shown, than are these elderly patients with prostatic hypertrophy.

The bladder can be more easily lacerated by the enucleating finger from below than can happen from above. No packing is used to cause pressure on the wall of the rectum with a resulting necrosis. Consequently, there is very little danger of rectal fistula, following this operation. No instruments are used, to drag either the bladder or the rectum down, as are used in the perineal operation; consequently, we are less apt to injure the bladder or rectum, and cause dribbling, which is usually due to injury to the compressor urethrae. There is no cutting nor dissecting of important muscles and fascia, as is the case with perineal prostatectomy, which are always followed by contraction of the cicatricial tissue.

The cicatrix of the wound is from above, and the resulting contraction lessens the sacculation of the bladder posterior to the urethrae. On the contrary, in the perineal operation the cicatrix is from below, and the resulting contraction draws the back-wall of the bladder down, thus increasing the sacculation of the bladder behind the ure-

thrae. The tissues we are working in are better recognized from above, and the enlargement of the median lobe easily recognized, also whether there is a ring or collar-like obstruction around the urethrae, In case of great gravity, the operation may be done in two stages, first doing a supra-pubic cystotomy and draining the bladder and proceeding with the enucleation of the prostate at some future period through the same incision, after the patient's condition justifies it. Lanz comments on the precarious condition of many patients with hypertrophy of the prostate. In eighty cases in his practice two of the patients died the night before the proposed operation. The slightest intervention in such cases is liable to be fatal. He regards perineal prostatectomy as altogether too severe an operation, and for two years has been using exclusively the supra-pubic route, as much safer and quicker. General anaesthesia is often contra-indicated in these old patients; also in those who are more or less septic, with their tendency to pneumonia. Lumbar anaesthesia rendered him good service in twelve cases, but even this is liable to injure the kidneys, and he has lately found that the operation can be done with local anaesthesia. In nine of his cases supra-pubic cystotomy was done under infiltration anaesthesia with one per cent. solution of cocaine.

I have two succesful cases in patients over seventy, with grave complications.

Case I. Mr. J. T., Irish, age 73, Purcell, Okla., admitted Jan. 22, 1909. F. H., father had bladder trouble for twelve years previous to his death. One brother died from dilatation of the heart. One brother and one sister died from tuberculosis. One uncle died from apoplexy, and one uncle from malaria. He has four children in good health.

Present complaint: He first noticed that the urine dribbled when passed, and then stopped and started again. This symptom has been very troublesome indeed since the previous June. He has a spasmodic jerking of the bladder after micturition, and lately he has suffered great pain after urinating; and he was obliged to use great force to start the stream. Since last June the bladder and bowels have acted simultaneously, and since Sunday, January 11, 1909, he has had to resort to the catheter entirely. He states that he has had nocturnal micturition for one and one-half years, and that he now has pain in the hypogastrium and anterior to the anus; also under the glans penis. He says there has been no bleeding except when the catheter was used, and that of late he has been very amorous. He is unable to stand from a neuritis of the lower limbs, due to uraemic poisoning. On examination we found a paralysis of the bladder from over-distension, a soft and large prostate, cystitis, mitral regurgitation, and the arcus senilis was very marked. His bladder was irrigated with copper sulphate, grains II to pints I, and a fifty per cent. solution of salol in oleum gaultherii was given in fifteen drop doses every four hours. Later this was changed to formin. A permanent drainage catheter was put in the bladder and allowed to remain until February 22nd, 1909, when I performed a supra-pubic cystotomy and found a large, ball like median lobe, acting as a ball valve over the opening of the urethra. I made a small incision over its summit, dissected it out, and snared it off. He made an uneventful recovery, and has written me since he- returned home that he was well and able to hoe in the garden.

Case II. Mr. S. J. F., American, 70 years old, referred to me by Dr. Scott of Crescent. F. H., father died from lung trouble. Mother died from erysipelas. Personal history: He has had dysentery at intervals for years, bronchitis, prolapse of the rectum and piles. About two years ago he had a sudden attack of bladder trouble, which the doctor said was prostatitis. Two years ago he had to get up three to four times every night and strain very hard to make water. His condition was much worse at night. He made about one and one-half pints of urine in the day, and complained much of bearing-down and weight in the rectum. Also a great deal of pain at every bowel movement. His urine started and stopped, and he had the other symptoms of prostatitis, such as pain under the head of the penis, etc. He had rheumatic pains elsewhere, buzzing noises in his head, a great amount of headache, eyes puffy in the morning, and limbs oedematous, and he complained of cramps in them. He was suffering at that time with enlarged prostate, chronic bronchitis, chronic interstitial Bright's, rectal prolapse and hemorrhoids, and adenocystoma of the testicle. He recovered from this attack under boric irrigations, salol in oleum gaultheriá, and massage of the prostate. When a year later he came to the hospital with the same symptoms and had been using a catheter ten days to relieve his bladder, I did a supra-pubic prostatectomy under chloroform. About ten days afterward he developed a suppurative epididymitis, and about a week later I did an orchidectomy. He made all his urine naturally, after the twelfth day, and is at present entirely healed, passes his urine naturally in a very large stream, with very little discomfort, and no effort needed. His rectal trouble has disappeared after results are in a much larger per cent. good than follow the perinal. I believe with a writer in the St. Louis Journal of Dermatology and Verneral Diseases that in the near future this operation will be the one generally performed, and that perineal prostatectomy will pass into history.

Bibliography: Cahn, Murphy, Moscou, Deaver, Stillman, Lydston, Ochner.

SOME NEW ORLEANS CLINICS

BY V. BERRY, M. D., OKMULGEE, OKLA.

During the past winter I had the pleas-ure of spending four weeks during the months of January and February attending clinics in New Orleans and I jot down a few notes hoping they may aid some one who contemplates special work. At the outset I wish to disclaim any intention of mentioning all the teachers doing good work in that city, but simply mention those in whose work I was particularly interested. I wish to emphasize the great wealth of clinical material available in New Orleans and also the fact that it is concentrated in such a small area, three-fourths or more being at the great Charity Hospital. There are about three thousand indoor patients treated here every year. There are over one thousand patients in the hospital at all times, and on account of New Orleans being a seaport town the variety of material is perhaps unexcelled any where in the world. The venereal and skin clinic is especially fine, and surgical material in all branches is abundant. There are eight major operating rooms in Charity Hospital, and Delgado Annex combined, and one can go the rounds and see almost any thing to his liking. The gynecological clinic, both medical and operative is supplied with abundant material.

In surgical work the visitor usually is interested in the clinic of Prof. Matas. He is truly one of the great surgeons of America. He is a plain, unassuming man, simple and kindly in manner, and a master of the principles of modern surgery. There are more rapid and artistic operators, but no better. He is an especially fine teacher as he knows the why of every thing he does, and knows how to tell it. He has that rare gift of making the humblest patient feel that he has a personal interest in his misfortunes. He is kind and considerate to the poor who fill up the great hospital where he has rendered service so long, which is in great contrast to some of the cruelties I saw perpetrated by one or two thoughtless young internists while there. When I saw the exhibition of kindness to these poor unfortunates it impressed me with the fact that a great man is usually a good man. Dr. Matas' work covers the entire list of general surgery so those cases are of practical help to the average student, for purposes of demonstration. I have seen him purposely reject an operation where a display of skill would have elicited the applause of the student and select a simple fracture, or some equally minor case, and put in the hour with a most interesting demonstration of those things that fill in the every-day life of the average practitioner.

Prof. Martin also conducts an interesting clinic in general surgery in the Charity Hospital. His work is done as simply as possible, with no effort at surgical carpentery, or slight-of-hand performances. He does good abdominal work, and very good plastic work.

The Younger Souchon also operates at Charity, and it is a real treat to see him do an amputation. He is rapid, accurate and artistic. He is one of the best men in technique, so far as I am capable of judging, that I saw operate during my stay. He is a son of the noted Edward Souchon, the veteran teacher of surgery in Tulane University.

In genito-urinary, and rectal surgery the clinics are especially good. Prof. Delaup is chief of this clinci, and is a splendid teacher. The material is so abundant that all of it can not be utilized. Delaup uses spinal anesthesia (stovaine) as a routine, and in the many cases in which I saw it used I never saw an untoward symptom; and in *his* clinic I never saw a failure to get sufficient anesthesia. I saw another operator use stovaine dissolved in about 40 minims of water, and choloroform had to be given to induce anesthesia, as the amount of fluid was so great as to get pressure paralysis instead of anstheseia. Prof. Delaup lays great stress on not using over twenty minims of water for the solution. He does all kinds of major rectal and genito-urinary work under stovaine, including prostatectomy, and operation for stone in the bladder, and the results are equally as satisfactory as with general anesthesia. He is a specially gifted teacher and I know of no place in this country where one can pursue this line of work with more benefit than in New Orleans.

In gynecology material is very abundant at Charity, and Prof. Miller is an especially skilled operator. His plastic work I think is unexcelled in this country. His perineal work is a real treat, and any man who wishes to post up along this line can get as good work under his teaching, I am sure, as any where in this country; and that means any where else. He does good abdominal work; in fact I have seen no better any where.

Prof. Cocram has a very interesting clinic in Charity, and his routine instruction in the examination and diagnosis of cases is very instructive. He also does good abdominal work in Delgago Annex. His assistant is especially accommodating, and is of great aid to the student desiring personal instruction.

In the domains of internal medicines i do not think there is a richer field in the world than the wards of Charity Hospital. Every form of disease known to man eventually turns up here, so I have been informed. Prof. Dock gives a very interesting

medical clinic in the Amphitheatre to the Senior students of Tulane. However, it is accessible to post-graduate students as well. He teaches all modern methods of diagnosis, as well as therapeutics.

However, it is to Prof. Lerch's out-door clinic, at Charity, I wish to direct the post-graduate student. Prof. Lerch is a master diagnostician. His work in physical diagnosis is the finest I saw while in New Orleans, for the post-graduate student. He is plain, thorough, accurate and enthusiastic. The material is far more abundant than can be used, at times; and every disease known to the average practitioner is constantly showing up. To the man who wishes special work on the heart and lungs the clinic is especially good.

For nose and throat work Profs. Lanfried and King have most excellent clinics. Prof. Lanfried operates at Charity, and he is one of the most skilled operators in America. Prof. King has an excellent and large clinic at the eye, ear, nose and throat hospital. There is a large eye clinic held here. Material is so abundant it becomes monotonous.

I will close by saying that there is one of the best skin clinics in America in the out-door department of Charity, and Prof. Menage is a master teacher.

I do not wish it understood that *all* clinics are good here, for there are some that are not. The chief criticism I think is that some of the work is not organized to a system as it should be. That will be corrected I think, in time. However the man who goes to New Orleans to "see things" can do so if he will keep his eyes open. The climate is mild in mid-winter, and living expenses reasonable, and the teachers have a professional spirit that makes it pleasant to come in contact with them.

THE EIGHTEENTH ANNUAL MEETING OF THE OKLAHOMA STATE MEDICAL ASSOCIATION, TULSA, OKLA., MAY 10, 11 AND 12, 1910

May 10th, 2:45 *P. M.*

Meeting called to order by the First Vice-President, Dr. C. L. Reeder, Tulsa, Oklahoma:

The Rev. Dr. Kerr of Tulsa opened the meeting with prayer after which an address of welcome was delivered by Honorable Loyal J. Martin, Mayor of Tulsa and this was responded to by Dr. LeRoy Long of McAlester in behalf of the State Medical Association.

Dr. G. H. Butler of Tulsa delivered an address on behalf of the Tulsa County Medical Society and this address was responded to by Dr. J. A. Walker, Shawnee, Oklahoma.

Dr. Walter C. Bradford, President, delivered the President's address after which the meeting was adjourned until 8:00 P. M.

May 10th, 8:00 *P. M.*

The House of Delegates was convened in executive session, Dr. W. C. Bradford, President in the chair.

The following credentials committee was appointed:

Dr. J. H. Scott, Shawnee.

Dr. D. A. Myers, Lawton.

Dr. C. S. Bobo, Norman.

A partial report of delegates entitled to seats was made.

A communication from L. H. South, Secretary of the Association of State Secretaries, was read, which in substance requested that the Secretary of this organization be sent to the Annual meeting of the American Medical Association for the purpose of taking part in the consideration of matters pertaining to the management of state journals, expenses, and such other matters of interest and connected with the affairs of state medical organizations. A motion was made that this request be complied with, which was put and carried.

The Council of the Association reported that they had audited the Secretary's books and statement of receipts and expenditures, and that they were correct; showing a balance on hand of $2,951.34.

Bills to the amount of $38.15 from members of the Council were allowed.

The Council recommended that county secretaries keep in close touch with their respective Councillors in order to promote the work of organization.

SCIENTIFIC SESSIONS.

Surgical. The following papers were read and discussed:

Post-Operative Exudates, W. E. Dicken, Oklahoma City.

Cause and Treatment of Inguinal Hernia, W. J. Frick, Kansas City, Mo.

Open Treatment of Fractures by Direct or Internal Splints, Herman E. Pearse, Kansas City, Mo.

Ileus, or Intestinal Obstruction, J. C. Watkins, Hallett.

Clinic, A. L. Blesh, Oklahoma City.

Concussion, Dr. B. F. Fortner, Vinita, Oklahoma.

Surgical Treatment of Bone Tuberculosis, L. H. Huffman, Hobart, Oklahoma.

Local Anesthesia, Leight F. Watson, Oklahoma City, Oklahoma.

Fractures and Dislocations of the Upper Extremities, M. E. Preston, Denver, Colorado. (Illustrated by stereoptican views.) This was a lecture and delivered from notes and not from written manuscript.

Management of Fractures of the Extremities. J. A. Foltz, Ft. Smith, Ark.

Some Interesting Observations in Connection with Appendicitis, Dr. LeRoy Long, McAlester, Oklahoma.

Ross Grosshart, Tulsa, Oklahoma, was elected Chairman of the Surgical Section for the next year, George W. West, Eufaula was elected Vice-Chairman.

SECTION ON GENERAL MEDICINE.

The following papers were read and discussed:

The General Practitioner. Esau Despised his Birthright, Chas. W. Fisk, Kingfisher, Oklahoma.

Poliomyelitis Anterior, J. Donohoo, Afton, Oklahoma.

Diagnostic Relationship Between Internal Medicine and Special Surgery, J. Block, Kansas City, Mo.

Prevention of Disease, T. F. Renfrow, Billings, Oklahoma.

Diagnosis and Treatment of Diabetes, Harry E. Breese, Henryetta, Oklahoma.

Malaria, Atypical Forms, R. K. Pemberton, Krebs, Oklahoma.

Thermogenesis, G. H. Thrailkill, Chickasha, Oklahoma.

SECTION ON PEDIATRICS.

The following papers were read and discussed:

Laryngeal Diphtheria, A. B. Montgomery, Muskogee, Oklahoma.

Cretinism, with Report of Case, J. E. Hughes, Shawnee, Oklahoma.

Cerebral Meningitis, F. B. Erwin, Norman, Oklahoma.

Disease of the Respiratory Tract, Winnie M. Sanger, Oklahoma City, Oklahoma.

The Hygiene of Infancy and Childhood, W. G. Little, Okmulgee, Oklahoma.

Empyema, D. E. Broderick, Kansas City, Mo.

Poliomyelitis Anterior, J. C. Mahr, State Health Commissioner, Oklahoma City, Oklahoma.

Report of Some Cases Found among the Dependent Children of Oklahoma, Dr. Carl Puckett, Pryor, Oklahoma.

Broncho-Pneumonia, Leonard S. Willour, Atoka, Oklahoma.

SECTION ON GYNECOLOGY AND OBSTETRICS.

The following papers were read and discussed:

Eclampsia, G. A. McBride, Ft. Gibson, Oklahoma.

A Case Requiring Herniotomy and Lipectomy, Charles Nelson Ballard, Oklahoma City, Oklahoma.

Obstetrical Surgery and Secondary Repair of Lacerated Perineum, J. M. Trigg, Shawnee, Oklahoma.

Extra-Uterine Pregnancy, Diagnosis and treatment, with Report of Case, I. B. Oldham, Muskogee, Oklahoma.

Causation of Insanity in the Puerperium, J. W. Duke, Guthrie, Oklahoma

The Trend of Modern Obstetrics, A. B. Leeds, Chickasha, Oklahoma.

SECTION ON EYE, EAR, NOSE AND THROAT.

The Prevention and Treatment of the Ophthalmias of the Newborn, Dr. Milton K. Thompson, Muskogee, Oklahoma.

Bacteria of the Eye, J. H. Barnes, Enid, Oklahoma.

A talk by Flavel B. Tiffany Kansas City, Mo.

HOUSE OF DELEGATES, MAY 12, 1910.

The following officers were elected:

President—D. A. Myers, Lawton.

1st Vice-President—C. L. Reeder, Tulsa.

2nd Vice-President—H. M. Williams, Wellston.

3rd. Vice-President—James L. Shuler, Durant.

Secretary-Treasurer—C. A. Thompson, Muskogee.

Councillor, 5th District—J. H. Barnes, Enid.

The following resolutions were introduced:

(*Amendment to the Constitution and By-Laws.*)

That within 30 days the President appoint a Legislative Committee, consisting of three members, one to be a resident of the capital, and one to serve one year, one two years, one three years; and one to be elected annually hereafter by the House of Delegates; the President and Secretary to be Ex-Officio members of this committee. Carried.

A resolution commending the Governor for his action in appointing a physician on the Board of Regents of the State University and suggesting that this Association be permitted to nominate men for such position as the Medical Department of said University is now the only Medical school within the State. Carried.

A resolution Commending the American Medical Association and Council on Pharmacy and Chemistry thereof for its efficient work in aiding in the enforcement of the National Pure Food Law. Carried.

A resolution appropriating One Hundred Dollars ($100.00) for the Davis Memorial fund. Carried.

Resolutions thanking the various civic bodies of Tulsa, Oklahoma, for their efforts in procuring entertainment of a splendid character never before equalled in the State. Carried.

The Committee on the study of Tuberculosis appointed May, 1909, reported through the Chairman, H. M. Williams, Wellston,

That it was the opinion of the Committee that the State provide State or county sanatoria for the treatment of this disease; that it should be the duty of the physicians of the state to promptly report all cases of tuberculosis as soon as diagnosed, together with the financial condition of the patient as far as can be determined to the County Superintendent of Health.

A resolution commending Senator Owen for his activity and work in presenting and urging the passage of a Law creating a Department of Health and calling attention to the right of the people to have such laws enacted, and asking all representatives in Washington to support the measure. Carried.

A resolution upholding the action of the Council and Secretary in arbitrarily separating the membership and subscription rolls was adopted.

There is an increase of membership; there being about 1,062 members as against 998 for 1909.

The attendance was about three hundred.

Muskogee was selected as a meeting place for 1910.

DELEGATES TO AMERICAN MEDICAL ASSOCIATION.

Charles R. Hume, Anadarko; Alternate, E. S. Lain, Oklahoma City.

Walter E. Wright, Tulsa; Alternate, Charles Blickensderfer, Shawnee.

THE BANQUET.

Those who attended expecting the ordinary features usually found at the Annual meeting were agreeably surprised and the most critical were delighted at the various phases of the entertainment provided.

The badges, which were the work of artistic thought, endeavor and expense had the wearers name plainly enscribed, so every one knew every one else at a glance.

The sessions were well attended and notwithstanding the many interruptions peculiar to our system of holding meetings of delegates, etc., more than the usual number of papers were read and discussed.

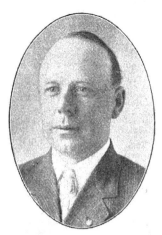

DR. DAVID A. MYERS, LAWTON, OKLAHOMA
President of the Oklahoma State Medical Association, 1910-11

The combined citizenship of Tulsa united their efforts to make the meeting the success it was.

Among the delightful events of the session was the musical given the Association by the Hyechka Club, a musical organization of artists, which Tulsa boasts and has good reason to be proud of. The musical was followed by one of the most elaborate banquets ever tendered any body in the state, over three hundred people being seated in the dining room of the Robinson Hotel.

The following toasts were proposed:
DR. FRED S. CLINTON, Toastmaster.
Mr. Chairman, Ladies and Gentlemen:

It is no idle boast to say that this occasion would be a splendid surprise to the most critical connoisseur of such affairs.

The pioneering and development of a vast empire is calculated to make or discover strong characters who will eventually become a part of its history.

Modern medical men do not regard their profession as the end of all living but a mere means to a loftier and more useful purpose. To be clothed with the full armour of citizenship is to be protected from the venomous shafts of a narrow specialization and given an increasing power in the philanthropic, economic and industrial as well as professional forces in life.

The speakers whom I am soon to introduce each have in their vocabulary of success such words as "Pioneers," "Optimism," "Aequanimitas," "Woman," "Tulsa," "Memory's Gallery," "Fads and Fancies," "Sunshine and Shadow," and know of the "Physician as a Packhorse for Reform and Sanitary Legislation," and that the County Society is the unit for membership in the State Association which is a passport to the National Organization.

The speaker has just received some important information through a little bird—a "Martin"—to the effect that Drs. Fortner and Bradford and Messrs. Connolly and Johnson were engaged in an animated conversation and one of them insisted that he knew of no parallel case where a "Reeder" would "Fite" or "Long" "Mahr" a banquet by having a "Butler" give "Bond" for a "Pigg" with which to feast the guests.

"Tulsa County Medical Society."
"What cannot art and industry perform,
    When science plans the progress of their
    toil."
DR. G. H. BUTLER.
Beattie—Minstrel Book I Stanza 13.

"Pioneers."

"pioneers;

Columbus of the land;
Who guided freedom's proud career
   Beyond the conquer'd strand;
And gave her pilgrim sons a home
   No monarch's step profanes,
Free as the chainless winds that roam
   Upon its boundless plains."

    Dr. B. F. Fortner.

"Oklahoma State Medical Association."

"The snows that fall on Mt. Washington are not purer than the motives which begot it. The fresh dew-laden zephyrs of the orange groves of the South are not sweeter than the hopes its advent inspired. Our own symbolic Eagle though he blew his breath upon the sun cannot be higher than its expected destiny."

    Dr. W. C. Bradford.

"Optimism."

"The evening beam, that smiles the clouds
   away,
And tints tomorrow with prophetic ray."

    —Bryon's Bride of Abydos.

    Dr. F. B. Fite.

"Opportunity."

"There is a tide in the affairs of men,
   Which taken at the flood, leads on to
     fortune;
Omitted, all the voyage of their life
   Is bound in shallows and miseries,
On such a full sea are we now afloat,
   And we must take the current when it
     serves,
Or lose our ventures."

—Shakespeare—Julius Caesar, Part II,
   Scene 3.

    Dr. C. L. Reeder.

"Memory's Gallery."

"Hail, Memory, Hail, in thy exhaustless
   mine
   From age to age unnumbered treasures
    shine.
Thought and her shadowy brood thy call
   obey,

And Place and Time are subject to thy
   sway."

—Rogers Pleasures of Memory, Part II,
   Line 429.

"Lull'd in the countless chambers of the
   brain,
   Our thoughts are linked by many hidden
    chain,
Awake but one, and lo, what myriads rise,
   Each stamps his image as the other
    flies."

—Rogers Pleasures of Memory, Part I,
   Line 171.

    Dr. LeRoy Long.

"Sunshine and Shadow."

"Behold him setting in his Western skies
   The shadows lengthening as the vapors
    rise."

—Absalom and Achitophel, Part I, J. Dryden.

    Dr. W. B. Pigg.

"Aequanimitas."

"Self reverence, self knowledge, self control,
   These three alone lead life to sovereign
    power."

    —Tennyson; Aenone, Line 144.

    Mr. Victor O. Johnson.

"Women."

"Tis woman's smiles that lull our cares to
   rest,
   Dear woman's charms that give to life
    its zest;
'Tis woman's hand that smooths affliction's
   bed,
   Wipes the cold sweat, and stays the
    sinking head."

    Mr. D. F. Connolly.

*"The Physician as a Packhorse for Reform
and Sanitary Legislation."*

"Had I served my God with half the zeal
   I served my king, he would not, in mine
    age
Have left me naked to mine enemies."

—Shakespeare, Henry 8, Act III, Scene 2.

    Dr. J. C. Mahr.

"Fads and Fancies."

"One of those passing rainbow dreams,
    Half light, half shade, which Fancy's
      beams
Paint on the fleeting mists that roll,
    In trance or slumber, round the soul."
      —From Lalla Rookh, Tom Moore.
DR. R. I. BOND.

"Tulsa."

"Our bosoms beat high at thy name,
    Thy health is our transport—
Our triumph thy fame."
HON. L. J. MARTIN.

"Goodnight, goodnight, a sweet goodnight
    And pleasant dreams and slumbers
      light."

PERSONAL

Dr. Frank Jackman of Cumberland and J. E. Reid of Madill are studying in the Polyclinics of Chicago.

Dr. C. E. DeGroot of Muskogee has been doing post-graduate work in New Orleans and New York.

Dr. T. A. Blaylock, County Superintendent of Health of Marshall County is doing post-graduate work in New Orleans, after which he will visit Havana and other points in Cuba. He is accompanied by his wife and son.

Dr. Walter B. Reeves of Wapanucka recently returned from the post-graduate schools of Chicago.

EDITORIAL

THE PROPOSED MEDICAL DEPARTMENT.

Senator Owen recently, of his own volition and initiative, introduced into the United States Senate a bill, which has for its object the consolidation of all existing health agencies of the National government, exclusive of the Medical Department of the Army and Navy, into a Department and whose head shall be a cabinet officer.

This move met with instant approval from a unanimous medical press and the great dailies and journals of the country recognize in it the efforts of a sincere man in office who wishes to do something more than vote yea and nay on measures up for action.

The move is practical and will entail less expense to the National Government in execution than does the now widely separated branches which the bill seeks to consolidate.

It is worthy of notice to call attention to the fact that one of the principal questioners of the bill, or rather questioners of the statements made by Senator Owen in referring to the results of epidemics and loss of life due to such epidemics was Senator Ballinger, himself a retired physician. It is ironical to have a man in public life who by training and fitness should support such a measure attempt to retard such an advance in the protection of the general public.

However, some of the Medical profession will doubtless recall that in 1904 it was charged that Senator Ballinger was responsible for the last two lines of the Act of Congress regulating the practice of Medicine in Indian Territory, which reads "and provided further, That osteopath, massage, Christian Science, and herbal treatment shall not be affected by this act."

After this no one can doubt that Senator Owen is a better fitted champion of the fight for reform and protection of the health interests than Senator Ballinger.

OUR NEW SYSTEM.

With this issue we begin the mailing of the Journal to subscribers only. Naturally in the change of a mailing list to subscribers from one that was formerly to members some errors will occur and some names are most surely to be omitted who are subscribers.

We ask that each physician who is entitled to receive the Journal or knows of some who is entitled to it and who fails to receive it call our attention to it at once and the matter will be remedied.

We believe each member should be a subscriber to his state publication and if you are not you are invited to become one.

CLEVELAND COUNTY MEDICAL SOCIETY.

Meeting April 1, 1910.

PROGRAM.

Symposium on Appendicitis, Anatomy and Pathology, W. L. Capshaw and L. A. Turley.

Ethiology and Diagnosis, R. E. Thacker.

Treatment, A. C. Hirshfield.

Leaders in Discussion, C. S. Bobo and R. D. Lowther.

The Spring Session of the Central Oklahoma Medical Association, held at El Reno, Oklahoma, Tuesday, April 12, 1910.

ORDER OF BUSINESS

Call to order at 10:30 a. m.

A. B. Cullom, President.

Reading Minutes of Previous Meeting.

Reports of Committees.

Miscellaneous Business.

Papers.

PROGRAM.

1. "Adenoids,"   W. A. Aitken, Enid

2. "The Conservative Treatment of Septic Infections Following Minor Injuries."
   Gayfree Ellison, Oklahoma City

3. "Malaria as an Obstetrical Complication." T. M. Aderhold, El Reno.

4. "Supra-Pubic Cystotomy".
   F .W. Noble, Guthrie

5. "The Present Status of Serum Therapy," A. D. Hatcher, El Reno

6. Remarks concerning Diseases of the Spinal Cord.
   A. D. Young, Oklahoma City

7. "Alcoholic Insanity,"
   J. W. Duke, Guthrie

8. "Squint,"   J. H. Barnes, Enid

9. "Tubercular Peritonitis,"
   A. A. West, Guthrie

10. "Diabetes,"   G. A. Boyle, Enid

11. "Ectopic Gestation,"
    F. H. Clark, El Reno

12. "Inmperfect Drainage in Relation to Diseases Demanding Surgical Intervention,"
    U. L. Russell, Oklahoma City

13. "Prostatic Hypertrophy,"
    W. J. Wallace, Oklahoma City

14. "Tuberculosis of the Fallopian Tubes."
    C. N. Ballard, Oklahoma City

JACKSON COUNTY.

The Jackson County Medical Society elected the following officers for 1910:

President...........J. W. Echols, Altus.
Vice-Pres. ....J. W. Wilson, Elmer.
Secretary-Treasurer..L. A. Hankins, Altus.
Alternate ....C. G. Spears, Altus.
Alternate ....R. H. Fox, Altus

OFFICERS OF THE OKLAHOMA STATE MEDI-
CAL ASSOCIATION.

President....................D. A. Myers, Lawton
1st Vice-President..............C. L. Reeder, Tulsa
2nd Vice-President.........H. M. Williams, Durant
3rd Vice-President............Jas. S. Shuler, Durant
Secretary-Treasurer........C. A. Thompson, Muskogee

COUNCILLORS.

1st District.................J. A. Walker, Shawnee
2nd District................John W. Duke, Guthrie
3rd District..............Chas. R. Hume, Anadarko
4th District..................A. B. Fair, Frederick
5th District.....................J. H. Barnes, Enid
6th District.............F. R. Sutton, Bartlesville
7th District.............W. G. Blake, Tahlequah
8th District..............I. W. Robertson, Dustin
9th District............H. P. Wilson, Wynnewood
10th District...................J. S. Fulton, Atoka

DELEGATES TO AMERICAN MEDICAL ASSOCI-
ATION, 1911-1912.

Charles R. Hume, Anadarko; Alternate, E. S. Lain,
Oklahoma City; Walter E. Wright, Tulsa; Alternate,
Chas. Blickensderfer, Shawnee.

ADAIR COUNTY.

Beard, D. A. ....Westville.
Barnes, C. O. ....Westville.
Farrer, O. W. ....Stilwell.
Lane, J. N. ....Westville.
Patton, J. A. ....Stilwell.
Robinson, C. M. ....Stilwell.
Williams, T. S. ....Stilwell.
Woodruff, P. A. ....Stilwell.
Robinson, J. A. ....Dutch Mills, Ark.

COAL COUNTY.

Briggs, T. H. ....Atoka.
Conner, L. A. ....Coalgate.
Clark, J. B. ....Coalgate.
Fulton, J. S. ....Atoka.
Goben, H. G. ....Lehigh.
Logan, W. A. ....Lehigh.
Long, T. J. ....Atoka.
Nelson, J. A. ....Wayne.
Spangler, A. S. ....Phillips.
Wallace, W. B. ....Lehigh.
Wilour, L. S. ....Atoka.

BECKHAM COUNTY.

Ballard, J. D. ....Sayre, (Shattuck.)
Gipson, H. H. ....Erick.
McComas, J. M. ....Elk City.
McCreery, R. C. ....Elk City.
Pinnell, G. ....Erick.
Speed, H. K. ....Sayre.
Standifer, J. E. ....Elk City.
Tedrow, C. W. ....Elk City.
Windle, O. N. ....Sayre.
Warford, J. D. ....Erick.
Wells, T. J. ....Erick.

BLAINE COUNTY.

Bell, Allen ....Geary.
Browning, J. W. ....Geary.
Buchanan, M. W. ....Watonga.
Campbell, J. L. ....Watonga.
Murdoch, L. H. ....Okeene.
Smith, I. T. ....Fay.
Stough, D. F. ....Geary.
Tracy, C. M. ....Canton.
Brandes, G. C. ....Okeene.
Blender, Henry ....Okeene.

BRYAN COUNTY.

Austin, J. L. ....Durant.
Armstrong. D. ....Mead.
Allen, J. R. ....Caddo.
Bradley, A. J. ....Albany.
Cain, P. L. ....Albany.
Clifton, W. F. ....Durant.
Grassham, R. H. ....Caddo.
Hagood, A. S. ....Durant.
Howard, S. H. ....Durant.
Kendal, W. L. ....Durant.
Kay, J. H. ....Durant.
Lively, C. O. ....Kemp.
Moore, L. F. ....Jackson.
McGregor, C. T. ....Caddo.
McCarley, W. H. ....Colbert.
Pate, John D. ....Durant.
Park, J. F. ....Durant.
Rushing, G. M. ....Durant.
Rappolee, H. E. ....Durant.
Smith, J. B. ....Durant.
Shuler, Jas. L. ....Durant.
Taliaferro. C. F. ....Bennington.
Woodward, A. M. ....Roberta.
Works, W. S. ....Matoy.
Wells W. M. ....Durant.
Yeats, H. W. ....Bokchito.
Yeiser, C. C. ....Colbert.

CADDO COUNTY.

Anderson, P. H. ....Anadarko.
Bird, Jesse ....Cement.
Brown. B. D. ....Apache.
Boyd, D. H. ....Anadarko.
Bailey, F. M. ....Carnegie.
Booth, Wm. E. ....Sickles.
Blair, S. ....Apache.
Colby. Geo. B. ....Gracement.
Campbell. Bertha H. ....Anadarko.
Campbell. Geo. C. ....Anadarko.
Downs Edw. W. ....Hinton.
Dinkler, F. ....Fort Cobb.
Dail, A. W. ....Cement.
Edens, M. H. ....Verden.
Gill, W. W ....Gracemont.
Henke, J. J. ....Hydro.
Hume, Chas. R. ....Anadarko.
Kerley, W. W. ....Anadarko.
Lane, C. W. ....Round Valley, Ind. Agency,
     Covelo, Calif.
McClure, P. L. ....Fort Cobb.
McCray, O. D. ....Binger.

Putman, C. E. ....Alfalfa.
Parrott, F. C. ....Oney.
Putman, Wm. B. ....Carnegie.
Rector, R. D. ....Anadarko.
Roland, M. M.....Oklahoma City, 203-5 Am.
  Nat. B. Bldg.
Russell, R. L. ....Anadarko.
Sanders, P. L. ....Carnegie.
Shadid, Michael ....Stecker.
Sims, John L. Jr., ...Lokeba.
White, D. O. ....Eakly.
Williams, S. E. ....Hydro.
Weiser, D. D. ....Alden.
Westermeier, Geo. W. ....Anadarko.
Waters, C. T. ....Hydro.
Willard, A. J. ....Cyril.

CANADIAN COUNTY.

Aderhold, Thomas M. ....El Reno.
Arnold, D. D. ....El Reno.
Brown, H. C. ....Okarche.
Clark, F. H. ....El Reno.
Dever, H. A. ....El Reno.
Fitzgerald, M. ....El Reno.
Hatcher, A. D. ....El Reno.
Hatchett, J. A. ....Eel Reno.
Kcons. R. F. ....El Reno.
Lane, Thomas ....El Reno.
L. W. Lynde, ...Okarche.
Muzzy, W. J. ....El Reno.
Miller, W. R. ....Calumet.
Runkle, R. E. ....El Reno.
Ruhl, N. E. ....El Reno.
Riley, Jas. T. ....El Reno.
Richardson, D. P. ....Union City.
Sanger, S. S. ....Yukon.
Taylor, G. W. ....El Reno.
Wolff, L. G. ....Okarche.

CARTER COUNTY.

Barnwell, J. T. ....Graham.
Boadway, F. W. ....Ardmore.
Booth, T. S. ....Ardmore.
Booth, J. E. ....Province.
Bogle, W. T. ....Ardmore.
Ballard, A. E. ....Lone Grove.
Clarke, C. B. ....Ardmore.
Denham, Thos. W. ....Oklahoma City.
Davis, A. B. ....Sneed.
Gillispie, L. D. ....Springer.
Goodwin, Geo. W. ....Ardmore.
Hardy, W. ....Ardmore.
Hargrove, J. H. ....Ardmore.
Hathway, W. G. ....Province.
Henry R. H. ....Ardmore.
Higgins, H. A. ....Glenn.
McNees, H. C. ....Ardmore.
Moore, R. D. ....Ardmore.
Parish, R. M. ....Ardmore.
Sullivan, C. F. ....Lone Grove.
Smith, J. H. ....Healdton.
Taylor, Don ....Woodford.
Von Keller, F. P. ....Ardmore.
Vaden, J. M. ....Ada.
Wh'tfield Jas. ....Beryn.
Willard Robt. S. ....Brock.
Booth, T. S. ....Ardmore.

CHOCTAW COUNTY.

Askew, E. R. ....Hugo.
Bonner, J. S. ....Ft. Towson.
Chandler, F. W. ....Hugo.
Ellis, J. C. ....Hugo.
Gee, R. L. ....Ft. Towson.
John, W. N. ....Hugo.
Miller, J. S. ....Hugo.
Moore, W. M. ....Sawyer.
Shull, R. J. ....Hugo.
Swearingin, C. H. ....Hugo.
Stephins, J. J. ....Boswell.
Vick, John T. ....Ft. Towson.
White, H. H. ....Hugo.
Wright, H. L. ....Hugo.
Lockett, B. L.................Swank.

CHEROKEE COUNTY.

Allison, J. S. ....Tahlequah.
Allison, T. P. ....Tahlequah.
Blake, Ed. W. ....Tahlequah.
Blake, W. G. ....Tahlequah.
Bewley, J. D. ....Peggs.
Coffman, LaFayettte ....Gideon.
Duckworth, J. F. ....Tahlequah.
Duckett, B. J. ....Hurlburt.
Hill, Israel ....Peggs.
McCurry, L. E. ....Tahlequah.
Peterson, C. A. ....Tahlequah.
Reece, Isaac ....Manard.
Thompson, Jos. M. ....Tahlequah.

COMANCHE COUNTY.

Alexander, C. W. ....Temple.
Angus, H. A. ....Lawton.
Burgess, W. C. ....Emerson.
Brashear, J. A. ....Lawton.
Clark, M. G. ....Temple.
Dunlap, E. B. ....Lawton.
Dunlap, P. G. ....Lawton.
Gooch, L. T. ....Lawton.
Gipson, T. J. ....Taupa.
Griffith, J. K. ....Randalett.
Hughes, A. R. ....Indiahoma.
Kirksey, R. L. ....Cache.
Knee, L. C. ....Lawton.
House, C. F. ....Hastings.
Lewis, J. L. ....Lawton.
Myers, D. A. ....Lawton.
Meredith, C. S. ....Lawton.
Mitchell, E. B. ....Lawton.
Milne, L. A. ....Lawton.
Mead, W. B. ....Lawton.
Meeker, E. D. ....Lawton.
McCallum, W. ....Randalett.
Stewart, A. H. ....Lawton.
Sanders, M. J. ....Temple.
Slaver, B. W. ....Temple.
Turner, W. M. ....Lawton.
Webb, G. O. ....Temple.

CLEVELAND COUNTY.

Bobo, C. S. ....Norman.
Burch, S. T. ....Norman.
Capshaw, W. L. ....Norman.
Childs, Henry C. ....Noble.
Clifton, G. M. ....Denver.

Capshaw, M. T. J. ....Norman.
Davis, J. A. ....Norman.
Griffin, D. W. ....Norman.
Hirshfield, A. C. ....Norman.
Hashall, J. L. ....Franklin.
Lowther, R. D. ....Norman.
Mason, W. J. ....Pocasset.
MacLaren, John Dice ....Norman.
Thacker, R. E. ....Lexington.
Walker, W. E. ......Lexington, R. F. D. 2.
Womack, J. L. ....Moore.

CRAIG COUNTY.

Adams, F. M. ....Big Cabin.
Pell. C. P. ....Welch.
Bagby, Oliver ....Vinita.
Bagby, Louis ....Vinita.
Craig, J. W. ....Vinita.
Clinkscales, A. M. ....Vinita.
Day. W. A. ....Big Cabin.
Hughson, F. L. ....Centralia.
Miller, G. E. ....White Oak.
Neer, C. S. ....Vinita.
Robinson, T. L. ....Bluejacket.
Staples, J. H. L. ....Bluejacket.
Stough, D. B. ....Vinita.
Wollard, Frank ....Welch.
Wimer, T. T. ....Welch.

CREEK COUNTY.

Ament, C. M. ....Sapulpa.
Avery, A. ....Sapulpa.
Bronaugh, J. W. ....Mounds.
Bone J. W. ....Sapulpa.
Coppedge, O. C. ....Bristow.
Croston, G. C. ....Sapulpa.
Chaney. J, F. ....Sapulpa.
Coppedge, O. S. ....Depew.
Fry, Melvin, ...Kiefer.
Groom. W. W. ....Bristow.
Garland, J. S. ....Sapulpa.
Hoover, J. W. ....Sapulpa.
Justice. H. B. ....Sapulpa.
Longmire, W. P. ....Sapulpa.
Mattoon E. A. ....Sapulpa.
McAllister, J. S. ....Sapulpa.
McCallun, C. L. ....Sapulpa.
Rutherford, Lafe ....Sapulpa.
Rentfro, J. L. ....Sapulpa.
Stafford, Gaylord, A. ....Kiefer.
Schrader. C. T. C..............Bristow.
Sweeney. R. M. ....Kellyville.
Soliss, J. P. ....Sapulpa.
Schwab, B. C. ....Sapulpa.
Wells, J. M. ....Newby.
Wetzel, G. H. ....Sapulpa.
King E. W. ....Bristow.

CUSTER COUNTY.

Baldwin, O. J. ....Weatherford.
Bolton, W. D. ....Clinton.
Frizelle, T J. ....Butler.
Gossman K. D. ....Custer.
Gordon, J. Matt ....Weatherford.
Hinson, T. B. ....Thomas.

Lamb, Ellis ....Clinton.
Murray, P. G. ....Thomas.
McBurney, C. H. ....Clinton.
Omer, W. J. ....Thomas.
Parker, O. H. ....Custer.
Parker, W. W. ....Custer.
Rogers, McLain ....Clinton.
White, N. P. H. ....Clinton.
Whitacre, F. S. ....Weatherford.

DEWEY COUNTY.

Adams, D. C. ....Taloga.
Leake, J. B. ....Taloga.
Leatherrock, R. E. ....Putman.
Marshall, J. G. ....Fountain.
Share, G. A. ....Seiling.

ELLIS COUNTY.

Craig, D. B. ....Stone.
Markley, W. F. ....Ivanhoe.
Newman O. C. ....Shattuck.
Sturdivant, John F. ....Arnett.

GARFIELD COUNTY.

Barnes, J. H. ....Enid.
Boyle, G. A. ....Enid.
Cotton, L. W. ....Enid.
Field, Julian ....Enid.
Hudson. F. A. ....Enid.
Jones, W. M. ....Enid.
Mahoney, J. E. ....Enid.
Smithe, P. A. ....Enid.

GARVIN COUNTY.

Burns, S. L. ....Hennepin.
Branum, T. C. ....Pauls Valley.
Callaway, John R. ....Mescalero New Mex.
Callaway, John R. ....Pauls Valley.
Hailey, E. L. ....Strafford.
Johnson, G. L. ....Pauls Valley.
Lain, F. H. ....Paoli.
Lindsay, N. H. ....Pauls Valley.
Lindsey, J. K. ....Elmore.
Morgan, J. B. ....Foster.
Morton, E. L. ....Hennepin.
Matheny, J. C. ....Lindsay.
Patterson, Price ....Maysville.
Roberson. M. E. ....Brady.
Shi A. H. ....Stratford.
Settles, W. E. ....Wynnewood.
Tucker, J. W. ....Purdy.
Webster, M. M. ....Stratford.
Wilson, S. W. ....Lindsay.
Wallace, J. C. ....Robberson.
Wilson, H. P. ....Wynnewood.
Young, J. A. ....Pauls Valley.
Bailey, H. C. ....Wynnewood.
Gray, A. W. ....Pauls Valley.

GRADY COUNTY.

Ambrister. J. C. ....Chickasha.
Bledsce, Martha ....Chickasha.
Beze, R. J. ....Chickasha.

Barry, Wm. R. ....Bradley.
Brown, C. C. : ....Chickasha.
Coulter, T. B. ....Chickasha.
Cook, Wm. H. ....Chickasha.
Downey, Dennis S. ....Chickasha.
Glenn, M. R. ....Chickasha.
Hume, R. R. ....Minco.
Leeds, A. B. ....Chickasha.
Owens, B. B. ....Minco.
Penquite, Walter ....Chickasha.
Peters, W. L. ....Oklahoma City.
Shippy, R. N. ....Chickasha.
Thrailkill, G. H. ....Chickasha.
Tye, R. P. ....Chickasha.
White, A. C. ....Chickasha.
Barker, C. E. ....Tuttle.
Finley, J. W. ....Rush Springs.
Gerard, G. R. ....Ninnekah.
Gordon, R. J. ....Ninnekah.
Hampton, P. J. ....Rush Springs.
Marrs, S. O. ....Chickasha.
Owensby, O. M. ....Chickasha.
Stinson, J. E. ....Chickasha.
Vann, Paul D. ....Chickasha.

GRANT COUNTY.

Hulen, C. R. ....Pond Creek.
Hulen, F. P. ....Pond Creek.
Antle, H. C. ....Renfrow.
Martin, J. F. ....Deer Creek.

GREER COUNTY.

Dodson, T. J. ....Mangum.
Dodson, W. O. ....Willow.
DeArman, M. M. ....Mangum.
Huffman, L. H. ....Hobart.
Jeter, O. R. ....Reed.
Norton, Porter ....Mangum.
Scarbrough, J. W. ....Mangum.
Tubbs, B. R. ....Russell.
Barr, J. H. ....Reed.
Pendergraft, W. C. ....Hollis.

HASKEL COUNTY.

Callaway, A. B. ....Stigler.
Davis, Ben ....Kinta.
Fannin, F. A. ....Stigler.
Henderson, Chas. F. ....Chant.
Mitchell, S. E. ....Stigler.
Turner, J. M. ....Hoyt.
Turner, T. B. ....Stigler.
Turner, C. A. ....Garland.

HUGHES COUNTY.

Adkins, W. D. ....Lamar.
Adams, J. C. ....Lamar.
Bentley, W. B. ....Calvin.
Bentley, J. A. ....Stuart.
Butts, A. M. ....Holdenville.
Cagle, T. J. ....Wetumka.
Denney, Z. C. ....Wetumka.
Davenport, A. L. ....Wecharty.
Evans, W. G. ....Stuart.
Edwards, J. J. ....Yeager.

Hicks, F. B. ....Raydon.
Hemphill, J. A. ....Wetumka.
Howell, A. H. ....Holdenville.
Johnson, N. J. ....Newburg.
Mitchell, P. T. ....Yeager.
McPherson, G. W. ....Spalding.
Martin, C. C. ....Raydon.
Melette, U. N. ....Holdenville.
Pope, A. J. ....Hanna.
Robertson, T. W. ....Dustin.
Scott, J. D. ....Holdenville.
Taylor, W. L. ....Raydon.
Tribble, E. T. ....Yeager.
Vanderpool, J. N. ....Calvin.
Wallace, A. J. ....Dustin.
Lowe, John W. ....Holdenville.

JACKSON COUNTY.

Clarkson, W. H. ....Blair.
Echols, J. W. ....Altus.
Fox, Raymond H. ....Altus.
Hankins, L. A. ....Altus.
Johnson, J. J. ....Martha.
Landrum, S. H. ....Altus.
Meredith, O. A. ....Olustee.
Miles, E. P. ....Altus.
Ralls, S. P. ....Altus.
Sanderson, W. E. ....Altus.
Spears, C. G. ....Altus.
Strothers, S. P. ....Altus.
Wilson, D. E. ....Hess.

JEFFERSON COUNTY.

Ashinhurst, T. E. ....Waurika
Baum, F. J. ....Waurika.
Cantrell, D. E. ....Waurika.
Clements, O. E. ....Hastings.
Cranfill, A. G. ..?.............Grady.
Derr, J. T. ....Waurika.
Ewing, F. W. ....Terral.
Ewing, L. D. ....Terral.
Garrett, S. S. ....Dixie.
Johnston, J. C. ....Waurika.
Lewis, A. R. ....Ryan.
Maupin, C. M. ....Waurika.
Moore, J. M. ....Addington.
Stephens, J. M. ....Hastings.
Sutherland, L. B. ....Waurika.
Walker, J. A. ....Fleetwood.
Wilson, W. A. ....Cornish.
Wilton, C. G. ....Ryan.

JOHNSTON COUNTY.

Stobaugh, F. B. ....Mannsville.
Looney, B. R. ....Mill Creek.
Reeves, W. B. ....Wapanucka.

KAY COUNTY.

Anderson, G. L. ....Newkirk.
Gearhart, A. P. ....Blackwell.
Johnson, W. M. ....Peckham.
Lowery, Allen ....Blackwell.
Miller, D. W. ....Blackwell.
Nieman, G. H. ....Ponca City.

Nuckels, A. S. .... Ponca City.
Panton, H. H. .... Ponca City.
Risser, A. S. .... Blackwell.
Robertson, W. A. T. .... Ponca City.
Waggoner, R. E. .... Ponca City.
Wood, V. A. .... Blackwell.
Hanna, J. W. .... Tonkawa.
Jones, J. A. .... Tonkawa.
Lively, M. M. .... Blackwell.
Lockwood, W. W. .... Ponca City.
Mathews, G. A. .... Braman.
Stricklen, H. M. .... Tonkawa.

KINGFISHER COUNTY.

Cavett, E. R. .... Kiel.
Cullum, A. B. .... Hennessey.
Fisk, C. W. .... Kingfisher.
Gore, Victor M. .... Kingfisher.
Gose, C. O. .... Hennessey.
Overstreet, J. A. .... Kingfisher.
Sloan, E. U. .... Kingfisher.
Rector, Newton .... Henessey.

KIOWA COUNTY.

Barkley, A. .... Hobart.
Beasley, A. ... . Hobart.
Beckham, H. F. .... Roosevelt.
Bonham, J. M. .... Hobart.
Chambers, M. E. .... Gotebo.
Dale, J. R. .... Hobart.
Hathaway, A. H. .... Mt. View.
Holland, A. W. .... Hobart.
Lloyd, H. C. .... Hobart.
Miller, Wm. M. .... Gotebo.
Muller, J. A. .... Snyder.
Ritter, J. M. .... Mondamin.
Richert, Peter .... Gotebo.
Stewart, G. W. .... Hobart.
Wagoner, A. L. .... Hobart.

LATIMER COUNTY.

Dalby, H. L. .... Wilburton.
Evans, E. L. .... Wilburton.
Horine, W. H. .... Wilburton.
Kilpatrick, Geo. A. .... Wilburton.
Kilpatrick, Garnett A. .... Wilburton.
McArthur, J. F. .... Wilburton.
Sackett, L. M. .... 122 1-2 N. Bdwy.
   Oklahoma City.

LEFLORE COUNTY.

Booth, G. R. .... LeFlore.
Moore, M. O. .... Braden.
Brown, W. W. .... Cameron.
Hardy, H. .... Poteau.
Hartshorne, W. O. .... Spiro.
Morrison, R. L. .... Poteau.
Riggan, C. E. .... Monroe.
Woodson, B. D. .... Monroe.

LINCOLN COUNTY.

Adams, J. W. .... Chandler.
Baird, W. D. .... Davenport.

Bilby, J. F. .... Stroud.
Cottrell, W. P. .... Kendrick.
Davis, S. O. .... Chandler.
Erwin, F. B. .... Norman.
Glenn, J. O. .... Sapulpa.
Hancock, J. M. .... Kendrick.
Hurlburt, E. F. .... Chandler.
Iles, H. C. .... Prague.
Marshall, A. M. .... Chandler.
Morgan, C. M. .... Chandler.
Norwood, A. H. .... Prague.
Williams, H. M. .... Wellston.
Williams, J. C. .... Chandler.

LOGAN COUNTY.

Barker, E. O. .... Guthrie.
Bowers, W. B. .... Guthrie.
Cotterall, C. F. .... Guthrie.
Duke, J. W. .... Guthrie.
Fulkerson, W. C. .... Marshall.
Hahn, L. A. .... Guthrie.
Hill, C. B. .... Guthrie.
Hodsdon, B. F. .... Guthrie.
Hamill, J. R. .... Guthrie.
Melvin, J. L. .... Guthrie.
Melvin, Elizabeth .... Guthrie.
Noble, F. W. .... Guthrie.
Overton, L. M. .... Guthrie.
Phillips, Lewis .... Seward.
Petty, C. S. .... Guthrie.
Rucks, W. W. .... Guthrie.
Rinehart, J. H. .... Meridian.
Stevens, David .... Guthrie.
Smith, R. V. .... Guthrie.
Underwood, E. L. .... Crescent.
West, A. A. .... Guthrie.

LOVE COUNTY.

Autry, D. .... Waunetta.
Beeler, C. A. .... Burneyville.
Batson, W. V. .... Marietta.
Batson, J. D. .... Marietta.
Crawley, J. J. .... Overbrook.
Friedsam, S. A. .... Leon.
Gardner, R. A. .... Marietta.
Gardner, B. S. .... Marietta.
Graham, E. F. .... Marietta.
Jackson, T. J. .... Marsden.
Looney, M. D. .... Burneyville.
Martin, A. E. .... Marietta.
Mathews, W. F. .... Bomar.

MAJOR COUNTY.

Davis, F. P. .... Enid.
Diemer, F. E. .... Enid.
English, C. C. .... Fairview.
Gleason, L. W. .... Fairview.
Johnson, B. F .... Fairview.
McCall, P. C. .... Fairview.
Specht, Elsie L. .... Rusk.
Smith, M. M. .... Fairview.
Townsent, B. I. .... Fairview.

MARSHALL COUNTY.

Blaylock, T. A. ....Madill.
Collins, J. A. ..:................Linn.
Davis, W. L. ....Kingston.
Gaston, J. J. ....Kingston.
Haynie, John A. ....Aylesworth.
Haynie, W. D. ....Powell.
Hornbeck, H. H. ....Kingston.
Holland, J. L. ....Madill.
Jackman, Frank ....Cumberland.
Robinson P. F. ....Madill.
Welch, J. S. ....Madill.
White, H. A. ....Madill.

MAYES COUNTY.

Hillis, J. E. ....Pryor.
King, F. S. ....Pryor.
Mitchell, J. L. ....Pryor.
Pierce, E. L. ....Salina.
Puckett, Carl ....Pryor.
Tilly, Geo. W. ....Pryor.

McINTOSH COUNTY.

Barton, A..H. ....Onapa.
Graves, G. W. ....Hitchita.
Lee, N. P. ....Checotah.
Montgomery A. B. ....Muskogee.
McCulloch, J. H. ....Checotah.
Nowlin, N. R. ....Eufaula.
Rice, J. F. ....Eufaula.
Tolleson, W. A. ....Eufaula.
Vance, B. J. ....Checotah.
West, G. W. ....Eufaula.

McCLAIN COUNTY.

Barger, G. S. ....Wayne.
Childs, J. S. ....Purcell.
Colby, J. H. ....Purcell.
McCurdy, T. C. ....Purcell.
Thacker, R. Emmett ....Purcell.
Tralle G. M. ....Purcell.
McCurdy, W. C. ....Purcell.

McCURTAIN COUNTY.

Denison, C. A. ....Idabell.
Graydon, A. S. ....Idabell.
Hooper, Z. ....Idabell.
McCaskill, W. B. ....Idabell.
McBrayer, W. H. ....Haworth.
Moreland, J. T. ....Idabell.
Moreland, W. A. ....Idabell.
Taylor, W. D. ....Haworth.

MURRAY COUNTY.

Adams, J. A. ....Sulphur.
Dunn, Robert ....Davis.
Ponder, A. V. ....Sulphur.
Powell, W. H. ....Palmer.
Slover, George ....Sulphur.
Slover, J. T. ....Sulphur.

MUSKOGEE COUNTY.

Aiken, S. W. ....Muskogee.
Brewer, A. J. ....Muskogee.
Ballantine, H. T. ....Muskogee.
Blakemore, J. L. ....Muskogee.
Callahan, J. O. ....Muskogee.
DeGroot, C. E. ....Muskogee.
Donnell, R. N. ....Muskogee.
Ellis, J. H. ....Muskogee.
Everley, A. W. ....Muskogee.
Fite, F. B. ....Muskogee.
Flamm, L. F. ....Muskogee.
Floyd, W. E. ....Muskogee.
Fryer, S. J. ....Muskogee.
Harris, A. W. ....Muskogee.
Hoss, Sessler ....Muskogee.
Howell, O. E. ....Oktaha.
Lemons, J. M. ....Muskogee.
Lightfoot, J. B. ....Muskogee.
Lee, J. E. ....:............Haskell.
McBride, G. A. ....Ft. Gibson.
Mitchell, P. S. ....Haskell.
Mitchell, M. C. ....Haskell.
Montgomery A. B. ....Muskogee.
Nagle, W. M. ....Muskogee.
Nesbitt, P. P.'............Muskogee.
Nichols, J. T. ....Muskogee.
Noble, J. G. ....Muskogee.
Norvell, B. P. ....Muskogee.
Oldham, I. B. ....Muskogee.
Rogers, C. T. ....Muskogee.
Rogers, H. C. ....Muskogee.
Shankle, H. D. ....Muskogee.
Thompson, C. A. ....Muskogee.
Thompson, M. K. ....Muskogee.
Tilly, W. T. ....Muskogee.
Vittum, J. S. ....Muskogee.
Warmack, J. C. ....Muskogee.
Winkler, C. E. ....Muskogee.
White, J. H. ....Muskogee.
Bacon, C. W. ....Warner.
Fuller, J. S. ....Ft. Gibson.
Howard, J. M. ....Ft. Gibson.
Sapper, E. J. ....Warner.

NOBLE COUNTY.

Brafford, S. F. ....Billings.
Coldiron, D. F. ....Bliss.
Emerson, A. V. ....Lucien.
Keller, F. L. ....Perry.
Kuntz, Lambertus ....Perry.
Lovelady, O. E. ....Red Rock.
Renfrow, T. F. ....Billings.
Watson, Bruce ....Perry.
Brengle, W. B. ....Perry.

NOWATA COUNTY.

Brookshire, J. Ed. ....Nowata.
Burns, H. B. ....Delaware.
Collins, E. F. ....Nowata.
Collins, J. R. ....Nowata.
Freer B. W. ....Nowata.
Howell, D. D. ....Nowata.
Hughes, Lawson ....Alluwee.

Lawson, D. M. ....Nowata.
Miller, C. L. ....Alluwee.
Russell, E. M. ....Nowata.
Scott, B. M. ....Delaware.
Strother, L. T. ....Nowata.
Suddeth, J. P. ....Nowata.
Waters, G. A. ....Lenapah.
Wilkerson, J. T. ....Lenapah.
Winget, W. W. ....Nowata.

OKFUSKEE COUNTY.

Baecht, F. C. ....Paden.
Bartow, A. C. ....Okfuskee.
Board, J. W....................Okemah.
Bombarger, C. C. ....Paden.
Davis, W. H. ....Castle.
Hilsmeyer, Fred E. ....Weleetka.
Lovelady, Benton ....Okemah.
McDonald, J. G. ....Okfuskee.
Reber, G. A. ....Okemah.
Stiles, G. S. ....Castle.
Pitchford, J. C. ....Morse.

OKLAHOMA COUNTY.

Andrews, Leila E.; 120 1-2 E. Robinson Oklahoma City.
Bevan, W. R. 114 Indiana Bldg ....Oklahoma City.
Bisbee, W. G.; 122 N. Broadway ....Oklahoma City.
Blesh, A. L.; Pioneer Bldg ....Oklahoma City.
Bradford, C. B.; Lee Bldg. ..Oklahoma City.
Boyd, W. J.; Security Bldg. ..Oklahoma City.
Buchanan, T. A.; Lee Bldg. ....Oklahoma City.
Camp, F. K.; Campbell Bldg. ......Oklahoma City.
Coley, A. J.; Campbell Bldg. ....Oklahoma City.
Cunningham, S. R.; Magestic Bldg. ..Oklahoma City.
Clement, W. R. ....Capital Hill Okla.
Cumings, W. C.; Security Bldg. .....Oklahoma City.
Cloudman, H. H.; Insurance Bldg. ....Oklahoma City.
Day, C. R.; Security Bldg. ....Oklahoma City.
Davenport, A. E.; Insurance Bldg. ....Oklahoma City.
Davis, E. F.; Lee Bldg. ....Oklahoma City.
Dicken, W. E.; Am. Nat. Bank, Bldg. ..Oklahoma City.
Dixon, W. E.; Security Bldg. ....Oklahoma City.
Edwards, R. T.; Lee Bldg. ....Oklahoma City.
Ellison, Gayfree; Am. Nat. Bk. Bldg. ..Oklahoma City.
Flesher, T. H. ....'.Edmond, Okla.
Fullington, W. A.; Security Bldg. ....Oklahoma City.
Fulton George; Campbell Bldg. ......Oklahoma City.
Ferguson, E. S.; India Temple ......Oklahoma City.

Foster, R. L.; Am. Nat. Bank Bldg. ....Oklahoma City.
Gay, Ruth A.; 209 1-2 W. Main ....Oklahoma City.
Hall, B. A.; 120 1-2 N. Robinson....Oklahoma City.
Hall, J. F.; 223 West 11th........Oklahoma City.
Howard, R. M.; Security Bldg. ....Oklahoma City.
Hartford, J. S.; Security Bldg. .....Oklahoma City.
Haas, Carl; ....Harrah, Okla.
Hunter, S. M., Baltimore Bldg. .....Oklahoma City.
Jolly, W. J.; Lee Bldg. ......Oklahoma City.
Johannes, A. D.; Security Bldg. .....Oklahoma City.
Kuhn, J. F.; 119 1-2 N. Broadway ....Oklahoma City.
Long, R. D; Lee Bldg. ......Oklahoma City.
Lain, E. S.; Am. Nat. Bk. Bldg. ....Oklahoma City.
LaMotte, G. A.; 209 1-2 W. Main ....Oklahoma City.
Langsford, William, 1st & Broadway ...Oklahoma City.
Looney, R. E.; Am. Nat. Bk. Bldg. ....Oklahoma City.
Lee, C. E.; St. Anthony's Hosp. ....Oklahoma City.
Messenbaugh, J. F.; 209 1-2 W. Main ...Oklahoma City.
McLean, G. D.; Empire Bldg. ......Oklahoma City.
Maxwell, J. H.;· 225 1-2 W. Main ....Oklahoma City.
Moorman, L. J.; Pioneer Bldg. ......Oklahoma City.
Meek, F. B.; Oklahoma Bldg. ....Oklahoma City.
Morgan, S. L.; 1025 West Reno ....Oklahoma City.
Martin, J. T.; Lee Bldg. ....Oklahoma City.
Neely, J. M.; Security Bldg. ....Oklahoma City.
Postelle, J. M.; Insurance Bldg. ....Oklahoma City.
Phelan, J. R.; 225 1-2 W. Main ....Oklahoma City.
Perisho, J. A. ....Luther, Okla.
Proffitt, J. H.; Security Bldg. ......Oklahoma City.
Rathbun, E. D.; 1301 W. 22d ......Oklahoma City.
Reck, J. A.; Lee Bldg. ....Oklahoma City.
Russell, U. L.; 120 1-2 N. Robinson ...Oklahoma City.
Riely, L. A.; Am. Nat. Bk. Bldg. ....Oklahoma City.
Rolater, J. B.; 200 1-2 W. Main ......Oklahoma City.
Ryan J. A. 209 1-2 W. Main ....Oklahoma City.
Reed, Horace, Pioneer Bldg. ...Oklahoma City.
Salmon, W. T.; 200 1-2 W. Main ....Oklahoma City.

Schaefer, R. F.; 120 1-2 N. Robinson....Oklahoma City.
Smith, M.; 209 1-2 W. Main ....Oklahoma City.
Sanger, Winnie M.; 120 1-2 N. Robinson Oklahoma City.
Stone, S. N.; ....Edmond, Okla.
Taylor, W. M.; Lee Bldg. ....Oklahoma City.
Todd, H. C.; Indiana Bldg. ..Oklahoma City.
Thomas, W. C.; Baltimore Bldg. ....Oklahoma City.
Walker, Delos, 316 W. Reno ....Oklahoma City.
Wall, G. A.; Lee Bldg. .....Oklahoma City.
West, A. K.; Majestic Bldg. ...Oklahoma City.
Watson, L. F.; 200 1-2 W. Main ....Oklahoma City.
Williams, C. W.; 219 1-2 W. Main ....Oklahoma City.
White, A. W.; 120 1-2 N. Robinson ....Oklahoma City.
Wier, W. M.; Bassett Bldg. ..Oklahoma City.
Will, A. A.; 120 1-2 N. Robinson ....Oklahoma City.
Wallace, W. J.; 122 1-2 N. Broadway ...Oklahoma City.
Wood, Ira J. ....Jones, Okla.
Young, A. D.; Security Bldg. ......Oklahoma City.
Roland, M. M.; Am. Nat. Bk. Bldg. ....Oklahoma City.
Westfall, L. M.; Security Bldg. ......Oklahoma City.
Buxton, L. H. ....Oklahoma City.
Clutter, W. S. ....Oklahoma City.
Pine, J. S. ....Oklahoma City.
Kelly, J. F. ....Oklahoma City.
Taylor, C. B. ....Spencer.
Norman Geo. R. ....Luther.
Wynne, H. H. ....Oklahoma City.

OKMULGEE COUNTY.

Bircaw, J. E. ....Okmulgee.
Breese, H. E. ....Henryetta.
Berry V. ....Okmulgee.
Cott, W. M. ....Okmulgee.
Culp, A. H. ....Beggs.
Hollingsworth, F. H. ....Okmulgee.
Little, W. G. ....Okmulgee.
Mitchener, W. C. ....Okmulgee.
Milroy, F. T. ....Okmulgee.
Newell, W. ....Okmulgee.
Oliphant, J. A. ....Okmulgee.
Perkins, H. ....Henryetta.
Stephenson, W. L. ....Henryetta
Weiskotten, W. O. ....Morris

OSAGE COUNTY.

Aaron W. H. ....Pawhuska.
Dewey, C. H. ....Pawhuska.
Houser, M. A. ....Pawhuska.
Meyrick, E. B. ....Burbank.
Speck, A. J. ....Pawhuska.
Walker, Harry ....Pawhuska.
Wharton, Divonis ....Pawhuska.

OTTAWA COUNTY.

Wormington, F. L. ....Miami.
Cooter, A. M. ....Miami.
Donahoo, J. ....Afton.
DeTaro, F. L. ....Miami.
Dean, F. R. ....Fairland.
Edwards, F. M. ....Fairland.
Harper, R. H. ....Afton.
McWilliams, W. L. ....Miami.
Rutledge, G. H. ....Afton.
Steadman, J. R. ....Wyandotte.
Troutt, L. W. ....Afton.

PAYNE COUNTY.

Anderson, Carl J. ....Perkins.
Cash, J. H. ....Glencoe.
Cleverdon, L. A. ....Stillwater.
Holbrook, R. W. ....Perkins.
Hughes, Eli ....Stillwater.
Janeway, D. F. ....Stillwater.
McQuown, H. ....Stillwater.
Murphy, J. B. ....Stillwater.
McHenry, D. D. ....Cushing.
Pickering, J. H. ....Stillwater.
Sexton, C. E. ....Stillwater.
Friedman, Paul ....Stillwater.

PAWNEE COUNTY.

Beitman, C. E. ....Skedee.
McCorl, E. B. ....Jennings.
Robinson, E. M. ....Cleveland.
Watkins, J. C. ....Hallett.
Weller, R. E. ....Pawnee.

PITTSBURG COUNTY.

Allen, E. N. ....McAlester.
Barnett, J. Z. ....Quinton.
Barton, V. H. ....McAlester.
Bond, R. I. ....Hartshorne.
Buffo, U. ....McAlester.
Brunson, C. J. ....Adamson.
Fowler, Wm. ....Alderson.
Gay, J. Paul ....McAlester.
Grubbs, J. O. ....North McAlester.
Gray, J. W. ....Quinton.
Graves, W. C. ....McAlester.
Griffith, A. ....McAlester.
Harris, A. J. ....McAlester.
James, Ed. D. ....Haileyville.
Johnson, P. S. ....Indianola.
Long, LeRoy ....McAlester.
Munn R. A. ....McAlester.
Mullins, G. C. ....Kiowa.
Mitchell, R. L. ....Dow.
Norris, T. T. ....Crowder.
Pemberton, R. K. ....Krebs.
Robinson, J. C. ....Chant.
Ross, S. P. ....Kiowa.
Sames, W. W. ....Harsnorne.
Street, Graham ....McAlester.
Turner, G. S. ....Krebs.
Williams, H. E. ....McAlester.
Watson, F. L. ....Alderson.

Wilson, McClellan ....McAlester.
Chapman, T. S. ....McAlester.
Lewallen, W. P. ....Canadian.
Rice, O. W. ....Alderson.
Troy, E. H. ....McAlester.

PONTOTOC COUNTY.

Runyan, J. R. ....Ada.

POTTAWATOMIE COUNTY.

Anderson, Robt. M. ....Shawnee.
Baker, M. W. ....Shawnee.
Baxter, G. S. ....Shawnee.
Ball, W. A. ....Wanette.
Blount, W. T. ....Asher.
Blickensderfer, Chas. ....Shawnee.
Butler. W. R. ....Maud.
Bradford, W. C. ....Shawnee.
Bence. F. ....Tribby.
Bradshaw, J. T. ....Shawnee.
Byrum, J. M. ....Shawnee.
Cannon, J. S. ....Shawnee.
Carter, J. S. ....Shawnee.
Carson, F. L. ....Shawnee.
Calhoun, C. E. ....Tulsa.
Campbell, H. G. ....Asher.
Clark, W. S. ....Byars.
Colvert, Geo. W. ....Tecumseh.
Cullum. J. E ....Earlsboro.
Ellis, J. B. ....Shawnee.
Farris, W. W. ....McComb.
Grey, E. J. ....Tecumseh.
Gallaher, W. M. ....Shawnee.
Hughes, J. E. ....Shawnee.
Henderson, W. E. ....Shawnee.
Kaylor. R. C. ....McLoud.
Mitchell, Ester ....Shawnee.
Mahr, J. C. ....Oklahoma City.
McAlister, E. R. ....Earlsboro.
Marshall, J. W. ....Shawnee.
McGee, W. N. ....Shawnee.
Rowland, T. D. ....Shawnee.
Rice, E. E. ....Shawnee.
Reynolds J. L. ....McLoud.
Reeder, H. M. ....Asher.
Royster, J. H. ....Wanette.
Sanders, T. C. ....Shawnee.
Scott, J. H. ....Shawnee.
Sanborn, G. H. ....Shawnee.
Trigg, J. M. ....Shawnee.
Taylor, J. C. ....Shawnee.
Wilson, H. H. ....Shawnee.
Walker. J. A. ....Shawnee.
Wingfield, W. C. ....Shawnee.
Wagner, H. A. ....Shawnee.
Warhurst, M. A. ....Shawnee.
Cone, H. L. ....Maud.
Applewhite, G. H..............Tecumseh.
Bloss, C. M. ....Tecumseh.
Cossey, W. A. L. ....Prague.
Dodson, S. D. ....Sacred Heart.
Nye, L. A. ....Okemah
Shipley, T. L. ....Shawnee.
Williams, W. R. ....Dale.

ROGERS COUNTY.

Anderson, F. A. ....Claremore.
Bass, E. Y. ....Talala.
Bennett, Geo. W. ....Talala.
Bassmann, Caroline ....Claremore.
Bushyhead, J. C. ....Claremore.
Caldwell, W. A. ....Chelsea.
Crabtree, J. S. ....Collinsville.
Dickson, T. B. ....Chelsea.
Hays, W. F. ....Claremore.
Hensal, T. W. ....Foyil.
Howard, W. A. ....Chelsea.
Lerskov, Andrew N. ....Claremore.
Means, J. F. ....Claremore.
Smith, J. F. ....Oolagah.
Strickland, Geo. ....Claremore.
Stemmens, J. F. ....Oolagah.
Smith, J. C. ....Catoosa.
Tinsley, B. S. ....Foyil.
Waldrop, J. G. ....Claremore.

ROGER MILLS COUNTY.

Allen, Frank W. ....Texmo.
Grant, V. V. ....Cheyenne.
Gregoire, J. A. ....Cheyenne.
Miller, J. P. ....Cheyenne.

SEMINOLE COUNTY.

Black, W. R. ....Little.
Harber, J. N. ....Seminole.
Harris, Chas. T. ....Konowa.
Knight, W. L. ....Wewoka.
Phillips, W. D. ....Seminole.
Turlington, M. M. ....Seminole.
Van Sandt, Guy B. ....Wewoka.

SEQUOYAH COUNTY.

Carnell, M. D. ....Sallisaw.
Cherry, F. T. D. ....Sallisaw.
Collins, M. D. ....Muldrow.
Hart, A. E. ....Sallisaw.
Hicks, A. A. ....Muldrow.
Hudson, V. W. ....Sallisaw.
Hunter W. M. ....Vian.
Jones, S. B. ....Sallisaw.
Johnson, S. P. ....Roland.
McDowell, M. T. ....Sallisaw.
McKeel, S. A. ....Sallisaw.
Morris, J. W. ....Sallisaw.
Morris, I. C. ....Vian.
Sosbee, J. W. ....Gore.
Wood, T. F. ....Sallisaw.

STEPHENS COUNTY.

Apling, J. S. A. ....Doyle.
Barnes, T. C. ....Marlow.
Bartley, J. P ....Comanche.
Brymer, W. G. ....Oklahoma City.
Conger, H. A. ....Duncan.
Christain, P. C. ....Bray.
DeMeglio, Eduardo........Oklahoma City.
Frost, C. E. ....Duncan.

Fuller, T. ....Devol.
Frie, H. C. ....Duncan.
Haraway, P. M. ....Marlow.
Harbison, J. E. ....:.....Alma.
Harrison, C. M. ....Comanche.
Howell, W. T. ....Duncan.
Holiday, J. R. ....Oklahoma City.
Long, D. ....Duncan.
Montgomery, R. L. ....Marlow.
Nickson, J. W. ....Loco.
Plunkett, B. J. ....Duncan.
Spears, W. S. ....Velma.
Williamson, S. H. ....Duncan.

TEXAS COUNTY.

Hayes, R. B. ....Guymon.
McMillan, James M. ....Goodwell.
Langston, Wm. H. ....Guymon.
Risen, Wm. J. ....Hooker.
Tucker, Wm. V. ....Carthage. R. F. D. 3.

TILLMAN COUNTY.

Bacon, Otis G. ....Frederick.
Comp, G. A. ....Manitou.
Collier, J. W. ....Manitou.
Fair, A. B. ....Frederick.
Gillis, J. Angus ....Frederick.
Hansen, J. H. .....:..........Grandfield.
Hays, A. J. ....Frederick.
Osborne Jr., J. D. ....Frederick.
Priestly, F. G. ....Frederick.
Ryan, J. N. ....Frederick.
Rosenberger, F. E. ....Grandfield.
Roberts, H. L. ....Frederick.
Spurgeon, T. F. ....Frederick.
Turpin, C. H. ....Mabton. Wash.
Van Allen, J. P. ....Frederick.
Wilson, Robt. E. ....Frederick,

TULSA COUNTY.

Ballance. R. A. ....:....Tulsa.
Brewer, F. L. ....Tulsa.
Brodie, W. W. ....Tulsa.
Bland, J. C. W. ....Red Fork.
Butler, G. H. ....Tulsa.
Clinton, Fred S. ....Tulsa.
Cook, W. Albert ....Tulsa.
Conway, W. Q. ....Tulsa.
Cosby, Jr., L. T. ....Tulsa.
Dart L. W. ....Tulsa.
Grosshart, Ross ... .Tulsa.
Hawley, S. DeZell ....Tulsa.
Hood, C. O. ....Dawson.
Jackman, J. A. ....Glenn Pool.
Jenks, E. E ....Skiatook.
Kernodle, O. P. ....Tulsa.
Kimmons, S. H. ....Tulsa.
Mohrman, S. H. ....:...Tulsa.
Mayginnis, P. H. ...|..........Tulsa.
Mayginnis, N. W. ....Tulsa.
Penny, T. A. ....Tulsa.
Reeder, C. L. ....Tulsa.
Rogers, W. H. ....Tulsa.
Wagner, R. S. ....Tulsa.
Webb, J. E. ....:..Tulsa.

Zink, H. F. ....Tulsa.
Wright, W. E. ....Tulsa.
Wiley, C. Z. ....Tulsa.
Wadsworth, D. U. ....Tulsa.
Wheeler, F. R. ....Manford,

WAGONER COUNTY.

Allen, R. L. ....Choska.
Adams, J. G. ....Porter.
Cobb, Isabell ....Wagoner.
Gordon, G. R. ....Wagoner.
Joblin, W. R. ....Porter.
Reich, J. L. ....Wagoner.
Ruble, G. W. ....Wagoner.
Shinn, T. J. ....Wagoner.
Smith, F. W. ....Wagoner.
Williams, J. M. ....Wagoner.

WASHINGTON COUNTY.

Athey, J. V. ....Bartlesville.
Curd, W. E. ....Copan.
Owens, A. P. ....Bartlesville.
Pollard, J. W. ....Bartlesville.
Pryor, R. E. ....Bartlesville.
Rammell, W. E. ....Bartlesville.
Sommerville, O. S. ....Bartlesville.
Sutton, F. R. ....Bartlesville.
Staver, B. F. ....Bartlesville.
Smith, Joseph G. ....Ochelata.
Weber, H. C. ....Bartlesville.
Wyatt, M. C. ....Bartlesville.
Woodring, G. F. ....Bartlesville.

WASHITA COUNTY.

Baker, J. C. ....Port.
Bungardt, A. H. ....Cordell.
Bennett, G. W. ....Sentinel.
Chumbley, C. A. ....Rocky.
Davis, S. C. ....Colony.
Dillon, G. A. ....Fose.
Farber, J. E. ....Cordell.
Harms, J. H. ....Cordell.
Jeter, A. J. ....Foss.
Jester, J. A. ....Cordell.
Kerley, J. W. ....Cordell.
Leverton, W. R. ....Cloudchief.
Lee, T. J. ....Rocky.
Mills, F. A. ....Foss.
McQuaid, J. M. ....Cloudchief.
Odell, I. H. ....Canute.
Sherburn, A. M. ....Cordell.
Tidball, Wm. ....Sentinel.
Weaver, E. S. ....Dill.
Weber, A. ....Bessie.
Sanburg, E. T. ....Cordell.

WOODWARD COUNTY.

Cockerell, J. C. ....Mooreland.
Patton, D. H. ....Woodward.
Pierson, O. A. ....Woodward.
Racer, F. H. ....Woodward.
Rose, W. L. ....Woodward.
Workman, J. M. ....Woodward.
Workman, R. A. ....Woodward.

MURRAY COUNTY.

The Murray County Medical Society elected the following officers for 1910:

President ....Dr. W. H. Powell, Palmer.
Vice-Pres. ......Dr. J. N. Brown, Davis.
Secretary ......Dr. J. A. Adams, Sulphur.
Censors ....Drs. Robt. Dunn, A. V. Ponder and George Slover. ·
Delegate ......Dr. J. A. Adams, Sulphur.
Alternate ....J. T. Slover, Sulphur.

FOR SALE.

$1,250 cash gets property consisting of three-room dwelling house, barn, stables, pair of horses, good buggy, office furniture and fixtures; $4,000.00 practice gratis; will introduce. Reason for selling—going to specialize in Texas. Address Dr. John T. Vick, Fort Towson, Oklahoma.

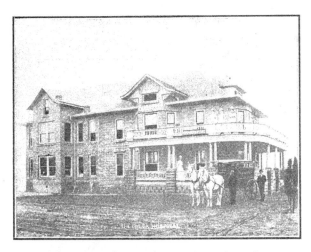

OFFICERS OF COUNTY SOCIETIES

COUNTY	PRESIDENT	SECRETARY
Atoka	J. B. Clark, Coalgate	T. H. Briggs, Atoka
Alfalfa	Z. J. Clark, Cherokee	O. A. Nylund, Helena
Adair	T. S. Williams, Stilwell	C. M. Robinson, Stilwell
Bryan	J. L. Shuler, Durant	D. Armstrong, Mead
Blaine	D. F. Stough, Geary	J. L. Campbell, Watonga
Beckham	J. M. McComas, Elk City	G. Pinnell, Erick
Coal	J. B. Clark, Coalgate	T. H. Briggs, Atoka
Choctaw	E. B. Askew, Hugo	J. C. Ellis, Hugo
Custer	J. Matt Gordon, Weatherford	O. H. Parker, Custer
Caddo	W. W. Gill, Gracemont	Chas. R. Hume, Anadarko
Cleveland	John D. McLaren, Norman	A. C. Hirschfield, Norman
Commanche	T. L. Gooch, Lawton	D. A. Myers, Lawton
Carter	E. A. Ballard, Lone Grove	C. B. Clark, Ardmore
Craig	C. P. Bell, Welch	Louis Bagby, Vinita
Creek	O. C. Coppedge, Bristow	C. L. McCallum, Sapulpa
Canadian	D. P. Richardson, Union City	Jas. T. Riley, El Reno
Cherokee	W. O. Blake, Tahlequah	C. A. Peterson, Tahlequah
Ellis	H. W. Hubbell, Arnett	John F. Sturdivant, Arnett
Garfield	J. H. Barnes, Enid	Julian Field, Enid
Grady	Walter Penquite, Chickasha	Martha Bledsoe, Chickasha
Garvin	W. C. High, Maysville	N. H. Lindsey, Pauls Valley
Greer	M. M. DeArman, Mangum	T. J. Dodson, Mangum
Haskell	S. E. Mitchell, Stigler	F. A. Fannin, Stigler
Hughes	A. L. Davenport, Holdenville	A. M. Butts, Holdenville
Jackson	J. W. Echols, Altus	L. A. Hankins, Altus
Jefferson	F. W. Ewing, Terrall	T. E. Ashenhurst, Waurika
Kay	W. A. T. Robinson, Ponca City	A. S. Risser, Blackwell
Kingfisher	C. W. Fiske, Kingfisher	C. O. Gose, Hennessey
Kiowa	G. W. Stewart, Hobart	J. M. Bonham, Hobart
Logan	E. O. Barker, Guthrie	R. V. Smith, Guthrie
Lincoln	C. M. Morgan, Chandler	E. F. Hurlburt, Chandler
Love	B. D. Woodson, Monroe	R. L. Morrison, Poteau
LeFlore	T. J. Jackson, Marsden	B. S. Gardner, Marietta
Mayes	E. L. Pierce, Salina	F. S. King, Pryor
Major	B. F. Johnson, Fairview	Elsie L. Specht, Rusk
Muskogee	H. C. Rogers, Muskogee	H. T. Ballantine, Muskogee
McIntosh	W. A. Tolleson, Eufaula	M. R. Nowlin, Eufaula
McLain	G. S. Barger, Wayne	G. M. Tralle, Purcell
Murray	W. H. Powell, Palmer	J. A. Adams, Sulphur
Marshall	W. L. Davis, Kingston	John A. Haynie, Aylesworth
McCurtain	A. S. Grayden, Idabell	W. B. McCaskill, Idabell
Nowata	L. T. Strother, Nowata	J. R. Collins, Nowata
Okmulgee	Wm. Cott, Okmulgee	W. G. Little, Okmulgee
Okfuskee	G. A. Reber, Okemah	Benton Lovelaly, Okemah
Oklahoma	A. A. Will, Oklahoma City	W. R. Bevan, Oklahoma City
Payne	C. H. Beach, Glencoe	D. F. Janeway, Stillwater
Pottawatomie	T. D. Rowland, Shawnee	G. S. Baxter, Shawnee
Pittsburg	R. I. Bond, Hartshorne	H. E. Williams, McAlester
Pontotoc		
Pushmataha		
Rogers	W. F. Hays, Claremore	A. Lerskov, Claremore
Seminole	W. L. Knight, Wewoka	M. M. Turlington, Seminole
Roger Mills		
Sequoyah	A. A. Hicks, Muldrow	M. D. Carnell, Sallisaw
Stephens	R. L. Montgomery, Marlow	D. Long, Duncan
Texas	Jas. M. McMillan, Goodwell	R. B. Hayes, Guymon
Tulsa	G. H. Butler, Tulsa	W. E. Wright, Tulsa
Tillman	F. G. Priestly, Frederick	A. B. Fair, Frederick
Washington	G. F. Woodring, Bartlesville	W. E. Rammell, Bartlesville
Washita	J. W. Kerly, Cordell	A. H. Bungardt, Cordell
Wagoner	F. W. Smith, Wagoner	J. L. Reich, Wagoner

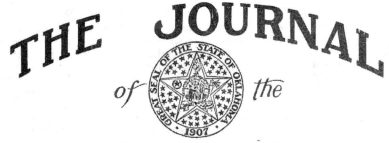

THE JOURNAL of the

Oklahoma State Medical Association.

| VOL. III. | MUSKOGEE, OKLAHOMA, JULY, 1910. | NO 2 |

DR. CLAUDE A. THOMPSON, Editor-in-Chief.

ASSOCIATE EDITORS AND COUNCILLORS.

DR. J. A. WALKER, Shawnee.

DR. CHARLES R. HUME, Anadarko.

DR. F. R. SUTTON, Bartlesville.

DR. I. W. ROBERTSON, Dustin.

DR. J. S. FULTON, Atoka.

DR. JOHN W. DUKE, Guthrie.

DR. A. B. FAIR, Frederick.

DR. W. G. BLAKE, Tahlequah.

DR. H. P. WILSON, Wynnewood.

DR. J. H. BARNES, Enid.

Entered at the Postoffice at Muskogee, Oklahoma, as second class mail matter, June, 1909.

This is the Official Journal of the Oklahoma State Medical Association All communications should be addressed to the Journal of the Oklahoma State Medical Association, English Block, Muskogee, Oklahoma.

INSANITY OF THE PUERPERIUM—CAUSATION, ETC.

BY DR. JOHN W. DUKE, GUTHRIE, OKLAHOMA

Apparently as far back into the annal. of time as the memory of man extendeth there has always been a popular fallacy, not only with the laity, but also with the medical profession, that childbirth was the cause of a certain kind of mental disease, characterized by a special pathological anatomy and symptomatology, diagnosed by the etiology, and a prognosis cautiously given in accordance with the severity of the symptoms manifested.

To say there is no such mental disease as puerperul mania, or insanity, I well know, is to invite surprise and opposition. There- fore, the purpose of this paper shall be an

(Read before the 18th annual meeting of the Oklahoma State Medical Association, Tulsa, May 10-12, 1910.)

endeavor to present the subject in such a light as to enable the general practitioner to readily recognize the exact cause of the mental alienation as he has been called to treat.

As a rule patients suffering from mental disturbance during the puerperium, because of the etiology, in the majority of the cases, are curable in from one to four months. The most frequently physical condition lead- ing to mental trouble during this period is exhaustion, consequently the exhaustion psychoses are the ones most apt to appear at the puerperium, and collapse delirium, and amentia, the most frequent of this class, the next in importance is a toxaemia, arising from an infectious organism, or from the destruction of tissue. Collapse delirium and amentia, although running a slightly different course, have many symptoms resembling each other. There is a marked disturbance of apprehension and coherence of thought, hallucinations, a flight of ideas, and psychomotor excitement.

Collapse delirium is characterized by an acute outset with confusion of consciousness, decided incoherence of thought, dreamy hallucinations, a changeable and emotional attitude, great psychomotor activity, and a fairly good prognosis.

This is a rare form of insanity, and childbirth is the most prominent exhaustion condition giving rise to it. As but few patients die from this trouble, but little is known regarding the pathological anatomy.

Following a few days of restlessness and insomnia. the patients soon become disoriented, and everything about them seems unnatural and changed. Many indefinite hallucinations and illusions are manifested. The furniture in the room assume, the form of menacing characters. The sunlight changes, people pass about in the room, they hear music, and pass through all kinds of strange experiences. They become very noisy and talkative, incoherent and confused, with a flight of ideas, they rhyme and repeat, which they sing as well as speak. Delusions are expressed which are incoherent and changeable, alternately depressed and exalted.

The emotional attitude is much more likely to be exalted than otherwise, though occasionally depression marks the whole course of the attack.

Some patients are irritable and inclined to violence and exhibitions of passion.

The motor excitement is very decided, patients constantly remove their clothing, rush about the room, upset furniture, beat on the door and walls and tear their clothing.

They are untidy and destructive, and reckless in their movements. They talk incessantly, often in a whisper, then shout at the top of their voices, at the same time gesticulating and clapping their hands. It is next to impossible to attract their attention, and they seldom answer questions. They are obstinate and contrary and almost never obey requests, resisting everything, even to dressing or bathing. There is great insomnia, if they sleep at all, it is only for a few moments at a time.

They take but little, if any nourishment, and it is often necessary to resort to forced feeding. The nutrition is bad, and there is a great and rapid loss of flesh, followed by physical weakness.

There is a tendency to acute bed sores, the reflexes are exaggerated, the pulse is weak and irregular, the temperature is unusually subnormal, and there are many muscular tremors. The duration is brief, often the disease does not last more than a few days, and seldom more tha a week or two.

The return to consciousness is often sudden, not frequently following a long sleep. It is to be differentiated from infection delirium by an absence of a flight of ideas, by greater cloudinesss of consciousness, more turbulence, and less pronounced hallucinations and delusions.

The catatonic excitement is recognized by the clear orientation, and the characteristic catatonic movements.

The delirious excitement of general paresis can only be recognized by the history of previous mental deterioration, and the presence of characteristic somatic symptoms.

The delirious mania of manic depressive insanity, in the absence of a history of a prior attack, can only be recognized by a greater disturbance of apprehension and the vivid hallucinosis-amentia by the longer course and the distractability of attention.

If the patients do not die from exhaustion they usually recover from the mental disorder.

Treatment.

The most important measures are to maintain nutrition and relieve excitement. The patients must recieve a sufficient quantity of liquid nourishment. In order to do this it will often be necessary to resort to forced feeding by stomach or nasal tube—milk, eggs, and alcohol constitute the best articles of diet for this purpose. Broths and peptoinzed meats may also be given. If mechanical feeding is not possible because of vomiting or hemorrhage of the mucous membrane, nutrient enemata may be given intsead. Failing in this, normal saline solution may be resorted to with fairly good results.

The prolonged warm bath is by far the most efficient means for controlling the excitement. The bath should be kept at ninety-five to ninety-eight degrees, all the time. The patients may be kept in the bath for hours, even days, without fear of harm. usually, however, they become quiet within an hour, when they should be returned to bed. When the excitement reappears, they should be placed in the bath again and kept there until the excitement is relieved. If because of great fear of the bath, it is impossible to keep the patient there, hyoscine hydrobromate gr. 1-100 to 1-60, or fifteen grains of vernol, or trional, may be given. Good results may also be had from paraldehyde, forty-five or fifty minims to the drachm.

Too much reliance must not be placed in sedatives, prolonged warm baths usually give much better results. In case of collapse strychnia and digitalis must be given by hypodermic injection. Constant attendance in an isolated place must be enfirced in order to get the best results and to prevent injuries.

Mechanical restraint must not be resorted to, a padded bed or room is better. During convalesence careful feeding, gradual exercise and freedom from excitement must be obtained. Recovery must be complete before the patients are permitted to resume their former duties or occupations. This does not occur until their normal weight has returned.

Acute Confusional Insanity (Amentia) is characterized by the rapid appearance of a multiplicity of illusions and hallucinations, clouding of consciousness and motor excitement, with an anxious expression. The chief cause of amentia is childbirth. This form of mental trouble constitutes about one per cent. of admissions to hospitals. The duration is from two to three months. At the beginning of the attack the patients are forgetful and confused, often stating that they have numbness in the head, and that they are unable to think. At this time they suffer from many hallucinations of the special senses. They see and hear strange faces and voices. Birds and insects are flying about. Lions and other wild beasts roar, poisons are placed in their food and thrown about the room, they are threatened with death and insulted by strangers. These hallucinations are the cause of many depressive delusions, incoherent, vague, and contradictory—They are to be burned, their children are dead, the home has been destroyed, and they are under some strange spell, which will destroy them. In a number of cases the delusions are expansive, they believe themselves exalted to high places, possessed of great power and wealth, will be queen of the world, and travel extensively. Their attention is attracted by their surroundings and they attempt to grasp what transpires. It is usually possible to direct the train of thought by holding objects before them, or by gestures and movements. This is only possible though, to a very limited degree.

The train of thought is greatly disturbed, they are unable to complete one idea before others occur producing a flight of ideas. They repeat words and phrases spoken by those about them. They often hold to definite delusions of persecution, and there is decided cloudiness of consciousness, with difficulty of arranging their ideas. Their emotions vary greatly, though they are more often happy than depressed, although they often alternate hilarity and sexual excitement with outbursts of temper and irritability, followed by dullness and stupidity. There is great psychomotor activity, they move about restlessly, crawl in and out of bed, but the movements are slow and performed without much energy; there are also intervals of complete quiet. The sleep is greatly disturbed, the appetite is poor and they sometimes refuse food. They also lose bodily weight, but not to the extent that they do in collapse delirium. The temperature is subnormal and the pulse is slow. The height of the disease is almost always reached within two weeks, but there may be remissions earlier than this, when they have a pretty clear insight into their condition. Permanent improvement comes on slowly, however, and after they have been clear for several days prolonged conversations or letter-writing has a tendency to again throw them into a state of confusion. After all the symptoms have disappeared, the patients are very easily fatigued, and for months mental shocks cause relapses. Death rarely occurs except by suicide, or collapse, during delirium at the outsetn, or heart failure,sepis, or tuberculosis. They almost always recover their mental health.

The treatment is the same as that in collapse delirium.

On account of the tendency to relapse they should not be allowed to enter their former occupations or environment until they have regained their bodily weight and their menses have reappeared, and the emotional attitude has become normal.

SOME INTERESTING OBSERVATIONS IN CONNECTION WITH APPENDICITIS.

BY DR. LeROY LONG, McALESTER, OKLAHOMA, PREPARED FOR SURGICAL SESSION OKLAHOMA STATE MEDICAL ASSOCIATION MEETING, AT TULSA, MAY 10, 11, 12, 1910

This paper will be devoted to some brief personal observations in connection with appendicitis. None of them, it may be, are original but the points involved seem to be of such a practical character that I feel they should be carefully considered.

I. Symptoms of Obstruction in Acute Cases:

1. Several months ago a physician living in a neighboring town telephoned me that the ten year old daughter of his partner was suffering of intestinal obstruction which had developed about thirty-six hours previous. He stated that cathartics had been administered in large doses, and a number of injections, high and otherwise, had been given without effect. The child was brought to All Saints Hospital on the first train and I saw her at 2 o'clock A. M. about forty hours after the attack had begun. At that time she had general diffuse peritonitis with great distention of the abdomen.

In this case the following history was obtained: She was seized with pain in the abdomen—the exact location not being very clear—about 10 o'clock A. M. while at school. Shortly thereafter she vomited and was sent home. Then the father; who was a physician, and his partner carried out the treatment referred to above without being able to cause the bowels to move. After consultation there was a diagnosis of probable appendicitis with rupture, and this was confirmed at the operation, which was done nearly forty-eight hours after beginning of attack. All that remained of the appendix was a gangrenous stump. The intra-abdominal picture was typical of a very pronounced general, purulent peritonitis. The child died on the fourth day. In addition to free drainage, Fowler's position and proctoclysis after Murphy were used.

2. On November 19, 1909, Mr. C. C., a young white man, twenty-two years of age was brought to Hospital by Dr. W., arriving about noon. This man became ill about 2 o'clock P. M. the day before while on the train enroute from Stigler to Atoka, about an hour after he had eaten a very heavy mid-day meal, consisting principally of pork chops. His first symptom was a violent pain in the epigastric region. He vomited about fifteen minutes later. The pain continued, but of a cramping character, and over the abdomen generally until he arrived at Atoka about two hours later. There was muscular rigidity over entire abdomen, and a feeling that the bowels should move. He had not had, so he told Dr. W. who was called, an evacuation for more than two days, his last movements having been produced by the rather drastic action of some pills he had taken several days before. To the mind of Dr. W. whom I regard as an excellent diagnostician, he presented the symptom of intestinal obstruction, and the ordinary means were resorted to in the efforts to relieve him, but being unsuccessful, a hypodermatic injection of morphine was finally given. When this young man reached the Hospital there was rigidity and tenderness over entire abdomen. I could not be sure that it was at one point more than another but was inclined to think it was a litle more marked in right lower quad-rant. His general condition was good. His temperature was slightly elevated. Remembering the emphasis which Murphy places upon the orderly sequence of the symptoms of appendicitis—first pain, second vomiting, third localized tenderness, fourth, fever,—I felt that this was a case of appendicitis, although the third symptom was not typical, the tenderness not being localized.

The operation was done about twenty-five hours after beginning of attack. In de-ference to opinion of Dr. W. the incision was made in median line. The gross appearance of appendix on outside was not bad—in fact, seemed almost normal: There was a slight swelling about the middle. After its removal a concretion was found at this point, surrounded by inflammatory material. There was a large hole near the margin of omentum, and a loop of small intestine had dropped through it. There was not the least constriction and I think had nothing to do with the symptoms. However, to prevent possible later trouble, this opening was obliterated.

An interesting sequela in this case was the development of an hepatic abscess, the first symptoms developing immediately after operation. This was operated by the trans-pleural route nearly three weeks later, the patient finally makng a good recovery. This abscess of the liver, it will be noted, de-veloped secondary to an appendicitis operated twenty-five hours after beginnig of first attack and in which there seemed to be only a mild degree of inflammation.

II. Pain and Tenderness in Children: The location I have found to be misleading.

A little boy, five years of age, was seen twelve hours after beginning of attack. There was history of diffuse abdominal pain The mother was not clear as to vomiting, but finally recalled that the child had complained of being nauseated, and had "spit-up" a little, but did not seem to vomit. Tenderness was more distinct on the *left side.*

I felt that sudden pain followed by nausea, and tenderness, even though the latter was in an atypical situation, indicated appendicitis. A consultant was of the opinion we had an ileo-colitis, and it was decided to wait. The result was a very large retro-caecal abscess.

III. Rapid Destruction of Appendix in Children:

It has been my observation that the appendix, on account of its low resisting power, breaks down very quickly in children. A little girl, five years of age, had initial pain at 5:30 o'clock P. M. I saw her at 7:30 P. M. The operation was done at 11:30 o'clock the next morning—eighteen hours after the initial symptom. The appendix was gangranous and ruptured. This had doubtless taken place during the night, as there was a sudden cessation of pain, and on the morning of operation the child was very comfortable.

IV. Haematemesis in Suppurative Cases: I have had one case—a nine year old boy operated for suppurative peritonitis fifty-four hours after beginning of attack. He did fairly well until the morning of the fifth day, when he had a large hemorrhage from the stomach. This recurred in smaller quantity several times during the day, and he rapidly sank and died.

This seems to be an accident unavoidable and, especially in cases already prostrated, usually fatal. A number of theories as to its cause have been advanced. Van Hook and Kanaval (Keen's Surgery, Vol. I V. page 630) sum up the matter as follows:

"It is well known that after various operations upon the body hemorrhages can take place, either in the stomach or bowels. After a study of the reported cases of this accident, Busse (Archiv-f-klin Chir, 76, 1-2) states that gastric and intestinal hemorrhages occur with about equal frequency in men and women after operations upon any part of the body, but especially after operations upon the abdomen. These hemorrhages occur from the direct or retrograde movement of thrombi in the arterial or venous stream. It is requisite that in the occurrence of these hemorrhages a further and additional moment of trauma shall occur. Usually such hemorrhages are multiple, and occur for the most part during the first week. The anatomic altera-

tions found consist of hemorrhages, erosions, and ulcerations, in the stomach and intestines. Anatomic alterations are frequently absent. Though the lesions are of such serious character and consequence, rendering the prognosis grave, it is best to follow a symptomatic course of therapy, abstaining from operative intervention."

V. Proctoclysis: I must confess that the efforts I have made to maintain continuous proctoclysis have not been rewarded with satisfactory results, especially in children. I hesitate to make this statement since I am aware that the method is in such general, and, apparently, satisfactory use by surgeons all over the country. The method I have attempted is that described by Murphy—the large, bent hard rubber tip with the three holes enlarged to 1-8 of an inch in diameter.

In my personal experience patients tolerate it with considerable distress, and usually the tip is expelled, or, if fixed, the water comes out around it. After repeated failures, I am at present injecting slowly the salt solution at intervals as I did formerly. There is no doubt however, that the continuous instillation is much superior if an apparatus can be constructed through which it may be caried out in an ideal and systematic manner.

VI. General Suppurative Peritonitis: These cases do not bear anesthetics or operative procedures to any marked extent. With ideal surroundings and facilities for operative work and after-attention, with an expert anesthetist and an expert surgeon, opening the abdomen, drainage, Fowler's position and proctoclysis would probably be the ideal procedure. In the absence of any one of these, the wiser and safer course would be, in my judgment, to sit the patient up in bed, give nothing by mouth, plenty of normal salt by rectum, in the hope that localization may take place in the lower abdomen, when an operation may be done with much less danger.

LARYNGEAL DIPHTHERIA.

BY A. B. MONTGOMERY, M. D., MUSKOGEE, OKLAHOMA.

Laryngeal Diphtheria, Membranous Croup, is an inflammation of the Larynx with membrane formation caused by the Klebs-Loeffler Bacillus. It is usually secondary to diphtheria of the tonsils or fauces, but may be primary. When secondary faucial or tonsilar diphtheria the laryngeal complication is usually indicated first by a dry, short, barking cough and a muffled quality of the voice.

(1.) Stenotic breathing becomes louder and leads to prolonged inspiration, followed by a pause and a short rapid expiration. The respirations are increased in frequency as the stenosis increases and dyspnoea becomes marked, calling into action all the auxiliary muscles. Pallor gives way to deep, cyanosis with threatening asphyxia. Evidences of carbon dioxide intoxication become marked. The patient becomes apathetic, sleeping with the eyes half open; the pulse becomes rapid and thready, and death closes the scene.

Primary Laryngeal diphtheria often develops very insidiously. May be very little, if any fever. It is first noticed that the child is hoarse. This hoarseness gradually increases and evidences of difficult respiration develop, and progress to a fatal termination from asphyxia to cardiac failure. Laryngeal diphtheria morbidity and mortality is greatest between the ages of two and five years. After ten years of age it is comparatively rare.

Diagnosis, Clinical, Bacteriological.

Clinical diagnosis is easy in secondary cases where laryngeal symptoms begin to develop after the membrane is fully developed in the throat. Inspection reveals the throat filled with membrane often necrotic and producing the horrible characteristic odor. Glandular enlargement is usually marked. The urine contains albumen. In secondary cases to the acute infectious diseases, measles, scarlet fever, whooping cough, the diagnosis is more difficult. Symptoms of gradually increasing embarassment of respiration such as hoarseness, rapid stridulous respiration and cyanosis are very suggestive of a diphtheritic involvement, while non-diphtheritic membranous laryngitis does occur, it is only in fifteen to twenty per cent of such cases that repeated bacteriological cultures fails to reveal the presence of the K. L. B. Practically all cases should be regarded as diphtheritic. When possible, bacteriological microscopic and cultural tests should be made.

Prognosis.

In the pre-antitoxin period over 80 per cent of cases were fatal. Under antitoxin treatment about 80 per cent recover and 60 per cent of such cases do not require intubation or tracheotomy. Prognosis is largely influenced by the time at which antitoxin treatment is begun, and vigor with which it is carried out.

Treatment.

Every young child with symptoms of laryngeal stenosis should be given antitoxin from 2,000 to 5,000 or 10,000 units, depending upon the urgency of the symptoms. Calomel should be given until it produces characteristic effects. Unless good effects of antitoxin as shown by easier respiration stay in progress of and exfoliation of membrane and fall of temperature occurs in eight to twelve hours, antitoxin should be repeated. (2.) Persistence of temperature unless due to complications always demands repetition of antitoxin. No case of diphtheria should be considered hopeless during

Read before 18th annual meeting of the Oklahoma State Medical Association, Tulsa, Okla., May 10-12, 1910.

the first stage. One reason for giving the large dose is that no one can calculate the amount of toxine that is present in the blood of a given case. (3.)

"The action of the remedy is the more intense and more certain the earlier it is used after the onset of the disease; four or five days after the onset of the disease it loses its action in a great number of cases."

Therefore, it is highly important that in all suspicious cases antitoxin should be administered at once, not waiting for the positive diagnosis by clinical or bacteriological methods.

The intrascapular region, abdomen, anterior aspect of the thigh, have all been recommended as sites for injection of antitoxin. The skin should be cleansed with soap and water first and then with alcohol. Strict asepsis should be observed. Antitoxin should be injected slowly and needle puncture sealed with flexible collodion or adhesive plaster. Mery advocates the use of repeated large doses of antitoxin and asserts that by this method he has saved many apparently hopeless cases. There need be no fear of anaphylaxis on this dosage. When the antigen is supplied in large doses, anaphylaxis does not occur. Muscular injections are more rapidly absorbed than subcutaneous. The gluteal muscles are a favorite point for injection. In cases seen early and properly treated, intubation or tracheotomy is rarely indicated. Even in the primary laryngeal cases over 60 per cent recover without intubation, (5) When antitoxin fails to check a progressive stenosis, the time for operative interference is at hand. The physician should not wait until the patient is cyanosed and the pulse intermittent.

Operative Technique.

The O'Dwyer tubes are generally used. The operation in itself is not difficult, but demands previous experience upon the cadaver. All the child's clothing having been removed, wrap the child securely in a sheet form the shoulders down. It should be held upright, facing the operator with its head against the nurses right shoulder who sits in a straight backed chair. The arms of the patient should be held firmly below the elbows, the legs are clasped between the knees of the nurse. The assistant stands behind the chair, holds the child's head firm between the palms of his hands, and when the gag is inserted includes it within his grasp. The operator now inserts his index finger, hooks up the epiglottis and inserts the tube in the funnel-shaped entrance to the larynx by elevating the handle of the introducer. The tube is then gently pushed home. The head of the tube is held by the tip of the index finger in the throat while loosening and withdrawing the obturator. When the tube is in the larynx and not blocked by detached membrane, a characteristic moisit rattle will be heard as the air is forced in and out in respiration. When tube is blocked with membrane and cyanosis occurs, the tube must be extracted and detached membrane expelled. Some children swallow liquids without difficulty with the tube in the larynx, others swallow semi-solid best, such as custards, scraped meat, ice cream, yolk of egg. Most patients swallow well in dorsohorizontal posture.

The air of the sick room should be kept moist, and in severe cases calomel fumigation should be used until antitoxin has time to produce beneficial effects. From 10 to 20 grains of calomel should be sublimed over an alcohol lamp under a croup tent, care being taken to give the child an occasional breath of fresh air if the vapor produces strangling. Cardiac weakness as suggested by arrhythmia or feeble pulse or vomiting should be met by administration of strychnine hypodermically with perfect quiet in the recumbent position. In cases of restlessness, with cardiac weakness, morphine hypodermically to effect continued for days may be of the greatest service. The use of an ice bag to the throat, and the swallowing of small pellets of ice is beneficial to the laryngeal process. The throat should be irrigated with a boric acid solution or some mild antiseptic. The post-diphtheritic paralysis is best treated with strychnine in full dosage, massage and electricity. Patient after severe attack of diphtheria should be kept in bed for two or three weeks, especially if there has been any evidence of cardiac weakness. People who have been ill with diphtheria and nurses, and those coming in contact with them should not be allowed to mingle with other people until two or three successive examinations by bacteriological methods show their throat to be free from K. L. B. E. E. Wuttke, of Halstead, Kansas, gives a study of forty-one cases of diphtheria. Of these cases there were twenty-eight in which there was no membrane in the throat, but in which culture showed the Klebs-Loeffler Bacillus to be present. The author believes that such cases are often overlooked on account of the absence of membrane, and that all cases of throat inflammation should be examined by culture.

(1.) Fruhwald & Westcott, Reference Handbook, Diseases of Children.

(2.) Forcheimer, Prophylaxis and Treatment of Internal Diseases.

(3.) Infections Diseases. Modern Clinical Medicine. (Baginsky, of Berlin.)

(5.) Caille, Diagnosis and Treatment.

(4.) International Clinics—Vol. 1.

DISCUSSION.

Dr. D. E. Broderick, Kansas City, Mo.

I enjoyed Dr. Montgomery's paper very much as being a conservative, scientific treatise on Laryngeal diphtheria.

I was very much elated to find the Docto speaking of anti-toxine and putting two thousand units as a minimum. He emphasized using five to ten thousand units of antitoxine. You will notice by the litera-

ture what is known as anaphylaxis, the disease following antitoxine injections but this is of such rarity and the results on the other side by giving big doses so great that we freely recommend big doses. In a hospital in Boston, it is the usual dose to give ten thousand units.

Dr. J. H. Scott, Shawnee.

I don't know as I have anything to add to the paper except to say that it is a good paper and a scientific production. The most difficult part of laryngeal diphtheria is in making the early diagnosis. I think when we overcome that difficulty, that we will overcome the greatest obstacle in our way. We don't have to be urged any longer to use antitoxine and use it in large doses. We are well convinced that it is the right thing to do. But the thing that we need impressed upon us most, and the thing that is the hardest for us to recognize is the early symptoms and making the early diagnosis. Personally I don't think we ought to wait to make the diagnosis. If any mistake is made about it being diphtheria a good dose of antitoxine won't hurt anything, and it will be a protection to the patient while we are waiting to form a conclusion as to what we have to deal with. I think that it is the supreme point of importance in laryngeal diphtheria, is to make an early diagnosis and give a good dose of antitoxine early.

By K. D. Gossom, Custer County.

I want to call attention to two points in connection with this subject. One is the low fever and the high fever. As a rule the lower the temperature the worse the case, and the higher the temperature, the better the prognosis.

And another thing I want to call attention to is a symptom that has been called to my attention by one of the physicians of Washita County; three of us have been calling it out for sometime and find that it holds good in most cases, and that is a blue line of demarkation. For instance, if the membrane is low in the throat, you will have the blue line of demarkation below that. Those of you who have diphtheria this next year take that up and let us have a report on it here next year. I am confident that there is something to that symptom. Attention was called to this fact at one of our Couty Medical Societies and we have found this to be present. A blue line of demarkation, and you never have it with tonsillitis.

I have had considerable expérience in diphtheria; probably as much as any man in the house that has had my experience of medicine. In giving antitoxine, I found it better to give large doses early and small doses late. I would like for that to be tested also. I find that that is an absolute fact. Give ten thousand units to a child of practically any age over six or eight months in the early symptoms and then drop down to about three thousand and we get our better results.

SOME STEPS TOWARDS THE PREVENTION OF POST-OPERATIVE EXUDATES.

BY WILLIAM EDWARD DICKEN, M. D., OKLAHOMA CITY, OKLAHOMA, LOCAL SURGEON FOR M , K. & T. RY. CO.; ATTENDING SURGEON ST. ANTHONY'S HOSPITAL; PHYSICIAN AND SURGEON TO OKLAHOMA STATE BAPTIST ORPHANAGE.

Post-operative exudates are of vast importance for the welfare and comfort of our surgical cases after operative interference. I have ben very much surprised, however, in investigating this subject, to find so little written about a subject, in my opinion of such vast importance to the surgeon.

The exudates that are thrown out after surgical intervention is in exact ratio of amount of tissue abrasion. There are several forms of exudates that we may mention in abdominal surgery, and I may say here that the exudates spoken of shall be confined to the abdomen and pelvis exclusively.

Owing to frequency of parametritic exudates and the great variety of physicial signs, to which they give rise, the differential diagnosis is supremely important.

Exudates may be mistaken for any kind of hard tumor in the neighborhood of the uterus.

Inspissated exudates, especially the spherical, intra-ligamentary masses with broad attachments to the uterus may closely resemble sub-seros myomata.

Intra-ligamentary peritoneal exudates are much less likely to be mistaken for myomata because the contents are fluid, and remain fluid for some time, but ultimately they became inspissated, the consistency more firm, and the outline at the same time more regular thereby greatly assisting the diagnosis.

Inflammatory exudates differs from ordinary transudates (limp and seros fluid) in its higher specific gravity and its definitly increased amount of protied matter, it is however in connection with seros surfaces, that fibrin characteristically tends to form, and its formation in this region is associated with the breaking down of leukocytes. It is to this fibrin that we owe the plastic aahesions in seros cavities, and these adhesions play a most important part in limiting the spread and generalization of many bacterial inflammations.

One has but to study the highly vascular and sensitive great omentum in connection with localized abdominal inflammations to observe how time and again a portion of it becomes firmly cemented over some infected area of one or other abdominal organ.

We have found such omental adhesions over danger spots on the walls of the stomach and abcesses about to burst into the liver, over ulcerated areas of the duodenum and on the floor of the pelvis, covering over the stump of a removed uterus.

Every one knows the constancy with which these exudates occur in connection with the inflamed appendix, but we must here point out and simultaneously recognize that it is not purposive that time and again these adhesions are productive of harm. As we may have by the presence of such exudates a prolonged plurisy, a kinking and obstruction of the bowels, torsion, internal hermia, etc. To repeat once again, the various phenoma of inflammation while tending to repair are not purposive, they are at most adaption and cannot and do not accurately fulfil all the needs of the economy.

The diagnosis of parametritic exudates as with other exudates is usually based upon the finding of a tumor in the pelvic connective tissue, presenting certain important characteristic determined by external and internal examinations.

In order of frequency post-operative exudates, are omentum, siginoid, small intestine and rectum. The intestines may become adherent to the abdominal or vaginal incisions. On account of the anatomic position of the omentum, it touching also every organ within the peritoneum including the pelvic floor, it may be seen how readily are produced abdominal lymphoctosis, circumscribed infected zones, and the covering of abraded surfaces.

The sympfoms are practically of no value in the differential diagnosis between myoma and exudate, even in an old exudate pain may be completely absent. On the other hand if the trouble began acutely with fever, this points to an exudate. Neither can we depend for positive information by a leukocyte count, for an old exudate has no influence on the number of leukocytes.

Frisch reports a case that illustrates the importance of this differential diagnosis.

"Many years ago," he says, "I did on ovarectomy on a patient who had come a long distince on account of a myoma as large as a fetal head with severe hemorrhage. The patient had no fever and left the hospital cured. Ten weeks later severe fever began and I discovered a peramentritis at the usual site above the pouparts ligament. The pus was discharged and the tumor disappeared. I had mistaken an old exudate for a myoma and the ovarectomy was entirely useless."

Experimentally adhesions of the peritoneum of dogs, may be produced by undue exposure to dry air; cold air; mechanical trauma, and culture of microorganism. Therefore in operating upon the human subjects these factors should be avoided, success is only achieved after careful and continued practice in the minutia of technic.

An operator may have great surgical judgement and extraordinary manipulative dexterity, and yet fail in the details of technic, as exhibited by himself or his assistant. Must we therefore take notice of the temperature and humidity of the operating room, is needless to say for on prolonged exposure of the peritoneum this is of importance theorectically, for the most suitable atmosphere is one that is very moist and of the temperature of the peritoneum. Practically this is never found, because operating staffs dislike to work under such conditions. An atmosphere charged with moisture at temperature of 90° F is perhaps the limit of endurance for prolonged surgical work. Defect in this respect in atmospheric conditions may to a great extent be made good by the avoidance of unnecessary exposure of viscera, protecting everything save the immediate area of operation, with gauze pads soaked in hot normal saline solution.

The next most important steps to pursue is the avoidance of trauma of the peritoneum; sponging should be employed as little as possible and al manipulations should be carried out with great gentleness, the injudicious use of retractors is likewise to be deprecated.

Care should be taken in removing tissue or separating adhesions that there be left no exposed areas, where it is possible to bury them under the peritoneum. Small areas on the parietal peritoneum, omentum, bladder, broad ligaments, mesenteries, may usually be easily covered with adjacent peritoneum by means of fine contigous catgut.

If we find it impossible to perform peritoneoplasty we can often bring down a portion of the omentum and with a few stitches of fine catgut protect the abraded surface. We have found it advisable in abrasions of the rectum to even cover the same with the uterus. We should also be very careful to avoid any raw surfaces in the closure of our peritoneal incision, thus to exclude any raw edge form the peritoneal cavity to avoid omental adhesions to the abdominal scar.

In the removal of the uterus, tumors or infected tubes and ovaries where extensive separation of adhesions has to be carried out, I have found it advisable to use what portions of the broad ligaments with the intervening uterine peritoneum, forming a flap across the pelvis, to be turned backward and stitched to the parieties and rectum, so as to form a new covering on the pelvic floor. Sometimes in extensive raw areas we stitch the utero ligamentus flap to the upper part of the rectum and its mesentery as it lies in an oblique direction across the pelvis. In this way the pelvic cavity may be entirely shut off from the general abdominal cavity and the latter may be often left without a single rawed area. In this way the general abdominal cavity is protected from the infected pelvis and our vaginal drainage may be kept up without any risk. Thus we can in most cases use the rectum and peritoneal flaps to cover the pelvis completely. And if a gap should be left in the right posteria half of the brim the caecum if

movable may be used (after removal of the appendix) to complete the deficiency, it being attached to the rectum and parietal peritoneum by a few stitches of fine catgut.

All operators in abdominal work have had some patients to complain for months and even years with pain and dragging sensations, even more so than their pre-operative pain, while on the other hand we have had patients to leave the hospital, saying they had never felt better, and able to go about their accustomed duties, with no discomfort. The former class however, suffering from extensive exudates which may in time be absorbed and their pain disappear, or they may become organized and firmly adherent, when the pain will never cease.

These pains are induced or exaggerated by excercise. It is dragging in character, indicating that the intestine or omentum is under traction.

I recall a typical case, Mrs. S., age. 38, which two years previous we did a retroperitoneal shortening of the round ligaments for the correction of a retroversion, and during this length of time the patient was never free from a dragging sensation and cramped like pain in the right iliac region, in fact the pain became so intense at times, that her family physician suspected an abscess formation; and later came back hoping for relief. Celiotomy was perfomed and upon careful examination of the viscera we found nothing abnormal except a slight exudate and adhesion of the end of the appendix to the perital wall. Appendictomy was performed and complete relief was the result.

Adhesions of the omentum cause less immediate trouble than those of the intestines, but the omentum has not the power of loosening itself so to speak, as have the small intestines. For this reason I give a laxative early after my abdominal operations, that the peristalsis may be re-established and adhesions broken up.

I have had patients to take horse back rides daily, for the purpose of breaking up post operative exudates with good results.

In conclusion, I wish to urge upon the surgical profession the importance of a proper technic, appreciating the significance of adhesions and so operate that they will not form again, or will not originate, de novo. 312-13-14 American National Bank Building.

Chairman Blickensderfer: "Gentlemen, Dr. Dicken's paper is now open for discussion.

Dr. Kuhn, of Oklahoma City. "I think the key note of the paper was struck in the last sentence, and I believe that post operative exudates are usually operative negligence. There isn't much occassion for post operative exudates if you are careful of your material; if your work is done under proper precautions, and if you have exercised that skill which your patients demand of you. There are certain times that it absolutely impossible to prevent adhesions, but in clean cases there is no occasion for post operative exudates. I believe this is a point that the paper should bring out very carefully. That it is usually an indication of a slip in your technic some place, and it is usually due to your own fault. I cannot help but think that that particular portion of the paper requires particular emphasis, because it is a fact. Physicians who are perfecting their technic are having fewer adhesions. The more we work the more we find that it is due to our own negligent work. I simply want to say again that I think the key note of the paper was struck in the last sentence. Post operative exudates are usually operative incompetency."

Dr. Cullum. I don't believe that post operative exudates are always a sequel of surgical incompetence. If we had no pathology in the beginning, it would not require a very skilful surgeon to leave a case clean. I have seen them follow the hand of such men as Murphy, and men of that class, and I do not think that it is strange that some of the surgeons in Oklahoma, where we are not rated as high as Murphy, would have some such results. The surgeon is correct at no time in saying that it is a mark of incompetence on the part of the operator."

Dr. Walker, of Shawnee. "This paper seems to be a paper that is well written and required a great deal of careful study and reading very fully the writing that has been written on this subject. As the essayist has said, there hasn't been very much written on post operative exudates. On this same line there is a condition that arises from the same cause, which is "post operative." In either case, as the gentleman has said, where we have a pathological condition to begin with, we cannot hope for as perfect results as we can where we have a condition without adhesions. If you handle your intestines a great deal, and expose them a great deal, there is necessarily more or less inflammation, and necessarily more or less likelihood of adhesions or exudates following. * * * * * * * * There is one part of the paper I would like to call especial attention to, with reference to the peritoneum. * * * Where the peretoneum is sufficiently loose to permit of it you can sew your peritoneum up with the gut sutures. sewing through and through, and that draws the edges of the peritoneum on the outside. It is not always practicable to do that because sometimes we find the periton. eum is too short. Another thing that I would like to speak of is, that the case that was reported, the abdomen having been opened. I believe, and the shortening of the round ligaments,—it is my custom and the custom at Shawnee, when we have the abdomen open to take the appendix out whether there is anything the matter with it or not. They said at Rochester, that an appendix in Rochester did not have any more show than a snowball down below. And that is the way we do down at Shawnee."

Dr. Blesh, of Oklahoma City: "I was very much interested when I read the caption of his paper, to hear what he would have to say upon the subject. In the post operative or any other type of exudate we may consider that there are of two classes, first the infective type, and second the noninfective types. The infective types may have their origin before the operation has been done at all—in other words what we call the pathology of the case. The surgeon is operating perhaps because of this exudate, and he will very likely have post operative exudates follow. · The noninfective types may be classed as hemorrhagic, and several other types, and that brings up another question in the matter of hemorrhage in operation. Another thing that bears deeply on this subject is the fact of operative rudeness. I believe the surgeon who operates the most successfully is the one who handles the viscera the least and the most gently. That can be demonstrated by taking a dog and simply pulling the intestines for a certain length of time and you will see an exudate actually occur. Now the handling of the viscera is one of the things that should be guarded against. Its exposure as dwelt upon by the essayist is another very important point. Jarring of the viscera will have very much to do with the exudate—that is to say with exudates that are non-infective in type. Exudates per se are not generally pathological in that they cause trouble of themselves alone. The trouble that they cause is secondary. Exudates may organize or they may liquify and dissolve. It is the organized style of exudates with which we have to deal and which causes us trouble. These may cause all types of trouble, vaginitis and those things which give rise to pain. I believe so far as technic is concerned the

essayist has said the right thing when he says as our skill increases in technical work, we will have less of it.

The covering of the Viscera is an important step, though it is possible it is not always advisable to cover the viscera following an operation."

Dr. Berry, of Okmulgee: "The subject is a very interesting to any man doing surgery, and it seems to me there should be no controversy over exudates. Any man who does surgery will have them. Exudates are either from infective or mechanical sources, and in doing an operation we are liable to do more or less mechanical work. However, as surgery is subject to a certain amount of accidents over which we have no control, such as post operative hemorrhage, it is impossible for any man to say that he never has exudates in his work. As I go along with my work I find that I have less trouble than I did ten years ago. And I attribute that to increased care in operation. Recently I have devised a method of drainage that I want to call the attention of the gentlemen to and they can take it for what it is worth. I take a piece of rubber dam about the size of this book and I cut it up in little strips about an eighth of an inch wide, and leave one little strip attached, and I have one long strip so that when I roll this up into a bandage I wrap the last strip of rubber dam around this. Now you can slip that clear down into the bottom of the abdominal cavity and when you are ready to take that out you can slip it right out, and the drainage is ideal. I don't claim that original at all. But the method of making it out of rubber dam so that you never lose one in the abdominal cavity is a very good idea. And you never have most of the strands clinging to the peritoneum as you do in gauze drainage. As you all know with gauze you have the granulations growing right onto the gauze and it is very difficult to take it out, and I have had several cases where I have had to open the abdominal cavity even a year or two after the primary operation. I have found in those cases where I have had no infection, in my first operation I have had no exudate or adhesion. But where I had an infection at the primary operation I have found an adhesion. Just two weeks ago last Tuesday, I had a second operation of a case of appendicitis at Okemah. We simply opened the abdomen and allowed the pus to drain out and put in proper drainage, and the man had no trouble at all for over a year. He was leading a very active life and had no pain in the region of the primary operation, but two weeks ago his physician phoned me that he had taken very seriously ill, and when I got there he was in a very desperate condition. On opening it we found about six or eight ounces of pus discharged from the wound and I found the bowel all matted with adhesions from the former operation. And it was entirely gangrenous except a little place at the top where it was adhering to the bowel. I deemed it advisable on account of the second attack to take the appendix out. Those adhesions were very tense and there were a great many of them. The point I want to make is this, that those adhesions caused no trouble and that this attack came on very suddenly. In some cases it may be lack of skill on the part of the operator, or it may be circumstances over which you have no control, but when we get down to the last analysis, we all have adhesions, and what we want to do is to find out how to avoid them, and the way to avoid them is to perfect our skill in operation. You take a uterus rising up and down and you will have adhesions there, and I care not how careful an operator is, who he is, or where he comes from, he is going to have post operative adhesions."

Dr. Mayberry, of Enid: "I want to congratulate the Doctor on his paper. I felt like it was an original paper, and that is where we get perhaps our greatest value in these meetings. I think a post operative exudate is a good thing. We might get the impression from the paper and the discussion that a post operative exudate is always an indication of rough handling or bunglesome surgery, which cannot always be the case. We have a pre-operative exudate from suppurative conditions. If you have a pre-operative exudate, why there is nobody to blame for that. You have only got to take care of it. Take a very fleshy person where you have operated cancer of the breast and you are going to get an exudate and is not going to be because you was not skilled in your surgery. It is going to be an exudate from your lymphatics. And that exudate is good and dangerous. We all understand the pathology of a cancer of the breast and we have an extension of that in the glands under the arms. An extension of that cancer from his lymphatic duct. Now you open this lymphatic in doing a clean operation for cancer of the breast, and you want a lymphatic exudate, and if you don't get it the chances are you are going to lessen your chances for a cure. My experience has been that when I got a great mass of lymphatic exudates I had better results.

When it comes to covering up all the surface of the bowel it is sometimes impossible. It is an interesting thing to get up and talk about folding the peritoneum over raw surfaces, but when you get to operating you find that lots of times you can't do it. The one that does it the best perhaps has done the nicest piece of surgery. But the trouble that I have had myself in exudates and am having now, is an exudate of the abdominal wall in itself. Rough handling of your muscular fibres, you have an exudate there that must be in itself a non-infective exudate. That kind of an exudate happenning I think we can blame ourselves for that, and make up our mind that if we have an infection of the sutures we have been a little awkward in our surgery. If you find that you have not been treating an infection as well as you might, which is of often greater moment, you had better take care of the exudate by a careful drainage, even if we operate on the non-infective cases.

The Doctor spoke of giving these operative cases laxative early in the case.

Chairman Blickensderfer. "If there are no further remarks Dr. Dicken will close the discussion."

Dr. Dicken: "I think a paper is successful to the extent in which it brings out discussion, and I was very much edified by the manner in which my paper has been discussed. I touched upon the thought that Dr. Walker brought out, and he completed it just as though I would have continued writing on that subject. The meth-od which he has in bringing the folds of the peritoneum together and sewing it through is being done by a great many surgeons with great success. That, as the Doctor said cannot always be done of course. The success of your operation is to the extent of the uterus adhering to the abdominal wall.

The great point I wished to bring out in the paper was the carefulness of our technic, and the result of the exposure of the contents of the abdomen, because the temperature in our operating rooms is largely below the temperature of the peritoneum itself, and the cold air itself will bring about adhesions. And then another thing is the closing of the exposed surface with the peritoneum. It does not adhere and is easily removed and does not block up and interfere with your drainage.

The cause of post operative exudates in my opinion is not always the fault of the physician."

AUTOINTOXICATION.

BY L. S. WILLOUR, M. D., ATOKA, OKLAHOMA.

According to Ewald, autointoxication is a poisoning of the body by normal or abnormal products of digestion, or of metabolic origin. The autotoxins are products always originating in the process of combustion of the proteids into their simpler forms. In this process any abnormality, either chemical or physiological, produces a discordant note in the harmony of digestion, and consequently arises some or all of the symptoms which we so often meet.

This discordant note results in excessive normal products, or in new abnormal products in the alimentary tract. These form in the intestine, intestinal autotoxins.

When in the stomach hydrochloric acid is not present, we are certain to have putrefaction, add to this the numerous micro organisms, lock up the intestines, and we have a veritable incubator for the production of autotoxins.

Some of the main causes for the appearance of autotoxins, are gastro-intestinal fermentation, lack of mechanical or physiological ability to rid the intestine of toxic materials, large burns, general psoriasis, and other conditions of the skin, not conducive to perfect elimination; disease or inactivity of the kidney, and, no doubt, the relation of diabetes to the pancreas, myxedema to the thyroid glands, Addison's disease to the suprarenal capsule, are cases more or less intimately related to autointoxication.

Autotoxins are always present in the body to a greater or less extent. When in small quantities, they are neutralized by antitoxins which Nature produces when the poisonous materials assert themselves, and speedily eliminate or render inert.

The symptoms are very variable, and present a veritable kaleidoscope of clinical pictures. The symptoms of greatest diagnostic value are nervous irritability, headache, fatigue, depression, vertigo, melancholia, disordered bowels, cold hands and feet, livid lips, etc.

The work of one organ may be thrown upon another, which necessitates over-activity of the imposed upon organ, and following sooner or later disease. The kidneys may suffer in order to rid the blood of autotoxins, as in lithemia, uric acid excess, etc.

The effect of autotoxins on the nervous system is most pronounced. The immediate effect upon nerve cells is that of lessening, retarding or preventing their power to transmit nerve impulses. When this action becomes chronic in character, the result will be trophic changes or organic lesions. According to I. Newton Snively, many conditions generally credited to autointoxication are primarily disturbances of the nervous system.

In conclusion, permit me to mention two points of particular interest: 1st, That intestinal autointoxication is more frequent in children, which is probably due, according to J. M. Anders, to the greater activity of intestinal absorption in childhood. 2nd, That symptoms of autointoxication may equal the symptoms of other toxemias, such as rigid spasms, paralysis, and ultimately, trophic or structural changes.

PNEUMOCOCCUS IN THE EYE.

BY DR. J. H. BARNES, ENID, OKLAHOMA.

The Pneumococcus is the most common germ the Nose and Throat man finds, for we find it in nearly all smears from even the normal throat and from this we would naturally suppose that we would find them in the normal conjunctival sack, it being so closely connected with the nose and throat. This is not the case, while we find them on the normal conjunctiva rarely they do not seem to thrive well in the normal secretions of the eye. The tears retard their growth and destroy their virulency.

The inoculation of animals with pneumococcus from the normal conjunctiva have not been successful owing to the lowered vitality of the germ. So wound infection of the cornea from the conjunctiva is not very probable, tho we do know that slight abrasions of the cornea may develop into a very severe hypopion ulcer. This germ which is usually the pneumococcus, may have been carried into the wound by the foreign body and not come from auto-infection.

The germ has no action at all on the unabraded epithelium of the cornea.

We will discuss three places of the eye where we find the pneumococcus; the conjunctival sack, the lacrymal sack and in the corneal tissue.

It produces a conjunctivitis in the new born baby in some cases almost like blenorrhea. It is most commonly a much milder infection, coming on after the fifth day. While gonorrheal ophthalmia is before the fifth day.

The infection runs a much milder course than ophthalmia neonatorium and is not so dangerous as far as the cornea is concerned. It may become chronic if it is not treated.

A microscopical examination should be made in all cases of ophthalmia neonatorium

Read before the 18th annual meeting of the Oklahoma State Medical Association, Tulsa, May 10-12, 1910.

for the parents protection as well as that of the child. There is only about 60 or 70 per cent of these cases due to gonococcus.

Pneumococcal conjunctivitis is an acute catarrh which develops very rapidly in both eyes with intense redness and swelling of the conjunctiva and the lids. There is a profuse discharge of pus which lasts only a few days when the redness and the swelling soon disappears. The whole course lasting four or five days in the adult while in the baby it is two or three weeks.

The germ rapidly disappears after the first day. There is litle pus after the second day.

I have had one case that was almost typical. A boy eight years old went to bed at night as well as usual, came down stairs about three o'clock in the morning crying and telling his mother that his eyes hurt him. I saw him at ten o'clock. The lids were swollen shut and a yellow pus runing down on his face. Elevating the lids the bulbar conjunctiva was lapping half way over on the cornea. It was very red. Lots of secretion and very sensitive to touch and painful to light. He kept his head burried in the pillow or his hands. The examination of the pus showed a great abundance of pneumococcus.

In two days the secretion had stopped, very little swelling, eye much better mother did not think it necessary to bring him back for treatment.

I saw two other cases in another family. The younger sister came to see me the second day after a severe attack of sore eyes as she said, complaining and giving nearly the same symptoms as the other case. There was some muco-pus slight redness of both eyes and photophobia.

On examination of the pus I found only a few pneumococcus. Not finding any other germs, I made a culture and confirmed the diagnosis which was not made till after the culture was made and the second case in the

family was seen and examined. She complained the same way just a few days after. I saw her in twenty four hours after the onset and found the germs more abundant but not so many as the first case who was seen early. They recovered in a few days.

The two sisters think they took it from a relative who had been visiting them. About seven days as near as I could figure it out.

There was one thing about all three cases, while there was no involvement of the cornea there was photophobia in every one and very severe in the boy where there was so much swelling and pus. The inflammation seems to be profound and involves the deeper structures of the eye.

In Dacryocystitis in more than one half of all cases the pneumococcus is found. They are very numerous and remain in the sack almost indefinitely in the chronic cases. The germ from the lacrymal sack is much more virulent than from the conjunctiva. Animals can be readily inoculated. Being cut off more or less from the tears and the increased temperature and the lack of drainage seems to be a culture media that grows an organism that is very infective.

The acute cases are more apt to become chronic than the other organisms that are found in the sack. These cases are harder to cure and is more apt to cause disease of the bone as it has been demonstrated that the germs will penetrate the walls of the sack.

Hypopion or purulent keratitis is most commonly due to the pnuemococcus. It may be due to the foreign body carrying the germ to the abraded cornea or to the secretion in the lacrymal sack after a slight abrasion. Not so apt to be from the germ in the conjunctival sack alone as it is proven that it is almost impossible to infect the cornea with these germs that have such a lowered vitality.

It is harder to demonstrate the germs in the cornea hence we are apt to find some other cause and send our patient away without much care to find the cornea almost destroyed in a few days. If we are careful to get some of the scrapings from the fresh ulcer of the cornea we will find the germ. When we do find it we do not want to lose any time in counteracting his progress, for it is characteristic of the pneumococcus to do its work quick. When it gets started on the corneal tissue it soon spends its force where it started and has invaded new tissue and the old is rapidly healing. It does not thrive well on the deep tissue where it is compacked. The germ dies and new tissue is invaded by fresh germs. So we find it making its way across the cornea not in any definite line which gives it the name of serpiginous ulcer. It many times spreads across or around the whole cornea.

In a very few days the inflammation is so pronounced that it produces a derangement of the deeper tissues of the eye.

To sum up. Some cases of ophthalmia neonatorium are due to pneumococcus. A microscopic examination should be made in all cases so as to protect the child as well as to free the mother from the suspicion of gonorrhea.

We need not be alarmed when we find severe cases of conjunctivitis resembling blenorrhea, when we find the pneumococcus.

All lacrymal sack cases should be examined so we can warn the patient against the pneumococcus infection should the cornea become abraded even from the slightest injury.

All cases of purulent keratitis should be looked on with suspicion and treated vigorously.

MEDICAL ETHICS.

ANDREW N. LERSKOV, B. S., M. D., CLAREMORE, OKLAHOMA.

It is true that this subject has been discussed with fevered interest at numerous times by the brainiest men of our profession, from the time of Socrates, Tubal Cain and the dawn of the Medical era though all the advancing ages to the present time but the question often comes home to me after a few years of hard experience; where should the principles and teachings of ethics begin? When should this great subject first be inculcated into the vocation of the professional pursuer? It is a given fact to a certain extent that locality and environment have some variations as to their rules but the broad principles are practically the same. Fees, modes of despensing drugs, social and financial standing and localities have their altered variations but the broad standard varies but a little. I think that the Medical College, the mother and birth place of every follower of medicine should be

the kindergarten and instructive institution for this important law and acknowledged fact. There is where this fundamental priciple of success should be instilled into the life of the beginner. It is as necessary to know how to deal justly with his senior colleague as it is to know how to diagnose or treat the deviation from the normal. During my lecture courses in different places I scarcely ever heard of this subject and in fact in most institutions no chair is included for its discussion, no lectures delivered for its benefit and no time devoted or but little attention paid to the respect of the important matter. We are ground from day to day through the fundamental principles and paths of our science which is perfectly right but we never take a halt to get out of the rut and consider other aspects of our duties and obligations that we justly owe to our fellow man. We are ushered out upon the great masses of the populace to mingle and intermingle with the many perplexing propositions, fresh from the green room and lecture halls, filled with theory, grit and a determination to gain prestige and practice at any peril or even at the expense of years of toil in the field of some other who is justly entitled to that field. We tread innocently at times on forbidden territory, criticise where agreement is indicated, divulge professional secrets where silence is demanded and very often offend and heat a temper not easily amenable to reconciliation and in some instances forever lose a friendship and then we ponder and ask ourselves in what manner and how this occured? We will in all probability have all respect due and sincerity for the brother and did the act of violation through ignorance and a free conscience. Then we will take a retrospection and ask ourselves the question if I ever were admonished of these facts or were these rules discussed at any time within the space of time occupied between the College walls? It is true that our mother organization the American Medical Association publishes its rules and codes of ethics but the student's limited area of thought and mind is clouded by numerous lectures and his time so limited that his attention is not vividly called to this essential subject and would not be appreciated, remembered or obeyed as much as if it were indelibly impressed and infused into his memory by the utterances of a fond and revered professor. The field of Medicine is so broad, its many subjects so complicated and marvelous details so numerous that the student at all times is striving only to absorb that portion dished out by his instructor. The minute details of ethics would not be necessitated but its great fundamental and most important parts and phazes thoroughly explained to the tender mind of the be-

ginner so that when he takes his part on the role of the drama and is delivered among his fellow practitioners he may be able to quote with higher ideals and make a right start and be saved of much trouble and embarassment. Taking into consideration the Medical College is only the foundation on which the Physician must construct his future structural career and only teaches him how and when to think and aids his mind to perform its function of growth and knowledge as his future problems increase in complexity as his experience widens and he needs all his theory coupled with common sense, deliberation, ethics and continual persistent study. And, too, looking at the proposition from another standpoint and phase we are not all saints or perfect and older practitioners who have had to gain their standing by such knocks should be willing to lay aside avarice, egotism, envy and jealousy and lend the beginner a helping hand. Assist him to overcome this obstacle and help him up when he falls and warn him of future pitfalls. At the present time I can look back into the past and see things that I have done that are grave wrongs or violations of ethics and had at most times thought that I was perfectly right and thought that I was doing what was right, but I was fortunately placed among some good broad minded men who were conscientious enough to admonish me of my wrong doings and I was and am now very appreciative of their efforts and kindness and will always stay with those good fellows. I would be grateful to them for those favors and probably simultaneously through ignorance of the law violate another of different rules unknowingly and again be turned right about face and put on the right road to success. And nothing like straight business and honest policies will win more for one both in financial and social standing to both laity and profession. By the many rectified mistakes and regretful violations, by the good advice of older practitioners who probably had experienced of many like problems, a purchase of a code of ethics and a thorough perusal and study of its pages I was able to begin to sit up and take notice and realize the pleasure and gratitude of being ethical, straight and clean with my brother co-laborer.

It is perfectly right to get business in a clean legitimate way and one will be respected and adored for it and can hold it without public advertisement, faking nostrums and dirty methods if his ability is sound and his motives conscientious. If a fellow competitor gets my business and my case in a clean legitimate way and his methods better and his results more successful I say "pat him on the back and say luck to you old boy I am with you" and it can be done without material injury to all concerned. And again if I got a business knowingly that I obtain illegally with malice a forethought and even my success be better I am rightfully not worthy and lose the confidence and respect of not only the local profession but the community in which I do my work and in turn the truth is imparted to other members of the profession in different parts of the State until I am branded as a reprobate and most times the profession wait and stand matters for a long time before those things are done. If I obtain a case and take charge of it and in any way unknowingly do the other fellow a wrong I appreciate it more if he will approach me and inform me of the mistake. I am always proud of him and am grateful and will guard myself thereafter, and in every way try and retrieve for the injury inflicted but if a man persists in continuing the practice of violating these rules of ethics knowingly and repeat the same act over and over after being informed, admonished and given time to consider them it is time to brand and ostracise him. We are probably one of the closest allied professions on earth, our interests should be more guarded and sacred than that of any other vocation. We should protect our brother not only at home but elsewhere and should ask him to protect us. We have all made mistakes and there have been places in our lives where another practitioner could send us to a profesional hell and we have probably been the other fellow in the same predicament and though it is not a violation of the moral law so much but should be respected and adored we maintain these rules the laity will be compelled to respect us and in order to obtain that goal, its teachings should begin with the teachings of that great art of medicine when the matriculant casts his lot and life's work in the corriders and lecture rooms of the Medical University.

"CHRONIC NEPHRITIS; ASSOCIATED CIRCULATORY CHANGES."

ARTHUR W. WHITE, M. D., OKLAHOMA CITY, OKLAHOMA, PROFFESSOR OF CLINICAL MEDICINE AND DIAGNOSIS MEDICAL DEPARTMENT UNIVERSITY OF OKLAHOMA.

There are many diseases resulting from affections of the circulatory system; there are many others which give rise to cardio-vascular changes, but in no case is the relationship so marked, as between chronic renal troubles and the vascular system.

Changes in the vascular system are practically constant in chronic nephritis, and especially are they seen in all those who suffer from the commonest form of kidney trouble, viz: degeneration of the interstitial tissue of the kidney followed by the formation of embryonic tissue and contraction of the whole organ, and classified by most authors as chronic interstitial nephritis.

The etiology of this form of nephritis is unquestionably hematogenous due to the presence of toxic material in the blood acting continuously over a long period of time, the sources of which may be metabolic or inflammatory. These forces act on the kidney substance to set up a marked irritation or inflammation as the case may be, also setting up a vascular reaction, which is primarily high blood pressure.

This chronic vaso-constriction together with the irritation or inflammation operating for a period, leads to the formation of new connective tissue which, like all fibrous tissue, undergoes cicatrization and contraction. The whole organ is pervaded with bands of scar tissue, radiating from the sites of the kidney stroma, which bands, by contraction, draw the kidney tissue together, literally reducing the size of the organ.

In the days when "deadhouse" pathology was *all* the pathology known (and, unfortunately, that day still exists, in degree) this was called the small contracted kidney. It has always been considered a fatal condition because our total knowledge has been that of terminal conditions.

Now, a true classification of kidney disease *must* be based on pathological knowledge; nevertheless it must still be, to a great extent, a matter of clinical symptoms, for, strange as it may seem, the kidneys which, after death, give the plainest evidence of change, oftentimes have produced the least apparent disturbance during life.

In studying these conditions, permit me to emphasize the circulatory phenomena; for in Bright's disease one cannot separate the circulatory apparatus from the kidneys, particularly in the chronic cases—they go hand in hand.

Chronic Bright's disease is essentially a disease of systemic scope involving the arteries and heart as well as the kidneys. Arterial Hypertension is one of its salient features, a fact long known and now strikingly demonstrated by blood-pressure readings with instruments of precision, notably the sphygmomanometer.

The heart and arterial symptoms frequently occur before there are any urinary symptoms. Often the first thing noticed is an increased arterial tension. Of the early manifestations this is the most important. It may be the only cardinal symptom in a congeries which includes headache, palpitation, bronchial cough, dizziness and a number of kindred phenomena.

The cause is mechanical, and originates in the action on the blood vessels of retained poison which should be carried off in the urine, but which, circulating in the blood, (the kidneys having failed to eliminate it) sets up an irritation to the muscular coats of the arteries, in consequence of which the vessels contract.

This must not be confounded with sclerosis of the arteries, which may follow prolonged arterial tension, or which may occur independently of renal disturbance and at about the same time in life with chronic interstitial nephritis.

High arterial tension, a resulting symptom in interstitial nephritis, is also a prominent causative factor in producing an hypertrophy of the left ventricle, as based on the following well known physiological law, i. e: "Any heart chamber which suffers an increase of pressure only during systole hypertrophies, i. e., corresponding to the greater amount of work, its muscles increases without an increase in the size of the cavity.

In these cases left heart hypertrophy is not determined so much by the absolute increase in the area of cariac dullness as by the marked accentuation of the second aortic sound of the heart and the gallop or pendulum rhythm of the heart's action.

These two signs are always diagnostic of left heart compensatory hypertrophy, without dilation. No murmur is heard so long as the heart is compensated, or unless the patient has been a sufferer from endocarditis, prior to the onset of his renal trouble; or to the latter itself, by long continuance, may have produced endocarditis and atheroma with an aortic systolic murur. As an associated condition of interstitial nephritis, per se, valvular disease does not exist.

The hypertrophy of the heart is conservative or compensatory, and so long as it remains so and is able to keep up its, work, all goes well; but when the left heart begens to fail and dilatation appears, the blood pressure falls and there begins a long chain of symptoms familiar to you all as "indications of failing heart," then there remains but one hope, i. e., compensatory hypertrophy of the *right* ventricle, which may avert the symptoms and support the patient for a time.

There are then two associated conditions of the cardio-vascular symptom in Bright's disease of primary importance to us, viz., high arterial tension and left ventricular hypertrophy.

If these be overlooked in the examination of the patient, in the great majority of cases of chronic nephritis the diagnosis will not to be made in time to be of any advantage, either to the patient or to the physician, for the urinary finding in the earlier stages of this disease are often misleading ·if not absolutely negative.

If, however, the condition is determined at a time before the resistance to the heart's action has become too great, and while there is still a compensatory hypertrophy of the *left* ventricle, much may be done for the patient. Hence, the necessity of making a careful examination,—in all patients of middle age or older, suffering from vague conditions, the symptoms of which are not prominent; especially in those individuals who present any urinary disturbances whatsoever,—first of the chest and second of the pulse and blood-vessels, for the purpose of determining whether there be hypertension.

Increased blood pressure is a difficult thing to determine. We have long attempted to do this by simple digital compression and palpation and no doubt these methods with some have some usefulness, but it is practically impossible for the unaided finger, no matter how skilled the observer may be in pulse reading, to determine with accuracy how much of the hardness and firmness of the artery is produced by high pressure of blood within the vessel and how much due to a thickening of the arterial wall.

The average systolic pressure, in an adult man, is usually considered to be about 115 MM, with the Riva Roca band (the one most commonly used) about 9 c c wide and a stanton sphygmomanometer.

It is practically impossible to fix a standard for any physiolgic phenomenon. In common with other physical processes, such as body temperature, respiration, etc., which are influenced by many conditions of every-day life, we find the degree of blood pressure affected by a great variety of circumstances producing transient, but comparatively wide fluctuations.

Due allowance for these things would, I believe, place the normal between 105 and 135 MM. Any persistent elevation above the latter figure may be considered a hypertension.

The clinical findings in left heart hypertrophy are a powerful, broad apex beat, displaced outward and sometimes downward; increased cardiac dullness in the left and upward; a booming low-pitched first sound and an accentuated second sound of a whistling character, heard best in the aortic area, although the last sound is heard in increased arterial tension when no hypertrophy exists.

The poisonous substances (commonly called urea) of which we have already spoken, circulating in the blood, cause a contraction of the small arteries; hence it is more difficult for the heart to keep pumping than normally; but the heart is wonderfully controlled by the nervous system and is regulated to give a sufficient blood supply to any part of the body as is required; so the heart works the harder as the blood vessels continue to resist, until the heart is no longer able to meet the requirements and cariac delitation results.

On the other hand, the reflex mediated by the depresser nerve comes into play so that either the vessels are dilated or the heart beats are retarded, but even if this reflex fails, there is an upper limit to the blood pressure, beyond which it cannot pass. The activity and power of the heart are not unlimited, and we have good reason for asserting that if the heart power is maintained and the high resistance remains in the vessels, the quantity of blood expelled in a given time actually diminishes, consequently the blood supply through the kidneys and other organs of the body is limited, and the kidneys, in their crippled condition, being the original cause for the increased resistance, the one influences the other, and a vicious cycle is established between the heart and arteries, and the kidneys.

In considering these cases we cannot help but be impressed with the limited, if not often times dangerous use of the much favored vaso dilators. All high blood pressure cases are essentially characterized by the element of systemic toxaemia for abnormal blood pressure is no more than a vascular reaction against the presence of toxins in the blood. In Bright's disease this vascular reaction is perpetuated by the continuous character of the toxaemia and is later enchanced by the uraemia resulting from inadequacy. The permanent and progressive character of the peripheral obstruction, and the limited powers of the heart for adjustment, lead first to an hypertrophy and ultimately to failure. On the other hand from a physiologic view point, it is perfectly obvious that the structural involvement and crippling of the kidneys must bring about increased force of circulation to compensate for the diminished excretion by increasing the blood current in the Glomerular vessels; so when we consider that the energy of the heart's force is used in overcoming resistance we can easily see why in high tension cases the heart hypertrophies. Clinically we know that the case of Bright's that maintains a high blood pressure and cardiac hypertrophy retains his vitality and activity the longest. Nevertheless, it is in the excessive high pressure cases that patients complain most of pains and the functional disturbances peculiar to Bright's disease.

Thus we have a happy medium in which to at least attempt to hold our patients. The temptation to reduce the arterial tension, when the sphygmomanometer shows it be high, is very great, and just when to use vaso dilators is a difficult problem, probably best decided by each individual case, e.g., a sustained high blood pressure of over 200 MM if accompanied by marked symptoms may render a course of vaso dilator medication advisable. The chosen drugs should, however, be given slowly and cautiously and the effects watched and should be stopped when the blood pressure has dropped 10 to 15 MM., as that is usually all that is necessary for the patient's comfort.

The employment of vaso dilators in the last stages of Bright's disease with cardiac dilitation, dropsy etc., is practically useless and were it not for the fact that the vasomotor control of the peripheral circulation is too much disturbed to respond, they might do harm.

Because the case was previously one of high tension furnishes no excuse for continuous use of these drugs.

THE ELIMINATION OF SECTIONAL LINES.

BY JAMES S. McALLISTER, B. S., M. D., SAPULPA, OKLAHOMA.

The elimination of sectional lines between different sects or schools of medicine, in the past decade is almost as marked with reference to the medical profession as it is with the denominational churches. In my short experience, I can remember when the war and strife between the different branches of the denominational churches was to the death. It was considered, by some, an unpardonable sin for a member of one denomination to attend the services of a different church, while the idea of a minister of one denomination occupying the pulpit of another was simply intolerable, and the only common meeting ground was for the purpose of a war in joint debate between two eminent divines on the all important subjects of pre-destination or mode of baptism, each side backing its individual Idol with all the enthusiasm of religious fanatics. So with the different schools or sects in medicine a few years ago. The division lines were so marked and drawn so taut that it was considered sufficient evidence to warrant social and professional ostracism for a so-called Regular, or Allopath to recognize or consult with a Homeopath or Eclectic or vice versa, and he was usually promptly expelled from any medical society to which he might belong for such a flagrant violation of the implied rules then laid down, under the caption of medical ethics. But thanks to a higher and a more liberal education of the profession and the pressure brought to bear by a more liberal public, sectional lines have become almost entirely obliterated, and we no longer hear the war cry of the Homeopath of the Allopath, the Eclectic or the Osteopath even, and some are liberal enough to let even the Chiro-Practic and the Magnetic healer live in the same world, while in the religious world, sectional lines have so far disappeared that we find in every city or community, ministerial associations, where the Jew and the Gentile, the Catholic and the Protestant, meet on common ground, not to wage war over non-essentials, but to band together for the common good of humanity, and sometimes we even hear whisperings of the "universal brotherhood of man and the Fatherhood of God," but the millennium is not yet.

As in the secret depth of our animal natures there is firmly implanted that indefinable something begotten, perhaps, by generations of savage ancestry, which ever and anon crops out and causes us to feel, in spite of successive generations of education and so-called civilization, that almost irresistable "Call of the Wild," so in our social and professional relations, the savage crops out at times, rendering us intolerable, not only with different sects or schools, but with reputable members of our own schools as well, no longer meeting on common ground as friendly competitors, but allowing hate and petty jealousies to come between us because of some alleged injustice or slight by a brother practitioner, and we feed this jealousy and hate until we almost bring ourselves to believe that we are the only honest and just person in the entire medical profession, and too often this feeling becomes so grounded and fixed in our jealous natures that we allow ourselves to, not only think but say hurtful things against an innocent brother practitioner, that makes the estrangement complete. Will Carlton has said that; "Thoughts unexpressed may sometimes fall back dead, but God Himself can't kill them when they're said." But thanks to our better judgement, and the influence of modern educational experience, these fits of jealousy and hate, with most of us, soon pass as a summer shower, and the sunshine of reason restores us to the normal, until we can again meet our brother on common ground, and realize that we after all, are no more perfect than he. But while we have become more tolerant with each other, and with different sects, and willing to concede a great deal that a few years ago would have been impossible, we are not quite ready yet to avail of every means at our command for the relief and suffering of our patients, regardless of the sources through which this knowledge comes. For instance, many of us hesitate to accept, and have a tendency to ignore and ridicule simple and valuable remedies if suggested by some old lady or grandmother, and especially has the profession hesitated and refused to recognize and accept the principle of Psycho-Therapy, which should be one of our principal axauliary batteries in combatting disease of both mind and body, but by our prejudice and a failure to grasp the true significance of these facts, we have left the door unguarded and allowed incompetents and charlatans to capture this strong hold thus permitting them to turn our own guns against us, and we often wake up too late, only to realize that some of our best friends and most appreciated patients have become discouraged and are flocking across the street to the Osteopath, Chiro-Practic, Faith Healer, or

more probably joining the ranks of so-called Christian Science, and why? simply because we are too narrow, too prejudiced to realize that just as sure as the sun moves, and "she do move," the people are thinking and observing for themselves, and realizing what many of us still try to deny, the effect of the mind over bodily disease, and failing to obtain relief from those in whom they have had most confidence in a professional way, like the drowning man they grasp at a straw, and when they obtain relief, which they often do, that relief from suffering, both mental and physical, which we have failed to give, no wonder they lose faith and confidence in all things material, and these are they, no matter how intelligent, how well educated, who fall an easy prey to so-called magnetic healers, spiritualism or go to swell the ranks of the famous Mrs. Eddy. The sooner we, as physicians and surgeons, realize that there is more to the practice of medicine than drugs and the surgeon's knife, and recognize that mysterious something, call it what you will, personal influence, magnetism, hypnotism, suggestion, telepathy or christian science, and its influence for good or bad both on mental and physical conditions, the better it will be for our patients and the sooner will these auxilary remedies be taken out of the hands of the dangerous charlatan, and placed in competent and safe hands, to be used, under the direction of the competent, conscientious physcian, for most of these so-called faith healers, christian scientists, etc., are totally incompetent to deal with organic or specific diseases as well as infectious and contagious diseases, thus often subjecting the patient and the public to grave dangers from infection or contagion, and causing directly much suffering and many deaths by delay in indicated surgical operations. which might have given permanent relief if done in time, for potent as properly directed Pschyco-Therapy may be, if properly directed, no matter by whom, it will not set a broken limb, remove an appendiceal abscess or relieve an ectopic pregnacy, and while these measures would be safe in the hands of the regular medical profession, they are often dangerous as dynamite in the hands of the charlatan or quack, and the physician who fails to realize this, and who does not in some way influence his patient so as to inspire that absolute confidence, so essentially necessary in the treatment of both the diseased mind and body, to such an extent as to make his presence involuntarially felt for good the instant he steps into the sick room, is a failure, and he will probably return the next day to find his patient worse or more often to find himself supplanted by a more diplomatic and successful, if not a more competent physician.

These are facts, gentlemen, facts that we as a profession have long ignored and ridiculed, because of the source from which they have originated, and not until they have been forced upon us by seeing many of our patients not only deserting us, but actually obtaining relief where we have failed. We, the medical profession of the great State of Oklahoma, have all realized this fact, that we have made great progress, since statehood, through organization both socially and professionally, and the noble band of physicians, composing the Creek County Medical Association, have not been found wanting. Let us improve this organization by cultivating that social and professional etiquet so essentially necessary in the protection of ourselves and the public, and thereby become a powerful unit and an integral part of the great state organization, which has already accomplished much in the way of valuable legislation for our mutual protection. But there is much yet to accomplish, and we, as a state organization should be able to present our claims so forcebly as to be irresistable, by presenting our claims, backed by an undivided profession, ready, as "Fighting Bob" said when he started on the famous world cruise of the battleship fleet, "for a fight or a frolic."

EDITORIAL

WHAT THE DAILY PRESS THINKS ABOUT THE MATTER.

The following is taken from the Editorial columns of the St. Louis Star and so thoroughly voices the sentiments and thoughts of the thinking end of the medical profession that it is reproduced:

A Department of Health.

Dr. William H. Welch, president of the American Medical Association, spoke in his installation address of the necessity for a Federal Department of Health, showing again the interest the medical profession takes in the prevention of disease. Two objections have been made to the creation of such a department. One is, that the President's Cabinet is already too large and unwieldy. This objection does not seem to be well-founded.

Foreign governments do not find large cabinets a weakness. On the contrary, they look upon a Cabinet officer to head any department representing any considerable national interest or governmental feature promotive of the general welfare. As to the President, he should be better served by a responsible Cabinet officer representing an important activity of the government, than by half a dozen chiefs of conflicting bureaus.

The other objection is that the creation of such a department is merely a scheme of what the objectors designate as the "medical trust" to control medical and health regulation matters in the United States. For this charge there appears to be little foundation. The association now meeting in this city, which must be the heart of this alleged "medical trust," if there be any such, admits to its membership all educated graduates of medical colleges of the various schools. The various bureaus of the government which deal with health matters are not exclusive in their attitude towards competent physicians of all but a single school of medicine.

To be sure, there are some "isms" and "ists" which none of these regularly educated physicians and surgeons of the scientific medical schools recognize, nor can they be recognized if any sanitary regulations are to be created and maintained, based upon the origin and nature of diseases as held by men of scientific attainments. All those object.

Those persons also object who desire less regulation of the character of medicines and of foods, those who find such regulations interfere with their business. A few others object on the general principle of the individual liberty of a man to do or not to do as he may please, no matter how much of a menace and a nuisance he may be to his neighbor.

The American people as a whole are sufficiently intelligent to understand the need of sanitary regulations and preventive measures of a public nature against the origin and spread of diseases. They have seen what such measures have accomplished, and they have seen the dire results of their absence. They have seen the country preserved from the pestilence of yellow fever, cholera and smallpox by such methods, and they believe what the medical profession tells them about twhat might be accomplished with regard to malaria, tuberculosis, contagious and infectious fevers, etc., by similar or allied precautionary regulations.

They have at last come to realize that one of the chief functions of government is the protection of the people's lives by prevention of disease as much as by maintenance of any army and navy against assault from abroad, or police forces against the thug and murderer at home. There is no more important function of government than the preservation of the health of the people governed and thus their pursuit of happiness. Man is of more importance in a government by the people than mere property. Bureaus in various departments are engaged in this work. What they are attempting to do could be better done by consolidating them into a department, where the effort to preserve the lives and health of the people would be given in equal standing with the effort to make farmers grow more corn to the acre.

We have no guide for the preservation of health and the prevention of disease save the results of scientific study and experiment. We must accept these results and act upon them, in spite of all those who object, whether merely from chronic opposition to all regulation and progress or from interested personal motives. As fast as any medical theory and regulations based upon it may be found to be wrong by new light discovered on the subject, we would act accordingly, but the only safe course for the welfare of all is to accept and act upon the best medical theories of the day, and not lag too far behind the procession of discovery and new knowledge.

THE VICTORY OF DOCTOR SIMMONS.

Never before in the history of the American Medical Association has there been such a unanimous feeling on the questions relating to the Secretary's office.

For some time the country has been flooded with literature from the pen of Dr. G. Frank Lydsdon of Chicago which called for a change in the present management of the Asociation's affairs and the Secretary's office; hinting at mismanagement, calling for certain reforms and forms of reports which already exist. That the attack was largely due to personal feeling rather than a genuine wish for a change in the present manner of conducting affairs and that the personal point of the whole attack was Dr. Simmons no one on the ground could doubt for a moment and the result when the House of Delegates finally spoke must have been gratifying to Dr. Simmons for not one voice of protest was raised on the floor and despite the fact that Dr. Simmons had resigned and placed his resignation in the hands of the House of Delegates and in good faith asked that he be relieved of the duties of the office, he was unanimously re-elected to the office he has so long held. The nomination was by Dr. Ira Carlton Chase of Ft. Worth, Texas, himself a man of intimate knowledge in the Association's affairs and one who is helping solve the troubles that constantly arise to bedevil the officers and embarrass them, when many of us are at sleep or on the seashore taking a vacation. Dr. Chase said in part that this was no time for any man to quit and that when the wolves of Charlatanism, Quackery and their ilk were snapping about we needed just such a man as Doctor Simmons and should retain his services. This was the sentiment of all and the vote was all that was necessary.

THE CARNEGIE FOUNDATION REPORT AND OKLAHOMA MEDICAL SCHOOLS.

The report of Dr. Abraham Flexner to the Carnegie Foundation aroused much interest and in some localities much resentment especially in those schools severely criticised.

Oklahoma was handled with very lenient hands; the report seeming to take into consideration that in everything we were yet in the making and that we were doing very well indeed when our resources and time were taken into consideration. It says: "The new commonwealth of Oklahoma may, if wise, avoid most of the evils which this report has described. * * * Immigration—of physicians, among others—has been so rapid that the state has easily three times as many doctors as it needs. They pour in from the schools of Kansas City, St. Louis and Chicago." The report foreshadowed the establishment of the clinical department in Oklahoma City, strange to say recommending that that step be taken in order to give the state the possession of the field and offering the opinion that the establishment and maintenance of a school was such a hazardous matter from the financial point of view that the state should do this. A high compliment is paid Oklahoma City in the folowing words: " * * * * * Its streets are of asphalt, its large buildings are fire proof, their plumbing modern; they have begun with enamel, not with tin or zinc, bathtubs. Why do they not in the same way avoid the costly errors in educational organization that the states about them have one after the other made? The older states are painfully correcting or paying for their blunders; should Oklahoma, to soothe the local pride of this little town or that, run up a bill of the same sort?"

The City Council of Muskogee has adopted an ordinance putting into effect the regulations of the State Commissioner of Health and the sections of the Oklahoma law applicable to sanitary regulations of cities of the first class; heretofore enforeament has been impossible on account of the present regulations not being in effect. The Council also adopted an ordinance prohibiting the sale and use of fireworks within the city.

The Muskogee Hospital Association is preparing to occupy their new Hospital on South Fourteenth street. This hospital is furnished throughout with the latest operating room fixtures and the furniture is all new.

DR. W. W. WINGET DEAD.

Dr. W. W. Winget of Nowata, died suddenly May 14th. Dr. Winget was a member of Nowata County Society. He was born at Strongtown, Ohio, in November, 1869; a graduate of Linsley Institute, Wheeling, West Virginia, and of Miama Medical College in 1893. He was resident physician in the hospital from 1893 to 1895, after which he entered the medical service of the government and was stationed at Missouri and Kansas points, locating in Nowata after this time, where he resided until his death.

A sad feature of his death was the fact that he had only recently married.

EUROPEAN LETTERS.

Dr. A. L. Blesh who sails from New York for a years stay in Europe on August 20th will from time to time give the Journal the benefit of his observations and study. Coming as they do from the pen of one of the ablest medical writers in the state these letters will be looked forward to with great interest by the profession generally.

Dr. Blesh will be accompanied by Mrs. Blesh and his two sons and daughter.

The County and City Boards of Health of Oklahoma City and County have notified all physicians in the city who have not regis-

tered to do so at once. After a certain length of time prosecutions will commence against all illegal practitioners.

AN IMPORTANT UTERO-OVARIAN SEDATIVE, ANODYNE AND TONIC.

While it is unquestionably true that many cases of pelvic diseases in women are amenable only to surgical treatment, it is quite evident that there are not a few in which, for some reason or other, operative measures are out of the question. Among these may be included the many cases of dysmenorrhea and ovarian hyperesthesia, for the relief of which recourse is too frequently had by the patients to alcohol, the narcotics, or some of the much-vaunted nostrums on the market.

It has been shown to be a mistake to suppose that substantial and lasting benefit cannot be obtained in these ailments by the internal administration of therapeutic agents, a number of which have been thoroughly tried, with results often satisfactory, sometimes brilliant. An agent of undoubted value in such cases is Liquor Sedans, a preparation introduced to the medical profession many years ago by Messrs. Parke, Davis & Co. and esteemed and prescribed by physicians to an extent, it is believed, not equaled by any similar compound.

Liquor Sedans is composed of three of the most important sedatives, anodynes and tonics to the female reproductive tract —namely, black haw, hydrastis and Jamaica dogwood—so combined with aromatics as to constitute a very acceptable preparation, being in this respect unlike some other agents of a similar nature which are ordinarily taken with great reluctance. It is of marked usefulness in the treatment of functional dysmenorrhea, menorrhagia, ovarian irritability, menstrual irregularity, etc. Parke, Davis & Co. also manufacture Liquor Sedans Rx 2 (without sugar), which is precisely like the older formula but for the omission noted, and which is available for use in cases in which sugar is contraindicated; also Liquor Sedans except that each fluid ounce contains 40 minims of the fluid extract of cascara sagrada, giving to the formula an important tonic-laxative value.

THE HAY-FEVER PROBLEM.

Again the physician is called upon to gropple with hay-fever, and a veritable army of sneezing, watery-eyed "miserables" come to him for relief. For a long time the idea was prevalent that litle or nothing could be done for these people. The patient dreaded the coming of the disease, and the physician dreaded the coming of the patient. The situation was one of ample misgivings and scanty faith. Now it is prety well recognized that medication, while still empiric to a certain extent, is nevertheless effective. The symptoms can be controlled or greatly minimized, and the patient may have the relief he seeks. And for this much he will be truly thankful, and the physician, in turn, duly thanked.

Adrenalin is perhaps the most effective agent. It antagonizes the symptoms and secures to the patient a marked degree of comfort. It allays the congestion of the mucous membrane, reduces the swelling of the turbinal tissues, controls the nasal discharge, cuts short the violent paroxysms of sneezing and the abundant lacrimation, and prevents depression by stimulating the heart.

The practitioner who desires to employ Adrenalin in the treatment of hay-fever has recourse to the product in a number of forms. Adrenalin Chloride Solution (1:1000) is doubtless the most widely used. It is first diluted with four to five times its volume of physiological salt solution, then sprayed into the nares and pharynx. Adrenalin Inhalant has many adherents. This is an oil solution, and is administered by spray. It may be diluted with olive oil—the inhalant one part, olive oil three to four parts. A third preparation is Adrenalin Ointment (1:1000,) which is effective either alone or in supplementing Solution Adrenalin Chloride. Another is Adrenalin and Chloretone Ointment—at once an astringent, antiseptic and mild anesthetic. The latest is Anesthone Cream (Adrenalin Chloride 1:20,000, para-amido-ethyl-benzoate 10 per cent. in a bland oil base,) an astringent, anesthetic ointment. The ointments and cream are supplied in collapsible tubes with elongated nozzle, which facilitates their application to the nasal mucosa.

Literature on any or all of the products above mentioned may be had upon application to the manufacturers, Messrs. Parke, Davis & Co., at their general offices in Detroit or any of their numerous branch houses. The company, by the way, issues an attractive brochure on the subject of hay-fever.

COUNTY SOCIETY

KAY COUNTY.

Paper—Cholera Infantum, Dr. H. H. Bishop, Tonkawa.

Discussion—Opened by Dr. J. H. Engles, Newkirk.

General Discussion.

Paper—Gonorrhoea; cause, course, treatment and sequelae, Dr. E. J. Orvis, Blackwell.

Discussion—Opened by Dr. G. H. Niemann, Ponca City.

General Discussion.

Business Meeting.

OKMULGEE COUNTY.

Henryetta, Okla., June 13.

PROGRAM.

Paper—"The Subliminal Scenes of a Doctor's Destiny," Dr. W. L. Stephenson.

Paper—"Eclampsia," Dr. Bercaw.

Paper—Dr. F. T. Milroy.

Delegates report of State Meeting, Dr. Brese.

Paper—Dr. Oliphant.

JOINT MEETING OF THE MEDICAL SOCIETIES OF WASHITA AND CUSTER COUNTIES.

Clinton, Friday, June 3, 1910.

PROGRAM, 11 A. M.

Selective.................Dr. J. C. Mahr
Discussion.
Banquet, 12:30 p. m.
Selective ....Dr. C. R. Hume
Discussion.
Selective ....Dr. J. S. Hartford
Discussion.
"The Duty of the Physician to Himself,"
Dr. J. H. Hottinan
Discussion.
"Washita County Fees,"
Dr. E. T. Sandberg
Discussion.
Clinical Cases.

CLEVELAND COUNTY MEDICAL SOCIETY.

Regular Meeting June 3, 1910.

PROGRAM.

Delegates Report of State Meeting, C. S. Bobo.

Paper—"The Clinical Significance of the Colon Bacillus," A. L. Blesh.

Paper—"Treatment of Rectal Sinuses, with report of Cases," R. M. Howard.

Leaders in Discussion—J. L. Hoshall, R. E. Thacker, J. L. Womack, G. M. Clifton.

BOOK REVIEWS

"Diseases of the Stomach and Intestines."

"Diseases of the Stomach and Intestines," by Robert Coleman Kemp, M. D., Professor of Gastro-Intestinal Diseases, New York School of Clinical Medicine. Octavo of 766 pages, with 279 illustrations. Philadelphia and London W. B. Saunders Company, 1910. Cloth, $6.00 net; half Morocco, $7.50 net.

This work is more profusely illustrated than any similar work on the subject of diseases of the stomach and intestines; the illustrations being especially applicable to the diagnosis and treatment laid down in the text.

In many of the conditions held to be amenable to both surgical and medical treatment the indications for surgical intervention are clearly given.

It will be found of value to the general practitioner for this reason alone.

The space allotted to examination, diet and treatment is accorded the prominence and volume it deserves.

No disease having any bearing on the stomach and intestines is excluded and the differential diagnosis is entered into in detail.

Practical Study of Malaria.

A Practical Study of Malaria. By William H. Deaderick, M. D., Member American Society of Tropical Medicine; Fellow London Society of Tropical Medicine and Hygeine. Octavo of 402 pages, illustrated. Philadelphia and London: W. B. Saunders Company, 1909. Cloth, $4.50 net; Half Morocco, $6.00 net.

A book of ten chapters every one of which are remarkable for their clearness and omission of theoretical problems.

More than one hundred pages are rightfully devoted to the etiology of malaria, which until understood thoroughly places the control of this disease beyond the profession and the locality which attempts its eradication.

No space is spared the prophylactic attention of this affection and the subject of prevention is profusely illustrated.

As most modern authors the book recognizes quinine as being "almost a specific" and the minute directions for its use in different conditions of malaria is worthy of close attention by those men who have given quinine all their lives and believe themselves familiar with its uses.

Dr. Deaderick lives in one of the worst malarial regions of the south, the Arkansas Valley, and adds years of practical experience in the treatment of the disease to an intimate knowledge of its technical understanding. His work is well named and should be in the hands of every physician in the south.

"Prescription Writing and Formulary."

"Prescription Writing and Formulary," by John M. Swan, M. D., Associate Professor of Clinical Medicine, Medico-Chirurgical College of Philadelphia. 32mo of 185 pages. Philadelphia and London. W. B. Saunders Company, 1910. Flexible leather, $1.25 net.

"Surgical After-Treatment."

"Surgical After-Treatment," by L. R. G. Crandon, A. M., M. D., Assistant in Surgery at Harvard Medical School. Octavo of 803 pages, with 265 original illustrations. Philadelphia and London. W. B. Saunders Company, 1910. Cloth, $6.00 net; half Morocco, $7.50 net.

"Pulmanary Tuberculosis and Its Complications."

"Pulmonary Tuberculosis and its Complications," by Sherman G. Bonney, M. D., Professor of Medicine, Denver and Gross College of Medicine, Denver. Octavo of 955 pages, with 243 original illustrations, including 31 in colors and 73 X-ray photo-

graphs. Philadelphia and London. W. B. Saunders Company, 1910. Cloth, $7.00 net; half Morocco, $8.50 net.

"Medical Electricity and Rontgen Rays."

"Medical Electricity and Rontgen Rays," by Sinclair Tousey, A. M., M. D., Consulting Surgeon to St. Bartholomew's Clinic, New York City. Octavo of 1,116 pages, with 750 illustrations, 16 in colors. Philadelphia and London. W. B. Saunders Company, 1910. Cloth, $7.00 net; half Morocco, $8.50 net. W. B. Saunders Company, Philadelphia and London.

International Clinics.

Volume Two, Nineteenth Series, by various authors, containing twenty one articles on different subjects.

J. B. Lippincott Company, Philadelphia and London.

PERSONAL

Dr. R. R. Smith, formerly of Kansas City, has located in Muskogee.

Dr. W. G. Bisbee, of Oklahoma City, is spending the summer in Tennessee.

Dr. M. J. Bartlett of Clarksburg, West Virginia, has located in Oklahoma City.

Dr. L. H. Huffman of Hobart will spend two months in the Chicago clinics this summer.

Drs. L. M. Sackett and W. G. Wallace, of Oklahoma City, have formed a partnership.

Dr. E. S. Lain is in the New York Skin and Cancer Hospital doing post-graduate work.

Drs. E. F. Davis and A. W. White of Oklahoma City are taking post-graduate work in Europe.

Dr. W. J. Wallace leaves this month for Europe and New York for the purpose of doing post graduate work.

Dr. A. L. Blesh of Oklahoma City sails for Europe from New York Aug. 20th. He expects to spend a year in the clinics of Vienna.

Dr. C. R. Phelps of Oklahoma City will leave July 3rd, for an extended trip through California, Yellowstone Park and the Northwest, he will be absent until fall.

Dr. L. T. Strother, president of the Nowata County Medical Society, received a fracture of the leg May 26. The accident was caused by his horse falling on him.

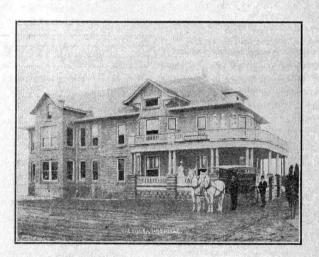

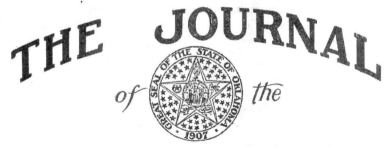

Oklahoma State Medical Association.

VOL. III. MUSKOGEE, OKLAHOMA, AUGUST, 1910. NO. 3

DR. CLAUDE A. THOMPSON, Editor-in-Chief.

ASSOCIATE EDITORS AND COUNCILLORS.

DR. J. A. WALKER, Shawnee.
DR. CHARLES R. HUME, Anadarko.
DR. F. R. SUTTON, Bartlesville.
DR. I. W. ROBERTSON, Dustin.
DR. J. S. FULTON, Atoka.

DR. JOHN W. DUKE, Guthrie.
DR. A. B. FAIR, Frederick.
DR. W. G. BLAKE, Tahlequah.
DR. H. P. WILSON, Wynnewood.
DR. J. H. BARNES, Enid.

Entered at the Postoffice at Muskogee, Oklahoma, as second class mail matter, June, 1909.

This is the Official Journal of the Oklahoma State Medical Association All communications should be addressed to the Journal of the Oklahoma State Medical Association, English Block, Muskogee, Oklahoma.

MODERN RESEARCH—A CRITICISM AND A SUGGESTION, WITH SPECIAL REFERENCE TO TYPHOID FEVER.

BY A. K. WEST, M. D., PROFESSOR OF MEDICINE, OKLAHOMA STATE UNIVERSITY.

It is not necessary to review in great detail the present status of our knowledge of Typhiod Fever. However, let us just touch the high points.

Notwithstanding the enormous expenditure of energy in research work, especially noticeable during the past few years, what is the present state of our knowledge concerning this subject? Let us strip it of preconception, surmise, hypothesis, and tabulate the facts and principles in terms of pure demonstrable science.

1st: Etiology: It is a demonstrable fact that the Bacillus Typhosus is always present in the body of the patient showing the clinical picture.

2nd: This organism is susceptible to a pure culture outside the living body.

This is the sum total of absolute knowledge. If we could only add the third proposition, of Koch's etiological triad, i. e., that the introduction of this pure culture into the non-immune body is always followed by the development of the disease, then we could say that we know the specific cause of Typhoid Fever. Unfortunately, the last proposition has not as yet been demonstrated. The pure scientist then may say, "I know that the growth and multiplication of Bacillus Typhosus in the body is a concomitant of and coincident with an attack of Typhoid Fever, but not indisputably the cause of the disease."

If the foregoing is true, and I think it may not be gainsaid, it immediately appears that our knowledge of the etiology of Typhoid is meagre enough, yet as compared with our knowledge concerning dissemination it is really voluminous.

How is Typhoid Fever disseminated? Of this we have no knowledge whatever. Of theories, hypotheses, surmises, all supported by a certain amount of evidence, there is no end. The water born theory, the contact theory, the agency of insects, especially the little "*Musca Domestic*," now become widely known as the "Typhoid Fly," infected milk, vegetables and other foods, and so on, but upon careful scrutiny we are forced to the conclusion that however much we may take upon faith, as a matter of knowledge we are still without a sure anchor. That the death rate from Typhoid Fever has been markedly lessened in a number of places by the improvement of the water supply is off-set by the fact in other places the improvement in the water supply has been followed by even an increase in the rate of mortality. These words from Dr. Welch are significant: "We should not make drinking water responsible for the disease without *conclusive* evidence. The evidence is strong, if not absolutely convincing that the drinking water at present plays no important part in the conveyance of Typhoid Fever in the City of Washington."

Now again, notwithstanding the prevalent opinion that flies play an important part in the dissemination of the disease, Dr. Lumsden found in a careful study of the subject that there was no relationship existing between the fly prevalency period and the Typhoid prevalency period on curve as shown by his chart. Likewise, no higher mortality in the districts of open privies and lack of screens, than in the districts of modern sewerage and protection against flies was apparent. Note

likewise this significant statement from Dr. Lumsden after his labors in Washington had concluded:

1st: "The possibility that the public water supply not distributing Typhoid Fever, does contain some agent which has to do with the establishment of the susceptibility to Typhoid infection."

2nd: "The possibility of there being peculiarly active in Washington, some entirely unknown cause or agent concerned in the dissemination of this infection."

Forest Dutton recently, (as he thought) was able to produce an attack of Typhoid Fever by confining a number of bed bugs upon the body of a father, taken from the bed of a child suffering from Typhoid Fever.

Now I only cite this short review as a basis for criticism of our present methods of investigation. All honor is due the men who are giving attention to this work, and all of the data collected will prove of value at no distant date, but in my opinion, until a radical departure from our present antiquated research methods has been made, little of any real value will be added to our store house of knowledge along this line.

As we know little of this subject, so likewise only a few years ago did we know little of Tuberculosis, of Diphtheria, of Tetanus, of Scarlet Fever, of Malarial Fever, of Yellow Fever, and other diseases, but especially of those mentioned we are at the present in possession of definite mathematical and demonstrable knowledge, so that we may truthfully use the term "Science of Medicine" when referring to these diseases.

By what method then was this scientific knowledge obtained? Apply the same methods of investigation to Typhoid, and we have every reason to anticipate a success which in its vast, far reaching beneficence will be equal to, or surpass any achievement in medical science. What then ıs the specific fault in the present method of research? Just this, the present methods do not preclude the. possibility of *MISTAKING COINCIDENCE FOR CAUSE.* Not only in medicine but in all the sciences, experiment—painstaking error eradicating experiment, has been the key to unlock the store house of knowledge, and give us the indisputable facts, principles and laws which constitute science.

By experiment, Pasteur laid the foundation for our knowledge of all the germ diseases. Following his lead the great Koch was able to demonstrate beyond per adventure the etiology of Tuberculosis. By experiment, Klebs and Loefler laid down a scientific law in regard to Diptheria. By experiment, Flexner threw a great light upon the etiology of Scarlet Fever. By experiment Walter Reed conferred upon humanity one of its greatest boons. By experiment, Astrology became Astronomy, alchemy became Chemistry, and Physics became science out of a chaos of misunderstood phenomena.

To make this criticism clearer, let us compare for a moment the work of the Yellow Fever Commission in Philadelphia rather more than one hundred years since, and the work of the Yellow Fever Commission in Cuba, with which we are all familiar. Please note that the methods used by Benjamin Rush are practically the methods being used at the present time in our attempts to throw light upon the subject of Typhoid Fever. His report in substance is as follows:

"That the cause of Yellow Fever is some unknown Miasm, originating out of decaying vegetable matter; that the cause of outbreaks of this particular epidemic is in all probabilities an amount of damaged coffee, brought in some trophical vessel, being unloaded on the wharf and allowed to putrify and fester during the hot months; that the disease spreads with the wind and

is therefore air borne; that many persons give a history of first feeling sick after smelling stench originating in the decaying coffee; that the disease is contagious, and that those nursing the sick would be afflicted, therefore accounting for the dissemination of the malady throughout all quarters of the City after a short period."

Now note the correctness of all these observations. Note also the lamentable failure to differentiate by error eradicating experiment between CAUSE and COINCIDENCE. Also note if you will the tremendous consequence of following the mistaken teaching of Benjamin Rush through the next hundred years, the appalling loss of life in epidemic after epidemic, the overwhelming cost in life and money, due to the throttling of commerce in our vain efforts at Quarantine to stop the spread of the terrible scourge, even to the extent of shot-gun patrols, and the fumigation of the mail sacks in our fear of the dreadful contagiousness of the enemy, and no man arose who doubted the observations of Benjamin Rush, and all were of one accord that Yellow Fever was due to a Miasm, and that it was a contagious disease.

Now look, if you please, upon the other picture, the work of Walter Reed, James Carroll and co-laborers who constituted the Yellow Fever Commission at Havanna in 1900.

·1st: A careful and scientific study of the then beginning to be realized cause of Yellow Fever, Bacillus Icteroides, or the Bacillus of Sanarella. After careful experiment and study, applying Koch's law, they were able to answer the question in the negative for all time that the Bacillus Icteroides is not the cause of Yellow Fever.

Taking up a thread which had been dropped some years prior by several observers, but notably Carlos Finley of Havanna, that Mosquitoes had something to do with the cause of Yellow Fever, or its spread, this was followed up in the same painstaking error eradicating methods of study, and the building and equipping of a station, by which both mosquitoes and experimental subjects were under absolute control, so that food, drink and all the details of environment were known quantities. The Commission was in a short time able to demonstrate to the Medical Profession, and to confer upon humanity one of the greatest boons of any age or any clime. They were enabled to show that Yellow Fever is conveyed by the Mosquito, indeed by a certain species of Mosquito, and that a definite term must elapse after it has bitten one afflicted with Yellow Fever, before the power of communicating disease is developed in the insect, i. e., about twelve days. That the possibility of communicating the disease is co-extensive with the life of the insect.

2nd: They were able to show that Yellow Fever is not a contagious disease; that the contact of individuals in the absence of Mosquito carriers was not in the least dangerous; that the bedding, clothing, fomites of whatever kind, might be used and handled with impunity and found quite impossible to convey disease to the non-immunes under control, except by direct inoculation with the blood of Yellow Fever patients, or the indirect inoculation of the bite of the Sxegomya Fasciata.

Note the difference now in the accurate observations of one as against the accurate observations of another, plus the painstaking eradication of all sources of error, by which not a hypothesis or a theory was promulgated, but a mathematical fact demonstrated. As to comparison of results, you know the story of Yellow Fever before and since the work of 1900.

Now then we approach the central, vital and only new thought in this paper. If present methods of research work have proven and are proving barren of results, surely a suggestion of change will not be resented. The departure from the beaten track may at first glance appear visionary, bizarre, and impossible of accomplishment, but after mature consideration I am thoroughly convinced that this new departure may be shorn of its objectionable features, and yield fruit in scientific findings of inestimable value to the human race. I refer to the establishment of an experimental station, patterned somewhat after the station established by Walter Reed and the Yellow Fever Commission, especially that feature which made possible his great discovery—*the use of human subjects voluntarily tendered for purposes of experimentation.*

This then is the general plan which I will now lay before you, subject as I well know to much criticism, many changes and improvements. The establishment of experimental stations for the study of diseases in the human being, by the State as a part of its Health Department, or by the Federal Government. Now the Federal Government, as well as several States spend thousands of dollars in the maintenance of Agricultural Experimental Stations, where the diseases of corn, wheat, cotton and potatoes are studied. Also departments for the study of diseases of hogs, cattle, sheep and poultry, the State paying for knowledge to save the farmer's hogs from Cholera, but not to save the farmer's wife and babies from Typhoid.

To meet the indications we could procure the whole time, the whole heart and the whole attention of a competent man to direct, to head, and to carry out this work. This a safe-guard against haste and superficiality.

2nd: Provide money for buildings, apparatus and equipment for the necessary accurate scientific experiment.

3rd: The most necessary, and the most difficult, but still quite possible, the supply of human beings for certain of the experiments, which without such subjects, must result in failure.

Now how could this last be accomplished without the charge of cruelty inhumanity and barbarism becoming applicable, and further, how could it be made legal? These are the real questions.

To answer the first question, I will ask others, if the experiments of the Yellow Fever Commission upon soldiers volunteering from the army, were not cruel, inhuman and barbarous? Why would experiments upon volunteers from among the inmates of our State Penal Institutions be such? Again, if it is legal for soldiers to volunteer this great service, why would it not be legal for criminals to do the same? If the State has a legal right to commute or pardon sentences on account of good behavior, or valuable services rendered, why has the State not the right to commute or pardon convicts for this service?

Now then you have the whole meat of this matter. That abuses might creep into the system is beside the question; that incompetent men might be appointed to head such institutions, as a matter of political preferment, rather than executive fitness; that influential and dangerous criminals might be fraudulently turned loose on society—these and other things may possibly occur, but what might be accomplished by the ideal is more to the point.

Let us see how an institution of this kind could and would be used for the study and solution of all diseased problems. Let us take as a hypothetical case, the study of Typhoid Fever, one of the undoubtedly preventable diseases as soon as we are in possession of all the facts.

1st: Note that those maladies which are now most nearly within the pale of true science, are those whose specific cause has been experimentally studied—Tuberculosis, Dyptheria, Tetanus and so on. Also remember what the Yellow Fever Commission was able to do by experiments upon volunteer soldiers. With these controls, it seems certain that facts of inestimable value not only could be, but would be established. The following questions, for instance could be answered in the positive or negative, and answered with a positive demonstrated trustworthy "Yes or No."

1. Is the Bacillus of Eberth the specific cause of Typhoid Fever? You may say that this is already an established fact, but remember, according to Koch's law, that only two-thirds of the proposition has been proven.

2. Will water contaminated with the germ, used in food and drink, give rise to an attack of fever? If so, in what percentage of cases?

This experiment could also answer the question of milk supply, raw vegetables contaminated oysters, etc., etc. In fact it would answer the broad question whether the germ taken into the Alimentary Canal will lodge and reproduce the typical clinical picture.

3. Can the disease be disseminated by insects? If so, how? By acting as an accidental carrier of contamination to food and drink, or may the infected blood suckers inject the virus direct into the blood stream?

4. Is the malady contagious? That is, can it be acquired by such contact as that usual and ordinary to nursing?

5. Is there such an anomaly as the Typhoid Carrier?

Now given the possibilities of an experimental station, such as outlined above, is there a cogent reason why all these questions may not be answered?

We now come to the really difficult part of the problem. How can such an experimental station be established? The first step would be undoubtedly to institute a campaign of education, first among physicians. This can be best reached by bringing the subject before the state and subsidiary societies for study and discussion—they in turn educating the intelligent laity—the men who influence legislation—the people at large. That this is no easy matter may be inferred from past experience. For example, after the destruction of the Alexandrian School of Medicine, the science of medicine was absolutely at a standstill, if there was not indeed a retrogression during the next thousand years, because of the prohibitory prejudice against dissecting the human body, and while a Papal Bull would probably not interdict the human experiments as it did the human dissections in the 13th Century, there would be much ignorant sentimentality to overcome. The Anti-Vaccinationist, Anti-Vivisectionist, opponents of the Serum Therapy in Diphtheria are cases in point. However, the outlook is by no means hopeless—the stone wall of unreasoning religious prejudice is a thing of the past. The whole people are better educated, better thinkers and more amenable to logic than in previous times.

Armed with the precedent of Walter Reed and his work, I believe that it is possible to overcome all objections to human experimentation, and the astounding possibility for good ought to be a sufficient incentive to command the respect of and enlist the sympathy and best effort of our best men.

For several years the matter of this paper, has been upon my mind. I have hesitated, partly from cowardice, for fear of criticism, and partly from a desire to give it more mature consideration before presenting it publicly to the profession. I ask you to give it careful consideration. If the idea herein contained be founded in truth, it will in time take deep and lasting root in the minds of my readers and eventually bear fruit. If only a vagary of an abnormal imagination, it will only be remembered in company with the inventors of Perpetual Motion and seekers after the Fountain of Youth.

MALARIA, ATYPICAL FORMS.

BY DR. R. K. PEMBERTON, KREBS, OKLA.

Malarial disease was recognized more than one thousand B. C. The early Roman writers were more or less familiar with the symptoms of malaria; for instance, Cato speaks of "black bile and swollen spleen." As to causation, Hippocrates speaks of the influence of rains, seasons, stagnant water, etc.

Morton in 1697 clearly described pernicious intermittent, and strongly advised the use of Cinchona. In 1717 Lancisi began microscopic investigation as to the cause of malaria. He was not the first to suspect that malaria was due to an animal organism, for we find that Varo, before the Christian era, held the opinion that malarial fever was caused by "animals so minute that they could not be seen by the naked eye, and which entered the body with the air through the nose and mouth." In 1849 Meckel and Virchow no doubt observed the malarial parasites, but it remained for that brilliant Frenchman, Laveran, in 1880, to recognize the parasite known as the plasmodium malaria as the true cause of malarial fevers. Among those in America first to accept this theory were Sternberg, Osler and Thayer.

The important role played by the mosquito in the dissemination of malaria had in

Read Before the Oklahoma State Medical Association, at Tulsa May 12, 1910.

many countries long been suspected. In 1848 Dr. Josiah Nott, of Mobile, in a paper on yellow fever, suggested that malaria was spread by the mosquito. After Laveran discovery of the parasite in 1880 a great impetus was given to the study of malaria, In 1884 Koch and Laveran, and in 1894 and 1896 Manson and Bignami, concluded that malaria was spread by the mosquito, but Major Ronald Ross, after three years of hard work, from 1895 to 1898, was the first to announce to the world that certain species of the mosquito were responsible for the dissemination of malaria, and for this he was awarded a Nobel prize.

In Deaderick's work on malaria, that author says: "The discovery by Ross of the role of the mosquito in the dissemination of malaria is the most startling achievement of modern medical science."

"Mosquitoes do not cause malaria; they carry it from infected to healthy persons. The parasites, sucked with blood from a malarial individual, undergo a cycle of development within the body of the mosquito, and are then innoculated into healthy persons. Man is merely the intermediate host of the parasite; the mosquito is the definitive host, and it has been said that man gives malaria to the mosquito, and not the mosquito to man."

"Not all species of mosquitoes are capable of serving as host to the parasites of malaria. It is only certain members of the sub family Anophelinae, that have been found to act in this capacity." This author names forty or more members of this family of mosquitoes, which he thinks are carriers of malaria.

Since malaria infection comes through the bite of the mosquito, a study of the life history, habits, etc., of that insect becomes necessary in order to thoroughly understand not only the many symptoms of malarial poisoning, but what is more important—its prevention. The Anaphelines deposit their eggs upon the surface of water, preferably fresh water of lakes, pools, marshes, ditches, etc. The eggs hatch in two to four days, but the larva remain from 10 to 26 days upon the surface and near the edge of the water. It has been estimated that one female mosquito, in one season, will produce five billions of mosquitoes. The male mosquito is a vegetarian, while the female is a blood sucker, and is consequently responsible for malarial infection. The biting usually done at night, and one feed in twenty-four hours is satisfactory. The mosquito cycle varies from eight to sixteen days, at the end of which time the sporozoits are injected from the salivary glands of the mosquito into the victim, where each soon enters a red cell and goes through its cycle. The malarial parasites belong to the animal kingdom, and there are three well defined species, viz: the parasites of tertian malaria; of quartan malaria; and of estivo-autumnal malaria. The latter is again divided into the tertain and quotidian. We are all familiar with the fact that the parasites of tertian and quartan develop uniformly in forty-eight to seventy-two hours respectively, and this sporulation causes what we know as second and third day chills; but the estivo-autumnal is not so regular in its development, hence the fever runs an irregular course with exacerbations causing the so called remittent malarial fever. Quoting Deaderick again, that author says: "The change of type of malarial attacks has been used as an argument for the unity of the malarial parasites. It is well known, however, that such occurrences are best explained by a number of different species. Quotidian malarial paroxysms, due to two generations of tertain organisms, may be tertain in character by the destruction of one generation. The quotidian paroxysms due to a triple quartan may become quartan or double by the death of two generations, or of a single generation of parasites."

It is nōt my wish to speak further of the typical and usual forms of malaria, but rather more to my subject—"Atypical Forms of Malaria."

One of the rare forms of malaria, formerly classed as the hemorrhage type of pernicous malaria, is now known as hemoglobinuric fever, and under this name is fully described by Deaderick in his recent work on malaria. This disease is known in different localities by the name of malarial hematuria, swamp fever, black water fever, bilious hematuric and melanuric fever. A few cases of this disease was reported from the Southern States in 1859, and Dr. E. R. Duvall, of Fort Smith, Arkansas, read a paper on black water fever in 1871.

The early American writers attributed the color of the urine to blood, and not bile. Corre in 1881 proved the condition to be one of hemoglobinuria, and not hematuria.

White men, aged thirty years, who have had repeated attacks of malaria, or who have long lived in malarial regions, are most liable to attack.

Authorities differ as to the nature of black water fever. Some claim that it is malarial, others that it is due to quinine poisoning, and still others that it is a disease suigeneris. Deaderick holds that malaria is, "Essentially and solely the predisposing cause, and that in some cases it may act as the exciting cause." The same writer says: "As favoring its malarial character are; (1) Geographic distribution. (2) Length of residene in endemic region. (3) Previous atacks of malaria. (4) Malarial prophylaxis is prophylactic of black water fever. (5) Blood findings: Parasites, pigmented leukocytes and monouclear leukocytosis. The fact that hemoglobinuric fever does not respond to quinine is one of the strongest evidences that it is not malarial per-se."

The objections to the quinine theory are: (1) It is restricted in geographic range, and is absent from some highly malarial localities, where much quinine is used. (2) It does not follow the administration of quinine for maladies other than malaria. (3) In a considerable number of cases the antecedent use of quinine can be eliminated with certainty. (4) The same individual may have an attack following the use of quinine, and later take it without harmful results. (5) The severity of the attack bears no relation to the size of the dose. (6) One dose of quinine could not cause intermittent hemoglobinuria. (7) The great majority of cases recover, even under the continued use of large doses of quinine."

In hemoglobinuric fever the pathology varies according to the severity of the attack. The body is deply jaundiced, the liver is saturated with bile, varying in color from yellow to brown. The spleen is congested, and in some cases immensely large, and the color may be gray or reddish brown. The kidneys are congested and soft, the cortex often yellow and the lumina frequently filled with hemoglobin. The condition of the stomach, bowels, heart and brain is pretty much the same as in other forms of malaria, except they may show evidence of hemorrhage and at times pigmentation.

The leading symptoms of black water fever are: fever, hemoglobinuria, icterus and vomiting. It has been my good fortune to see not more than three or four cases of hemoglobinuric fever, and in presenting the symptoms I must necessarily follow more or less closely the authorities, of whom I find Deaderick decidedly the best.

After a severe chill the fever rapidly rises, and the patient soon passes a large amount of red or black urine, containing hemoglobin, albumen and urobilin, and this last symptom may be the first symptom noticed. Bilious vomiting and jaundice soon set in. The patient has severe pains in the head, loins and epigastrium. These symptoms rapidly pass off, and the patient recovers in a few hours, or a day or two; or, the symptoms may become severe, suppression ensue, and death rapidly follow. The bowels may be constipated or there may be a bilious diarrhoea. At times the passages are thin and watery, and of a reddish brown color resembling the urine. The patient is thirsty and the tongue heavily coated. The pulse is first full and bounding, later feeble and compressible. Respiration is increased and dyspnea, from edema or congestion of the lungs, may follow. Anemia rapidly develops, and it has been estimated that one-half of the hemoglobin is often reduced one-half or to one-fourth. This is not a painful disease, but extreme prostration is rapid. There is a low delirium in some cases, though at times the mind remains clear until just before death, when coma supervenes. Plhen is quoted as calling one a "black water fever candidate" when he has lived in a black water fever area for six months, had repeated attacks of malaria, been treated improperly, and shows a depressed condition, mental apathy, restlessness, jaundice of the sclera and skin, and albumen in the urine. Black water fever may be confused with the socalled bilious remittent, but if we remember that in the latter the attacks come on more slowly, jaundice is mild, parasites usually present, albuminuria not constant, and urine colored by bile, while in black water fever the attack is sudden, with intense jaundice, parasites not always present, albuminuria constant, and urine colored by hemoglobin, the diagnosis will be made easier. The danger is in proportion to the amount of urine voided. Suppression nearly always means a

fatal termination. The mortality is usually about twenty-five per cent when quinine is used, but in 1,000 cases treated without quinine the mortality was eleven per cent.

Now a few words as to masked malaria, some times called biliousness, or latent malaria. When we get into a tight place for an exact diagnosis these terms are too often used as a cloak for ignorance. Latent malaria is atypic malaria, and its frequency varies inversely with the care employed in diagnosis.

A great many diseased conditions and obscure symptoms are, in this southern country, attributed to malaria. It is a fact that quinine often works wonders in the relief of these symptoms. Many gastro-intestinal symptoms, and nervous and neuralgic conditions are speedily received by the use of quinine, thus proving their malarial origin.

There is a difference between chronic malaria and malarial cachexia. In chronic malaria the vitality of the host is equal to the attack of the parasites, while in malarial cachexia the parasites have gotten the best of the host in the struggle. Chronic malaria is an active disease condition, while malarial cachexia is a sequel of the malarial infection. In the latent state of chronic malaria the patient may seem practically well. However, there is usually present malaise, loss of appetite, aenemia and enlarged spleen. Malarial cachexia is said to follow the estivo-autumnal infection more often than that of tertain or quartan. The patient is aenemic and the spleen very much enlarged. The red blood cells are no longer manufactured as fast as they are destroyed and are consequently reduced in number. The pulse becomes small, weak and irregular, and there may be palpatation and an aenemic murmur, dilatation, or even myocardatis. Dyspuea, bronchitis and pulmonary oedema may develop. There may be no fever, but there is often diarrhea or dysentery, and the urine is scanty and highly colored. The liver and spleen are usually enlarged, and the malarial cachectic is a fit subject for most any complication.

The term Typho-malaria is usually a compromise diagnosis and should never be used unless a careful diagnosis has determined the presence of both the malarial parasite and the bacillus of typhoid fever. Most of the cases are pure typhoid fever.

Atypic forms of malaria are frequently seen in children. The rigor is often absent, and the fever is inclined to go higher than in the adult, often causing convulsions.

Malaria frequently shows some peculiar or unusual features in the negro race. In the first place, the negro is more immune to malaria, especially black water fever, than the white. The spleen is rarely so large, nor does the negro suffer such severe gastro-intestinal symptoms. However, the negro, when suffering from malaria, is more subject to such complications as pneumonia, tuberculosis and nephritis.

The treatment of malaria in any and all forms naturally divides itself into two divisions: (1) Phophylaxis. (2) Cure of the infection.

Taking up first the subject of prevention, we must acknowledge the great debt of gratitude we owe to Ross for his discovery of the role the mosquito plays in malaria. Thousands of lives and millions of dollars have already been saved in the last few years through this discovery. The fight, then, is largely one against this particular family of mosquitoes—the anophelines.

Our efforts must not only be directed against the prevention of bites of the mosquito by gauze, wire netting, etc., but we must endeavor to eradicate the mosquito. This may be done by destroying their breed-

ing places, or by directly attacking the mosquitoes. Ross' motto was: "No stagnant water." Swamps must be cleared, stagnant pools and ditches drained, and no water allowed to stand exposed to the air. The march of civilization has unconciously done much to eradicate malaria by draining low lands, reclaiming marshes and building levees to prevent rivers from overflowing. As illustrating may be done along this line, the death rate annually from 1885 to 1902, in a town of a few thousand inhabitants, situated on the Suez Canal was eighteen hundred. In 1902 the President of the Canal Company had Ross and two other experts to come and investigate as to the hygeinic surroundings. They began their campaign against the mosquito, and in 1903 the deaths from malaria were two thousand and fourteen, in '04 ninety, and in '05 only thirty-seven. Witness also the wonderful results obtained by Gorgas and others in Panama. Thousands of men have lost their lives in this canal zone, which is only about fifty miles long, but now there is something like fifty thousand men on the zone at work, and it is said that the death rate at present is not greater than that of New York City. This has been brought about by cleaning up and draining the low lands, and where draining was impossible, the small ditches were concreted; and then the people had their houses screened, slept under mosquito bars, and were furnished quinine free by the government, and urged to take it in three grain doses daily. Where water can not be gotten rid of, then our efforts must be directed towards destroying the larva.

To Howard belongs the credit of first using oil successfully for this purpose. Common furnace oil is the best. One ounce will cover about fifteen square feet, or a barrel ninety-six thousand square feet. It may be sprayed on, though it is best allowed to drop about twenty drops to the minute from a small hole in the bottom of a barrel, elevated three or four feet above the surface of the water, in order that it may spread well, and this is repeated every two or three weeks. The oil destroys the larva and sometimes the young mosquito, but will not effect the adult mosquito. When it is necessary to attack the grown mosquito, this is best done by the fumes of burning sulphur. Two to five lbs. of sulphur should be burned in a tight room for every one thousand cubic feet of space; or, pyrethrum powder is quite as effectual as sulphur. A few ounces to one lb. to the thousand cubic feet should be used. It may be burned by first moistening with alcohol.

In attempting to destroy the parasites in the human body by the use of quinine, which we recognize as a specific for malaria, we have also to use the specific as a prophylactic to prevent the completion of the incubation stages of the parasites when a healthy person is inoculated.

The greatest danger to the public is from latent and atypical cases of malaria. These cases harbor the malarial parasites for months, and are a constant source of infection, whereas, an acute attack is usually promptly treated and cured. Quinine as a prophylactic is best given by the Koch or Plehn methods. The Koch method consists of giving fifteen grains of quinine every sixth and seventh days, while Plehn gives seven or eight grains every fifth evening. One of these methods should be used so long as one is exposed to malarial infection, and for two months after he has removed from a malarial district, if he would be sure of escaping malaria.

If each case of malarial infection could be isolated, protected from the mosquito, and vigorously treated, then it would not be long until malaria could be stamped out.

Quinine may be given by the mouth, per rectum, endermically, hypodermically and intravenously. For quick action, fifteen grains of bimuriate dissolved in two and one-half drachms of water, and injected deeply into the muscles is probably the best mode of administration. In order to avoid ulcers and necrosis, thorough asepsis must be had, and the quinine well diluted. Some authors advise a single large dose of quinine before the expected paroxysm, others, a single dose in the decline, and still others, fractional doses. The latter is probably the best method of administration, owing to the many different forms of the infection.

Some patients claim they can not take quinine, but this advice should usually not be heeded unless the symptoms produced are such as depression of the heart, or dyspnea. One salt of quinine is some times well borne, when others are not. Equinine is a new preparation of quinine that may sometimes be substituted in these cases.

Methylene-blue was first used in 1891 as a substitute for quinine, and is perhaps more efficient than any other substitute. It is best given in capsules, one and one-half to three grains each, every three hours, until fifteen grains are taken, this to be given daily for a number of days. Experience teaches that this remedy is probably more efficient in chronic malaria than it is in the acute attacks.

Carpenter has used powdered splenic extract with success, but I have no experience with this remedy. He gives it in capsules of five grains each, every two to four hours. He says, "In more than six years experience, and in the treatment of hundreds of cases of malarial infection of all types and complications, not a single case has been met with which did not yield to this remedy."

Quinine is a true specific, and will destroy the parasite, provided it is absorbed, and is not prevented by thrombi from reaching the parasite, as is sometimes the case in pernicious malaria.

In the treatment of hemoglobinuric fever, to give or not to give quinine is the question. Where quinine is given as a rout. ine practice, the mortality is greater. Thayer's rules are: (1) If the attack occurs spontaneously with a malarial paroxysm, the blood showing parasites, quinine should be given freely. (2) If there are no parasites, abstain from giving quinine. (3) If an attack arising in the middle of malarial infection, after using quinine, do not give more. (4) If an attack after quinine, parasites continue to develop, give the quinine.

Deaderick says: "Give quinine where the parasites show no tendency to disappear after forty-eight hours from the onset, and also give it in intermittent hemoglobinuria where the outbreak corresponds with parasitic sporulation." There is no specific for black water fever. Keep the patient quiet in a warm bed, and use only liquid nourishment. The bowels should be kept open with, preferably, small doses of calomel.

Quennic treated fifty cases without a death by the chloroform treatment. One and one-half drachms of chloroform was given, a sip at a time, in emulsion daily. Calcium Chloride is recommended, one to one and one-half drachms daily. Cardamatis has used with apparent succes one drachm doses of ether every three hours. It is very important to prevent suppression, and for this, water is the best diuretic. The patient should drink as freely of water as possible, and normal salines should be given per rectum as the best means of preventing and combating anuria. Stimulation and supportive measures should be resorted to when necessary. If quinine has not been given during the attack; then small doses should be given during convalescence, watching closely its effect upon the urine. In the treatment of masked or latent malaria, chronic malaria and malarial cachexia, fifteen grains of quinine on two successive days, twice a week, should be given. Tonics of iron and arsenic should be used, and the hygienic surroundings improved, and in malarial cachexia a change of climate is often an absolute necessity.

R. K. PEMBERTON, M. D.,
Krebs, Oklahoma.

DIAGNOSIS AND TREATMENT OF TYPHOID PERFORATION.—REPORT OF THREE CASES.

BY DRS. J. HUTCHINGS WHITE AND I. B. OLDHAM, MUSKOGEE, OKLA.

Since the suggestion by Lyden, and the successful termination of a case of abdominal section by Mickulicz for Typhoid perforation in 1884, the number of operations for typhoid perforations have been on the increase. While the success of this work is still far from gratifying, the reduction of a mortality of 100 per cent is decided strides in the fight for longevity. In 1904 Hart and Ashhurst collected 8,881 cases of typhoid fever with 225 perforations, or 2.54 per cent.

Quoting from paper by Dr. J A. Scott, New York Medical Journal of February, 1907.

"Since January, 1903, to October, 1906, there have occurred 29,873 cases of typhoid fever in Philadelphia, with 3,257 deaths. Considering that at least one third of these deaths were due to perforation, we have had 1,085 perforation cases to deal with in this city."

Scott claims the general mortality of Typhoid is 8.05 per cent—that is, in 3,006 cases 242 deaths occurred. The perforation mortality of 2.59, or 78 cases in 3,006. The proportion of perforation to the total number of deaths is 32.2 per cent, or one perforation in a little over three cases.

According to Brown (Journal A. M. A. February 27, 1906), based upon statistics collected by Taylor, some 25,000 deaths occur annually in the United States from intestinal perforation during typhoid fever. In this large number of cases it is surprising to find, according to Harte and Ashhurst, (Annals of Surgery, January 1, 1904,) that up to January, 1903, only 362 cases had been reported.

Whiting (Annals of Surgery, May, 1910,) cites 2,053 cases of typhoid occurring in the German Hospital at Philadelphia between 1900 and 1909. Of this numbr 206, or 10 per cent, died from various causes. In 180 of the 206 deaths there was no suspicion of perforation noted. Of the remaining 26 deaths 17 were due to perforation, found either at operation or post-mortem, and in 9 cases death was due to peritonitis —probably perforation, the diagnosis not being confirmed. Giving a mortality of 1.26 per cent. from perforation, this is the lowest percentage of death from typhoid perforation we have seen, and reduces the ratio of 1-3 of Osler and Scott to 1-8.

Perforation is most common in cases of moderate or severe type. None are, however, to be excluded from the possibility. They occur most frequently between the fourteenth and twenty-first days. Perforation may, however, take place as early as he eighteenth day or as late as the sixth week. They may be single or multiple. Seventy-three per cent occur within the last twelve inches of the ileum. They may be found in the colon, appendix caecum or Meckels diverticulium. They vary in size from a pin point to a dime or even larger where the base of ulcer sloughs. The per-

foration is usually situated opposite the mesentery or the fundal line where the blood supply is least and where the lymph follicles are situated. It may, however, occur near the mesenteric attachment, as it was in one of our cases.

The signs formerly relied upon for a diagnosis, such as presence or absence of liver dullness and leucocytosis, are practically without value. Often times pain and tenderness are not more prominent than they have been throughout the disease. Scott says: "I am convinced that the important things to keep in mind in making a diagnosis are, to exclude pneumonia and pludisy, retention of urine even though there seems to be no physical signs to call our attention to such a condition (a catheter must be used); ilies or femoral thrombosis; and peritonitis. Either peritonitis and appendicitis are operative, and need not bother us in making a differential diagnosis." He cites twenty cases diagnosticated as perforation, but, upon operation, proved otherwise.

Whiting claims perforation should be suspected in every instance where the regular course of the typhoid infection in that individual case has been interrupted by some untoward mishap. Perforation should be diagnosed in all such cases, when the mishap cannot be traced directly to some complication other than perforation. The physician in charge of the case, who has closely watched his patient from day to day, is certainly in a better condition to note this mishap than the surgeon, who has seen the case only once. While it is true there are no pathognomonic symptoms, the picture is so complete in about seventy-five per cent. of the cases that one is justifiable in doing an abdominal section even though an occasional mistaken diagnosis is made.

It is very important that an early diagnosis is made if we are to expect a reduc-

tion in mortality. To this end we would recommend, where accessible, the hospital care
of these cases. Where not available, an experienced nurse should be placed in charge,
with instructions to report immediately any
sudden change in the condition of the patient.

Pain which is sharp and stabbing, with
point of maximum tenderness in the right
iliac fossa is present in seventy-five per cent.
·of the cases. Tenderness and rigidity, respectively, are present in from 75 per cent.
to 65 per cent. of all cases and are usually
combined.

Murphy of Chicago claims vomiting is
constantly associated with perforation, peritonitis and typhoid fever. It was absent in
a number of cases reported by Whiting.

A fall in temperature usually follows
perforation, but may be easily overlooked
unless the temperature is taken often. A
rise shortly follows, due to peritonitis. Collapse and sweating are found in many of
the cases. The pulse is rapid and weak, the
facial expression anxious.

A. J. Brown (Journal A. M. A., February 27, 1909,) describes two new signs of
perforation. The first he designates as
"dipping crackle" sign, and is present for
only a short time after perforation and disappears with the accumulation of gas. On
placing the bell of a stethoscope over the
right iliac fossa dipping suddenly with it
as in dipping palpation, a very fine crackle
is heard which sounds much like a fine
crepitant rale, or as if two sticky surfaces
were being drawn apart. The author considers this a valuable confirmatory sign, as
it seems to be due to the fact that in dipping suddenly the visceral and parietal layers
of the peritoneum come in contact for an
instant and, apparently, the inflamed surfaces stick together for a moment and then
pull apart. He has never found the sign
present over an area of more than two

inches in diameter, and never later than four
hours after the initial symptom.

The second sign of perforation: The patient was examined immediately and a small
area of tenderness found low down in the
right iliac fossa. He was turned on his left
side and in half hour the area of tenderness
had moved toward that side about two
inches.

The diagnosis made there is only one
treatment—Abdominal section and repair of
the injured gut. The mortality rate according to Allabin's collection of five hundred
cases was 62 per cent.; in Deaver and Whiting's collection of 33 cases the mortality
was 1.1 per cent. Hart and Ashhurst's
tables show that during the first twelve
hours after perforation the mortality is 73
per cent.; the second twelve hours 73.8 per
cent.; during the third twelve hours 93 per
cent.

While it is unnecessary to go into all
the details of the operation, dispatch is of
great importance, and the question of
drainage is yet a mooted one. In three
cases here reported soft split drainage tubes,
inclosing strip of iodoform gauze, were
used.

Greaves raises objections to drains in the
lower abdomen:

1. The drain is acting under the mechanical disadvantage of the patient lying
upon his back, forcing all the fluid to pass
up hill;

2. Whereas, perfect rest is greatly to
be desired in any case of general peritonitis, but especially in typhiod fever, the presence of the drainage tube adds to the difficulties of nursing, and must be constantly
emptied by a suction syringe;

3. The drainage tube provides an open
path for the intrusion of germs from without;

4. The drainage tube, if flexible, is
easily occluded and so rendered useless; if

rigid, it may by its pressure injure the intestine or bladder. A fecal fistula has resulted from such pressure;

5. On withdrawing the tube some portion of the bowel, such as the appendix, Meckels diverticulium an appendix epiploica or part of the great omentum may have entered the tube and be withdrawn also.

Drainage should be reserved for the most septic cases, and then applied to the most dependent parts, such as the lumbar regions, rather than to the abdominal incision. The abdominal incision should be closed in layers and the sutures should be interrupted.

To guard against infection of the subcutaneous fatty tissue it was suggested that a small drain should be inserted into the wound at the lower end of the incision after the peritoneum is completely closed, removing one of the interrupted sutures when necessary. It seems to us that a peritoneal cavity containing portions of fecal matter which are decidedly septic should certainly be drained. The Fowler position with a soft split rubber drainage tube of large calibre containing a strip of idoform gauze inserted into the pelvis will come about as near giving complete drainage as anything we can use.

Case No. 1.

Joe B., aged 16, entered hospital 7:00 p m. on December 5, 1909, temperature 103.6; pulse 120; had been ill one week from history given, which was very meager from fact that patient had been sent to hospital from distant town without an attendant, and was unable to give accurate history. On December 7, at 11:00 p. m., had profuse intestinal hemorrhages; hemorrhages occurred daily until December 10th.

December 10th, at 6:00 a. m., temperature 102; pulse 104. At 7:45 a. m., complained of severe pain in lower abdomen, pain referable to the region of the bladder

extending to end of penis; temperature dropped to 97; pulse rose to 112; patient was catherized, bladder was found empty: much tenderness over abdomen, more over right lower quadrant.

Diagnosis of intestinal perforation was made, patient taken to the operating room at 2:00 p. m. On opening the abdomen two perforations were found in ilium within eight inches of cecum, which were closed by linen purse string suture; abdomen drained through wound with soft split rubber tube with iodoform gauze wick; drainage tube removed on tenth day, leaving sinus which discharged until January 25, 1910. Patient left hospital on February 6th, fully recovered.

Case No. 2.

W. F. M., about 30 years of age, was admitted to Baptist hospital under care of Dr. O. C. Klass during second week of typhoid, and on December 17th temperature was 103; pulse 100; abdomen distended. Patient had several hemorrhages between the 17th and 31st. On December 31st at 6:00 a. m. temperature was 99; at 12:00 o'clock same day temperature was 97.6 F; pulse 88; some distension of abdomen. The symptoms not being clear enough for a diagnosis of perforation, we decided to wait, instructing the nurse to watch for hemorrhage. For the next three days temperature run from 98.6 F to 101.7 F; pulse 84 to 100. On January 3, at noon, patient complained of severe pains in abdomen, temperature 99.4 F; pulse 90. At 3:00 p. m. temperature was 101 F, pulse 116; at 3:15, temperature 102 F., pulse 126. Distension of abdomen about the same as for several days. Saline enema returned with much gas and small amount of blood. Operation at 4:00 p. m. A loop of the ilium was found in an old hermal sac within the abdomen with a perforation near the mesentery and plastic adhesions to the other side of loop. A good deal of free fluid was also encountered. Gut repaired, split rubber drainage in pelvis, and wound partially closed. At 9:30 p. m. temperature 100, pulse 130, from which time temperature and pulse gradually rose to 103.4 F and 170 by 3:30 p. m. January 5th, from which time both temperature and pulse gradually subsided, reaching 99.8 F. and 116 on January 6th at 7:30 a. m. At 11:30 a. m., temperature 102 Rectal, pulse 125, respiration 40. A pneumonia developed, from which patient died on January 13th.

Autopsy showed three large yellow spots on the ilium near seat of repaired perforation which proved to be the base of typhoid ulcers. Pneumonia of lower lobes of right lung.

We regret that we cannot give full details of the third case, which was seen in consultion by Dr. White with Dr. Laws, of Broken Arrow. Patient presented a picture of general peritonitis, perforation having been diagnosed by Dr. Laws. Delay in operation, due to failure to secure consent of patient; operation forty-eight hours after perforation; abdomen filled with fecal matter; a perforation one-fourth inch in diameter repaired; abdomen mopped out with saline sponges. Split rubber drains inserted and abdomen partially closed. Death at 3:00 a. m., five hours after operation. No autopsy.

LOCAL ANESTHESIA.

BY LEIGH F. WATSON, M. D., OKLAHOMA CITY, OKLA.

Whenever the choice of anesthetic is possible, local anesthesia should be selected in preference to general narcosis, because of the greater safety and comfort afforded the patient. To those using the cocain method its advantages are apparent, and the field continually enlarges as the technic improves.

The importance of local anesthesia has never been sufficiently appreciated in America. Mitchell has said, this may be due to American hurry, but more probably to inexperience in the method and a certain deep rooted fear of poisoning traceable to the days of strong cocain solutions.

The strong solutions are equally or more dangerous than general anesthesia, while the weak solutions are the safest of all methods of analgesia. Reclus says, cocain, when properly and prudently administered is the least treacherous of all anesthetics, and when local anesthesia is possible I prefer it to ether or chloroform because I believe it less dangerous, from observations on its use during the last 23 years in over 10,000 operations not only without a death but without any disturbance of the "equilibre physiologic" of the patient.

A. E. Barker, of London, in a personal communication, says, I use local anesthesia whenever time permits, as I have strong objections to using general anesthetics which involve risk, whenever a local anesthetic can be employed which involves no risk.

Reclus states that the reason dentists have frequent mishaps with cocain is because of their faulty technic: (1). The use of too strong solutions. (2). They inject the cocain with the patient sitting up. (3). They permit the patient to stand up, walk around and go away too soon after operation. This accounts for the frequent occurrence of fainting, nausea, malaise, and vertigo. He reports over 70,000 extractions according to his technic without a single accident.

Halsted was the first to emphasize the importance of the intradermal use of cocain, and the first American surgeon to employ it as a local anesthetic (1884). The importance of using the weak solutions was first urged by Corning (1885), Reclus (1886) and Schleich (1888). Their subsequent adoption did much to extend the scope of local anesthesia.

Schleich suggested the extreme dilution of 1:20-1:100 per cent. Reclus says, anesthesia with Schleich's weakest solutions is tardy in appearance and fleeting in effect.

Familiarity with the technic and the employment of the weak solutions has given cocain a wide range of use in the hands of Matas, Crile, Bodine, Cushing, Mitchell, Gilday, Horsley, Samuell and a few other American surgeons. Schleich has stated that 90 per cent. of his operations are completed under local anesthesia, Mitchell has 50 per cent and one third of the operations of Bodine and Gilday are completed under cocain.

Untoward or poisonous symptoms have never been observed following the use of the weak solutions. The weaker the solution, the greater the amount of cocain that can be injected without producing toxic symptoms, twice as much can be injected with safety in a one fourth per cent than in a one per cent solution. Upon the strength of the solution depend the rapidity, intensity and duration of the anesthesia. With the strong five per cent solutions anesthesia is complete as soon as the injection is made, with the two per cent solutions anesthesia is almost immediate, while with the solutions weaker than one half per cent a longer wait is necessary, usually two to three minutes, the time required to prepare the field of operation.

Mitchell states that cocain is a protoplasmic poison, forming with protoplasm an unstable compound that breaks down slowly, after which the tissues return to their previous condition and resume their normal function; cocain which has exerted its an esthetic action and entered into this combination can not be absorbed into the circulation, and, therefore, poisoning can only be due to absorption of an excess.

Reclus says, cocain first excites and then paralyzes protoplasm. It anesthetizes all nerve fibres, both motor and sensory.

When applied locally to mucous or serous membranes or injected subcutaneously, cocain reaches the terminal nerves and produces analgesia.

Water will produce temporary anesthesia if a sufficient amount is injected to paralyze the nerves from pressure, as soon as the water is absorbed and the pressure removed the sensibility to pain returns.

Schleich first noticed the pain and irritation following the injection of plain water, the "anesthesia dolorosa" of Liebrich, and suggested the use of normal saline solution.

Ethyl chloride has a very limited field as a local anesthetic because of the pain caused by the freezing, the pain of the tissues thawing out and the hyperesthesia that always follows the use of freezing mixtures.

Corning (1885) was the first to employ elastic constriction to prolong and intensify the anesthetic action of cocain. The constriction also prevents rapid absorption and toxic symptoms when the strong solutions are used. Elsberg and Barker first suggested the addition of adrenalin to the cocain solution to confine it to the area injected and limit absorption.

Pressure anesthesia, according to Braun, can only be obtained by sufficient pressure to injure the nerves. Victor Horsley believes that the ordinary Esmarch bandage often injures the nerves of the extremities and should never be used except when absolutely necessary, and always removed as soon as possible.

Eucain and Novococain have been widely employed as substitutes for cocain, to avoid the toxic symptoms. Eucain is only one-fourth as toxic as cocain but the effect is obtained more slowly, anesthesia only lasts one-half as long and is never as deep as that with cocain. Pouchet has proved experimentally that Eucain is not as harmless as at first supposed. He found that in the beginning the symptoms were not as marked as those of cocain, later it is more dangerous because the accidents it causes appear suddenly and unexpectedly without prodromal symptoms, the animal dying suddenly without a chance for resuscitation.

More hemorrhage follows the use of Eucain because it produces a hyperemia of the superficial vessels while cocain produces a vaso-constriction. Eucain infiltration is more painful than cocainization because the anesthesia appears more slowly. After a thorough trial of novococain, Bodine says, it does not add to the safety of the patient nor is the anesthesia as satisfactory as with cocain.

Novococain, according to Braun, is a strong but fleeting local anesthetic and is useless unless combined with adrenalin, the effect appears in twenty minutes. Lennander also states that Novococain is unsatisfactory unless combined with adrenalin, and he emphasizes the importance of always waiting thirty minutes after injecting the Novococain before proceeding with the operation in order to obtain complete anesthesia.

Urea and quinine hydrochloride was suggested as a substitute for cocain by Thibault, the effect is obtained more slowly than with Eucain but the anesthesia lasts longer than cocain. It was employed in the clinics of Wyeth and Bodine soon after Thibault's report, but was later discarded in favor of cocain. The principal objection was the slowness of the anesthesia appearing after the solution had been injected. This unnecessary loss of time proves very annoying to a surgeon accustomed to the immediate analgesia following cocainiza-

tion. Recently Hertzler, Brewster and Rogers reported their results with urea and quinine hydrochloride and particularly recommend it for tonsillectomy, hemorrhoids and fistulae because of its prolonged anesthesia.

Stovain, according to Pouchet, Billou and Goyanes, is two to three times less toxic than cocain but hypodermically it sometimes causes sloughing of the tissues.

Bodine has remarked, so long as cocain fulfills all the requirements of the ideal local anesthetic it is a waste of time to experiment with others of doubtful value.

The technic of the injection is always delicate; it varies with each region, each operation and in each patient. The technic must be learned with a knowledge of its application and adaptation to each individual case. Success in the use of local anesthesia depends on patience, special training in the technic and an intimate knowledge of sensory nerve distribution. Because of the slower appearance of complete anesthesia with the weaker solutions, surgeons that begin operating as soon as the injection is finished will often fail with local anesthesia.

The sensation of pain is confined to the skin, nerve trunks, parietal peritoneum, periosteum and synovial membranes of joints.

There is no sensation of pain in bone substance, bone marrow, cartilage, tendon, articular surface of bone covered with cartilage, lungs, heart, bladder serosa, kidney, pelvis, ureter and bile ducts.

Lilienthal was one of the first to note the absence of sensation in the intestine.

Lennander has demonstrated that all internal organs obtaining their nerve supply only from the sympathetic and vagus, below the branching of the recurrent nerve, have no sensation, for this reason the abdominal and pelvic viscera are insensitive that heat, cold, pain and pressure, both in health and disease. In operating for a depressed fracture of the frontal bone under cocain anesthesia Bodine noted an absence of sensation in the dura and brain substance of the frontal region.

Braun states the dura is sensitive beneath the occipital bone.

Lennander has observed sensation to pain in the dura beneath the zygomatic arch, elsewhere he claims it is insensitive.

A slight twinge of pain is felt when blood vessels are divided.

Traction on the ligaments of the thoracic, abdominal or pelvic viscera will cause pain, traction on the mesentery besides producing pain will cause nausea and if traction is severe vomiting may occur.

The operator must gain and maintain the confidence of the patient by engaging him in conversation during the entire operation, and so far as possible keep his mind occupied.

Where retraction is necessary, as in abdominal work, the diversion of the patient's attention gives greater relaxation of the muscles and allows the operator a better view of the field without causing pain.

Nerves, no matter how small, should never be handled previous to cocainization, to do so will lessen the confidence of the patient in the method, cause unnecessary pain and a certain amount of shock. For a similar reason lacerated and contused wounds of the extremities should not be prepared for operation previous to cocainization.

Without the absolute confidence of the patient work under local anesthesia will tax the patience of the most skilful surgeon, therefore, it is very important to always proceed slowly during the early stages of an operation under cocain.

Bodine impresses on the patient the less solution used the quicker the healing; by this method it is possible to make every drop count.

With a nervous patient a drop of carbolic acid or ethyl chloride spray may be used to deaden the slight pain of the first injection.

The addition of adrenalin to the cocain solution gives a bloodless operative field, and by limiting absorption it prolongs the effect of the cocain and prevents toxic symptoms from the strong solutions.

I consider the addition of adrenalin unnecessary to prevent poisoning when the weak solutions are used, besides it increases the tendency to secondary oozing of blood into the tissues.

Along the line of incision a series of small wheals (about one-third tto one-half inch in diameter) are produced by thrusting the point of the needle just beneath the skin surface and injecting until the area turns white. The needle is then withdrawn and reinserted at the furthest edge of the anesthetized area and the procedure repeated until the entire line of incision is cocainized.

With proper cocainization the anesthesia of the skin incision will remain for an hour and a half, or longer. A subcuticular stitch will make the secondary suturing painless when sensation has returned to the skin wound after a long operation.

The point of the needle should always be in sight (intra-epidermal), otherwise an unnecessary amount of solution will be required to anesthetize the sensory nerve terminals. It is impossible to insert the needle too superficial. The subcutaneous tissue can be more easily infiltrated and less solution is required if it is injected before the skin incision is made.

Usually one-fourth to one-half grain of cocain is all that is required for major operations, including herniotomie, although one or two grains can be safely employed by using dilute solutions and distributing it over one to three hours time. Bodine states that there has never been a case of death reported following the use of two grains or less of cocain hypodermically.

Epigastric discomfort, transient pallor and sweating frequently occur at the beginning of an operation under local anesthesia, even with the most dilute cocain solutions. These are not symptoms of cocain poisoning and should be disregarded as they disappear in a few minutes when the operation may be continued and more cocain used with the assurance that they will not recur. Bodine says they are purely psychic, the strangeness of being cut even without pain is responsible, and as surgery under cocain becomes better known to the people these psychic phenomena will become less frequent.

Reclus insists that it is very important to always have the patient in the horizontal position so as to keep plenty of blood in the head, the first effect of cocain is one of vaso-constriction both local and systemic.

He says in speaking of "idiosyncrasy," I certainly admit that certain individuals are more "sensibles" (sensitive) than others to cocain, and while one is able to tolerate large doses, in others weak doses will produce toxic symptoms: this idiosyncrasy is not confined to cocain alone but is common to other alkaloids as well. We have seen grave symptoms follow one-twenty-fourth grain of morphine, while it is well known that one-sixth to one-third grain are ordinarily perfectly tolerated.

Reclus and Legrand state that the inhalation of three or four minims of Amyl Nitrite is the most effective antidote to relieve the vaso-constriction of cocain poisoning.

Advantages. While it adds to the comfort and safety of the young and robust. in the presence of old age, shock, hemorrhage, pulmonic, cardiac and nephritic lesions local anesthesia is especially indicated.

There is an absence of the fear many patients have for a general anesthetic and its after effects. While children and nervous patients are not the most favorable subjects, this factor alone is not sufficient to exclude local anesthesia; although it requires more time to gain their confidence and much care to maintain it, when they finally become convinced that the method is absolutely painless they are usually model patients.

The nervous, frightened patient is the one that suffers most from shock under general anesthesia and for that reason alone an effort should always be made to employ local analgesia.

I have never seen a patient that has went through an operation under local anesthesia that regretted the selection of the method, nor one that would consent to general anesthesia for a second operation. This is well illustrated in patients with double herniae who usually desire both operations at one sitting and invariably refuse to even consider general narcosis for the second operation. It is not at all unusual for the patient to fall asleep during the latter part of an operation under local anesthesia, especially when the work is necessarily long and tedious.

As there is no necessity for hurry, fewer assistants are required than when general anesthesia is employed. Bodine believes that the gentler handling of tissues under local anesthesia, the avoidance of cutting nerve trunks, the use of as few ligatures as possible and the absence of nausea and vomiting favor an early repair without infection and in cases of herniae lessen recurrence.

Besides the absence of nausea, vomiting and shock the post-operative pain is less than that following general anesthesia. Reclus states that twenty-five per cent of the cases having cocain anesthesia sleep the night following operation, while only seventeen per cent of the cases receiving chloroform sleep the first night. The first thought of every surgeon is to provide the minimum operative danger with the maximum post-operative comfort for every patient.

Disadvantages. The most serious disadvantage of local anesthesia is that its application is limited to those parts of the body where the nerve supply can be controlled. Much more time is required than when operating under general anesthesia; there are so many advantages, however, that the question of time will seldom have to be considered, except in large clinics.

Vein anesthesia has been suggested by Bier, with this method complete analgesia of a limb can be obtained so as to allow resection of joints and other extensive bone operations. The blood is expelled from the part by means of an Esmarch bandage and a tourniquet applied above and below the field of operation and the limb anesthetized by injecting the cocain into a superficial vein between the tourniquets, anesthesia is complete in a few minutes and remains until the tourniquets are removed.

I have reported a case in which an infected wound of the foot was freely incised under vein anesthesia without the knowledge of the patient. A tourniquet was applied just above the knee and fifteen c. c. of a one-fifth per cent cocain solution was injected into the external saphenous vein in the upper third of the leg. Anesthesia was complete in thirty minutes extending as high as point of injection. Sensation reappeared as soon as the tourniquet was removed. No uptoward symptoms were present at any time. Freeman has recently reported a case successfully operated on with vein anesthesia

Bier, in a personal communication, states that he has employed vein anesthesia in 220 cases without harm to the patients, he injects 100 c. c. of a one-half per cent Novococain solution, vein anesthesia is contradicted in children, senility and diabetic gangrene.

Hartel has recently described Bier's technic in detail.

Arterial anesthesia was first employed by Goyanes. In a communication to the Madrid Academy of Medicine and Surgery Nov., 1908, he says, about a year ago we had occasion to practice a series of experiments on dogs in studying the anesthesia and toxic action of certain drugs. From a previous study of the surgery of the blood vessels we were already familiar with the traumatic experimental lesions of the arteries and veins, and we now endeavored to find a new method of conducting the anesthetic to the central nerves and other regions of the body that could be utilized in the clinic. The first case, an amputation of the arm, was operated upon Nov. 7, 1908.

In this latest communication, he states that he has performed over twenty amputations and dissections on the extremities with excellent results.

Goyane's technic is as follows, the extremity is exsanguinated by means of an Esmarch bandage and a tourniquet applied above and below the field of operation. The most important artery of the region is selected and opened under infiltration anesthesia and fifty to one hundred c. c. of a five per cent Novococain in normal salt solution injected slowly and gently through a very fine needle. By introducing the needle obliquely into the artery there will be no subsequent hemorrhage.

Methylene blue is added to the solution so that the operator may observe the penetration of the tissues by the anesthetic. The anesthetic passes into all the vessels in five minutes, the skin is colored a light and the arteries and veins a dark blue. In five to ten minutes the anesthesia is complete.

After conservative operations (resection of joints, excision of tumors, cureting bone, sequestrotomies etc.) the distal tourniquet is first removed to permit the arterial circulation to flow while the venous return is impeded, this produces a venous hemorrhage that carries the anesthetic out of the circulation, finally the peripheral tourniquet is removed. Partial anesthesia persists for several hours and the patient is free from post-operative pain.

Oppel states that cocain solution is eight to ten times safer injected into the aorta than into the inferior vena cava, injected into the aorta the cocain is neutralized and diluted, while in the veins it almost immediately comes in contact with the cerebral and medullary centers producing symptoms of intoxication. Cocain is twice as fatal in the aorta than in the femoral artery.

Petrows states that the toxic dose of cocain was two to three times and the fatal dose seven to nine times greater without than with the use of a tourniquet on the limb.

Oppel says he was sure from the start that vein anesthesia was not the last word on local analgesia, but that it would be necessary to consider the feasibility of arterial anesthesia.

Bier states, it is very probable that better local anesthesia will be obtained through the arteries than through the veins.

Goyanes says, in conservative operations our experimental work and practice in the clinics up to date has demonstrated that the method is harmless to the vessel, and it is easy to understand that the diffusion of the anesthetic through the region is much better and more physiologic when injected into an artery than the injection into a superficial vein.

Ransohoff has recently reported several amputations successfully performed under arterial anesthesia. He uses a 1-10 per cent cocain solution.

Solutions. The cocain solutions should always be freshly prepared for each operation and of a definite strength, so that the operator may at any time know the exact amount of cocain that has been used. The cocain should be sterile and dissolved in sterile normal salt solution.

Cocain can be sterilized by heating to 212 degrees F., but a temperature above this, as well as repeated sterilizations, are injurious.

Reclus states that cocain solution left exposed to the air begins to lose strength by the end of the first week and at the end of thre weeks almost ceases to be analgesic. If sterilized and kept in sealed tubes it does not deteriorate, he has performed gastrostomy with a one-half per cent solution four and one-half years old and was unable to note any loss of strength in the solution.

The most convenient form of cocain on the market is put up in sealed glass tubes as suggested by Bodine. Each tube contains cocain hydrochloride .06 gm. and sodium chloride .18 gm., they are sterilized by the manufacturer. The contents of one tube dissolved in one ounce of warm sterile water makes a 1-500 cocain in normal salt solution; to make a 1-1000 solution this is diluted with an equal amount of sterile normal salt solution. Mitchell recommends a tablet containing cocain hydrochloride .05 gm. and adrenalin .00016 gm. These are sterilized by dry heat an hour on three successive days. One tablet dissolved in fifty c. c. of normal salt solution gives a 1-1000 solution; this he uses for infiltration. One tablet to five c. c. gives a one per cent solution; this or a one-half per cent he employs for nerve blocking.

Eucain and Novococain can be boiled without injury.

Barker employs Eucain one-fifth per cent or Novococain one-fourth per cent with adrenalin. Braun and Lennander prefer Novococain. The strengths recommended by Braun are.

	I.	II.	III.	IV.
Cocain hydrochloride	.1	.1	.05	.05
or				
Novococain.	.25	.25	.1	.1
Normal salt solution 100.	.50	.10	.5	
Adrenalin	m.V	m.V	m.V	m.V

Strength;

Cocain	1-1000	1-500	1-200	1-100
Novococain	1-250	1-125	1-150	1-125

Urea and quinine hydrochloride (equal parts) in strength of one-fifth to one-half per cent gives complete anesthesia, stdonger solutions will cause sloughing of the tissues. It is most conveniently dispensed in five grain capsules. One dissolved in an ounce of normal salt solution makes a one per cent solution. Sterilize by boiling in a test tube just before using. This can be further diluted as required with sterile normal salt solution.

An all-glass syringe that holds one or two drams is most convenient for infiltration and nerve blocking; the X-Ray and Sub-Q are two of the best. The needles must be kept sharp and clean and the smallest size should always be used for infiltrating the skin.

A one-fifth per cent cocain solution is used for the skin and nerve trunks; elsewhere a one-tenth per cent solution is employed.

Matas prefers massive infiltration of all the tissues, using a very dilute solution which is rapidly injected under pressure with a special apparatus, then ice bags are applied over the infiltrated area to intensify the analgesia.

When extensive and tedious dissection is required in an area well supplied with nerves, as the breast, Matas' method should be employed.

Preliminary treatment. The same aseptic and antiseptic precautions should be carried out as for any major operation. An extra cushion should be placed on the operating table so as to make the patient as comfortable as possible during the operation. A soap poultice should be applied for six hours preceding the operation, or the ten to twenty per cent oleate of mercury in lanolin dressing used, as recommended by Bodine.

This softens the epidermis and facilitates the skin infiltration.

When time does not permit the application of a preliminary dressing the surface should be prepared, dried and an application of tincture of Iodine made to the field of operation.

A dressing of scarlet red in lanolin is very useful to promote the rapid healing of skin wounds as well as chronic ulcers and burns, besides being mildly antiseptic it stimulates the epithelial cells which results in the formation of new epithelium and a rapid epidermization over the raw area.

As a rule, all patients should receive a dose of morphine (gr. one-sixteenth to one-fourth) one hour before operation. This allays any restlessness or nervousness that may be present and takes the edge off of the slight pain the patient may experience during the operation. It also lessens psychic shock and prevents toxic effects in patients with an idiosyncrasy for cocain.

Patients who are very nervous or excited should receive a preliminary dose of morphine and hyoscin hydrobromate sufficient to produce drowsiness, thus effectually preventing pyschic shock. Psychic shock alone has been known to cause death before operation as well as during convalescence. Bodine and Gilday have obtained excellent results in treating morphine poisoning with large doses of cocain and vice versa.

The addition of hyoscine to the preliminary dose of morphine also makes possible the completion of operations under local anesthesia that have heretofore been regarded as only suitable for mixed or general anesthesia, as large umbilical and ventral herniae and selected cases of acute appendicitis.

Mixed anesthesia. By combining local with general anesthesia less of the general anesthetic is required, the period under general narcosis is greatly shortened and the liability to post-operative complications is reduced to a minimum. The shock of major amputations is avoided by the cocainization of large nerve trunks previous to their division, as first suggested by Crile.

The intraspinal use of cocain or tropococain has not been considered because its field is constantly narrowing as the technic of local anesthesia is perfected.

There are ten per cent failures to obtain anesthesia in the hands of experts. The after effects are more frequent and serious than following general narcosis and the mortality is higher. Gabbett reports a case in which he injected Novococain .1 gm. and strychnine .001 gm. between the eleventh and twelfth dorsal vertebra. Death followed in one-half hour with tonic spasm of arms and chest. Gabbett believes death was due to strychnine poisoning.

This is the technic recommended by Jonnesco, the addition of strychnine to prevent poisoning from the anesthetic.

Local anesthesia can be employed in any part of the body where the nerve supply can be controlled. With a proper selection of cases the majority of surgical operations can be performed under local anesthesia.

Hernia. All forms of hernia can be operated on under local anesthesia, while the radical cure of inguinal hernia is the most successful major operation in the entire field of local analgesia, "the triumph of cocain" (Reclus.)

In inguinal hernia a general anesthetic is never indicated, and in strangulation the lowered vitality and shock make cocain a

necessity to eliminate the additional shock of general narcosis; besides it allows ample time to ascertain the viability of the gut, and if resection is necessary the radical operation can be performed. Whereas under general anesthesia it is often only possible to establish a fistula at the first operation, and do an anastomosis at a subsequent period.

The first herniotomy by the neuro-regional method was performed by Cushing.

The technic preferred is Bodine's modification of the Halsted operation, as recently described in detail and illustrated with forty-seven stereograms in Dr. H. A. Kelley's Stereo-Clinic.

With a one-fifth per cent solution inject the line of incision over the most prominent part of the hernia (3-5 inches) parallel with and about one-half inch internal to Poupart's ligament and extending higher than is usual with general anesthesia, at least two inches above the site of the internal ring and extending well down on the scrotum below the external ring. Be careful not to make the incision too far from Poupart's ligament or difficulty will be experienced in getting sufficient retraction to place the deep sutures, because strong retraction here will cause the patient pain.

The painful areas in this operation are the skin, nerve trunks and parietal peritoneum.

The subcutaneous tissues are infiltrated and the incision carried down to the deep fascia at the upper angle of the wound. The fascia is injected, caught up with thumb forceps and carefully incised. The Ilio-inguinal nerve is found lying immediately beneath the external oblique aponeurosis, or upon the internal oblique muscle. The nerve is infiltrated with a one-fifth per cent solution until it turns white. The ilio-hypogastric is found above the ilio-inguinal and is also injected. If the ilio-hypogastric is not readily found time should not be spent in searching for it, as the ilio-inguinal supplies nine-tenths of the sensation in this area. The higher up the nerve trunks are infiltrated the more thorough will be the anesthesia of the operative field. These nerves occasionally divide higher than the line of incision, so it is always advisable to inject all small nerves that can be found, provided the two large trunks are not readily recognized or the ilio-inguinal is of small size.

The incision is now completed through the subcutaneous tissues down to the external ring.

Two or three veins will be encountered at the lower angle of the wound, and occasionally the superficial epigastric artery will be divided.

The vessels should be exposed and clamped simultaneously on either side by operator and assistant before cutting. This gives one twinge of pain where otherwise three would be felt. No ligatures should ordinarily be used, but the bleeding controlled by twisting the vessel before the clamp is removed. Cocain one-tenth per cent is now infiltrated around the margin of the external ring and into the tissues over the sac in the line of the incision. No more cocain is required until the sac is ligated. The nerve trunks should never be cut, but dissected free and retracted to the inner side of the wound. The preservation of the nerves lessens recurrence and prevents a subsequent relaxation of the scrotum.

The patient is told to cough, the sac located, picked up with thumb forceps and freed by sharp dissection with scissors. Sharp dissection is painless, but blunt dissection with scissors or gauze pads will cause considerable discomfort and some pain. Painful swabbing of the wound should be avoided and the instruments handled quietly. The clicking of the scissors may be prevented by placing a piece of rubber tubing on one shank. Care must be

exercised in separating the sac from the cord not to cut the vas deferens. If it is accidentally divided the ends may be reunited by slipping them over a piece of plain catgut and uniting with a suture on either side, as suggested by Chetwood. The sac is dissected free up to the neck, then opened and the contents returned to the abdominal cavity. If there is a large amount of omentum present a portion of it may be ligated and excised, but as this causes a certain degree of shock it should only be done in selected cases. Cocain one-tenth per cent is injected beyond the neck of the sac before it is ligated and excised.

If the appendix is in the sac it should be removed, being careful not to make traction on its mesentery.

It is not necessary to transplant the cord except in very large or recurrent hernia, although Bodine has shown that transplantation does not add to the difficulty of the operation.

Suture the conjoined tendons and internal oblique to Poupart's ligament. Then the upper edge of the aponeurosis of external oblique is sutured to Poupart's ligament beneath the lower edge of the aponeurosis.

The overlying edge can be sutured or left free. The sutures must not be tied too tightly lest they cut out from constriction, nor placed too close together, and should be of medium size, preferably of medium kangaroo tendon or No. 2 chromic catgut. It is important to carefully exclude nerve fibres in suturing because of the liability of producing a neuritis that may persist until the suture is absorbed.

Use a small gutta percha wick drain in the subcutaneous tissues for forty-eight hours where there is much fat and in large herniae.

During the entire operation the fingers of the operator or assistant should not touch the wound—the tissues and pads are handled with thumb forceps. This lessens the chance of infection.

Recurrent herniae and those that have been subjected to the injection treatment are much more difficult to dissect out and in these cases it is necessary to prolong the incision higher than that of the previous operation so as to find the nerve trunks above the scar tissue.

In femoral herniae the nerve supply is controlled by injecting the inguinal branch of the ilio-inguinal and the genital branch of the genito-crural above the field of operation.

With umbilical herniae the Mayo operation can be satisfactorily performed by simple infiltration, this is also sufficient for ventral herniae. The addition of hyosin to the preliminary dose of morphine relaxes the abdominal muscles and facilitates the reduction of the contents of the sac in large umbilical and ventral herniae.

An early cathartic with an intestinal and urinary antiseptic administered while the patient is confined to his bed will prevent intestinal and bladder disturbances.

Bodine has operated on 1,114 cases of herniae without infection and less recurrences than when he was employing general anesthesia.

Laparotomy. Infiltration anesthesia is sufficient for the abdominal incision. Care must be exercised that traction is not made on the parietal peritoneum or mesentery. Breaking up adhesions will usually cause some pain. The abdominal operations most frequently performed under local anesthesia are appendectomy, cholecystotomy, exploratory for typhoid perforation and intestinal obstruction, supra-pubic cystotomy and drainage in peritonitis. Other operations that have been completed under cocain are gastrotomy, resection of pylorus and intestine, gastroenterostomy, colostomy, ventro-suspension and fixation of the uterus, salpingo-oophrectomy, shortening

the round ligaments and removal of ovarian cysts.

Cushing, in a personal communication, says that he was the first to perform laparotomy under cocain anesthesia for typhoid perforation, Sept. 13, 1899. He states that exploratory laparotomy with cocain does not increase the danger to life nor add to the shock already present and is without effect on the temperature, pulse and respiration.

Appendicitis. Interval cases with history of mild attacks in a patient with a thin abdominal wall can be operated on under local anesthesia. Acute cases should have general anesthesia unless contraindicated.

Bodine believes the best method for acute cases is cocain plus a few whiffs of general anesthesia, preferably nitrous oxide gas, for freeing and treating the appendix.

Operations on the skull. Trephining, mastoidectomy, exploratory craniectomy and removal of depressed fractures can be performed under cocain. The sensation of pain is confined to the skin and periosteum, while the bone, dura and brain substance are insensitive.

Ligation of arteries. All the arteries of the extremities and neck can be ligated under local anesthesia.

Thyroidectomy. The collar incision should be used, simple infiltration is all that is necessary, although Mitchell suggests blocking the cervical nerves at the side of the neck behind the sterno-mastoid to eliminate the dragging pain caused by the delivery of the gland.

Wyeth and Kocher recommend cocain for all goitres unless strongly contraindicated. Dunhill states that operations on the thyroid are without danger if performed under local anesthesia.

Tracheotomy and Laryngotomy. Simple infiltration is sufficient.

The sensitive mucous membrane should be previously cocainized by a spray or as soon as the incision is made, to avoid the reflex irritability caused by the inspiration of cold air.

Cervical Glands and Tumors. Solitary glands and benign tumors can be removed with ease. With tuberculosis or malignant disease the deep glands must also be removed. This requires patience and gentleness in dissecting. Simple infiltration is all that is necessary.

Inguinal Glands. These can usually be removed "en masse" with simple infiltration.

Amputation of the Breast. Simple amputation is best performed with massive infiltration anesthesia. Cocain is contraindicated in malignancy where the axillary glands are to be removed.

Benign Tumors. These can be removed either with simple or massive infiltration.

Operations on the Extremities. It is unnecessary to use a tourniquet if the weak solutions are employed and adrenalin added to prolong the analgesia. Nerve blocking was first employed by Crile in 1897, and independently suggested by Matas early in 1898 while unaware of its prior use by Crile. Matas advocates nerve blocking at a distance for all extensive operations on the extremities, although the infiltration method is sufficient in thin subjects. For operations on the forearm, wrist and hand, the median, musculo-spiral and ulnar nerves can be blocked at the elbow. For the shoulder and arm, block the brachial plexus in the supraclavicular fossa. In the lower extremity block the sciatic and long saphenous nerve below the knee; above the knee block the sciatic, external cutaneous and anterior crural nerves.

Young was the first to cocainize the external cutaneous to obtain skin grafts from the antero-external surface of the thigh.

All amputations can be performed under local anesthesia. Cocainization at a distance from the operative field should be employed whenever possible in preference to infiltration at the site of operation, the cutting and handling of tissues tends to diffuse the cocain solution and hasten the return of sensation.

Dislocations can be reduced and fractures reduced and wired by previously controlling the nerve supply.

Diseased bone can usually be removed without difficulty if the nerve trunks and periosteum are thoroughly cocainized.

Arterial and vein anesthesia will probably be the most satisfactory of all methods for amputations.

In dislocations, fractures and amputations of the fingers and toes simple infiltration, either on both sides or around the base of the digit is sufficient for complete anesthesia.

Abscess. Braun and Hackenbruch recommend infiltrating a ring around the abscess, keeping outside of the inflamed area, then inject the subcutaneous tissues before incising.

Fractured Patella. Simple infiltration is ample to allow an approximation of the bony surfaces and suture of the capsule and periosteum.

Varicose Veins. Small varices can be easily removed under local anesthesia, but cocain is not usually to be recommended where the entire external and internal saphenous veins are to be removed.

Perineorrhaphy. The Hegar operation can be performed without difficulty by infiltrating around the triangular area to be denuded.

After this is removed the deeper tissues are injected and the levator ani exposed on either side and sutured in the usual manner.

Edema of the vulva may follow if an excessive amount of the solution is injected. All the classical operations on the vulva, vagina, perineum, cervix, uterus and opening the cul-de-sac for pelvic suppuration have been accomplished under local anesthesia.

Hemorrhoids and Fistulae. Local anesthesia is sufficient for all cases but it requires a very thorough infiltration to anesthetize all the nerves supplying this region.

The hyoscin-morphine preliminary treatment, as suggested by Tuttle, is especially useful in these cases to prevent post-operative pain.

Give hyoscin hydrobromate gr. one hundredth three hours before the operation and repeat the same dose of hyoscin combined with morphine sulphate gr. one-sixth-one-fourth on e hour before operating. When the morphine is given with both doses of the hyoscin untoward symptoms as- syanosis with slow, shallow breathing have been frequently observed, but do not occur when only one dose of morphine is administered.

The most satisfactory infiltration technic is that suggested by Reclus: A small pledget of cotton is saturated with a weak cocain solution and the patient requested to strain, the pledget is now introduced into the anus and the contraction of the sphincter as the patient relaxes draws the tampon up inside the sphincteric ring. This procedure is repeated with pledgets of increasing size until the sphincter is partially relaxed and the mucosa completely anesthetized.

The needle is now introduced into the anesthetized mucosa and the skin around the margin of the anus infiltrated.

After cocainizing the muco-cutaneous margin, the index finger of the left hand is introduced into the rectum to guide the needle while cocainizing the sphincter, this step is painless if the needle is introduced at a right angle to the skin surface. Six punctures are made at equidistant points around the circumference of the sphincter and each time about one-half dram of the solution is injected into the sphincter and surrounding tissues. The sphincter can now be painlessly and completely relaxed in a few minutes by digital dilatation.

Urethotomy. A one-fifth to one-half per cent solution is strong enough to anesthetize the urethra. Adrenalin may be added to prolong the analgesia.

Circumcision. Retract the foreskin and anesthetize the inner surface of the prepuce by local application of a one-fifth per cent solution. Inject a few drops of a one-tenth per cent solution into the frenum, and encircle penis near the base with a series of small wheals, only injecting the skin. The skin beyond the ring of infiltration will be completely anesthetized in five to ten minutes.

The advantages of this technic are: it permits an accurate approximation of the edges of the wound, the healing is more prompt, there is no edema and less scar tissue after healing.

Hydrocele. Infiltrate at the point trocar is to be inserted. If the injection method is used a small quantity of one-half per cent can be injected previous to the carbolic acid. If the radical operation, simple infiltration can be used or the inguinal branch of the ilio-inguinal can be blocked through the high incision.

Varicocele. The high operation is to be preferred. After the skin is injected the subcutaneous tissues are freely infiltrated before incising. It is not necessary to look for the nerve trunks, although it is important not to cut them or a relaxation of the scrotum may follow the operation. A small amount of cocain is injected above the upper ligature before tying. It should always be tied and cut before the lower, so as to give only one twinge of pain.

Operation on the Testes, Epididymis and Vas. If the high incision at the upper part of the scrotum just below the external ring, is used, it is only necessary to block the inguinal branch of the ilio-inguinal; at the lower part of the scrtum the genital branch of the genito-crural will be encountered.

Bibliography.

1. Crile: Transactions Ohio Medical Society, 1897.
2. Legrand: L'anesthesie Locale, These de Paris, 1899.
3. Cushing: Annals Surgery, Jan., 1900.
4. Matas: Phila. Medical Journal, Nov. 3, 1900.
5. Bodine: N. Y. Medical Record, April, 1905.
6. Reclus: L'anesthesie Localisee par La Cocaine, Paris, 1903.
7. Bodine: Annals Surgery, July, 1907.
8. Mitchell: J. A. M. A., July 20, 1907.
9. Barker: J. R. A. M. C., Aug., 1907.
10. Horsley: Southern Medical Journal, July, 1908.
11. Mitchell: J. A. M. A., Nov. 7, 1908.
12. Bodine: N. Y. Polyclinic Journal, Febr., 1909.
13. Thibault: Jour. Ark. Med. Soc., Sept., 1907.
14. Watson: J. A. M. A., July 31, 1909.
15. Ransohoff: Lancet-Clinic, Aug. 7, 1909.
16. Watson: Okla. Medical News Journal, Aug., 1909.
17. Braun: Die Lokalanesthesie, Leipzic, 1907.
18. Bier: Archiv fur Klinische Chirurgie, Berlin, LXXXVIII, No. 4.
19. Bodine's Operation for Inguinal Hernia: Stereo-Clinic, 1909.
20. Goyanes: Revista Medica, Madrid, Jan., 1909.
21. Bier: Berliner Klinische Wochenschrift, Mar. 15, 1909.
22. Lennander: Keen's Surgery, 1909.
23. Oppel: Munchener Medizinische Wochenschrift, Aug. 31, 1909.
24. Goyanes: El Siglio Medico, Madrid, Oct. 2, 9, 16, 1909.
25. Samuell: Texas State Journal of Medicine, Oct., 1909.
26. Hertzler, Brewster and Rogers: J. A. M. A., Oct. 23, 1909.
27. Watson: Texas State Journal of Medicine, Dec., 1909.
28. Freeman: Denver Med. Times anl Utah Med. Jour., Jan., 1910.
29. Gabbett: Indian Medical Gazette, Calcutta, Febr., 1910.
30. Ransohoff: Annals Surgery, April, 1910.
31. Wyeth's Surgery.
32. Hartel: Wiener Medizinische Wochenschrift, No. 35, 1909.
33. Schley: N. Y. Medical Record, Febr. 5, 1910.

EDITORIAL

THE PROPHYLAXIS OF TYPHOID.

Constantly recurring cases of typhoid fever in one locality following an initial attack would seem to indicate that too little attention is being paid to the prevention of this disease by proper precautionary measures.

There is now traceable to one case in Muskogee County ten others, with the possibility of others not yet developed. Of the eleven cases one died with the further possibility of more deaths. There were four children and seven adults in the list.

A diagnosis of malarial fever was made in two of the cases and stubbornly held to despite all evidences to the contrary.

This condition only emphasizes the absolute necessity of the health authorities taking uniform action in the presence of this infection for the assistance in the diagnosis in doubtful cases and uniformity in the prophylactic features as well.

Some system should be developed by which every case of typhoid should be investigated by the health authorities as to cause, destruction of cause and prevention of its spread by proper isolation.

A simple direction as to destruction of excreta, care of the patient and his surroundings and safeguarding of the water and food supply should be in the hands of every family where the disease prevails and energetic steps taken demanding the enforcement of such regulations.

There is no good reason for Oklahoma becoming a typhoid center when the carelessness and ignorance of the attending physician and family are eliminated.

Fire and crude carbolic acid will do a great deal.

DOCTOR McCORMACK COMING TO OKLAHOMA.

The news that Dr. McCormack is coming to Oklahoma for the month of October will be gratifying to those of the profession interested in organization work and in having the laity have a better understanding of the relations that exist between the physician and the public.

Dr. McCormack and his work need no introduction or word of commendation to those who are familiar with the man and his accomplishments.

For this trip a regular itinerary will be arranged and from this plan there will be no deviation, as the organization department of the American Medical Association understand from wide experience the steps to be taken and the futility of attempting a tour of the state without first having a full understanding as to dates and places of appearance.

Necessarily he will be able to visit only the larger centers.

The plan generally followed is to have an afternoon meeting of the medical society and in the evening a meeting for the profession and the public. For this purpose it will be necessary to appoint a committee on arrangements for the purpose of advertising the time and place to all concerned.

THE ASSOCIATION OF STATE SECRETARIES AND EDITORS.

One of the useful wheels and inner workings of the American Medical Association is the above body whose object is to devise plans for aiding organization work and improving the various medical journals now in operation by state societies.

This body met in tS .Louis at the annual meeting and much interesting work was accomplished. Perhaps the most considered phase before the meeting was the plan in operation in some states for Physicians Mutual Defense. The concensus of opinion and the statements made by those who know was that this work is the most valuable being done by state societies and it is practical and more economical than any one not familiar with the subject would believe. It was here brought out that Pennsylvania met all damage suits against its members during the past year for the sum of ten cents per capita. This statement seems incredible until one hears it from the man who has charge of the matter; other states get their protection from malpractice suits for the sum of twenty-five cents per capita and near that figure.

Oklahoma physicians should certainly organize in this manner and thus secure legal aid at a nominal figure.

Another feature of the work is the closer attention that association will enable the editors to give to medical advertising. Many of them start in new at the work and cannot have adequate ideas of just what houses should have access to their columns and unwittingly allow space to unworthy causes.

It is to be hoped that this organization shall be perpetuated and meet annually with the parent body.

BOOKS RECEIVED

THE PRACTICAL MEDICINE

SERIES, comprising ten volumes.

Volumes One, Two and Three.

Volume I. By Frank Billings, A. M., Head of the Medical Department and Dean of Rush Medical College, Chicago, and J. H. Salisbury, A. M., M. D., Professor of Medicine, Chicago Clinical School.

Volume II. By John B. Murphy, A. M., M. D., L. L. D., Professor of Surgery in the Northwestern University, Attending Surgeon and Chief of Staff of Mercy Hospital, St. Joseph's Hospital, Wesley Hospital, St. Joseph's Hospital and Columbus Hospital, Consulting Surgeon to Cook County Hospital and Alexian Brothers Hospital, Chicago.

Volume III. By Casey A. Wood, C M., M. D., D. C. L. Consulting Opthalmologist to Cook County Hospital; Attending Ophalmic Surgeon St. Lukes Hospital. Chicago, and,

Albert H. Andrews, M. D., Professor of Otology, Rhinology and Laryngology, Chicago Eye, Ear, Nose and Throat College; Occulist and Aurist to the Chicago, Rock Island and Pacific Railway; etc., and,

Gustavus P. Head, M. D., Professor of Otology, Laryngology and Rhinology, Chicago Post Graduate Medical School. Chicago, Ill.

1910 THE YEAR BOOK PUBLISHING COMPANY, CHICAGO, ILL.

While primarily intended for the use of the general practitioner who will find these works of great value, the volumes are so classified by subjects that they will be found of use by the specialist.

The subject of the work is to place before the profession the advances in medicine and surgery and allied lines and in doing this much is eliminated from the usual text book style.

The physician wishing to have the latest information and deductions on questions before the profession today should be the possessor of this work. The entire he retails at $10.00, but may be purchased at a slight advance over this price by the single volume by those wishing special volumes.

"LANE'S CONCEPTION OF CHRONIC CONSTIPATION AND ITS MANAGEMENT."

BY A. B. COOKE, M. D., NASHVILLE, TENN.

In his monograph entitled "The Operative Treatment of Chronic Constipation." Mr. Lane first defines the scope of the treaties by stating that the term, chronic constipation, as he employs it includes all those conditions which are the consequences of the accumulation of material in the intestinal tract for a period sufficiently in excess of the normal to produce on the one hand alteration in the gastro-intestinal tract and in other viscera, and on the other hand toxic changes from absorption.' The fact is emphasized that while constipation is usually marked by infrequent hard stools, there may be a daily evacuation, and inexceptional cases the motions are loose and frequent.

Abstract from the Transactions of American Proctologic Society, St. Louis, Mo., June 6 and 7, 1910.

The two chief pathologic factors in the production of chronic constipation, according to the author, are enteroptosis and acquired mesenteries or adhesions, the latter resulting not from inflammation, but being developed to opose the displacement of viscera, the tendency to which exists whenever the erect posture of the trunk is assumed. The displacement and fixation of the several portions of the colon in faulty positions result primarily in defective drainage, and secondarily in auto-intoxication and pathologic changes both in the gut itself and in the other abdominal viscera.

After describing these changes in detail, the author proceeds to discuss their immediate and remote effects, advancing the idea that in many cases diseases of the appendix, gall-bladder, stomach, duodenum, pancreas, kidney, ovaries, etc., must be regarded as sequellae of chronic constipation. In addition the phenomena resulting from toxic absorption are graphically described and the importance of their recognition stressed.

With reference to treatment Lane states that 'in no circumstances should operative interference be contemplated till the surgeon has satisfied himself that every means of treatment has failed, whether medical or mechanical.' The surgery indicted depends upon the conditions present. In mild cases in which non-operative measures have failed, division of the adhesions and constricting bands may be effective. Severer cases call for more radical surgery consisting either in dividing the ileum and anastomosing it with the sigmoid or upper rectum,

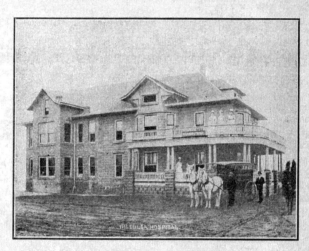

thus short-circuiting the fecal current, or, when pain is a prominent factor in the case, removal of the colon in addition.

The writer of the paper, after personal observation of Lane's work, regards his conception of the nature and management of the malady with much favor and thinks it entitled to serious consideration at the hands of the profession.

PERSONAL

Dr. J. L. Blakemore, Muskogee, is taking an extended trip to Colorado. A novel feature of this trip is that it is not by Pullman and summer hotel, but by wagon, tent and all the glories of tent life, which includes the bugs, dirt and heat.

Dr. I. B. Oldham of Muskogee will spend the summer months visiting in Minnesota where he has a summer home, and incidentally taking in the Mayo clinics.

Dr. A. L. Blesh was operated upon for appendicitis July 20th and rapidly recovered from the effects of the operation. Dr. Blesh sails for Europe August 20th.

Dr. E. S. Ferguson of Oklahoma City has returned after a six months trip to the clinics of Vienna and Berlin.

Dr. J. A. Ryan, Oklahoma City, is taking an extended trip through Yellowstone Park and the Northwest.

Dr. P. P. Nesbitt, Muskogee, will spend a part of the summer in the Ozarks on White river.

Dr. O. C. Klass, Muskogee, will spend several months in Vienna during this summer and fall.

Dr. A. D. Young, Oklahoma City, is spending the summer in the East and New York City.

Dr. R. H. Wilkin, Oklahoma City, is spending the summer in Colorado.

Dr. H. T. Ballantine, Muskogee has been appointed City Physician.

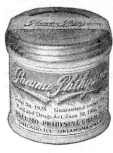

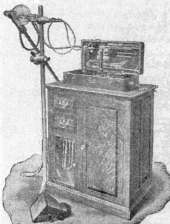

STANDING COMMITTEES OKLAHOMA STATE MEDICAL ASSOCIATION.

Public Policy and Legislation—Dr. David A. Myers, Chairman, Lawton; J. H. Scott, Shawnee; J. A. Hatchett, El Reno; F. S. Clinton, Tulsa; Claude A. Thompson, Muskogee.

On Medical Education—Drs. B. J. Vance, Checotah; A. K. West, Oklahoma City; E. O. Barker, Guthrie.

On Scientific Work—Drs. Floyd E. Waterfield, Holdenville; P. A. Smithe, Enid; Claude A. Thompson, Muskogee.

On Necrology—Drs. C. S. Bobo, Norman; H. M. Williams, Wellston; M. A. Warhurst, Remus.

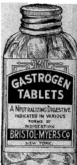

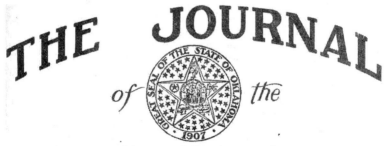

THE JOURNAL of the

Oklahoma State Medical Association.

VOL. IV.   MUSKOGEE, OKLAHOMA, SEPTEMBER, 1910.   NO 4

DR. CLAUDE A. THOMPSON, Editor-in-Chief.

ASSOCIATE EDITORS AND COUNCILLORS.

DR. J. A. WALKER, Shawnee.
DR. CHARLES R. HUME, Anadarko.
DR. F. R. SUTTON, Bartlesville.
DR. I. W. ROBERTSON, Dustin.
DR. J. S. FULTON, Atoka.

DR. JOHN W. DUKE, Guthrie.
DR. A. B. FAIR, Frederick.
DR. W. G. BLAKE, Tahlequah.
DR. H. P. WILSON, Wynnewood.
DR. J. H. BARNES, Enid.

Entered at the Postoffice at Muskogee, Oklahoma, as second class mail matter, June, 1909.

This is the Official Journal of the Oklahoma State Medical Association All communications should be addressed to the Journal of the Oklahoma State Medical Association, English Block, Muskogee, Oklahoma.

DIAGNOSIS AND TREATMENT OF DIABETES.

BY HARRY E. BREESE, M. D., HENRYETTA, OKLA.

Diabetes ranks with rheumatism as being the least understood diseases, yet when we compare Tyson's Practice of 1899 with this paper on diabetes at the American Medical Association of 1907, we can note that many clinical experiences and laboratory tests have proved an encouragement. He deserves no more credit than numerous other writers to whom I am indebted.

If I were able to do the title of this paper justice, it would be an imposition on your time. Each paragraph must answer for a long chapter on its respective topic.

There is great confusion in the minds of many on the symptoms, food values,

"Read Before the Annual Meeting of the Oklahoma State Medical Association, Tulsa, Okla., May, 1910."

different stages, urinalysis, acidosis, childhood and old age forms and prognosis.

It is well known that an excess of sugar in the urine is no proof of a decided diabetes. Glycosuria may be caused by traumatic and non-traumatic neuroses; by Graves disease; gastro-intestinal and hepatic disorders. The spontaneous transitory type may appear after injury, extirpation of important organs, chloroform anesthesia, and after administration of drugs and chemicals like phloridzin, mercuric-bichloride, chloral, morphine, acetanilid, arsenous, salicylic, dilute hydrocyanic and sulphuric acids, excessive use of tobacco, thyroid and adrenelin preparations and during the luetic process and after infectious diseases, especially typhoid.

Non-diabetic glycosurias are usually the result of intoxications, that are of more or less grown disturbance due to influence coming from without or to such rising from within.

I had a case illustrating these manifestations. Family history gouty and of a rheumatic diathesis. Patient was 25 years old; at sixteen she had inflammatory rheumatism during January and February of 1909 she had the muscular and nervous forms of influenza. The latter simulating typhoid except that the temperature was normal a great deal of the time. This resulting in a severe neurasthenia and a 1 per cent. glycosuria. The rest treatment completely relieved both conditions. Soon after good health and normal weight had been gained, last September, she fell on the arm of a chair and severely contused the perineum and the coccyx, resulting in an abscess in the perineal body; while planning to leave home for an operation, the abscess ruptured into the vagina and made a spontaneous recovery, except the glycosuria which lasted after all soreness was gone. Patient developed an abnormal appetite for sweets and meats eating both to the appetite's satisfaction, and at the same time losing weight and strength. I was consulted for swollen lips. Urine examination showed less than 2 per cent. of glucose. A strict proteid diet was directed with cream and wine. At the end of two weeks urine test gave less than one-half per cent. The next week oat meal was allowed; at the end of which the test was negative. Potatoes fried were added, followed gradually by anything she wanted, except sweets with no bad results. And the last month she has used loaf sugar in tea and coffee, and on fruits with no signs of glycosuria.

This illustrates that some transitory glycosurias may attain a certain state of chronicity, if the underlying cause persists. True diabetes exists long before sugar excretion, and with rare exceptions it still continues, when for the time being glycosuria has ceased. Perhaps this patient had also a physilogical glycosuria.

Dr. Ripperger (*New York Med. Jour.* 7-13-'07,) states that this may be true quite constantly in healthy persons, but only in a slight degree rarely exceeding 0.05 per cent. sugar. Also that an alimentary glycosuria may become a true diabetes.

Two deleterious manifestations are known in glycosuria, the loss of sugar and through the hyperglycemia always associated with it. So long as the diabetic excretes sugar above normal so long will there be a hyperglycemia. And what causes this, I refer you to Dr. Harper's paper in our State Journal of January, 1910.

Suffice it to say that there seems to be cases of a functional inactivity that can be repaired or a neuroses needing care for a relief. Therefore, the aim should be to study each case separately. The scientific justification of the dietetic treatment may be said to be established without a doubt.

We must look for further results than urine examination. A cessation of glucose in the urine is no proof of a cure. Cases are reported with patients gaining weight, especially the disposed corpulent and yet the metabalic processes were destructive. This teaches us that it is absolutely necessary at the start, to study the systemic conditions of which the glycosuria alone is capable of but little harm.

Then how shall we begin? The laboratory students would have us not differ in kind; but in degree the different forms.

The clinician classifies his into several different forms. In the mildest it is a contusion, a drug, an anesthesia, or a neurasthenia, with the patient gradually improving in strength and perhaps weight, and the excretions also improving. Then, for such cases, we do not diet or medicate for diabetes.

A further advanced degree is a cessation of glucose after a gradual reduction of corbohydrates to a proteid diet for a few days. And upon a gradual, resumption of the carbohydrates, a tolerance may be noted. Some cases may take quite a lot of carbohydrates in small allowances at a time, but they cannot take a full meal at a time safely. It is easy to prescribe a Von Ncordon diet list in these cases, but it is not justifiable.

A popular method for determining the mild from the medium is to give the test meal. This may have two portions; carbohydrate-free composed of meats, eggs, meat soups, cheese, cream, spinach, asparagus, tea, coffee, saccharine and burgandy or claret wine. The other portion four ounces common wheat bread, a part of the bread for the morning and the remainder for the afternoon. If no sugar is found after being on this small allowance of bread, we may know that the case is mild. If sweets are allowed three days with this same diet and the test finds glucose, we will know to eliminate candies, preserves, etc. It may be possible that sugar could be allowed in tea or coffee. This could be called a medium form.

If sugar persists with said small amount of bread and nitrogen appears in the urine, the food albumin must be reduced, this would be called a case of medium severlty.

If the proteids have to be reduced too low for the required caloric value for sustenance and ten grains of nitrogen is found in the 24 hours urine, we are then dealing with a case of severe diabetes. Fortunately, these cases are very rare, but the mild cases can be transformed into the severe by injudicious living and diet.

The diabetic is robbed in a nutritive way, because of the great loss of sugar, a valuable heat and energy producing material. And he compensates for this by

destruction of body tissue. In the severe grades there exists a breaking down of body albumin, forming collaterally organic toxins of a poisonous nature that disturb the cell protoplasm. A diminution of the body fat is the result on a diet restriction, which may be desirable in the obese.

Proteids are the only foods that are reliable for repairing and building tissue and at the same time produce heat. Fat is a condensed form of energy and has twice the caloric value of proteids; besides it has the advantage of not being avoidable as a sugar source, as proteids are, and it cannot add to the hyperglycemia or glycosuria in any statge or form of diabetes.

It would seem from these two that we have a carbohydrate substitute. But a multitude of difficulties arise. Fats are hard to digest and not palatable and are poor absorbers. Proteids may over stimulate the nitrogenous metabolism and produce acetone. B-oxybutyric and other acids and toxins.

All patients can take some form of the carbohydrates with proteids, fats and alcohol, the latter, at least one to two ounces per day, placing the patient on a restricted diet two or three times a year for two to three weeks at a time; provided the sugar is in excess and in order to give the metabolic process a rest. But cases are reported that too much restriction has caused a lack of tolerance for the carbohydrates after a return to them. And coma has been occasioned by a sudden restriction. It then becomes apparent that too close a restriction will avail nothing. The weight of authority is opposed to a too rigid diet in all forms of diabetes for reasons already stated.

Diabetes should, therefore have some form of carbohydrates, but how much is the great question. If sugar is excluded, the organism is compelled to form the catabolism of fats and albumins. And a certain proportion of carbohydrates is required for the body nutrition. ·

Many patients may not feel very sick nor lose in weight till consultation establishes a too strict routine diet that slowly but unceasingly robs them of the reserve vitality they may possess.

The only real symptoms of the disease are emaciation and weakness, other symptoms are secondary to sugar in the blood, or conditions occasioned by the necessity for ·its elimination. The glycocaemia effects are neuritis, cataract, perforating ulcer and retinitis, and by excretory symptoms we have polyuria and thirst. Sometimes the saccharated blood sems to be a good culturia media for the microorganisms of boils, gangrene and tuberculosis. All diabetics should have their chest examined and phthisis cases their urine for glucose two or three times a year.

Henry L. Shively (*N. Y. Med. Jour. May* 6-'08), gave an excellent article on these phthisis complications. It is only the grave cases that are unable to utilize sugar at all. Therefore, it is wrong to draw a diet list of permissibles and non-permissibles, prior to our having determined his assimilative power.

We are to determine, whether the patient may have more or less bread daily allowing so much; say four ounces a day for three days and testing for glucose, and so on till the right amount has been established, testing for only one food at a time, but at the same time allowing the use of the foods already tested. If the bread cannot be used sufficiently to satisfy the craving for butter spreads, etc., then it's time to use the "Gluten flour," which is the flour that has been washed to rid it of starch to a lower per cent. White flour is from fifty to eighty per cent. starch. And the so-called gluten flour three to forty per cent. and

some unreliable at that. The best of them may vary from time to time.

Herriman Barker, Sommerville, Mass., is reported to make a reliable gluten flour of three grades 2, 6 and 10 per cent, starch with each labeled. Also Steward, Collard and Watt, of London, who have a branch house in New York, made a casoid flour.

A few years ago potatoes were not allowed. It is now known, that they may help to mitigate and not instigate trouble, especially if fried as that method of cooking deprives them of more starch. It is true that some individuals have a tolerance for certain starches and rebel against other foods containing them.

Especially described by Victor C. Vaughan, (*N. Y. Med. Jour.* 2-26-1910.) 'Amongst other things he says. "In many persons the capacity for assimilating carbohydrates is largely determined by the time of day when the food is taken. Glycosurics who cannot metabolize carbohydrates when taken for breakfast may dispose of 100 grains of bread when taken at six o'clock dinner."

The literature universally finds no bad effects from the use of soccharine unless used in excess causing gastric irritation. Drug treatment is more easily carried out than is the dietary. The majority take medicinal advice, but sooner or later become arbitrarily stubborn against the dietary.

When this occurs, make urine examination more frequently, bringing the patient in closer touch and perhaps a discovery that the diet may be changed, which keeps up the encouragement of both the advised and advisor. However, frequent consultations in some way is the only means to keep the patient faithful by criticising excess in eating, in exercise, in rest and in mental endeavor and worry. I must repeat: What is excess to one is not to another.

Opium has been found more reliable than its alkoloids, beginning on one-fourth grain t. i. d. and it has been increased to twelve grains a day. But when possible to control the sugar by diet avoid all use of opium as the dose has to be too large and when necessary to stop, the patient may rapidly decline.

Medical Records (May 23-1905) Translated, German writer who claimed that 88 per cent. of the cases taking 35 grains or over, of loaf sugar daily did not decrease or increase the glucose in the urine while the general condition of the patient was improved. The sugar was given in water or coffee; the rule being no sugar without exercise and no exercise without sugar.

J. Rudisch (*Jour. A. M. A., Oct. 2-1909*,) reports two and one-half years experiments with atropine and proved a reduction in the amount of sugar excreted and an increase of carbohydrate tolerance in cases unselected. The methylbromide has the advantage of being less toxic. The initial dose of the methylromide of atropine for adults was 2-15 gr. t. i. d. increased to 8-15 gr. t. i. d. The sulphate he used 1-60th gr. gradually increased to 1-20 gr. t. i. d. Appearance of toxic symptoms marked dryness of throat. The atropine was either stopped or the attempt to increase the dose temporarily abandoned.

Medicines, like solol, aspirin, salipyrin and autipyrin perhaps are efficatious only when the glycosuria belongs to a gouty or rheumatic diathesis. They should not be used in cases complicated with albuminuria. Unfortunately these symptoms antagonize each other with reference to diet. A methodic use of glycogen beginning on 15 grains a day has been found to eliminate these conflicting symptoms.

Dr. S. G. Soules of Quebec (*N. Y. Med. Journal, Nov.* 16, 1907) wanted to go on record curing a doctor 62 years of age with fluid extract of chimaphelia two dram doses with milk at each meal. He gives arsenic some credit and got good results from the use saw palmetto, and grindelia robusta.

We note that this case was of eight years standing, that he also dieted, that he used diuretics, and diaphoretics and tonics, the very same thing we often do in men of that age whether there is diabetes or not.

In my opinion this happened, as it were, a selected case. And it only proves that if we are fortunate enough to know the case, especially if over 45 years of age, we can be optimistic and that we can help the middle life as easily in proportion to the nature of the disease for the different ages, its being rather discouraging before puberty. Yet we note reports of cures from the use of proprietory medicine, but I am inclined to believe that said reports, if true, are those of alimentary glycosuria. This is an age of tremendous sugar consumption, and often times the glands become tired and need a rest.

In the severe cases, we must look out for coma; constantly keeping in mind at each consultation the probability of a B-oxybutyric acid and its allies. If a few drops of perchloride of iron solution turn the urine a dark port wine color, then the patient is always in danger of coma. Then the carbohydrates are gradually reduced and one-half to two ounces of bicarbonate of soda given daily. In this way a sugar free diet may be reached, or the patient may weaken and keep on losing weight and coma threaten. For the latter mix the diet. Abandon the rigid proteid diet allowing not over 500 grains per day. Give plenty of olive oil, animal and fish fats with brandy, whiskey or sour wines to digest the fats, green vgetables, oat meal, fried potatoes, cream, salad with oil, saccharine and gluten bread, etc. Acidulated water to quench the thirst; fresh fruits are allowed, dried fruits never, nuts are good for their oil, chestnuts excepted.

If the perchloride test is negative a more strict diet may be enforced gradually increasing till a tolerance is found what can be assimilated. Remembering that it is not the sugar in the urine that hurts but the cause of its being there. Its being understood that the bowels must be kept as nearly as possible in a state of normal activity. That from time to time bowel antiseptics may be needed.

The latest American as well as Foreign specialists still insist that bicarbonate of soda 3 to 5 per cent. solution, a quart in quantity should be injected into the veins, during a state of coma, if strength regains sufficiently to swallow, he should be given a teaspoonful of sodium bicarbonate every hour and encouraged to drink large quantities of milk and mineral waters.

DISEASES OF THE RESPIRATORY TRACT.

BY WINNIE M. SANGER, M. D., OKLAHOMA CITY, OKLA.

Beginning with the nose, the other parts functioning in respiration are the throat, larynx, bronchial tubes, lungs and pleura, the diseases of which, belong to this subject.

Since my colleagues have papers on pneumonia and empyemata we will omit those of the respiratory diseases, from this discussion.

Among all classes, the largest number of deaths the first year, is from gastro-enteric diseases, and in second rank, are the acute respiratory diseases.

This order, aside from the acute infections of diphtheria, scarlet fever, measles and pertussis is noticeable until puberty. Even in Oklahoma of mild climate, in winter, we note in the Vital Statistics, for March, a rate of 37 per cent. of all cases reported, from deaths, of pneumonia, and of tubercular cases, 55 per cent. death from tuberculosis.

Either of these is a higher proportionate rate than of all others combined, at this season of the year in the list given. We can not, then, make too close a study of the causes, lesions, diagnosis and treatment of respiratory diseases.

"Read Before the Annual Meeting of the Oklahoma State Medical Association, Tulsa, Okla., May, 1910.

All our knowledge on the subject, however comprehensive and carefully chosen, requires a retentive and active memory to be of value and effective when needed, so that the papers of a State Medical Program, should besides the new ideas refresh us in details and data, that would require much time to look up in reference books. A long while ago, Marcus Aurelius remarked to us:

"Nothing has such power to broaden the mind as the ability to investigate systematically and truly all that comes under thy observation in life."

The frequency of inflammations of the respiratory tract is due to the tendency of the cells of the mucus membrane to undergo proliferation from slight or unusual irritation, and the habit of irregular innervation, modifies, in children, the many symptoms as manifested in adults.

In America, we are all so prone to "catch a cold," that the English speak of it as "American catarrh."

The predisposition is due to heredity, and environment, also, adds to the chance of infection. Anything causing mouth-breathing, puts in abeyance the nose function of filtering; this in turn makes a new demand upon the protective functions of the lower sections of the respiratory tract.

Some times the etiology of cold is a weakness or loss of tone of the mucus membrane, resulting in increase of mucus from faulty digestion. This has a close relation to our food and nutrition, causing faulty metabolism and deterioration of health. But we will consider only the microbic infection at this time.

Exposures of weather and improper clothing do not increase resistance of tissues.

The Germans tell us of the Process of Abh artung, or hardening, which is to reduce the vaso-motor reaction, of the skin, to sensitiveness of themal changes, which causes a contraction of bloodvessels and a sudden hyperemia of internal organs.

The savage who tosses his new born baby into the cold flowing stream, understood this causative factor of cold, and began his early immunizing processes.

Of the bacterial infections, we should protect the others and prevent further auto-intoxication. The serum treatment for this phase is yet in its infancy for immunization.

The function of the nose giving us the sense of smell is lost in enlarged turbinals and atrophic rhinitis. In infants the first nasal disturbance we treat is coryza, "snuffles," or nasal stenosis, which in mild form lasts a few days, in severe a few weeks, and repeated attacks lead to chronic form. It often causes difficulty in nursing. Though rarely, if ever, fatal, the remote sequels lead us to use care in their prevention; deafness, otalgia, otitis, laryngitis and bronchitis being the common ones.

If this catarrh persists, we suspect syphilis, and treat accordingly.

The rapid proliferation of glandular tissue in children causing glandular activity, and a purulent discharge, later manifests as hypertrophy of tonsils, and adenoid growth. .

Since fever is the commonest symptom for which the laity ask our attention, we remember that diminished alkalinity of the blood is found in fevers and we give a soda.

Knowing that the pneumococcus, streptococcus and staphylococcus albus and aureus, may be found in any nose, we have the mother, or nurse, use the normal salt solution or the modified Dobells, viz: equal part salt, soda and borax, as a spray, for the part must be kept clean, then protected with an oil. When necessary to give further remedies, the rhinitis or coryza tablet is a favorite with all of us. This for the five year old.

I am not at all partial to adrenalin, as so often mentioned in our texts. In proportion of 1-4,000 it reduces the hypertrophy temporarily, but loses its effect after a while. It is not curative. It is in the chronic cases that we should be most concerned, though we do not regard this as the disease, but only one of a variety of pathological conditions.

Excluding syphilis, the nasal and pharyngeal growths or chronic enlargements, should be early removed, and I am not so sure that they should not be removed in syphilis. I feel this, since losing this winter my first baby patient, at eight months old of broncho-pneumonia, which I had under treatment for several months previous for catarrh, both systemic and local, for I knew it was syphilitic. The Iodine of iron, mercury inunction and local sprays seem to accomplish little and I believe of the adenoids and hypertrophied tonsils had been removed, it would have had a better chance than the five days from broncho-pneumonia. This is the youngest of my experience so afflicted.

Neither have I much respect for cod-liver oil as a tonic treatment. For very young children cream, gravies, and sugar supply enough carbo-hydrates. Excess of sweets often cause catarrh

The wooden voice and reflex cough, should not cause us to send the patient to the specialist, as some text books tell us, but to be prepared ourselves with the galvano-cautery, or wire snare to remove the hypertrophied tissue so commonly found in the nasal passage or in the pharynx.

In rhinitis, the possibility of a primary nasal diphtheria, should not escape us, ror a membrane, gray or white, may occlude the nares, and a sero-mucus discharge be present. It is not necessary to wait for a culture to prove the Klebs-Loeffler bacillus, for we give the antitoxin, regardless of the doubt. No harm results from its use, should we be mistaken.

Another disease most common to young infants, is croup or catarrhal spasm of the larynx, coming most often after six months to the third year. Again we learn that adenoids and enlarged tonsils are exciting causes in a majority of cases. The daily remissions, mildness of inflammation and spasmodic character of the dyspnoea teach us to distinguish catarrhal spasm from membranous croup. Give us syrup of ipecac, calcium iodide or apomorphine and we can quickly relieve any spasmodic croup.

Catarrhal laryngitis is much more serious than croup whether it is primary or secondary to infectious diseases. The slight amount of inspiratory dyspnoea, which is constant, the constitutional disturbance, pain or coughing, perhaps suffocation and cyanosis, are prominent symptoms. The cough is dry, hard and severe in the early stage, and inhalation of medicated steam is a favorite method of relief.

The use of cold applications are highly recommended by some on account of the reaction, but I prefer a counter irritation, but not to blistering, of mustard, and hot applications, for heat relaxes to a reaction from cold. As yet, I have not had to use intubation, but I would do so if the dyspnoea increased, and cyanosis and pallor were present.

The same applies to membranous laryngitis, true croup and laryngeal diphtheria, now known to be nearly always due to the Klebs-Loeffler. Sometimes to the Streptococcus.

The membranous inflammation may be assumed if there is severe, constant increasing dyspnoea, with aphonia, and here again we give the antitoxin on the clinical diagnosis.

Calomel fumigation stands first as to remedies aside from antitoxin or intubation, which has almost displaced trachetomy, but this would lead to the discussion of diphtheria, an infectious disease.

Tonsillitis and Pharyngitis, when adenoid vegetations are present, are classed by Holt, as diseases of the digestive system, but since deformities due to lymphatism, interfere with pulmonary expansion, they could well be considered under respiratory conditions.

However, the acute inflammations are easily treated and chronic hypertrophies, should be surgically treated by the family physician, himself.

In lung troubles, we keep in mind that young children breathe at a rate of 35 at birth 27 per minute first year, diminishing by two or three up to twelve years at 20 (Uffelman) and this is increased during waking hours, and the rythm easily disturbed up to 2 years, so that we have "peurile breathing."

The child's bronchial tubes are relatively longer, the air cells smaller and interstitial tissues more abundant and chest walls thinner, because the muscular development of the thoracic framework, is feeble. The air vesicles being small, acute congestion, may interfere with their function as completely as consolidation. Inflammation easily tends to spread to the smaller bronchi. Respiration rapidly increases on account of the child's rapid metabolism.

The large size of liver, and comparitively greater proportion of size of heart to lungs, tell us to be careful in diagnosis of pneumonia, of lower right lobe, or enlarged heart. The percussion note, can not always be depended upon since consolidation spots may be surrounded by healthy lung. An auscultation of a child's healthy lung, gives a low, pitched intense vesiculor sound.

This brings us to the mention of acute catarrhal bronchitis, of which we have all had liberal experiences with children of all ages, as it accompanies influenza' or measles, in almost every family at some time of the year.

A bilateral inflammation of the bronchial mucus membrane of the larger tubes, the trachea often affected at sometime. If this extends beyond the smaller tubes, we have capillary bronchitis. All stages show congestion, hyperplasia, and exudation of mucus, pus cells, the walls of the large tubes showing infiltration, with leucocytes.

Expectoration in younger children is absent but the cough may be severe. The chest sounds dry, sonorous, or sibilant rales heard every where, but especially between the scapula and the clavicular regions.

Given severe dyspnoea, with chest recession, increased respiration to 50 or 80 a minute, then we watch that the feeble pulse, rapid superficial breathing, clammy, cyanotic skin, which tells us of lung collapse and resulting carbonic acid poisoning.

There is so much to do in cases of this kind as to make the heart of the internist glad as he makes his plans. Counter irritation 2 to 8 times a day. Steam inhalations of lime water, containing turpentine, creosote, eucalyptol or Tr. benzoin serve to relax the tissues and also are anti-baceterial. An expectorant, not truly named in young children, for the class of medicines we employ, opiates are best entirely omitted, but first to liquify the secre-

tions, best are calcium iodide, ammonium muriate, citrate potassium, and ipecac, which we use as emetic unless slight stupor, or weak pulse forbid.

We are often hastily summoned for the suffocation and respiratory failure, which we have warned the mother might present in any severe case.

The active massage of back and chest with an occasional hot and cold, douche, alternated to the diaphragm, to get reaction, all mothers can do, as well as the hot mustard bath, the brandy, strychnia and atropine usually left for us to use therapeutically, on our arrival. For bronchitis, following measles, a creosote antiphlogistic poultice does well.

Bronchial croup strikes terror to any observer, though fortunately, lime water, or any alkali dissolve the casts, which makes the diagnostic sign.

In chronic bronchitis, rather rare in children, intratracheal injections have brought good results in the hands of trained experts, though broncho-pneumonia from the foreign body so introduced has resulted.

In treating the cough, we must educate in the inhibition of the cough reflex, and use mild alkalin drinks. If severe, to cause loss of sleep, we *must* then *resort* to opiates. A prolonged use of iodides, physical chest training, passive movements by massage and electricity or special apparatus is recommended, but often a history of rheumatism being present, we will get excellent results from a combination iodide, the salicylates, ammonium chlorides; *asthma*, rare in infancy, common in older children, is a vaso-motor neurosis of the respiratory tract, characterized by severe spasmodic dyspnoea. It begins in a large number of cases before the seventh year; some cases simulate capillary bronchitis, others follow it; hay fever, or Kopp's asthma occuring in summer, and the nervous type, as in ordinary adult asthma.

Some authors mention another type in children, known as ˙asthma dyspepticum, due to gastric irritation of the terminal filaments of the pneumogastric nerve. Too heavy proteids of a milk diet often cause it. Excluding cardiac, renal and typhoid asthma, the characteristic sputum and "perles of Laennec" and blood, with the usual physical signs, make it not difficult to diagnose.

In speaking of the reflex causes of asthma from the rhino-pharynx, most authorities fail to mention defective eyes. I learned this in one of my earliest cases. A boy of eight suffering severely from asthma, even after a change of climate ordered by his physician. I found the symptoms very easily mitigated after he had been fitted with glasses, whether permanently cured I know not, for the family removed to another town.

We first examine the rhino-pharynx, and treat any pathological condition there found, as indicated. The serum treatment

for cure of asthma in adults, I have not seen used in children for the reason that a simple nose and throat operation and treatment, or removing other causes of the reflex condition, I have not had to rely on it.

As a summary, I would emphasize first, a removal in every case of abnormal nasal and pharyngeal growths when causing reflex disturbances. Second, a very careful and thorough examination, clinical, and bacteriological, when not certain that the diagnosis in true, to determine the *causes* of *chronic* cough, the majority being due to diseases of larynx, bronchi, lungs or pleura. The non-respiratory coughs are persistent, dry and spasmodic without pulmonary signs. Our physicians should teach our future mothers more about healthy respiratory conditions in prophylaxis, by overcoming sensitiveness to "cold," by out-door living and fresh air bedrooms and hygiene of diet, clothing, etc. And then, having done our best, we may feel that "Angels could do no more.": If the patient dies it is not our fault.

PREVENTION OF DISEASE.

BY T. F. RENFROW, M. D., BILLINGS, OKLA.

I have selected this subject, not for the reason that I in any way consider myself an authority on the great and all important subject, but it is a subject that appeals to me as does no other subject connected with our profession.

While we take great pride in trying to cure, and give relief to our unfortunate patients who (as well meaning, but I sincerely hope, somewhat mistaken old lady remarked), are powerfully unfortunate if Dr. Renfrow was treating them. We

Read Before the Annual Meeting of the Oklahoma State Medical Association, Tulsa, Okla., May, 1910.

should and I am sure would take far greater pride in preventing altogether as far as possible the preventable diseases. To steer him or her, as the case may be, clear of physical misfortune, suffering, anguish and death. Granting that it is possible for us to relieve our brother of all his physical ailments, it is quite possible that he would not appreciate the greatest of all blessings, good health.

We often observe that happiness follows sorrow, rest fatigue, and poverty may follow great riches. All these are trivial as when untimely death results from what we believe to be a preventable disease. We also too frequently observe that good health may not follow disease.

We can, in a measure, reconcile ourselves to the passing away of the aged and infirm, but the babe, the youth, the father and the mother, in the prime and glory of manhood and womanhood, these, O these,. are the ones that rack our brains and tear our hearts when we think of what might have been. These thoughts, my brother practitioners, hang on me as the weight of a millstone about my neck as all the stubborn facts force themselves on me that that preventable, yet insidious, so tenacious, so stubborn and fatal disease, the white plague, has like some cruel monster, attacked the child of my father and mother, my sister. Yet through the hazy and sad fact, that our mother, three uncles and one aunt was taken, as it appears to us, ruthlessly away from us by this arch enemy of our homes, I have yet hopes through the invaluable aid of our modern care and treatment of the once formidable disease, I may yet see my dear sister enjoying life and training her boy in the paths of righteousness, as well as consoling and making happy her deserving husband. I mention this sad personal case, not to cause you sorrow, but that I may be the means of causing you to take more interest in this great and beneficent subject. "The Prevention of Disease," and further I earnestly hope you will be able in the near future to keep not only your own families free from the dread "White Plague," but your neighbor and your neighbors families not only free from the white plague, but a host of its kindred in mortality.

The good mechanic, wishing his machine to run smoothly, yield him, or as in most instances, his employee, a nice profit, that it may endure long, and that it may be as the wonderful "One Horse Shay," each part lasting as long as the other, and have a record for service and useful age. These aspirations of our mechanical brother might well be the highest ambition of our nearer brother the practitioner of medicine and surgery.

What is true in avoiding accidents in man made machines holds true in the greatest of all machines, God's masterpiece, man.

Man, today, as he has been through all the ages, wishes to avoid pain and suffering, which are but subjective symptoms of disorder and disease. And it is well that he wishes to avoid disease, not only to be free from pain and suffering, but that his physical makeup may work efficiently, naturally and normally.

Some writer has said that health is man's greatest heritage. It is the main source of his wellbeing. It aids in character building and is most essential in mental development. It is the gift that makes life worth living. Another has said, "My wealth is my health," and another, "My health is my wealth."

Seeing that health is the thing most to be desired, more precious than rubies, yea. than fine gold, it behooves us as guardians of our brothers most precious gift, to keep our eyes open to all things that will help him to retain in full measure this most precious gift, health, not only for his own special benefit, but first, for his posterity, second, for the benefit of society and we would place third, for his own benefit, as one might suffer for the benefit of others But in disease one suffers and his posterity with him.

Your children and your grandchildren through many generations suffer also. "Weep, and you weep alone," will not apply as an illustration in disease, but. the phrase, "Laugh and the world laughs with you" will more aptly apply, but not so charmingly.

While disease may play a prominent part in the higher development of mankind, was the belief of the ancients, (and some not so ancient,) that disease was providential and the unfortunate ones were possessed of devils, these are problems for the gods to solve and man to meditate and ponder over. But realizinz that self preservation is the first law of nature we feel that we, as the Great Medical Fraternity, in relieving the suffering of "the least of these" may be among the true worshipper of the "Lowly Nazarene."

In meditating upon disease we can comprehend little, if any, good coming to us as a result of it, and can in a measure understand how our ancestors regarded disease as coming from the evil one.

We, most of us, would agree with the noted Ingersoll, when it was said he was asked critically if he thought he could suggest any improvement on God's laws, the great man jestingly remarked that he would gladly change the laws in regard to health and disease. Just turn it around as it were and make good health catching instead of disease.

You have doubtless wondered why I have not told you ere this, some ways of preventing disease. I will answer by saying that I have excellent reasons. First, I do not know as many as I should. and you. already know more than I do. And I will repeat that my reason for choosing this subject was, as far as it is possible for me to do so, to impress the great good to be acomplished along this line. I will read to you some of the encouraging words that some of my more worthy and better qualified brothers have said on the prevention of disease.

When we realize that the death rate in the United States to the 100,000 of the preventable disease is first Tuberculosis, 90, Typhoid fever, 33.7, Diphtheria, 35.4, Cholera Infantum, 47,8, Diarrhoeal diseases, 85.1, we may feel that we have a greater work to do, and greater benefits to bestow on mankind by actually preventing the diseases mentioned as well as a legion of other things and conditions to avoid, which prepare the system for the ravages of disease.

One way we can do a great service to humanity is to help push through the Bill introduced by Senator Owen to create a department of health. This would be a great move in the right way. Senator Owen, in introducing this bill, said that the plan is to concentrate in one department the various bureaus of health, Biology, and Sanitation which are now strung through the separate branches of government. The question of health, while of supreme and final importance to the nation, has been tabled heretofore by the consideration of politics and commerce, but Senator Owen contends that even more essential than the conservation of natural resources is the conservation of national vitality. Mr. Owen in offering this act to the Senate stated that the people of the United States suffer from preventable causes the loss of six hundred thousand lives per annum. These deaths result, he declared, from polluted water, impure and adulterated food and drugs, and epidemics of various preventable diseases, as Tuberculosis, Typhoid and Malarial fevers, unclean cities and bad sanitation. If the life of an American citizen may be computed in money, at an average of $1,700 the loss would amount to one thousand million a year. This is as much as the entire income of the government. In addition there are three million persons in the nation sick from preventable diseases, and as one million of these are in the working period of life the financial forfeiture at an average of $700 per annum reaches five hundred millions. To this may be added five hundred millions for drugs, medical attendance and care, making another thousand million of pure economic drain.

The pension roll of the United States exceeds on hundred and fifty millions a year, but three-fourths of it, said Senator

Owen is due to illness and death which might have been entirely avoided. A wiser policy in the past would have saved the government one hundred and twenty-five millions in pensions, and the people themselves over two billions in money, together with much human misery and pain. In New Zealand, largely on account of rigid state care and protection of health and well-being of the individual there averages a fraction over nine deaths per thousand as against 16.5 in the United States, an extra loss of seven to the thousand or from the ninety million population, six hundred thousand needless deaths every year. Appropriations of almost fifteen million dollars has been made for the health activities of the government during the present fiscal year.

Another great help in the prevention of disease is the educational department of the American Medical Association. In Volume 5 of January 15, 1910, Doctor Arthur Dean Bevan in his address as chairman of the Association, among other things, said, "To prevent disease is to begin with the babe, proper nursing, diet, clothing, hygiene, and environment, to eat right, sleep right, and live right according to the best methods requires instruction and education along these lines. To prevent pneumonia one of our most dreaded, also one of our most fatal diseases, is in most instance only necessary to avoid taking cold, and if not able to avoid the cold, a double dose of quinine, a good physic, a warm bed and a good sweat is sufficient.

To avoid a great many of the most fatal diseases it is only necesary to keep the system at 100 per cent. par. Good health is the best safeguard against diseases. The contagious disease does attack one in good health, but by proper care and good nursing will bring one through with but little injury.

In my little town and surrounding country we have had few cases of Typhoid fever in seven years. Only cases who have contracted the disease other places. Our town has no sewer or water system. Our neighbor towns with both these systems have typhoid every year. I have had only two cases in seven years that I had reason to believe contracted the disease in our own part of the country. These were living near a small stream. With the knowledge that we have now, and with what the future will bring, we may hope that typhoid will also in the not too distant future be in a great measure prevented.

The importance of modern medicine to the community can hardly be estimated. The advances made in the last thirty years in determining the germ cause of many diseases; in the prevention of disease by scientific methods of hygiene and quarantine; in the accurate diagnosis and investigation of disease by rational methods of treatment, have changed what was formally a mass of empiricism into a science.

Today medicine is a science, and it is the most important of all sciences both from the standpoint of the individual and the welfare of the community. The practical application of the known facts of modern medicine by efficient national, state and local boards of health would save this country thousands of lives and millions of dollars each year. A small fraction of the money appropriated to the great national undertakings like the panama canal and the projected deep waterway in the Mississippi Valley would, if properly used, insure efficient boards of health throughout the country, would be of enormous benefit in the prevention of suffering and disease and would bring to the community much greater benefit than could be obtained by any other national movement.

Great improvements have been made in care of the sick by modern scientific methods, our great public hospitals, insane asylums, and infirmaries for the blind are gradually being molded by scientific methods into institutions where the unfortunates receive the kindly care of good nursing, the benefits of modern hygiene and the best medical treatment. The individual if he is wise can secure for himself and his family the benefits and protection of modern scientific medicine by securing the services of a well trained scientific physician He is foolish and unfortunate who selects for his medical adviser the poorly trained medical man, the pathist, the pretender or the charlatan, who cannot give him the benefits of modern medical knowledge. Many of us here know the difference between the modern intelligent medical care and the ignorant charlatan care of the sick. We have seen the woman dying of child bed fever which might have been prevented by the intelligent aseptic care of her confinement. We have seen the child dead from unrecognized and untreated diphtheria which might have been prevented by early labratory, or intelligent clinical diagnosis and the proper use of antitoxines. We have seen the pinched and dusky face of the man dying of peritonitis which could have been prevented by early diagnosis and proper operative treatment. We who are medical men know the great difference between in-

telligent and ignorant, between trained and untrained medical care. But the great public does not know; it does not understand. The public does not as yet realize the importance of public health measures and of measures aimed at securing properly trained medical practitioners.

Millions of dollars have been given to endow colleges and theological schools, but comparatively little has been given to medicine. Certainly one of the best investments John D. Rockefeller ever made was the money given to the Rockefeller Institute, which resulted in finding a cure for cerebrospinal meningitis, and the most far-reaching and beneficial investment the state or a rich philanthropist could make would be in money given to medical research and medical education.

It is the duty of the medical profession to educate the public in these matters, since the public should know the great value and the great possibilities of modern medicine. Public opinion will then demand the creation of efficient boards of health, the adoption of effective public health laws and thorough training medical practitioners in the science of medicine. Further, the public must be shown that, either through state or private endowment funds must be provided for the development of strong medical schools, where men can be properly trained in modern scientific medicine and where thorough research work every effort can be made to add to our present knowledge.

ETIOLOGY AND TREATMENT OF INGUINAL HERNIA.

BY DRS. W. J. FRICK AND R. D. IRLAND, KANSAS CITY, MO.

With one important exception, the principles of the etiology of inguinal hernia are essentially the same as those which underlie the etiology of all other hernia. Therefore

Read Before the Annual Meeting of the Oklahoma State Medical Association, Tulsa, Okla., May, 1910.

we have chosen to confine ourselves in this paper to a consideration of hernia of this type, as they occur with vastly greater frequency than do any others.

A variety of conditions are important in the causation of hernia, most prominent among which are age, sex, certain nutritional disturbances, habit of life, pathological conditions which increase intra-abdominal pressure, long mesentery, congenital defects and faults in post-natal development.

Age is an undoubtedly important factor. Statistics show the incidence of inguinal hernia to be greater in the early and late years of life. In our own experience the majority of cases come to operation between the ages of twenty-five and fifty years; but almost invariably they give a history of the existence of the hernia for three to ten years or longer. The youngest case in our series was seven months; the oldest eighty-two years.

It is conceded that inguinal hernia is operated much more frequently in males than in females. The anatomical differences between the sexes suggest a plausible reason why this should be so. But, on the other hand, it is altogether likely that many small inguinal herniae exist in women without causing any inconvenience or symptoms, and therefore are never brought to the attention of the surgeon.

Nutritional disturbances are not to be disregarded though their importance is slight in a majority of cases. In poorly nourished individuals the tissues are dificient in tone, and consequently the natural weaknesses of the abdominal wall are increased by so much.

The habit of life is quite important. Those individuals whose occupations require great muscular effort are subjected to frequent sudden changes in intra-abdominal pressure and are often the subjects of hernia. This doubtless is significant in connection with the greater frequency of hernia in middle aged males, than in females and in older males who naturally lead more quiet and more shielded lives.

Pathological conditions which increase intra-abdominal pressure, such as coughs, vomiting, constipation, abdominal tumors, pregnancy are to be credited with value as casual factors of hernia.

A long mesentery, in our opinion, is of little importance. Tandler of Vienna has shown that entehoptosis is a congenital, not an acquired condition; and in none of our cases has enteroptosis existed. Moreover, having given certain faulty anatomic conditions and a suddenly increased intra-abdominal pressure, a mesentery of normal length is no bar to the formation of a hernia of the gut. It is therefore logical to consider a long mesentery as a negligible etiologic factor of inguinal hernia.

Though there is something of importance in most of the conditions suggested as possible causes of hernia, yet after a careful observation of the cases in our experience, and after consideration of the published reports of other surgeons, we are impelled to agree with those who say that the basic element of the etiology of inguinal hernia is a localized weakness in the abdominal wall which usually, if not invariably, is congenital in origin. If these weaknesses are not to be considered as congenital, they must be regarded as faults in the post-natal development of the individual. But in either case the weak spot is conceded to exist before the hernia can occur, and that is the point which is essential to our thesis.

Of inguinal hernia, the indirect variety is much more common than the direct. Therefore let us consider them before taking up the less frequent direct hernia.

In early embryonic life, before the descent of the testis begins, the processus vaginalis is formed from the peritoneum and projects itself towards the genital swelling at that spot in the lower anterior abdominal wall which later on becomes the internal abdominal ring. Attached to the processus vaginalis, and accompanying it in its progress toward the genital swelling, is the inguinal ligament, known also as the gubernaculum testis. As the processus vaginalis elongates, it and the inguinal ligament push before them a part of the transversalis fascia which then assumes a funnel-like shape, and which for this reason is called the infundibuliform fascia. This is the first step in embryonic development which produces a natural weak spot in this region of the abdominal wall.

As the testis descends it reaches the abdominal wall at the infundibuliform fascia, and progressing obliquely downward it gradually produces the structure commonly called the inguinal canal, though the name is not precisely descriptive of it. Coincident with the descent of the testis, the processus vaginalis becomes further elongated and accompanies the testis to its adult position in the scrotum. Here, shortly after birth, the lower portion of the processus approximates itself to the testis to form the tunica vaginalis testis. Then the cavity of the upper part, or neck, of the processus is gradually obliterated by a fusion of its walls, becoming a fibrous band or cord (1). Sometimes ony a portion of the neck is obliterated, the rest remaining patent. Sometimes no obliteration takes place. In either of these departures from the normal development there is a diverticulum of the peritoneum extending to some extent into the inguinal canal or scrotum, according to the degree of obliteration which has taken place (2).

These embryologic and anatomic facts give us the following steps in the formation of the weakness in the abdominal wall which makes possible the occurence of an indirect inguinal hernia:

1st: The pushing out of the transversalis fascia to form the infundibuliform fascia;

2nd: The formation of the inguinal canal by the elongation of the processus vaginalis, and by the descent of the testis;

3rd: The imperfect obliteration of the neck of the processus vaginalis.

Of these three steps, the last is of very great importance. It is our belief that in indirect inguinal hernia, almost invariably this is the chief etiologic factor. In other words, if the obliteration of the processus vaginalis is complete, the natural weakness of the abdominal wall at the internal ring would not alone cause the formation of hernia. This is of much importance in the theory of the treatment for the radical cure of hernia.

While in surgical phraseology the term "congenital hernia" is reserved for only those cases in which no obliteration of the neck of the processus vaginalis has occurred, and in which the cavity of the tunica vaginalis testis remains in direct communication with the peritoneal cavity; yet in a strict sense, if a hernia occur into the patent remnant of the processus, it should be considered as being of congenital origin.

The direct hernia are never congenital; their sacs are never preformed by a fault in the embryonic development of the individual. Nevertheless they have as the chief factor of their etiology an anatomic weakness in the abdominal wall.

Almost without exception these herniae occur within the triangle of Hesselbach. Only a few cases are reported in which a viscus has pushed its way betwen the fibres of the rectus muscle into the inguinal canal or between the layers of the abdominal wall. Hesselbach's triangle is in relation with the middle inguinal fossa and the lower external angle of the internal inguinal fossa. The middle inguinal fossa is a notoriously weak spot. Rodman and Bonney state that in only a small percentage of the cadavers examined by them have they observed a well developed conjoined-tendon of the transversalis and internal oblique muscles. And, furthermore, that even in those instances when a well marked tendinous union between the aponeuroses of these two muscles exists, the lower portion of Hesselbach's triangle is protected in front by only the transversalis fascia and the aponeurosis of the external oblique muscle (3). It is reasonable to infer that in the relatively small number of cases presenting hernia of this type, this natural weakness has been exaggerated by abnormal post-natal conditions.

The diagnosis of inguinal hernia seldom offers serious difficulty to the experienced surgeon. In this region only a few conditions simulating hernia occur with sufficient frequency to merit detailed differentiation. Inflammation of the inguinal glands, hydrocele, and varicocele are perhaps the commonest of them, and each presents certain well known characteristics which usually make a differential diagnosis easy. So that, at this time, we shall not enter upon a discussion of this phase of our subject.

Treatment: Stated broadly, the proper treatment of inguinal hernia is operative. Only those cases which because of age, debility, lesion of the heart or lungs would not bear well a general anaesthetic or the shock of an operation, should be made exceptions to this rule. The injection method for obliteration of the sac is to be condemned without qualification because of its dangerous uncertainty. The truss is to be considered only in selected cases offering contra-indications to operative interference. A simple truss made from a knotted hank of yarn is often serviceable in retaining inguinal herniae in infants. Frequently as the child develops, an apparent cure follows the use of this contrivance. At least it usually controls the defect until the child becomes more fully developed and is better able to withstand an operation. But, in a general sense, the use of trusses is not advisable for a two-fold reason: first, they are uncertain, and a sudden failure to do

what is expected of them may result in a fatal strangulation. Second, the pressure they exert is frequently the cause of adhesions within and surrounding the sac, which seriously complicate later operative measures. One recent case in our series offers a striking instance of this fact. The adhesions about the sac were so dense that in breaking them up the sac was so badly torn that the operator was unable properly to tie it off. The opening into the peritoneal cavity was closed as well as was feasible and a flap of the sac was sutured to the transversalis fascia just inside the outer margin of the internal abdominal ring.

In repeating that operative treatment should be employed in the great majority of all cases of inguinal hernia, we would say that our opinion is in consonance with that of the surgical authorities of today. All cases of strangulated hernia are operative, in spite of conditions which would be contra-indications if this complication did not exist. In all uncomplicated cases it is decidedly the method of choice. Furthermore, the sooner operation is performed, the better are the results to be expected.

The choice of the operation to be done is the next consideration. The technic of all the modern operations for inguinal hernia is based upon that of the Bassini method, which has as its chief features the obliteration of the sac and the transplantation of the cord.

In view of the etiology of the indirect hernia, the obliteration of the sac is by far the more essential part of this operation and of any of its numerous modifications. We firmly believe that if the sac is properly treated the cure will be complete, no matter what is done by way of narrowing the inguinal canal and transference of the cord.

In our work we have used with satisfaction for many years a modification of the

Ferguson-Andrews operation. The incision is made over the hernia parallel to Poupart's ligament down to the aponeurosis of the external oblique muscle. This structure is carefully opened from the external to the internal abdominal rings, and the cord exposed. By gauze dissection the sac is freed from the cord and loosened from the abdominal wall well beyond the internal ring. The sac is caught by two hemostats and carefully opened between them by nicking with the knife, enlarging the opening with scissors. If the hernia has not, by this time, been reduced it is probably adherent to the inner wall of the sac. The adhesions are sought for, broken up, and the viscus, usually the omentum, returned to the peritoneal cavity. If the peritoneum has been well separated around the internal ring, it is now possible to draw the sac down bringing its junction with the peritoneum plainly into sight. Its walls are then transfixed and tied with No. o iodized catgut, the sac cut off and the stump dropped into the abdominal cavity. This step in the operation must be thoroughly well done or the result is likely to be disappointing. The following steps are of lesser importance. If the internal ring has been greatly widened, as is usually true especially in old hernia, a few stitches with No. o iodized catgut are taken in the transversalis fascia. The lower fibres of the internal oblique and of the transversalis (if present) muscles are then sutured with No. I iodized catgut to the shelving portion of Poupart's ligament. To avoid the likelihood of puncture of the femoral or external iliac arteries, which has occurred a number of times with unpracticed hands, an assistant grasps the shelving portion of the ligament in two Halsted forceps and lifts it well up from the underlying vessels; the suture is passed on a curved needle first downward through the muscle, then upward through the ligament. Interrupted sutures of No. I iodized catgut

are employed to close the wounds in the external oblique aponeurosis and in the deep layer of the superficial fascia. The skin is closed with interrupted sutures of No. o iodized catgut. Tincture of iodine, full strength, is applied to the line of incision, and a simple sterile dressing placed.

It will be noted that in this operation the cord is not changed from its original bed; and that the only attempt at narrowing the inguinal canal lies in the suturing the transversalis and internal oblique muscles to Poupart's ligament, and sometimes the narrowing of the internal ring. Iodized catgut is used throughout, No. I being the largest size employed. The rational simplicity of its technic, and the satisfactory results obtained with it are the chief arguments which recommend the operation as above described.

The sac of a direct hernia is tied off in the same manner as that of the indirect type. The opening in the transversalis fascia is closed with No. I iodized catgut. If the fascia is much relaxed the edges are overlapped. The other steps in the operation are about the same as those of the operation for indirect hernia.

Local anaesthesia is employed for hernia operations by some surgeons. The results claimed are good. The method is especially serviceable in those cases presenting contraindications to general anaesthesia. Its disadvantages lie in a tedious complication of the technic, and a failure to secure complete relaxation of the structures involved.

Bibliography

(1)   J. P. McMurrich. "The Development of the Human Body," pp. 387-388-390. P. Blakiston's Son & Co., Philadelphia, 1903.
(2)   Wm. Hessert: "Congenital Sacs in Oblique Inguinal Hernia." Surgery, Gynecology and Obstetrics, Vol. X, No. 3, p. 252.
(3)   Rodman and Bonney: "Etiology and Pathology of Inguinal Hernia." American Journal of the Medical Sciences, Vol. CXXXVIII, No. 6, p. 853.

W. J. Frick, M. D., and R. D. Irland, M. D., 418 Keith and Perry Building, Kansas City, Mo.

THE DOCTOR OF WASHITA COUNTY AND THE NEWLY ADOPTED SCHEDULE.

BY ERIK E. SANBURG, M. D., CORDELL, OKLA.

Gentlemen:

This subject presented itself to my mind a few days ago, when I was requested to sign an agreement whereby we bound ourselves to charge certain fees and to refuse to attend certain people who are delinquent. I have very little to say as regards the office consultation fee or the fee for day or night visits except I think there should be no iron-clad rules laid down. It would be better, to my mind, to say prescription and advice from 50c up, than to fix a minimum fee of $1. So also I think we ought to leave the old fee of $1.50 and upwards for visits in town, depending on the part of the county where we live and how far we have to go. I wish to call your attention to the fact that I am considering conditions in Washita County for here we have no large towns and no boom towns with a large floating population, but our county is settled by substantial farmers and of these 95 per cent. pay their bills, a fact to which I can testify after nine years experience in the county.

The fee of fifteen dollars and mileage for obstetrics originated in the larger towns and cities and to my mind is an excessive fee for an ordinary obstetrical case in a farming community. This fee is meant to include one or more visits to a patient prior to confinement, urinalises, attendance during delivery and at least a visit once a day for the first three days after confinement. All this is out of the question in country practice for we are frequently never called to the house until labor has set in and consequently the physician is not called upon to make either visits or urinalises prior to

Read Before the Custer and Washita County Medical Socities at Clinton, Okla., June 3, 1910.

the birth of the child and unless it is convenient he may never pay a second visit. Therefore I say that for an ordinary obstetrical case, $15.00 and mileage is too high a fee and we should be content with $10.00 and mileage and I think that no reasonable person would object to the paying of $1.00 per hour after 6 hours under those conditions. But if we expect city fees the public is entitled to city service and it is our duty to give it.

Regarding the clause pertaining to ministers, I know that excepting two or three denominations, their remuneration is absolutely inadequate to furnish even the necessaries of life, and if there are any people deserving of charity it is the ministers and their families. Of course if a man is engaged in other business and preaches on Sunday, he should pay his doctor. Such a man does not come properly under the classification of ministers, since he might as well be classed as a farmer or merchant or whatever occupation he pursues. The point is this however that I do not think it wise to allow the medical society to interfere with our private affairs, and certainly not in the dispensing of charities which is the greatest privilege granted to us by an All Wise Providence and one which we as christians and gentlemen should recognize as such.

We come then to the consideration of the delinquents and here I am free to confess that I hold views entirely contrary to the agreement as it has been adapted. In the first place we must always remember that the practice of medicine is not a business nor an exact science, but a profession and an art, and that our success or failure depends not so much in our skill and learning as it does on the opinion of the people among whom we live and the esteem in which they hold us. It has been argued that because the bakers, carpenters, blacksmiths, barbers and other crafts have formed unions and established higher prices and shorter hours, we should do the same, but I can not see how that argument pertains to us as physicians. They are laborers who are paid by the day to do so much work, whereas we are professional men and should be living on a higher plane, engaged in a mission of rescue and mercy for which we are entitled to an adequate fee, it is true, yet one who of necessity must be very flexible to meet all requirements. We can not guarantee anything we do, and our stock in trade, if I may use that expression, is simply our knowledge and our judgment in which we ask our patients to trust implicitly.

In this enlightened age, we must give the public credit for possessing, at least in a limited degree, some knowledge and judgment in medical matters, and if you will stop and reflect, you may find that some of your uncollected accounts have not been paid because in the judgment of the people your services were not proportionate to the fee charged. For instance, you may have made a mistake in diagnosing a case of pus in the appendix as acute indigestion and have not used the proper tact in explaining conditions and a great many people object to pay for anything unless they get value received, or think they do. Of course it may seem hard to lose an account even of this kind, but the fault lies primarily with the physician, because he lacked the necessary amount of tact to deal with the collecting end of that particular case, and considering that the physician is only a man, and no more honest than other men, how many accounts will he pay that he considers unjust? It seems to me that it would be a far better policy in these kind of cases, to present a bill, and if it is not paid within a reasonable length of time,

simply credit it to your profit and loss account and forget all about it. If you push these bills you will certainly make an enemy instead of a friend of the party, it may finally have to be settled in a court, and no matter how it is paid, you will eventually reap more harm than good from such procedure, because every man has a certain influence and a certain number of friends and you will have lowered yourself in their esteem.

There is a class of people who seem to be born with an adverse disposition towards paying their doctor. What are you going to do with them? Someone must look after them in case of sickness and even though there may be no law to compel us as physicians to attend anyone, unless we feel so disposed, there is an unwritten law which is just as powerful, and its name is PUBLIC OPINION, that compels us to look after them, whether we feel like it or not, if we wish to hold the love and respect of our friends. The man most dispised on earth is the hard hearted miserly man, with no pity and no feeling for his fellow man, and if you refuse to go to see anyone who is sick, and let him die for want of care because he does not pay his doctor bill, you will soon find that your practice has left you for people care very little for a doctor who refuses calls. Certainly they would think it strange if you refused to go simply because the man owed a bill to another physician. You may consider this a poor argument, and yet I do not believe anyone here is anxious to try the experiment just to prove the strength of the argument.

There is also an other class of poor pay but of this it is needless to speak, because no self-respecting, honorable gentleman who calls himself a physician, will refuse to attend them, because they are the unfortunate poor who can not help themselves.

At the first glance it would seem that a "blacklist" or to use the less offensive and more refined term, the "delinquent" list, would be an excellent arrangement to make people "come across." But on second thought I see some dark spots appearing here and there. I begin to wonder how it is that we all at once become so solicitous about each others outstanding accounts. It is truly a gladsome sight to observe so much brotherly and fraternal love oozing out as it were, on all sides, and it only remains that we tithe ourselves and create a fund for the deserving brother physicians who have been compelled to spend their lives and their substance attending the deadbeats of Washita County, Okla. But when we analyze this feeling further we find that it is not love at all, but pure and simple selfishness that underlies the whole arrangement. Of course physicians are too highminded to ever allow themselves to be spiteful, you know.

There is nothing more unfair than blacklisting, because it is a too one-sided affair and we are liable to allow our personal grievances to hold the upper hand, and we may report people whom we know are good pay ordinarily, but who for some good and sufficient reason in their mind, refuse to pay us. It follows then, that this person **being prevented from employing any other** physician, he perhaps will fall out with the whole profession, and so we may eventually still hold a patient who otherwise would have drifted into the hands of a competitor. Again you may have listed a person whom I consider good pay because he has always paid me. Yet how is it he is blacklisted? Surely you do not expect me to refuse to go to see him, when I know from past experience that he will pay me every cent he owes me. Then where is the fairness of blacklisting to the public or the profession? A blacklist may be admissible if we limit ourselves to simply placing the person on a list, but leave it to every members judgment whether he will attend him or not.

Therefore I say again, I think we make a mistake when we allow the medical society to interfere with our private affairs, to the extent that we pass any prohibitory measures, knowing as we all do that they will hinder us in our work, are contrary to our ideals that we held while yet young in the profession, and are bound to redound to our hurt instead of our good.

The American Medical Association has lately been branded "The Great Medical Trust" which is a term absolutely unjust and false as pertaining to that great organization, yet if we as members of the County, State, and ultimately The American Medical Association allow ourselves as an association to raise fees, and designate who is, and who is not permitted to be attended by the members, the public and the yellow journals will not be very far wrong after all. Hence the statement that blacklisting will eventually redound to our hurt instead of our good.

Again is it not possible that we would have to amend our code of ethics to meet this condition? The physician who would attend anyone who is indebted to any other physician would be considered un-ethical?

Medical societies were instituted that we may have an opportunity to meet and become acquainted with each other, where we could discuss medical topics and exchange views and experiences which would be helpful in our work and eventually to be a benefit to our patients, but they were never intended to become collecting agencies for doubtful accounts. If we lose sight of this fact and allow ourselves to become mercenary, we are no longer physicians in the true sense of the word, but simply traders in pills and mixtures and perhaps, human lives.

I dare say if we could hear what people say while we are holding this meeting, it would be something like this: Better look out the doctors are holding a meeting.

Or, did you see Dr. So and So go to that medical meeting? I used to think he was a pretty good man and a friend of mine, but I must have been mistaken. These k'nd of remarks do not raise the doctor in the esteem of the people, but I will tell you what they do. They drive them into the hands of midwives and quacks, osteopaths, chiropractors and patent medicines, and it remains with us to get them back again.

Gentlemen, let us consider these matters and resolve to remember always that we are physicians, first, last, and all the time, and that to attain success in our chosen field whether we be rich or poor is our highest aspiration, and I am convinced that we will never see an epitaph over the grave of any of us:

Here lies Dr. Sawbones, who died an extreme and abnormal death, in abject poverty, as a result of failure to collect his bills from deadbeats of Washita County, Oklahoma.

WHAT THE WOMAN'S CLUB CAN DO IN THE CAMPAIGN AGAINST TUBERCULOSIS.

BY MRS. J. M. BYRUM, SHAWNEE, OKLAHOMA

Much of the present work in the campaign against tuberculosis is educational. The people do not realize nor know all the rules and regulations of the public health authorities nor do they appreciate the full importance of a close observation of the hygienic measures necessary to combat effectively the germ of tuberculosis. If it be required that the unfortunate one use his own drinking cup or that he refrain from promiscuous spitting, he and his friends and relatives usually consider it more of a punishment for being sick than as a sanitary measure to protect others from the selfsame deadly disease. It is not necessary to tell this audience of Doctor's Wives that tuberculosis is an infectious disease due to a very active and persistent germ found in the sputum of the one affected and transmitted by particles of this sputum in the dust or on the clothing or drinking vessel or other agency acting as a carrier from the one to the other. It is perhaps a divine provision that sunshine is the great enemy to the germ and protects us from the infec-

Read Before the State Meeting of the Ladies' Auxiliary to State Medical Association at Tulsa.

tion of the street dust to a great extent, since the germ cannot live many days in the sunshine.

It is easily within the function of the Woman's Club to so mold public opinion that this erroneous idea will no longer be held by those in the radius of our activities. If the sick ones are too debased or are too ignorant to have thought for the public good it is still within our power so to educate his community of relatives, neighbors and friends, of their dangers and by this means put them on their guard against the infection. We can make this so strong when working in connection with the health authorities that these neighbors and friends will become wrought up to the point where they will demand of the family of the sick ones that there be a proper observance of the precautions necessary to limit the spread of the disease. In this connection it will not be amiss to say that the woman's club exerts a greater influence on the public community in general than any other agency or organization. When this influence is directed along the avenues here in mentioned, the campaign against tuberculosis an impetus not otherwise obtainable.

One of the literary, clubs of Shawnee recently had a lesson or program on Public Affairs of the day and papers were read on tuberculosis and other diseases of an infectious or contagious nature. This proved one of the most interesting meetings of the year. If the Federation in each town should arrange programs for each club at stated intervals, this in itself would be a good work, there are many ways of doing this but the essential feature is to get in touch with that element of people that we do not meet every day. At these meetings, each club woman should be requested to ask the attendance of some woman who has no time to read or who can not read, some one who has a member of her family sick with tuberculosis or some one who has not considered this subject seriously, or who has had no opportunity of knowing the dreaded situation as it really is unfolded to us. At each of these meetings each club should be represented by a paper on some phase of the topic under consideration such as "Necessity of Fresh Air," "Well Ventilated Sleeping Apartments," "Absolute Necessity of Individual Drinking Cups in the Schoolroom and in Traveling," "The Unsanitary Condition of the Back Yard and Alley," "Proper Ventilation of the Moving Picture Show," "How to Breathe, Stand and Walk," all these are subjects which are of every day importance to us. For instance, with reference to the moving picture show, where the attendance is made up of all classes of people whether they be afflicted with tuberculosis or not, are crowded together in one room with scarcely any ventilation at all. Can you imagine the consequence if only one of this number be tubercular and is expectorating on the floor or if not spitting, he is exhaling the germs with particles of sputum into the already vitiated air of the room. How many of us would knowingly enter such a dangerous place? Yet this is what some of us are doing every day. I suggest that our clubs appoint committees to call upon the managers of these shows and ask them to fumigate the rooms at least once a day and to provide for more scientific ventilation. "How to Breathe" is a splendid subject. We all breathe but do we get the full benefit of breathing? Exercise in breathing makes the voice flexible and deep. "How to Stand and Walk" is something we should also notice. Some one has said that "Man is differentiated from the lower animals in two great physical respects: He can stand erect and has power of speech." No two things does man do worse!

The club woman can use her influence in the public schools. What are your schools doing? Are they educating the children to be healthy citizens or are they feeding the mind and denying the body its necessities? Twenty million children attend school in this great country—are they worth saving physicially as well as mentally? When the child enters the modern school room, his physical education begins. He has already, perhaps, learned to live without fresh air in his unventilated home and is thereby so poorly developed physically and mentally that it requires years and years of training to over come it. Tubercular children come from such home but if physical culture is practiced daily, which it will be in the ideal school, this means an overcoming of this tubercular taint or weakness generated since birth. If the school children of this generation are properly taught, both physically and mentally, how to live and how to prevent tubercular diseases, the next generation will be remarkably free from such affections. If you have an athletic league in your school, offer your assistance in its organization and maintenance and feel sure that you are doing a deed that will not only be appreciated by the student but will redound to your glory in years to come by the development of those strong physiques that we so much admire.

An other way to assist in this promotion is to teach the poorer people among our acquaintances to appreciate and make use of the city parks. I suggest that each club give a series of picnics through the summer time to the children who are not otherwise permitted or invited to such events. Can you imagine what it would mean to their little starved bodies to enjoy such outings?

Of course we wage war against the common house fly as the greatest carrier of disease germs. We should go farther. We should refuse to purchase from the grocer who places his wares on exhibition in an uncovered state and exposed to the fly. It is not enough that all displays of fruits and vegetables be placed inside the store with screened doors, but we should demand that the rules of the State Board of Health be complied with and these articles be placed beneath individual screens. On the contrary imagine yourself eating vegetables or fruits from a display on the sidewalk subjected to the continuous visitation of the fly coming from places you know not where. The mere thought is too revolting for further development.

The Club Woman of Oklahoma can do a lasting work in this particular cause as well as in any other, for the club woman has a determination that has no equal and she must succeed.

EDITORIAL

THE OCTOBER MEETING OF THE MEDICAL ASSOCIATION OF THE SOUTHWEST.

The fifth annual meeting of the Medical Association of the Southwest will be held at Wichita, Kans., Oct. 11-12. From all that can be learned regarding the plans in preparation this will be the best meeting the society has ever held.

The program will include many of the best known men in the district and as there is nothing of a business character to come before this body practically all of the time can be given up to the scientific work.

The local committee are looking well to the social side of the meeting and are planning not only for the men but are making special plans for the ladies as well, so just set aside these two days as sacred to the cause and tell your wife about the plan early and don't fail to attend this meeting and get good and help to do good.

TROUBLES IN THE STATE BOARD OF MEDICAL EXAMINERS.

After a long continued fight within the State Board of Medical Examiners, Dr. E. T. Hensley, a member of the Board resigned upon request of the Governor. The investigation upon which the resignation was brought about was due to charges filed with the Governor by Dr. W. T. Tilly, President of the Board. The Journal has been unofficially informed that the resignation was not asked for on the strict ground of the charges filed, but upon the finding that there existed irreparable incompatibility among members of the Board.

About the time this was occurring Dr. Frank P. Davis, of Enid, Secretary of the Board was asked for his resignation. He asked for an opportunity to be heard in refutation of any charges that might be filed against him. This request, which the Governor considered fair, will be complied with and Dr. Davis will be given an opporturity to defend himself.

THE DEATH OF DR. MIHRAN KAS-SABIAN.

The recent death of Dr. Kassabian in Philadelphia, from cancer as a result of continued X ray exposures over a long period of time adds another name to a long list of heroes whose memory will be indelibly carved on the tablets of memory in the medical profession.

Dr. Kassabian was one of the pioneers in this class of work and did great service in developing and perfecting technic along unknown lines and making our knowledge what it is today, of this hitherto little understood science and in doing this work he gradually received injuries from which he never recovered.

While such a death is deplored by the profession the warning it gives to others is worthy of notice and while the dangers of this work are being gradually eliminated and controlled by a better understanding of the mysteries of radioactivity there is still enough danger to warn amateurs to go carefully in their experiments.

ACTIVITY OF THE OKLAHOMA PUBLIC HEALTH LABORATORIES.

The State Laboratories situated at Norman have taken a step recently that will be of great benefit to the state generally and to physicians individually who will co-operate with the officers in the proposed work.

Each County Health Officer and any individual who may wish them has been and will be sent specific directions and data for the forwarding of suspected specimens of water, sputa and typhoid infection and these specimens will be given prompt attention on their receipt and an immediate report made to the sender.

This is certainly a step in the right direction. There is no longer an excuse for a physician to plead lack of time, equipment or ability in the diagnosis of infectious troubles dangerous to the general public health.

This work is under the direction of Professor Louis A. Turley, State Bacteriologist and A. M. Alden, the Assistant; both of these men are able and the physician who is enabled to have their assistance should congratulate himself as should the Oklahoma Municipality who calls on them for an opinion.

A CITY UNDER ARREST.

Muskogee is probably about the only city on earth who has its entire set of city officials under arrest. The city officials are charged by the County Superintendent of Health with violating the sanitary regulations of the state by permitting its sewage to flow into Coody's Creek without proper and scientific treatment. The sewage proposition has long been a vexatious one in Muskogee, many thousands of dollars have been spent in the construction of septic tanks and sewage disposal projects that do not dispose of or render inert the sewage. The health authorities feel that sufficient time has been given the city to correct the evil and finding other means unproductive have placed the matter into the courts by arresting practically all the city officials.

EXCHANGES

Appendicitis.

L. G. Guerry, Columbus, S. C. (*Journal A. M. A.*, January 1), reports his experiences with a consecutive series of 545 cases of appendicitis operations with only 2 deaths, these occurring in the first 100 patients operated on. This experience proves, in his opinion, that there is a factor in the surgical mortality that is not fully appreciated or provided against. In this total of 545 there were 240 chronic cases calling for an interval operation, with no deaths, as might have been expected. Of acute cases, 92 patients were operated on within 36 hours. His rule so far as he has one, is, he says, to operate as soon as the diagnosis is made, provided it can be made within 36 hours. After that the pathologic conditions are different; the third and fourth day cases are the ones that furnish the mortality statistics. Guerry holds that there is a definite tendency to localization in cases of appendicitis complicated with suppuration; there were 213 cases of this kind in the series; 68 of these were first seen on the third or fourth day of the disease. The pulse in most cases was .135, temperature 104F., vomiting, distention, pinched features and some delirium were also present. None of these patients was operated on at once, but all were treated according to the Ochsner method which he thinks is life saving, at least in the practice of the ordinary surgeon and practitioner. Guerry emphasizes the fact that none of these patients was operated on immediately and none died. It must, he says, have been genuine insight in Ochsner to recognize that the chief factor in dissemination of the peritoneal infection is the vermicular movement of the small intestine and that physiologic rest is the rational treatment of the diseased process, thus enabling Nature the chance she seeks to localize the disease. Gastric lavage, also is rational as it carries off the regurgitated contents of the small intestine and favors the attainment of physiologic rest of both organs. Guerry does not wish to be considered extreme but

he desires to emphasize the importance of ultizing and aiding the natural forces, and of using surgical discrimination and judgment in these cases. In almost all cases, he operated through the McBurney incision when drainage is needed he drains through a stab wound to one side. The rule is to remove the appendix but there are exceptions to this rule. He believes it better to enter the peritoneal cavity by Ware's modification of McBurney's method, pack off the infected area and remove the diseased tissue. One of his patients who died had renal tuberculosis and succumbed on the eighth day with postoperative anuria. The other fatal case was that of a child who had been ill 10 days and died of a continuation of the peritonitis.

Serum Diagnosis of Syphilis.

Howard Fox, New York (*Journal A. M. A.*, August 27), gives a comprehensive detailed review of the literature of the serodiagnosis of syphilis during the past year from June, 1909, to June, 1910. He summarizes the results of his critical review as follows: "1. The various precipitation tests for the diagnosis of syphilis are too unreliable to be of much practical value. 2 The Schurmann color reaction has been extensively tried and found to be worthless. 3. The favorable results that have been claimed for the intradermic reaction are at least encouraging, as the performance of the test seems to be simple. 4. Excellent results have been claimed by Richard Weil for his cobra-venom test. They are, however, somewhat lessened in value by the fact that very considerable experience is required to perform the reaction. 5. Further investigations are required to show whether the leuko-diagnosis, the antitryptic index or the meiostagmin reaction can be used as diagnostic aids in syphilis. The results obtained with the Muck-Holzmann reaction appear to be of no value. 6. The artificial antigens of Sachs and Rondoni, and of Schurmann for the Wassermann reaction have not succeeded in replacing the use of organ extracts. 7. The use of barium sulphate suggested by Wechselmann to remove the disturbing complementoids from the patient's serum has apparently given greater proportion of positive reactions than those obtained by the original Wassermann method. 8. The use of urine in place of serum for the Wassermann reaction is not to be recommended. 9. No single modification has as yet entirely replaced the original Wassermann method. The modifications of Hecht and of Stern have apparently given good results abroad, while the Noguchi test has received almost universal recognition in America. The methods of Bauer and of Tschernogubow second test appear to be of much less value. 10. To the list of non-syphilitic diseases which at times give a positive Wassermann reaction, must apparently be added acute lupus erythematosus. It has also been found that many individuals give a positive reaction following ether narcosis. 11. The diagnostic value of a positive reaction is generally recognized. There is no general agreement as yet regarding the value of the test as a guide for treatment. 12. From recent serologic investigations it would appear that syphilis plays a very important role in the etiology of aortic insufficiency. Syphilis is probably of more importance in the causation of nerve-deafness than has been previously supposed. There is apparently little or no relation between syphilis and ozena. 13. A new field seems to have been opened by the Wassermann reaction for the discussion of the problem of the inheritance of syphilis and of the interpretation of the laws of Colles and Profeta. 14. In the field of pathologic-anatomic diagnosis the Wassermann reaction seems to be of considerable value.

15. Serologic examinations have shown that the percentage of syphilitic infections in prostitutes is extremely high."

PERSONAL

Dr. J. C. Ambrister, of Chickasha, is spending the summer in Colorado.

Dr. W. F. Hays, of Claremore, spent his vacation in the mountains of Arkansas.

Dr. J. Hutchings White of Muskogee, has been doing Post-graduate work in Boston.

Dr. W. L. Kendall, of Durant, is taking Post-graduate work in Rochester, Minnesota, with the Mayo's.

Dr. Milton K. Thompson, of Muskogee, is suffering from an attack of infection due to an abrasion of his finger.

Dr. W. L. Gleason, of Fairview, spent the month of August in the Chicago Polyclinic doing post-graduate work.

J. C. Ellis, of Hugo, who has been in Europe attending the Vienna Clinics for three months contemplates extending his stay for another three months.

Dr. J. C. Mahr, State Commissioner of Health has received reports of a case of Infantile Paralysis in Major County and a death from the same disease in Woods County.

Claremore is to have a hospital, the building now being under construction and practically ready for patients. It is owned and controlled by local physicians of Claremore and Rogers County.

Dr. C. E. DeGroot, of Muskogee, and Miss Edna Shinn, of Russelville, Arkansas, were married in the latter place August 22nd. After a short trip to St. Louis and New York they will return to Muskogee. Here's happiness and prosperity to them.

The Medical Department of the Kansas University will give their annual course of surgical and medical clinics during September in the Hospitals at Kansas City, Mo. These Clinics are becoming of importance and will draw a large attendance from the Southwest.

DR. BUFFO DEAD.

Dr. Umberto Buffo, of McAlester, died August 22, 910. Funeral services were held from St. Johns Catholic Church on August 26, interment was had at the Catholic Cemetery in North McAlester. Dr. Buffo's death is mourned by a large circle of friends and acquaintances.

STANDING COMMITTEES OKLA-HOMA STATE MEDICAL AS-SOCIATION.

On Public Policy and Legislation.

Dr. A. L. Blesh, Chairman, Oklahoma City.

Dr. J. C. Mahr, Oklahoma City.
Dr. C. S. Bobo, Norman.
Dr. D. A. Myers, Lawton.
Dr. C. A. Thompson, Muskogee.

MEMBER OF THE NATIONAL LEGISLATIVE COUNCIL OF THE AMERICAN MEDICAL ASSOCIATION.

Dr. J. M. Byrum, Shawnee, Oklahoma.

COMMITTEE ON NECROLOGY.

Dr. E. S. Ferguson, Oklahoma City.
Dr. L. T. Gooch, Lowton.
Dr. Chas. Blickensderfer, Shawnee.

Dr. J. N. McCormack, National Organizer for the American Medical Association, will spend the month of October in Oklahoma at the following places:

Vinita	October 3
Muskogee	October 4
Eufaula	October 5
McAlester	October 6
Atoka	October 7
Durant	October 8
Hugo	October 9
Ardmore	October 10
Pauls Valley	October 11
Norman	October 12
Oklahoma City	October 13
Chickasha	October 14
Duncan	October 15
Waurika	October 16
Lawton	October 17
Anadarko	October 18
Hobart	October 19
Clinton	October 20
El Reno	October 21
Watonga	October 22
Cherokee	October 23
Enid	October 24
Guthrie	October 25
Shawnee	October 26
Holdenville	October 27
Okmulgee	October 28
Sapulpa	October 29
Tulsa	October 30
Bartlesville	October 31

It should be borne in mind that some slight change may be necessary in the above program on account of delayed trains, etc., and if for any reason, Dr. McCormack cannot reach a place on the date he is scheduled to appear in that place the meeting at that town will have to be cancelled and the regular meeting held in the next town on the fixed date.

SURGICAL MISTAKES IN CHILDREN.

S. W. Kelley, Cleveland, Ohio, (*Journal A. M. A.*, September 3), calls attention to the necessity for caution when operating on children, and gives examples, coming under his observation or to his knowledge, of fatalities from unexpected hemorrhage and bad effects from operations performed when unsuspected or overlooked disease like rhinitis, whooping cough or pharyngitis existed. It is a mistake to perform an operation on a child when a fever temperature indicates the possible onset of an acute disease. A case of the bad effects of neglect to promptly remove foreign bodies from the larynx is reported. There is no safety until such are removed. Mistakes of diagnosis in children are not uncommon. Many a case of retropharyngeal abscess has been mistaken for tonsilitis, and he reports a case in which it was taken for uremia. Other instances of diseases liable to cause mistakes are mentioned, such as empyema, intussusception and appendicitis diagnosed instead of pneumonia. The article is full of striking instances, too numerous to be given in an abstract, of diagnostic and surgical mistakes in treating children. Many conditions are present in the child which never or seldom occur in the adult, and it is a great mistake to consider that we can be guided by the surgery of adults in the surgical treatment of children.

FOR SALE.

For $2,000.00 in cash I will sell my nice new 7-room dwelling, two room office in yard, good barn and stables, office fixtures and household furniture, all new and turn a $5,000.00 practice in a good farming country, good town 2,000, ethical competition, reason for selling going to Texas.

DR. JOHN T. VICK,

Fort Towson, Okla.

BOOKS RECEIVED

The Practical Medicine Series, Volume IV, devoted to Gynecology, Edited by Emilius C. Dudley, A. M., M. D., Professor of Gynecology Northwestern University Medical School; Gynecologist to St. Luke's and Wesley Hospitals, Chicago. And C. Von Bachelle, M. S., M. D., Assistant Professor of Obstetrics Chicago Polyclinic and College of Physicians and Surgeons; Gynecologist to the German Hospital, Chicago. Series 1910. Chicago. Bound in cloth, Price, $1.25.

THE YEAR BOOK PUBLISHERS, 40 Dearborn Street, Chicago.

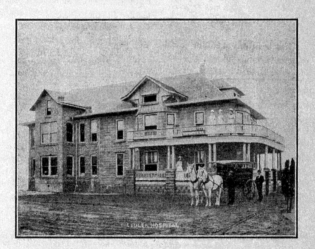

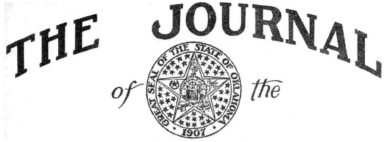

Oklahoma State Medical Association.

VOL. III.	MUSKOGEE, OKLAHOMA, OCTOBER, 1910.	NO 5

DR. CLAUDE A. THOMPSON, Editor-in-Chief.

ASSOCIATE EDITORS AND COUNCILLORS.

DR. J. A. WALKER, Shawnee.

DR. CHARLES R. HUME, Anadarko.

DR. F. R. SUTTON, Bartlesville.

DR. I. W. ROBERTSON, Dustin.

DR. J. S. FULTON, Atoka.

DR. JOHN W. DUKE, Guthrie.

DR. A. B. FAIR, Frederick.

DR. W. G. BLAKE, Tahlequah.

DR. H. P. WILSON, Wynnewood.

DR. J. H. BARNES, Enid.

Entered at the Postoffice at Muskogee, Oklahoma, as second class mail matter, June, 1909.

This is the Official Journal of the Oklahoma State Medical Association. All communications should be addressed to the Journal of the Oklahoma State Medical Association, English Block, Muskogee, Oklahoma.

THE HYGIENE OF INFANCY AND CHILDHOOD.

BY DR. G. W. LITTLE, OKMULGEE, OKLAHOMA.

Oliver Wendell Holmes has said, "To properly train up a child in the way he should go, you should begin with his grandmother." The prenatal influences may be vicious and beneficent and the training of the progenitors would be to eliminate the vicious and preserve the beneficent. Obviously such training in the individual is beyond attainment but is to be reached only in the mass and by systematic, concerted effort on the part of all classes and professions, and especially under the leading of the medical, the sociologic and religious workers.

Every child has a claim to a good birthright. Of course he can not enforce such a demand for he is a passive agent in the matter. But society generally must safe guard

such a claim for the race, while individually the family must stand for the health and well-being of its own offspring. This is a matter of too little thought. The raising of people has less thought and care than the raising of blooded stock.

The old adage that "The God of love is blind" and the other one that "Love laughs at lock-smiths" may still be true, and yet admit the choosing of mates for life wisely, and with some scientific foresight, with a little help from the conservitors of social progress. But as to the immediate care that prenatal forces may combine to the best advantage so that the individual child may claim his birthright of being "well born" a few hints may not be amiss.

THE MOTHER.

Physical well being on the part of the mother is a condition to be sought for; enough work to employ mind and hand; too little to engender constant fatigue; enough sleep, but not too much; good reading and a good mental outlook on life, and the conditions for good birth are about ideal, and such as should be striven for in every home, where a child is expected.

THE INFANT.

The baby is usually the object of much congratulation on his arrival, but whether this is deserved may depend on his future career, which would have a brighter promise if he is allowed to lead a very simple life during these initial months of his puzzling career. At the best he will enter the turmoil of life soon enough. He should be allowed to sleep—to rouse and eat; to sleep again, and on each morning of his life enjoy the luxury of a bath with its exhilaration and stimulus. He needs no entertainment; neither is he a "pink doll" that every neighbor woman should kiss and handle and fatigue him because he is helpless. Warmth, food, and air are all he needs, with cleanliness, and the exercise he will get for himself as he kicks and squirms and rolls on his bed. At the proper time and in his own way the greater activities will assert themselves.

FOOD AND DRINK.

For his nourishment nature has provided sustenance, and unless there is some reason for doing otherwise, the mother's breast should be the source of the food supply for the infant at least six months of its existence. Added to this at frequent intervals water boiled and cooled, should be given in abundance. Food should be given at regular intervals to the baby and the clock should determine these times. And water should be given to relieve thirst and to satisfy the cravings of the child at any time. These simple rules will obviate much illness on the part of the child in its early years and teach it proper habits of life at an early period in its existence. I recently heard another reason for giving the child water, viz: "That it should be given some water as soon as born, so it would not get "three months colic." If this rule appeals to you sufficiently to warrant its use, it will be only along the right lines, but not for the reason given in the rule itself. Even among intelligent people, queer things have credence, and our removal from superstition is not always so great as our wisdom indicate when we smile at the man who plants his potatoes in the dark of the moon; or carries a buckeye in his pocket to ward off rheumatism.

So I say food and drink and sleep are the three elements for the young child that are essential.

Besides these clothing for protection and warmth.

CLOTHING.

Any soft, porous, seamless material is best for the baby with its tender skin. Starched, ruffled furbeloes and be-ribboned garments are an abomination from a hygienic stand-point and should have no place in baby's wardrobe. Mothers should refrain from torturing their little ones with these, even though the fashion papers may abound with the fancy pictures and they, themselves, may wish to be incarcerated in these "fancy doins' " to the banishment of comfort and the invitation of many ills.

EARLY HABITS.

The formation of habits should be started early. The child should never be rocked to sleep—or walked to sleep; or those means used which are so common with the mothers. Every child has a desire to exercise his lungs by crying, and if nothing hurts him, let him cry. Every child has a right to kick and wiggle and twist and squirm on the bed and not sleep if he wishes to do so. Moreover, if he is put on the bed to sleep and taught that from the first much weariness of the flesh and annoyance of the mind will be avoided. The child should sleep in the open air as much as possible, and his daily bath should not be neglected. Constant and early acquaintance with water is a feature too often neglected in the homes of our country.

SHIELDING FROM DISEASE.

The infant should be shielded from all approach of disease. If he can be kept from having the usual childhood diseases, the better off will he be. It is a popular fallacy that the child is better to have these diseases and be over with them than to have them after he is grown up. They never reckon that he may not "grow up," or grow up and be afflicted all his after years because of his childhood trouble, which the ignorance or criminal heartlessness of his parents allowed him to have. The old proverb "An ounce of prevention is worth a pound of cure" today is the slogan of medical research, and is a basic and rational scientific principle, one that should be applied to the present day care of children. For the strength, hope and purity of the race of tomorrow will depend on the care, health and moral fibre of the training today, and other things being equal, a sound, strong body is more apt to shelter a sound mind and stalwart moral stamina than a weak body.

NEW DANGERS.

As the child grows up new dangers arise, due in most part to the fast age in which we live, and the artifical life with which we are surrounded. It is an age of raising dollars rather than of raising children. The more luxurious air tight houses gives rise to more exposure to disease and physical infirmities which even the warning of science and medical education cannot overcome, and which the sanitary engineer is unable to combat.

THE MODERN SCHOOL.

The school of today is a menace to the health of the child. During the years he should be growing and developing physically he is penned in the school. The school men of today are the most popular, who can get some new fad, no matter what, or how nonsensical or useless, and add it to the already burdened system in the schools. It does not need to have a basis in reason. Hence the old rational system is subverted and the child is made over into an old person before he has reached the age where reason and judgment are active.

The industrials are added in even the kindergarten, so that the child of today has no childhood, and at the time when he should be entering the real life of the school, he is in the midst of the industrial turmoil which makes up the business of life with its struggles.

SCHOOL AGE.

The child is put into school too young. It is essentially wrong to put children at tasks at the age of 3 or 4 years, and especially indoors. If they must be cared for in the kindergarten let it be in the open air. The foundation for future nervous breakdown is laid in these early years when the child should be developing the physical instead of the mental. I say this notwithstanding the published statement of the Honorable. James Bryce, Ambassador from England, who two weeks ago in Kansas City, speaking of the schools, said: "The children in America are not put into school early enough. They should be started at the age of four years."

The parents, generally, in this country are intelligent enough in this generation to teach their children at home, the little beginnings of the educational life and if they are given their free childhood rights of home and parents till they are eight or nine years old, and are then put to school, they will outstrip their fellows before the sixth grade is reached, and will have greater freedom from nervous and other troubles.

TOO MANY STUDIES.

Again there are too many studies. A smattering only of most of them is obtained anyhow, and it would be better for teacher and for children, if only the essentials were taken up, leaving the technical and manual studies for the high schools and colleges.

MUSIC.

The teaching of music in the schools may be all right, but for parents to put their little tots at the piano in these early years is but inviting ills of many kinds; as eye strain, nervous troubles, headaches, and heartaches, as in after years, the women are nervous wrecks, traceable to this added, heavy burden imposed upon them as children by parents enthusiastic for a musical accomplishment, and at the behest of some music teacher whose purse will be richer for this same enthusiasm for music. Even those great masters who are musical geniuses from childhood paid the penalty in wracked nerves, terriffic headaches due to eye strain, and by robbing the world of years of brilliant and beautiful melody because of graves filled early in life. How many a little girl, after a day of nervous strain in school goes home, not to play or rest, but to hear her mother say, *her* mother who should protect her, to hear that mother

say "Now you must practice your lesson on the piano. Miss Jones will be here tomorrow to hear your lesson and you will need to practice it for a long time." But mamma, "I am so tired and I want to go out and play a little." But mamma is inexorable, and the little girl, that needs the out doors and the relaxation of exercise and freedom, is driven to the practice.

Too soon will the children be ushered in to the strenuous life without our hurrying them into it. N. P. Willis too clearly saw all this when he wrote, seeing a child tired of play:

"Tired of play! Tired of play!
What hast thou done the livelong-
day!
*   *   *   *   *   *
There will come an eve to a longer
day
That will find thee tired, but not
with play,
When thou wilt lean as thou lean'st
now,
With drooping limbs and an aching
brow,
And wish that the shadows would
faster creep,
And long to go to thy quiet sleep."

IMPROVEMENTS.

Improvements in these things are suggested as follows:

Parents to show some humanity in caring for their children with a look at their future that is not measured by dollars. Some common sense will help in this. Fewer studies at school and a longer time for work. Also more individual attention and care that only fundamental work be given in the lower grades. The "fads" should not be practiced on the helpless children. The present system is wrong, largely due to the "fadists," and on an unreasonable basis for work. The address of Jenkin

Lloyd Jones, the genial, big hearted, promoter of that mighty force in Chicago known as Lincoln Center, is on the right course. He says in part as follows:

"This is the day of "practical education." "Domestic science" for the girls and "Manual training" for the boys. The saw and hammer, the dough-board and the chafing dish are deemed as necessary tools for the proper education of our boys and girls, as are the spelling books, the slate, the diction. ary and the masterpieces of the bards. I quarrel not with this insistent so-called "technical education." Let it be tried. No knowledge or skill can come amiss. But give me the girl for a farmer's wife who is an intimate of Shakespeare's Portia, has suffered with Pompilla and who knows her Romola. These preparations will make the lore of the barnyard, the skill of the kitchen easy and sure. Not but that the knowledge of breadmaking and stocking darning and setting hens is important. It is a case of not loving Caesar less, but Rome more. Let the young lady at school learn how to build, furnish and occupy the "Castle in Spain" and I will trust her to make beautiful and happy the coal miner's cabin in Pennsylvania or the sod house in Nebraska. It is important that the boy preparing himself for the business of the world should know his multiplication table, understand the mysteries of the day book and the ledger, be competent to harness a horse, drive a nail without hitting his thumb, and when needs be, sew on a button dexterously; but it is far more important that the young man who is to enter business should have the fine discrimination of the difference between "meum" and "teum"—between the "mine" and the "thine;" that he has caught sight of the Gospel of co-operation, that he believes with Emerson, in

"The identity of the law of gravitation, with purity of heart, and that the ought, that

duty is one thing with science, with beauty and with joy."

McCormick and the other reaper builders made the complex industrial life of the Mississippi valley possible, but it took an Emerson and a Lincoln to make that complex life tolerable and to save the big farm and the great granaries from becoming a blight and a curse, a mill stone around the neck of the body politic that will drag it down into the deep sea of oblivion."

MEDICAL INSPECTION.

Medical inspection of all schools with an adaption of work to the needs of the pupils and a careful oversight of all pupils having defective health; errors of refraction should be corrected; throats examined and treated; nervous and backward children cared for in the proper way are among the things we need.

Individual Drinking Cups are already here.

Sanitary Sweeping should be enforced in all public and private schools and as far as possible in the homes. This may be had as soon as school boards and janitors can be taught to do so, a matter of no easy accomplishment.

Proper Ventilation with open windows and doors, with clothing suitable to such a mode of life, and with sunshine accessible to as much of the room as possible, should all be provided for by the school of the near future.

PUBERTY.

As the age of puberty approaches the girl should be instructed concerning herself by the mother in the home, if the mother can do so in a proper spirit and with good judgment. The father should see to it that the boy has suitable teaching for his guidance at this period of life. This presupposes fathers and mothers of proper moral and mental habits that they will appreciate the vast importance of this question. In the schools this might be taught to the boys and girls separately if there is a teacher especially adapted to such work. It is a problem of no small import, not only to the physical and intellectual development of the children, but also for their future welfare, and value to the state.

HABITS.

Habits are of value from a hygienic standpoint. Habits of eating, sleeping and work may determine much of the future man or woman. Sleep should begin before 10:00 p. m. and for the young child much earlier. The boys and girls of eight to sixteen should eschew late hours, street loafing and flirting. Smoking is a detriment to all—young and old.

Alcoholic stimulants are needed only on rare occasions as a medicine, never otherwise.

This is a discursive paper and I hope a suggestive one. You can get statistics from your text books and magazines. The future of our citizens is wrapped up in the child of today; he is our great national asset.

DISCUSSION .

Dr. G. R. Gordon, Wagoner:

I think that was an excellent paper and ideal, and I would like to only make this little addition, and that is with regard to the idea of not too highly seasoning the pastry we usually have. And another thing, so many mothers and fathers rush their children into the fashion of society. We should be very careful and hold our children back.

Dr. Gossom, Custer City:

I want to say it was a very fine paper and voices my sentiments.

Dr. Coons, El Reno:

I would like to mention something that I think was omitted, and that is the use of opiates for young children. The doctor didn't mention that, and I think that is one of the worst things of mankind today.

Dr. J. J. Hardy, Poteau:

It is unfortunate that the laity can't get such a paper as that. I wish we could get it in every home in the State.

SURGICAL TREATMENT OF BONE TUBERCULOSIS—REPORT OF TWO CASES.

BY DR. L. H. HUFFMAN, HOBART, OKLAHOMA.

The almost universal prevalence of Tuberculosis, the enormous death rate together with the possible prevention and cure, have focused the attention of the world on this disease. Physicians, Philanthropists and Educators are all doing an active part to control the spread of the disease. The opportunities for infection are so frequent that the education of the people in every way to raise the standard of vitality becomes the first step in active warfare to blot out the disease. At no time in the history of the world has there been so much hard work to arouse the public interest in the subject of health. The treatment of bone tuberculosis has an important place in surgery. After the correct diagnosis is made of the diseased bone or joint the surgical treatment will either stay the progress of tuberculous disease or remove it. Tuberculous inflammation of the bone is usually a subacute process not as rapidly destructive as an acute osteo-myelitis. The process oftentimes going on without pain or discomfort to the patient. Tuberculous ostitis however is often converted into an acute infectious process by becoming a mixed infection. The profession has come to look upon these lesions as surgical rather than medical. There is no surgical disease in which well considered promptness in regard to treatment is more signally rewarded than in tuberculous affections of the bone.

We may draw the following conclusions in regard to the various forms of infections in generalized tuberculosis:

1. It is impossible to gain any knowledge as to the point of entry from either the location or the degree of development of the tuberculous lesions.

2. Fetal infection is proved but not common.

3. Infection through the mouth, tonsils and pharynx is of frequent occurrence and may be produced by inhalation or ingestion.

4. Primary infection does occur by inhalation through the lungs.

5. Infection through the intestinal tract is definitely proven.

6. Bones may be infected through the intestinal tract as well as through the respiratory tract.

Secondary infection of the lungs occurs but rarely after tuberculosis of the bones or joints. In tubercular arthritis almost any joint may be involved. Knee, ankle and elbow are probably most often affected. The disease is more frequent in males than females and more frequent in children from one to five years of age. The fact remains however that the study of statistics prove that old people do not have as great an immunity from tuberculous bone disease as might be supposed. The children inherit a predisposition which is most marked as a rule, as in this case to be reported, when the mother is the tuberculous parent, to overcome a tuberculous predisposition to benefit the child, the treatment should begin before the birth in a general way. The best hygienic enviroment, freedom from

care and worry, good food, systematic respiratory exercises are the best means for the mother to overcome tuberculous predisposition of her offspring. In almost all families where you find the children infected the mother is so situated that she has to do hard work. Municipal philanthropy should aid such mothers. The newly born child should likewise have the best hygenic environment. These children especially should be watched carefully as to adenoids and other obstructions to free breathing.

While congenital tuberculosis is considered extremely rare there is no doubt that a tubercular mother may infect the fetus by the bacilli gaining entrance to the fetal circulation through the placenta without any placental lesion. The chances for infection of the fetus is much greater where the placenta has a local lesion.

The placenta is not a perfect filter for micro-organisms. In the first case I report, the tubercular arthritis is surely the result of placental transmission and it must be borne in mind as a definite possibility in all cases in which the question of marriage and pregnancy of tubercular women come up for consideration. We are forced to recognize heredity. The factor of hereditary predisposition outranks any of the approximate causes, such as contagion, bad sanitation, overcrowded tenements, alcoholic and other excesses. The first undertaking in the campaign waged for the extermination of tuberculosis is to put a stop to the propogation of human beings who bring with them to this life the peculiar liabilities or susceptibility to the disease. Too much stress can not be placed on the hereditary nature of the malady and less thought on the contagious factor. In spite of our wishes to the contrary we are in a measure what our progenitors were and there is no escape from the laws of nature that the characteristics of the fathers and mothers are indelibly stamped on their offspring. The public is in need of educators along this line.

Public schools should receive lectures pertaining to the laws of health covering this subject. The present advancement in civilization requires a stronger race of men, mentally and physically than at any time in the past. Physicians in their close contact with the home should impress the young people of the danger of the marriage of consumptives.

In the treatment of tuberculosis of bones and joints outdoor life night and day is as essential as in the medical cases. Early diagnosis is important to prevent deformity and ankylosis. Many cases are treated for rheumatism. Treatment by sunshine, fresh air, rest and proper mechanical and surgical procedure will prevent and cure without deformity many patients with hip-joint disease or tubercular arthritis at the knee and smaller joints. Many thousand doses of pure air in twenty-four hours is far better than three or four doses of nauseous drugs that disturb digestion. It has been shown that 90 per cent. of bone and joint cases come from the poorer classes. We can do much in conquering the disease by building up the resisting power of the patient. In children the majority of these patients are fed on artificial food, and this becomes the most serious question to confront the physician. The surrounding conditions especially in the cities make it almost impossible to have mothers' milk for food. The vitality of these patients is far below par, consequently more trouble to manage the feeding than in a normal healthy infant.

The housing of patients with surgical tuberculosis in tents is unsatisfactory. Buildings with roomy porches for beds connected with private rooms or with wards which have moveable window sashes that the beds may be either out-doors or indoors giving when needed the advant-ages of a warm room for surgical dressings, are preferable. The same precaution is required however to care for the cast off dressings in an aseptic manner as in the case of pulmonary tuberculosis to destroy the sputum. The protection from cold, and the use of good food are two essential items in the care of these patients.

The surgical procedures in all cases where the point of infection is accessible the indications are exposure of part affected by incision as free as possible and a thorough removal of all diseased bone. For instance, exsections of the joints to remove the diseased ends of the bones to destroy the established focus of the disease.

It is not my purpose in this paper to discuss the operative procedures on the different bones but to view the tuberculous lesions of the bones from a surgical standpoint. Omitting all reference to Potts Disease, and to abbreviate an extensive subject, will state briefly that in the treatment of hip-joint disease the most common of all tuberculous bone trouble, the injection of mixtures used early in the disease often give good results. A favorite mixture consists of creosote three parts, iodoform 7 parts, and ether 25, olive oil 50 parts. Repeating injections every three to five days for a period of one to two months. Beck's Bismuth paste injection may be used in sinus tracts.

Weight bearing with short spica bandage facilitates the employment of out door life and shortens the time of treatment. In the treatment of this form of tuberculosis as in all other forms we can hasten recovery and influence the final results by vaccine therapy.

I believe that a great majority of patients with bone tuberculosis would secure nearly perfect functional and anatomic results if they would come to the surgeon early enough, and they could be placed under proper hygienic conditions, with suitable measures adopted for the prevention of secondary infection, the joints be perfectly immobolized for sufficient length of time and by the use of vaccine therapy.

The first case I wish to report is one of unquestionable placental transmission of tubercular bacilli.

Case 1. E. F. A male patient born August, 1908, was of normal size and weight, was fed on mother's milk. The family history showed that both parents were living, father normal. State of health mother pulmonary tuberculosis, seven children in family, four living, oldest son died in his sixteenth year of typhoid fever, son nine years of age died of intestinal tuberculosis, May 2nd this year, one child died in infancy.

I saw the patient first when it was fourteen days old, he had a slight elevation of temperature and very fretful. On the seventeenth day it was noticed that there was swelling at the ankle joints. No particular change was noted from this time until he was placed in the hospital for treatment when 31 days old.

Physical Examination. Both hip-joints both ankle joints were swollen also the left wrist. There was some redness around the joints and at the ankle and soft on palpation. The muscular atrophy a marked feature in tuberculous joints had progressed rapidly from the time the baby was first seen at two weeks of age up to this time. The muscles were in a more or less constant condition of contraction. The abscesses grew rapidly and there may have been mixed infection on account of the abscesses coming out so near the skin. The patient was fed on diluted cows milk with the addition of a small amount of milk sugar at intervals of four hours

Operation. A free incision was made into each hip joint. The left hip was opened on the lower external portion of the buttocks, the right was opened on the internal side at the groin, the incisions were made through a good thickness of healthy tissue, the cavities lightly curetted and wiped out with iodoform gauze. Tube drainage was left in for two days with great care used to keep the cavities sterile, after the drainage was removed sterile saline solution was used twice daily to cleanse the cavity. At the ankles two openings were made, one on either side of the joint, no drainage was left in the wound, but the saline cleansing solution was used in the same manner as at the hips. The acute symptoms were relieved almost immediately. At the end of thirty days the patient was dismissed from the hospital, and continued to improve making final recovery without any ankylosis.

No splints nor plaster paris has been used up to the present time. The patient however has a typical tuberculos deformity of the right hip which began to show as early as he was able to stand. The foot is slightly inverted and the leg is shortened. This is a case of double-hip joint trouble, with an infection at each ankle to complicate matters. With the present existance of deformity at the right hip, the treatment resolves itself into the proper appliances to prevent shortening of the limb. The ambulatory treatment has proven to be the most satisfactory and efficient method in cases where the acute symptoms have subsided. The general health of the patient at this time is good. He has a normal weight, with good digestion, and perfect development of the muscular system.

In the treatment of this class of cases we cannot consider constitutional measures nor local treatment. Open air treatment, sanitation, good nourishing food and the administration of certain drugs may show beneficial results and are necessary following the surgical procedures.

It is evident that the problem of the reduction of the mortality from tuberculosis is to a great extent a question of improving the environment in which individuals live who are predisposed.

The bacillus is important, but not any more so than the unfavorable conditions under which people live. By laboring to improve the unfavorable conditions the natural immunity will be strengthened, which will aid much in the success of the crusade against tuberculosis.

Case 2. L. T. A male 24 years of age, born in Missouri, a farmer by occupation. His family history showed that his father had died of cancer of the tongue at sixty years of age, mother died in her thirtieth year of pneumonia. No history of pulmonary tuberculosis. About three years before I first saw the patient he had an operation done in Kansas City for tubercular ostitis of the tibia, of a traumatic origin. The second operation was made on the same bone two years later. During this illness he had suffered pain of a mild character.

When I first saw the patient about three years after the first operation, there was a marked muscular atrophy between the knee and ankle and destruction of bone. The disease had spread from the cancellus bone at each end of the tibia to the articular cartilage, producing arthritis with abscess of the knee, also at the ankle of a milder form. The characteristic fusiform enlargement of the knee and the attitude of flexion was present. The head of the tibia was thrown backward and the limb shortened.

There was a slight increase in the heat in the joint, restriction in the movement, and considerable pain. The abscess pointed intra-articular. The constitutional state of the patient was not good. There had been slow and constant loss of body weight from the time of the first operation. As a complication tubercular disease had already made its appearance at the left wrist.

The prognosis was unfavorable and against conservative treatment. There was but little hope to preserve the function of the joint, and the danger of a mixed infection was greatly increased by the abscess. Under these circumstances the chances for good results by excision of the joint are greatly diminshed.

Ordinarily the operative treatment of the knee joint requires very careful consideration. If the tuberculous tissue is localized, an operation to eradicate the disease may produce a perfect functional result. In this case considering the fact that there had previously been two operations to eradicate the trouble, more radical measures were decided upon this operation.

Operation. A circular amputation of the long anterior flaps and short posterior flaps was done in the usual manner at the middle third of the thigh. The patient now has an artificial leg, is much more comfortable than any result that we may have obtained by excision at the knee. He gained strength and weight from the time he was dismissed from the hospital until he is now a little better than the average size. There are no symptoms of any secondary infection, the point at the wrist has been restored to a normal condition through nature's efforts.

I present this case to prove the efficiency of amputation in cases of this character to completely eradicate the focus of infection. It presents no new principle, but I feel the experience I have had with this case may be helpful to you in similar cases.

DISCUSSION.

Dr. Walker, of Shawnee, made the following remarks: "That paper forces to mind that the movements, especially in Oklahoma within the last few months, are for the betterment of the general public with relation to tuberculosis. We have read a great deal about tuberculosis in Oklahoma, and we are going to hear a great deal more, in the next few years. The ladies in Oklahoma, and especially the association of the doctor's wives have taken this subject up, and you know when the women get to talking about anything they never stop till they get results, and so we are going to get results on this tuberculosis in Oklahoma. The propriety of opening up tuberculous abscesses I doubt very much. The tubercular abscess opened up don't seem to do nearly so well as if they are left closed up and injected with some of the numerous injections that are being used now. I believe the doctor was in error when he stated that they were only using these pastes in tuberculous cases. I know Murphy is using one of his solutions for the purpose of injecting in the tuberculous joints and in his clinic he shows subjects continuously that are doing excellently well under that treatment. The Beck's are showing subjects that are even getting well under a treatment of aspiration, and are injecting them with bismuth's paste. My experience in that line has been very pleasing to me. Take these old tuberculous abscesses and drain them and keep the air from them just as much as you can and fill them all of Beck's paste, it doesn't matter how large they are, ordinarily fill them full, and maybe one injection will cure that abscess, maybe two or three, but if you don't make your opening too large you will get excellent results. He is doing the same thing with acute emphysema. He drains an ordinary chest cavity of the pus and injects it with bismuth paste with excellent results.

Dr. Smith, of Oklahoma City. The subject of bone tuberculosis is one that I think of paramount importance, not only to the surgeon, but to the man in the general practice of medicine as well. As a rule the man in general medicine is the man that sees the case first, and upon him rests the responsibility of diagnosis. It is a subject of such vast importance and vast interest, that it is next to impossible to discuss it intelligently in the limited time of four or five minutes. But in the past ten or twelve years if you will pardon me, I have had perhaps as much as ten or twelve cases of bone tuberculosis in all of its different forms and the treatment of these cases has been very well gone into. Open air, and all that we thoroughly understand, and as the doctor said that canvass is on to a finish, and will reach results a little later on. I think myself that even to the medical profession, when they want anything done and done right they turn it over to the ladies. And it is generally done right. Now when it comes to the treatment of these cases an early diagnosis is of paramount importance. That is the first thing in the treatment of any disease, is to know what you are treating and then the next thing is to know how to treat it intelligently. Beck's paste was quite a revelation to me. I want to say that the more I treat these cases the less I open them up. We have now reached a point that we are almost positively sure that we can cure these cases without making an incision into it, except where there is dead bone in it. Clean your cavity out, put in your paste, and you will have the extreme pleasure of dressing your patient about once every seven or eight days, when you had been accustomed to dressing these cases about once or twice every day. I have treated them for months and months and finally they come back to me with the same old story. We cut that short now by the method that the doctor had reference to awhile ago. Now a word in regard to the bismuth preparation the doctor referred to. I have used that in the last six or eight months. I want to say this, before I go any further, that I never undertake to treat a case of bone tuberculosis without having a picture taken of it so that I can see the extent of the disease, and what I am doing. And then from month to month, or week to week as the case may be I have another picture taken. Tuberculosis of the bone, in a vast majority of instances, commences in the embryo. I wish I might dwell on this subject a few minutes and the mode of transmission of that germ, and so on. It is a physiological fact that we ought to study more. As the doctor stated in his paper the prevalence is from one to three, and a little above that, I rather say from three to thirteen has been my experience and observation, corresponding with the statistics. Now the injection of the formalin glycerine does what. It has a physiological action to perform. It destroys the tubercular germ and as a result you have a normal condition instead of the pathological condition that previously existed. I usually inject, according to the condition of the patient, anywhere from one to three or four ounces and in every single instance it has been with the most satisfactory results. I have one patient that has a tubercular knee that I treated in the old way and she did not get any better. I injected three times with formalin glycerine and she is walking up town every day with comparatively little effort. Stay out of the tubercular abscess just as long as you can possibly, and nature will do a great deal more than you can accomplish with the surgeon's knife.

Dr. Grosshart: This is a subject that we can all get up and talk some on, I reckon. My experience has been that the treatment of tubercular joints and tubercular bone trouble has been along the line with the doctors paper and the doctor that has just talked preceding me. And my opinion is that the least amount of surgery that can be done, is best for the patient. If you are not satisfied with your diagnosis the next step that I pursue is to put on this jar of paste. After I get my reaction

from the paste, and I believe if you will use it and use it right you will all diagnose your cases easier; you will get a reaction almost every time. If I make up my mind that that is a tubercular condition, I use the bismuth paste. After the case has progressed to the point where it has formed an abscess, the treatment that has given me the most satisfaction has been with Beck's paste.

Dr. Frick: I wish to thank the doctor for this excellent paper. There is very little left to say. I never heard a better paper on the subject. I have not used Beck's paste in abscesses. I have only used it in very few cases. It has acted very well in those cases.

Dr. Huffman: I wish to thank the doctors for their discussion of this paper.

Dr. Pearse. May I ask a question? From where do you get your authority for the statement that the hereditary tendency to consumption outweighs all other factors? That is to me a mistake so far as I know.

Dr. Huffman: In answer to that question I think the case that I have given, the first case that I reported, answers the question very clearly, from the fact of the age of the child at the time that the infection was in the child before it was born.

Dr. Pearse: One swallow does not make a summer.

Dr. Huffman: I know that is disputed to some extent. Evidently it must be a fact from the experience that men have had in treating cases of this kind, especially in the states where we find a great many of these cases. With regard to the opening of the joints in the first case that I reported, the joints were opened there from the fact that there was a possibility of a mixed infection. That it was not purely tubercular. The symptoms were acute and there was considerable redness around the joints, and the baby suffered intense pain. In fact you could hardly touch the child and the child lay in the cot with its muscles all in a state of constant contraction. And of course as it would move the joint and the muscles contracted it would suffer more pain. In regard to Murphy's method, I have seen him use it frequently myself, for two or three years, and I think that is all right. It is a very successful way to treat tubercular joints.

ANTERIOR POLIOMYELITIS.

BY DR. J. C. MAHR, STATE COMMISSIONER OF HEALTH, OKLAHOMA CITY, OKLA.

From the fact of my having been assigned to furnish a paper upon this subject, I naturally infer from my selection that you would be more interested in such information as I could give you relative to this disease, as a preventable disease which is frequently epidemic.

The Board of Health records throughout the United States show that during late years much attention has been paid to this particular disease. A number of the New England States, as well as others, in the northeastern part of the U. S. have found it necessary to class this disease among the infectious and contagious diseases, requiring that the same be reported to the local health officers. In some epidemics it has been found necessary to establish quarantine, isolating the sick from the well, maintaining this quarantine for a period of 21 days. There were a few cases of this disease reported in Oklahoma during the year 1909, in several localities near us it was a prevailing epidemic. In Marshall County there were some 11 or 12 cases during the months of August and September, while just across the river in Texas, there was a much greater number. Bryan County, which adjoins Marshall County, in the east reported some 8 cases. There were 2 cases reported from Beaver County, and 3 cases reported from Osage County, this will give you some ideas of how wide spread and far apart these cases were.

In Massachusetts, Vermont, New York, Michigan, Wisconsin, and Kansas they have had quite extensive epidemics of this disease. In examining their records as to the probable cause, we find that they have all agreed that the agency bringing about this condition of affairs could not be located. They were at a loss to know, (as had been the history of other epidemics of this disease) the cause of its origin.

Leegaard, in Norway, investigated an epidemic of 54 cases and wrote: "The disease is plainly contagious and spread along lines of communication."

Harbitz reports: "1,053 cases with 145 deaths, a mortality of 13.3 per cent in the years of 1905 and 1906," and further states: "There can be no doubt that acute polio myelitis is an infectious disease dependent upon a specific micro-organism.

Wickman, who so carefully observed an epidemic in Sweeden, reported: "That the disease appeared to spread from school houses being often carried by individuals who were not themselves affected."

Dr. Darlington, of New York, in referring to the epidemic in New York that occurred a few years ago, reported that the schools were not in session and, therefore, this could be a factor in the spread of this disease.

Dr. Harper, Secy. of the State Board of Health for Michigan, in a paper read before the National Conference of State and Provincial Health Officers, spoke of an epidemic at Eau Claire, Mich., and states that there could have been no infection as sociated with school houses as the schools were closed at that season of the year. Many other epidemics having been investigated with similar reports recorded, but it appears that we are, as yet, at the beginning of the solution of this problem. Not knowing the method of transmission of the infection, all we can do is to direct isolation for the patients as well as attendants, with thorough disinfection of all excreta and of the premises, quarantining the same should the isolation be incomplete. A few years ago Dr. Colvert, of Shawnee, reported 3 cases, as well as several others that he had observed during that season. One point Dr. Colvert brought out, was that all of these cases had occurred in a certain valley. Upon examination of the report of the epidemic that occurred in Vermont recently, attention is called that all of the cases there had occurred in a certain valley, but upon comparing the report of Dr. Harper, of Michigan, we find that the observation of the physicians there were the reverse they report that the disease was more prevalent on dusty, unsprinkled streets. Dr. Harper's investigation verified this observation. Now if you will recall the past summer, you will remember that during August and September there was a drouth in which there was practically no rain fall, it being very hot, very dry, and very dusty, and during this time an epidemic prevailed in Wisconsin and in Kansas and we had a few cases in Oklahoma. The symptomatology is about the same in all of these reports. The ages of those afflicted running from less than 1 year of age to young adult life, 20 or 21 years. The largest per cent being under five, and possibly as much as 20 per cent between 5 and 15 years of age. Male children seem more predisposed to this disease than females. A child is generally taken sick with an acute gastro intestinal disturbance, fever ranging from 100 to 105, accompanied by muscular pains in the limbs,

and head, with symptoms of convulsions. In a few days the painful and distressing initial symptoms would usually subside when there would be a day of ease, and apparent convalescense on the part of the patient, except soreness and stiffness in the limbs. This is invariably followed by paralysis of some of the extremities, and not until this time, is a positive diagnosis made. The fatal results usually depend upon the degree of paralysis. Death nearly always following when the respiratory muscles are involved. The mortality for this disease is about 15 3-10 per cent. This was the rate of mortality in Michigan, and is about the average. Dr. Harper reports a fatality of 54 and more than 300 young people made invalids by paralysis, the permanency of which cannot be definitely stated.

There was reported during the year of 1909, in Oklahoma, 117 cases of Meningitis, classified as follows:

Tubercular Meningitis	- 24
Cerebro-Spinal Meningitis	- 90 .
Infantile Paralysis	- 3

We cannot tell definitely, how many cases of acute polio myelitis we have had in the State of Oklahoma. We do not know how many of these deaths reported as Tubercular Meningitis; Cerebro-Spinal Meningitis, may have been acute anterior polio myelitis, for the reason that most of the deaths occurring from this disease, happened most too early for the attending physician to make a positive diagnosis. But this we do know, that there were 90 deaths from Meningitis; that there were more cases of acute anterior polio myelitis than was reported to the Board of Health for the year 1909.

Dr. Works, of Bryan County, reported 4 cases between July 26th and Sept. 1st. The symptoms in Dr. Works' case were fever, restlessness, vomiting, distended abdomen, symptoms of convulsions; as they have a great deal of malaria to deal with in

Bryan County, and especially at that season of the year, the doctor reports that his first diagnosis of these cases was Malarial fever not knowing the real conditions of these cases the diagnosis was made Malaria, until the appearance of the paralysis. In Marshall County, the doctors experience was about the same as that of Dr. Works.

Now to recapitulate, acute anterior polio myelitis is an acute infectious and contagious disease, frequently epidemic in character. The etiology of this disease is not well understood and unfortunately I cannot present anything on the subject. The agency bringing about this condition of affairs has not been located, such has been the history of other epidemics of this disease. I have avoided taking up etiology and pathology and only lightly refer to the symptomatology of the disease. It is the opinion, however, of the Massachusetts State Board of Health, that the cause of this disease is to be found in the intestinal tract. Investigations are being continued along this line. Prof. Theo. Smith, feels quite certain that the cause, when found, will be shown to be a bacterium of the intestinal tract. Prof. Barber, of the Medical department of the Kansas State University, made a number of experiments last fall, endeavoring to learn a specific cause for this disease. In answer to a letter I wrote him about this time, he advised me that they had not been able to make much progress for the reason that none of the cases brought to the college had been brought early enough.

As to the treatment employed, clean out the intestinal tract, keep the temperature down. Massage and electricity, in connection with strychnine are of a great deal of benefit after the acute symptoms have subsided.

'As a preventative,' a complete and thorough sprinkling of streets have been practiced in Michigan, since the epidemic of this disease. Fruits and vegetables have been ordered cooked or thoroughly cleansed before being consumed, and general cleanliness in eliminating the debris from streets and alleys is put in vogue. And, in conclusion, I desire to state that last June at the Annual Conference of the State and Provincial Health Officers in Washington, D. C., a committee was appointed to investigate and report upon this disease. Their report was made the latter-part of April of this year, and will more than likely be in print in a very short time; this will probably give us some definite information.

DISCUSSION.

By Dr. Bland, Red Fork, Okla.

The paper is well taken. He said, I believe, the prevalence of the disease is between the ages of five and twenty years and 20 per cent cured, and the prevalence of the disease is with children younger than five.

I had three cases, each leaving a marked paralysis each in one of the lower extremities. Had one occurring in the spring of the year, and all of them in the country and scattered widely apart, and they were at the age of eighteen to twenty-five months.

Now, as to the fatality of the disease, from what I have read upon it, it looks as though the prognosis as to life is usually good, but as to cure, there is little promise.

As to diagnosis, you can't hardly diagnose it until the paralysis occurs.

DIAGNOSIS AND TREATMENT OF EXTRA-UTERINE PREGNANCY WITH REPORT OF CASES.

BY DR. IRA B. OLDHAM, MUSKOGEE, OKLAHOMA.

While this subject has been so thoroughly developed within recent years it will be difficult for me to offer you anything new in diagnosis and treatment of such conditions, still it will be my effort in this paper to bring to mind some of the important points as to diagnosis and treatment that may be of value to the general practitioner and surgeon, at the same time with the hope of bringing out a thorough discussion of the subject.

Extra-uterine pregnancy is one of the pelvic conditions that we should ever bear in mind when called upon to diagnose and treat any pelvic disease in married women, especially those who have borne no children or who have had long intervals between births of children. Diagnosis of ectopic gestation is rendered often difficult before death of foetus. We have to differentiate between ovarian cysts, ovarian fibroid, pyo-salpinx, hydro-salpinx, sub-mucous fibroid, retroverted uterus and abortion. The principal difference in diagnosis between pyo and hydro-salpinx and ectopic is history of absence of previous menstrual period with other symptoms of pregnancy, also shape and size of tumor, that of ectopic corresponding in size to the approximate age of foetus with irregular outline, while the size of mass in hydro and pyo-salpinx may be larger or smaller, at the same time of elongated oval shape and smooth in its outlines; also, in pyo-salpinx we have history of previous infection, often accompanied with elevation of temperature and pain.

Sub-mucous fibroid simulates ectopic in that we have irregular bleeding, slight enlargement of uterus, absence of extra-uterine tumor except when complicated ovarian tumors and diseased tubes. In such conditions an operation often is necessary before diagnosis can positively be made. We also have premature deliveries accompanying retroversion of uterus giving rise to symptoms of ruptured tube with escape of blood in cul de sac, disappearing after uterus has been emptied.

Cases of rupture are accompanied with severe pain in the lower abdomen corresponding with affected side followed by shock, collapse, rapid pulse, subnormal temperature, rapid accumulation of blood in abdomen, on examination pelvis often found filled with doughy mass. Unfortunately this condition is more often the one which we are called upon to treat. Often giving history of symptoms indicating pregnancy, nausea, vomiting, absence of menstrual flow, usually six to eight weeks. Often before rupture occurs patient has irregular bleeding, passing shreds of membrane, sometimes entire casts of uterine cavity often mistaken for premature delivery and treated as such. We should never attempt to curette uterus in cases of supposed early abortions without first thoroughly examining pelvis for ectopic gestation, as it often occurs that rupture of tube is caused by manipulation in attempting to empty uterus. In advanced cases where the foetus has survived rupture of tube it is often difficult to make diagnosis until full term, when after false labor pain has lasted for some time and examination will reveal a large tumor on outside of uterus, uterus being about the size of three months gestation, being pressed forward against the pubis or pressed downward filling pelvic cavity; also cases of twins, one being in uterine cavity, other extra-uterine after delivery of first uterus contracts, revealing remaining foetus in abdomen. In diagnosis between ruptured tube and tubal abortion the principal points of difference are, shock and collapse more profound consequent to more profuse hemmorrhage in rupture than tubal abortion. Also mass less liable to be absorbed on account of haematocele following accumulation of blood in pelvis resulting from ruptured tube. Shock following tubal abortion very rarely if ever accompanied by sub-normal temperature, lasting shorter time, reaction more prompt than in rupture.

As to the value of vaginal puncture for differential diagnosis between pelvic abscess and ruptured tube. I shall only mention it to condemn it, as the difference in the history of the case should be sufficient to differentiate besides the loss of much valuable time in taking such steps.

TREATMENT.

Prompt surgical treatment, in my opinion, is the safest and at the same time the most conservative treatment for ectopic gestation. The so-called conservative treatment by delay after death of foetus until recovery from shock and maternal circulation is cut off, relieving danger of hemmorrhage, has many advantages; at the same time many dangers stare the patient and surgeon in the face, while waiting for such conditions to take place. We have the additional danger of secondary rupture, and infection, followed by all symptoms of first rupture, often exaggerated; also danger of extensive adhesions involving all pelvic organs as well as intestines, making operation more difficult and dangerous to patient. The delay treatment requires long confinement to bed, the average time in cases reported by Dr. Kelly being those of Fehling 54.6 days with report of ninety-one cases without a death. A majority of our patients are not able to lose the time required for such treat-

ment; at the same time the dangers above mentioned, added to the loss of time in following the non-operative course, in my opinion, would be far in excess of benefit derived from same. As to choice of operative procedure, it is my opinion that we only have one safe and rational operation for ectopic gestation, laparotomy. I shall only mention the vaginal route to condemn it, as dangerous and iftimes incomplete, the operator being often unable to complete the operation having to resort to laparotomy after failure, at the same time subjecting patient to danger of secondary hemorrhage and infection, as his troubles are only begun when operation is completed. Oft times after gauze is removed from vaginal opening hemorrhage follows; at same time if patient escapes secondary hemorrhage infection often occurs consequent to dressing abdominal wound through un-sterile openings, while laparotomy has the advantage of allowing the operator to survey entire field of operation to secure all bleeding points, remove all pathology, at same time being able to close abdomen in non-infected cases without drainage. When ectopic is complicated by infection of tube of opposite side it is better to wait for second operation where possible to do so, than to attempt to remove diseased tube and risk infecting abdominal cavity. Cases where the foetus has survived rupture and gone to full term make operation more difficult and dangerous to the patient on account of adherent placenta which may cover entire pelvis, involving broad ligaments and sigmoid, making danger of hemorrhage very great. In such cases where no particle of placenta is detached it is well to remove foetus, attach sac to abdominal wound, pack with gauze and allow placenta to escape through the wound piece by piece. But if at operation placenta is partially detached giving rise to severe hemorrhage, it is better to entirely enucleate placenta, checking hemorrhage by suture and hot packs.

CASE REPORTS.

Case No. 1. Mrs. T. Referred by a specialist for pelvic examination for supposed pregnancy on April 1st, 1907. History: Age twenty, married two years. No history of pelvic disease. Menstruation regular, last appearing about 10th of March. Slight tenderness over breasts, no vesicle irritation; examination revealed slight engorgement of uterus, soft cervix, no tumor could be found at that time. Diagnosis of probable pregnancy made, patient kept under observation till April 29th. Called April 29th about 7.30 p. m. History: Patient dressing for supper, attacked sudden pains lower left side and abdomen, followed by fainting. Condition present, pulse rapid, 160, temperature sub-normal, patient suffering great pain, severe shock; evidences of impending collapse. Examination revealed large doughy mass in pelvis; diagnosis of ectopic made, immediate operation recommended. Patient taken to hospital, operation delayed on account of light until three a. m. Laparotomy performed, mass size of walnut, rupture on left side with accompanying blood clots removed, abdomen closed without drainage, patient made uninterrupted recovery; after eighteen months giving birth to healthy child.

Case No. 2. Mrs. O. Age forty, married sixteen years, mother of four children, youngest two years old. Was seen about 7:00 a. m., February 29, 1908, by Dr. Bosley, who made diagnosis of ectopic, advising consultation and operation. Called to case about 1:30 p. m. same day. Following history given: Patient had been well up to one month prior to present attack. History of previous menstruation negative. One month ago had severe pain in lower abdomen, accompanying uterine hemorrhage, slight shock; patient confined to bed about

one week, afterward being up and around doing household duties until the morning of February 29th while getting breakfast had sudden attack of pain followed by fainting and collapse. At time I saw patient she was practically exsanguinated. An operation was advised as last resort, patient removed to hospital, laparotomy performed at 3:30, mass the size of lemon in right side, showing previous rupture and secondary rupture; abdomen filled with blood, patient very weak, and in bad condition when removed from table, did not recover from shock, died one hour after operation.

Case No. 3. Mrs. M. Age thirty, married ten years, one child nine years old, no history of pregnancy since birth of child. History of pelvic trouble diagnosed ovarian cyst. Operation advised but not done. On December 2nd, 1908, while dressing for supper patient attacked with violent pain on right side. No shock, no collapse. History: Some months before menstruation delayed for ten days, accompanied by extreme nausea and vomiting, since which time menstruation had been regular. Diagnosis ectopic was made on account of sudden sharp attack of pain associated with enlarged tube and ovary. In this case consultation was had, the consulting surgeon disagreeing with me as to diagnosis of ectopic, but agreeing that an operation was necessary to relieve existing conditions, supposed by him to be pyso-salpinx; my conclusions having been the physician to the patient for three years previous and having during that time gotten no history of infection of tubes, absence of temperature led me to believe that present condition was due to ectopic. Following day operation revealed double hydro-salpinx with tubo-ovarian pregnancy. Mass about the size of a hazelnut having ruptured at time of pain, the specimen which I will exhibit for your opinion. Patient made uninterrupted recovery.

The above cases are interesting inasmuch as they vary in history and clinical aspect, the first demonstrating the good results following prompt operative procedure; the second demonstrating the danger of delay and consequent secondary rupture, endangering the life of patient; the fourth demonstrating error in diagnosis between uterine abortion and ectopic gestation. The three points I would like to impress are prompt surgical interference, abdominal operation route; also grave danger in use of stimulents and saline solution before operation following rupture of tube. We have at this time patient with overworked heart, bleeding vessel. If salines and stimulants are administered to relieve shock before bleeding point has been secured we dilute the blood, stimulate the heart action, thereby assisting the patient in bleeding to death. On the other hand, would recommend hypodermic of morphine, elevation of hips, ligation of extremities, absolute quiet until operation is begun and bleeding point secured, after which the administration of stimulants and saline solutions.

ECLAMPSIA.

BY DR. G. A. McBRIDE, FORT GIBSON, OKLAHOMA.

The word is synonymous with convulsions and epilepsy which occur at any age and in either sex, being derived from a Greek word meaning "brilliancy." Hippocrates learned that epilepsy is often accompanied with "flashings of light" and gave to the disease the name Eclampsia; but for our purpose in this short paper we shall confine ourself to Eclampsia Gravidarum, or convulsions of pregnant and parturient women. So many hypotheses have been advanced for the causation of this disease that it has been called "one of theories." It truly seems strange at this age of scientific advancement and progress along medical lines that the absolutely true cause of this disease is yet to be discovered, inasmuch as this is the most dangerous puerperal condition with which obstetricians have to deal. Without taking up your time in referring to the probable causes of Eclampsia advanced by different obstetricians of note, we shall refer only to one or two which seem to us the most probable. An Italian physician first put forward the theory that Eclampsia was an auto-intoxication resulting from the heaping up of some substance in the system during pregnancy, holding that its presence was indicated by an increase of toxins in the blood serum. Continuing along this theory, later German obstetricians declared these toxins are attached to the molecules of albumen which is derived from the placenta connected only with a live foetus. I call your attention to the live foetus, as we may again refer to that important feature of the subject. Whether the throwing off of these toxins is a normal condition in pregnancy, or whether if normal, their presence results in no danger to the woman, provided they are neutralized by anti-toxins somewhere or somehow in the placenta and not allowed to escape into the maternal circulation. This theory is the most generally accepted, as evidently some intra-uterine toxin must be produced and non-eliminated or non-neutralized during the life of the foetus and escapes into the maternal circulation, finding lodgment in the brain, liver and kidneys, in which organs this poison seems especially to accumulate.

Still further and continuing along the same line, the disease claimed by some is due to some poisonous substance in the blood which has the power of attacking its fibrin and producing a thrombosis of the smaller veins, causing an oedema noticed first in the extremities, and further these toxins seem to have the power of producing an inflammatory condition in the cells of the kidneys and thus interfering with the function of that organ and resulting generally in a suppression of the urine. I do not believe, however, that the disturbance in the function of the kidneys is ever so severe as to produce the convulsions, *per se,* but that the convulsions occur more likely as the result of an arterial cramp in the brain. My experience is that eclampsia occurs most frequently in the primipara, and in the primipara most fatal. Perhaps a fair ratio would be six to one. Neither does one attack render the woman immune from subsequent attacks, but rather predisposes.

The following cases came under my observation: Mrs. R., age 17, primipara; family history, negative; was seized with violent convulsions January 17, 1908, at 4 a. m. At 10 a. m. the following day, thirty-hours after first convulsion, I saw her and found she had had about thirty convulsions. She was comatose; pulse 140; axilliary temperature, 101 1-2; had been given quinine, the labor pains had been frequent, but not hard during the preceding twenty-four hours; os dilated to the size of a silver dollar; neck almost obliterated; membranes not ruptured. Under chloroform os was hastily dilated; forceps applied and delivery accomplished. Child has been dead but few hours. She lived twenty-four hours after delivery, during which time she had four more convulsions and coma continued until time of death. This woman had thirty-four convulsions; her condition was not improved by delivery. The further treatment instituted in this case was subcutaneous injections of saline infusions and two drop doses of croton oil; repeated once; no reaction of any kind noted.

The conclusions in this case are that had some treatment been instituted during the latter months of pregnancy, having its object the correction of the oedeatous condition of the entire body and had delivery been effected at the beginning of confinement, the termination would have probably been different; but after having had thirty convulsions and waiting twenty-four hours from the first and finding her in deep coma, no reaction could be induced even after instrumental delivery.

Case No. 2. Mrs. R., sister of above woman; same husband; primipara; age 19; weight about 160; limbs, face, hands, eyes extremely oedematous; was seized with convulsions March 10, 1910, at 5 a. m. I saw her one hour later; pulse 130; axiliary temperature 101; semi-conscious; pupils dilated threatened with another convulsion; os firm and undilated; under chloroform with some difficulty, the os was dilated and version (head was presented) was attempted, failing, and she having had another convulsion, forceps were applied to the head and delivery affected. During the following twenty-four hours she had four more convulsions, at the end of which time she became semi-conscious, in which condition she remained for twenty-four hours longer, when consciousness returned. Croton oil was given twice in two-drop doses, producing free evacuation. Post partum hemorrhage was free and no effort made to check it until after a very large quantity of blood had escaped. Subcutaneous infusion of saline solution was repeated every four hours for the first twenty-four after delivery. After second day recovery uneventful. Child lived. Kidneys required repeated stimulation for first week, after which they became normal in function.

Case No. 3. Mrs. B., age 38; primipara, with following family history: 4 brothers, 2 sisters living, all healthy; father died with Brights disease at the age of 68; time of confinement due; had slight convulsion two hours before I saw her; found her extremely oedematous; very weak, able to speak only in a whisper; respiration 30; pulse 150 had had six or eight light labor pains; asked if I thought she would live. Soon afterward had a convulsion and died. Believing that the child was alive I hastened to dilate the os and applied forceps, and thirty or forty minutes after her death delivered her of a live posthumous child, which still lives, now about six years old.

Case No. 4. Mrs. B., age 30; primipara; family history good; nothing untoward in personal history; up to the present time had always been healthy; had had the usual diseases of childhood; strong, robust; weight about 150; no oedema, no epigastric pain; no albumen in the urine and the quantity of urine normal; in fact, her physical condition in every respect appeared normal. During the first stage of labor the nurse noted a slight staring with eyes temporarily fixed for a brief space of time, perhaps three seconds. This was not followed by coma or unconsciousness. The second and third stages of labor progressed satisfactorily; no chloroform was administered. Forty-eight hours after confinement she was seized at 11:30 p. m. with a convulsion from which she passed into a deep coma and died twelve hours later. This presents unusual interest from the fact that no premonitory symptoms appeared before the convulsion occurring forty-eight hours after confinement save a slight fixedness of the eyes during the latter part of the first stage of labor, and as I was congratulating myself on the satisfactory condition of the patient, like a "bolt from a clear sky" the eclamptic convulsion appeared.

This interesting case further teaches us that fatal eclamptic convulsions are not always preceded by premonitory symptoms indicative of the toxaemia of pregnancy such as oedema, headache, epigastric pain, disturbances of vision, scantiness of urine, etc.

It seems that in these cases we would frequently have a jaundiced condition. Personally I have never seen such a condition exist, but should I find a patient becoming markedly jaundiced, either during or just after the convulsive seizure, I would regard it as indicative of serious hepatic lesion and the prognosis would be extremely grave.

In all cases there should be frequent examination of the urine and immediate institution of appropriate treatment and diet as soon as any abnormality is detected or symptoms appear which indicate that the eliminative processes are at fault. Cases that do not improve under these precautionary measures and become progressively worse under treatment should have premature labor terminated promptly. Prophylactic treatment, while productive of much good, is not always successful, for eclampsia is not a preventable affection under our present knowledge of its cause, and can never be regarded as such until its aetiology is perfectly understood and we are in possession of more accurate and reliable methods of foretelling the outcome in cases of toxaemia of pregnancy.

Treatment under the head of curative embraces chloroform to be administered during convulsive attacks, after which comparative large doses of morphine be given hypodermically, beginning with 1-4 grain and repeating if necessary until three doses are given. When convulsions have once occurred the pregnancy or labor, as the case may be, should be terminated as soon as is consistent with the safety of the patient. The question as to the advisability of early operative interference can be decided by determining the proportion of cases in which convulsions cease after the birth of the child. A safe conservative estimate is 85 per cent. in favor of the immediate emptying of the uterus, resulting in a cessation of the seizures, as against a mortality of 28 per cent. under expectant and 11 per cent. under active treatment. It is my practice to give a strong cathartic as quick as possible, preferably one or two drops of croton oil. Diuresis should be stimulated by means of a hot pack and. further favored by the subcutaneous injections of large amounts of salt solution. If improvement is not noted shortly after delivery large amounts of blood should be withdrawn. Pilocrafine should never be used on account of its tendency to produce oedema of the lungs. With veratrum viride my experience is limited.

Eclamptic women seem to be more liable to infection than those whose confinement is normal; hence all operative procedure must be conducted in the most rigid apestic manner. After the birth of the child I never attempt to hasten the third stage of labor, as a moderate loss of blood should be encouraged rather than checked.

The writer of this paper has not attempted to enter into detail the many various questions that are still debatable as to the aetiology of this subject, as that question is still unsettled; but we trust that our remarks will at least furnish suggestions that will prompt a most liberal discussion of our subject.

CONCUSSION.

BY DR. B. F FORTNER. VINITA, OKLAHOMA.

Like many another hackneyed theme this is one which can never cease to be of interest to the industrious physician. In our haste after the new, we are inclined to relegate the old. But their ghosts will return to vex our souls. The history of brain concussion represents many an ill waged cinflict. Spinal concussion even more. The two are distinct and should be studied separately. Concussion is a fact, that of the spine a fallacy, in the usual sense. The theory of Erichson was founded upon a speculative hypothesis of molecular construction. Microscopy of today, far in advance of that of his day, has failed to discover a molecular structure of either brain or cord. Hence it must not be expected that he should have formulated a theory that would hold good today.

There has been given no better definition of concussion than this—"a violent shaking." This is both ligitimate and convenient. But since we usually think only of brain and spinal concussion, our investigations and our interpretations of symptoms are apt to begin and end there. It is however true that the term applies with increasing importance and force to other tissues and organs of the body. For instance it is known that one of the most fruitful sources of paralysis agitans is this concussion of the body organs. Baily, a recent author says, "That the disease often appears and becomes permanent soon after a severe shock, without any physical injury, there can be no doubt; but more frequently there is an injury as well. Cuts, stabs, and even fright produce the disease. In Walz's analysis of 21 cases of paralysis agitans, 6 were caused by concussion of the body alone, and 8 by body contusions. Baily further says. "When the injury is general, such as a concussion of the whole body, the symptoms begin in one or both of the upper extremities, thus acting similarly to progressive muscular atrophy when it occurs in those parts which had previously

Read Before the Annual Meeting of the Oklahoma State Medical Association, Tulsa, May 10-12, 1910.

been affected through spinal injury." Thus in a case described by Walz: "Male aged 61 years, laborer. No syphilis or alcholism. Heredity negative. Was struck on the back of the head by a package weighing about 65 pounds, which had fallen from a fifth-story window. The patient was knocked down and rendered momentarily unconscious. After ten minutes he got up and walked home. For two weeks he was in bed with pain in the upper extremity from the neck to the fingers, with rythmical movements of both hands and of the head. The patient recovered sufficiently to be up, but he could not work, and he was granted a pension, in accordance with the German law, for "paralysis agitans which was the direct result of injury." This patient died from spasm of the respiratory muscles four years later. The autopsy report says: "There are no local findings, and certainly no hemorrhages of old or recent date; no marked atheroma, nothing abnormal in the dura or the bones." This can be the more readily understood when we reflect that all life is from an egg, otherwise expressed, all life is the expression of the complex of cell life. Violence to the delicate elements of our body structures may be such as to individually and prejudicially modify their vital affinities and appropriations. The softer the structures, other things equal, the greater the degree of damage. On this account nature has well provided for protection of the vital organs of this nature, notably the brain and spinal cord. Except for the globular shape of the head, the firm bony spinal column, the numerous ligamentous guys, and the admirable water bed of the brain and spinal cord, casualties would be far more frequent within these organs.

I desire to lay special stress upon that feature of my subject pertaining to *other* structures than the brain and spinal cord. To the application of force directly or indirectly to such organs as the liver, kidneys, stomach, and even the heart under certain circumstances. It is sufficient for a time at least to stop them from their normal function, so that the recuperative powers of the system as a whole are materially lowered. I have been especially impressed with many of these cases occurring in the railway hospital during my service in that institution, and less frequently in private practice. A recognition of this principle is of the greatest importance in the treatment of ordinary wounds, for an important reason among others, that suppuration the entrance, multiplication and invasion of pyogenic bacteria is greatly facilitated by this lowering of the vitality of the tissues environing trauma. This is saying nothing about the mental shock which usually attends such experience as falling from great heights.

Ordinarily when we speak of concussion the mental trend is toward railway injuries and railway surgery, because of the frequency of the condition in that service. And this idea has crystalized in the establishing in some schools of a separate chair of railway surgery. I believe this both premature and unwise; for the reason that there is nothing in railway surgery to distinguish it as a separate branch of the science. Wherever machinery of great weight and momentum is being used, the same sort of injuries, requiring the same sort of treatment, are being sustained. Surgery is surgery. A broken head is a broken head, whether its possessor acquired it falling from a tree or a box car. Concussion follows a rule. It requires a given amount of force and a given amount of resistence to cause concussion, whether these conditions are met in a runaway buggy, a runaway car, or in an automobile casualty. The difference is one of degree.

Cerebral localization and its surgery has not made their expected advancement. The interpretation of its symptoms has been far more inexact and unsatisfactory than that of the spinal cord. By a careful study of the pathologies and trauma of the latter much of the mists of error have been cleared away, and our deductions are much more nearly correct. With it so-called "railway spine" has ceased to be recognized.

If we accept the definition of cerebral concussion to be a "severe jar" to the brain, causing temporary unconsciousness, nausea, and often vomiting the usual signs of shock, accompanied in many cases with capillary hemorrhage, we see why a more or less severe cerebritis frequently follows. Then if we go a step further and consider contusion to be an exaggerated degree of hemorrhage resulting from a greater lasceration of brain substance and blood vessels contained therein, we are in position to recognize their intimate kinship, and the consequences of the two conditions as described in books. Really they are one. The two extremes are, upon one hand small hemorrhagic points with moderate symptoms, and upon the other, large points with symptoms exaggerated. The subsequent and resultant symptoms go hand in hand with the pathological changes and are to be interpreted by the rules laid down in the books.

Of late years our profession has not been satisfied with speculative deductions, but in the dead room have sought to unravel the mysteries of cerebro-spinal injuries, and have found that the laws of pathological physiology have not been tresspassed; that a lesion at a given point will, except for special mechanical reasons induce a given set of symptoms. The great difficulty attending the diagnosis of brain lesions, more particularly, is dependent upon the closeness to each other of the centers of innervation, and the irregularity of the surrounding bony walls, the partitions and shelves of resistant dura which present different plains of resistance to encroaching hematomata and other forms of compressing and lacerating force. For instance, we have the tentorium cerebri widely expanding between the cerebral lobes and the cerebelum. The falx cerebri separating the two hemispheres. The irregular basins and their sharp bony brims defining the boundaries of the fossae for the anterior middle and posterior lobes—all contributing to the confusion which must come from this variety and of inclination of resisting planes. If this view of the confusion of signs be correct, we may reasonably conclude that perfection in cerebral localization is not likely to be accomplished very soon.

When we descend to the spinal cord we may repeat in brief, that there is no such thing as concussion of that structure. True, around it we may have subdural hemorrhage, into its structure very rarely, and never as a result of a jar, we may have hemorrhage as a result of fractured bone, projectiles and dislocations. All of these conditions produce definite modification—if not paralysis, of motion or sensation in a definite region. This is because the cord is largely a conducting medium and only in a minor degree an initiating one. So that whatever compresses or completely severs these conducting tracts puts out the light and leaves the field of distribution in darkness. The language of cord distress is voiced by the principles of anatomy and physiology.

DISCUSSION.

Dr. Pearse, of Kansas City. In interpreting the damage done to the blood vessels which are within reach of surgical assistance, I have found more trouble from overlooking hemorrhage in the presence of concussion, than I have in under-estimating the extent of the concussion as a complication. Not long ago my friend Dr. Hyde, of Kansas City, called my attention to a man lying in my service, who was comatose, and asked me why I didn't operate on him. I told him because I could find no symptoms that indicated to me a blood clot within the reach of the surgeon's knife. The man had stepped into a room or closet hung up his coat and hat and slipped and struck on the cement floor. He was simply sleeping and had been when I saw him for twelve hours. Beyond a slight dilation of the pupil on the opposite side from which the blow occurred, there was no symptoms of paresis or paralysis to guide me. I told the doctor I could not see any signs why I should operate, but if he would show me any I would operate. He simply pointed to the bruise on the side of the man's head and said, "Operate there." I didn't and later the man died, and we had a post. At the post there was no clot on the side of the bruise, but on the other side there was a blood clot some four inches in diameter and nearly an inch in thickness, and I should have operated upon my man, not only upon the side of the injury but upon the opposite side of the head. About a month later, when I had finished smarting under the criticism of my colleagues when I reported my failure as I always like to do to my associates, I found another comatose man in a ward one day and the card on his bed bore Dr. Hyde's name. And I called him up and asked him why he did not operate. He said "I am thinking about operating." Well, I said, it is as you told me, operate to-day. The next day I found the man in the ward still comatose, and he died that day. We held a post and again we found a large blood clot. This time on the same side of the head as the injury.

Dr. Grosshart, of Tulsa. In regard to this subject, the doctor's paper has voiced the sentiments, of all of us, I guess, that have had any experience. And in regard to the treatment that Dr. Pearse has outlined, and the administering of an anesthetic, I just want to add one little mode of treatment of that condition that can be pursued without any material danger to your

patient—without any shock to your patient. The patient is in a comatose condition and suffering from the shock at the time you see him. With the exception of the nerve ending in the skin you can take out the bone material on one or both sides of his head without an anesthetic, with ten drops of a solution of cocaine. And it has been a rule that I have adopted, if a man comes in to the hospital that is suffering concussion and shock of the cerebrum, to not administer an anesthetic to that man, but do it under cocaine. You will be surprised when you do it.

Dr. Fortner: One object I had in presenting this paper was to call attention away from the brain and spinal column to the concussoin of the body organs and I wish to stress that. If the important body organs have been seriously damaged and their function interfered with, the vital processes are interfered with, and your patient is not in a good condition to recover from an operation. In fact that in any case is to be well considered, as well as in concussion of the brain. I was very much interested in the case that Dr. Pearse reported, and I am glad that it has taken a sort of practical turn, because I feel sure that we overlook cerebral hemorrhage in many of these cases. A doctor told me of a case in the St. Louis Hospital which reminded me very much of the case which the doctor reported. The patient was in a comatose condition, and that was about all. Nothing could be learned of the condition except that he had concussion. He went on and finally died, and when they came to examine him, the anterior lobe of the brain was almost entirely covered by a clot. Now I remember—and I want to make this remark before passing—that different portions of the brain will tolerate growths, for instance. and clots, a great deal more readily than others. For instance, if a tumor is on the cerebrum if it is pressing upwards it may travel over that direction of the brain and present very little symptoms, but if it be below it and the pressure is down, you will frequently get localization and sudden death. Tumors often grow up high, and before we find any localization or focalization, that points to the character or the nature of the trouble our tumor is very large, and as we cut in now, through the nose, we find that we have got a much larger tumor than we expected. We do well to consider the anatomy of the head when we begin to consider the possibility of a local hemorrhage. Speaking about the operation, I remember there came into our service at the hospital a man who had concussion of the brain. There wasn't any focalization, except that one pupil was a little dilated. We opened the temporal muscle and let the blood out from under the anterior lobe and the man was well in a very short time and began to improve immediately, and in a few days he began to articulate a little, and his eyes began to get in line, and he began to improve in every way and gradually these things all got in line and the man got well. A few years ago we would not have thought that possible. I believe and most heartily concur in the doctor's suggestion to trephine. Why not? What harm can it do? We once thought if we touched the heart it would cause death. Now we sew it up. If you don't find it there, go over on the other side and hunt for it. Keep hunting. I know a man who had so much of the bone taken away that his head caved in. That man has been running a delivery wagon for the last six or eight years since that operation. And so if we do these things, in a clean way I think there is no danger. I concur in the idea of the doctor in hunting for it.

EDITORIAL

McCORMACK, THE GUEST OF THE OKLAHOMA PROFESSION.

While this is going to press Dr. McCormack, National Organizer for the American Medical Association is making a rapid tour of our state.

In many places he and his work are known already and need no introduction and it is unnecessary to say that he will be welcomed by all who hear him.

The work he undertakes consists in first meeting and talking with the physicians and then lecturing to the people and physicians in the evening. Owing to the amount of territory to be covered a limited amount of time only can be given to each place, the schedule in most towns calls for an arrival in the morning or early afternoon, an afternoon meeting of the profession and an evening meeting with both profession and laity and an immediate departure for the next place.

In this connection it is especially requested that no attempt be made by the local committees of arrangements to have banquets or receptions of any character as every moment of the time will be consumed with matters pertaining to the trip. The necessity of this request will be understood when one considers that Dr. McCormack enters the state on the morning of October 3rd, delivers two lectures that day, two each succeeding day, including Sunday's until October 31st. It is to be regretted that more places cannot be visited but we should feel that we have had our share when we have had him with us for one month.

THE DOCTOR AND POLITICS.

Elsewhere appears a letter from Dr. J. M. Postelle, who was recently a candidate for Lieutenant Governor in the Democratic primaries.

The Editor ordinarily assumes the position that politics and the State Journal have nothing in common and that as far as possible political questions should be kept from its columns, but the letter contents have a direct meaning to the profession in this state and for that reason is published. Dr. Postelle while not officially endorsed by the state medical association was endorsed by its officers and many of the "Old Guard" and men who have made their names well and favorably known in the professional annals of the state and the tone of his letter indicates that he is appreciative of their support.

A physician usually has his mind so thoroughly occupied with his work, and to attain success, his mind must be at all times on his work, that he has no time for politics and if he has time for such matters his professional attainments and laurels are almost sure to suffer sooner or later from the division of effort necessary, but it must be admitted that the medical profession is becoming active when questions involving its politics and principles are in question and as previously mentioned in this journal they have a right to demand better laws and more law enforcement for they are a valuable part of the states citizenship from a moral and financial standpoint as well as professional and when it is observed by politicians that the profession or their representative is observant of their vote and acts on questions affecting the profession they will hesitate before doing some of the undoubtedly fool things some of our alleged legislators are said to have done with reference to medical legislation. Illinois, through the eminence of some of its profession and its activity has recently received a great deal of good by medical legislation and there is much yet to be done and the Illinois State Journal of Medicine has undertaken to show every member of its profession just how the candidates for office, irrespective of party affiliation, stand on questions affecting the profession. Wherever a man has previously been in office his vote and action on medical matters is listed so that the Illinois physician will have no trouble in seeing who his friend is. In some instances a warning is plainly sounded that this man is unfit for office and gives the grounds upon which the statement is made.

Such work can have but one effect and that is to make legislators study very closely all proposed acts and to weigh very carefully the demands of the regular profession before turning a deaf ear to them.

We want no favoritism shown us, we want no protection not accorded to others, but we do want all physicians, i. e., all who treat the sick to be qualified to treat them and to be qualified means years of endeavor which the regular medical profession insists is necessary to make a physician. A profession so qualified has a right to a voice in the political transactions of the state.

ERLICH'S 606.

It seems we are to have a new specific for syphilis and if the reports are not misleading, as they sometimes are, with reference to the new discoveries of medicine, Erlich's 606 will revolutionize the treatment of syphilis. The name seems to come from the fact that the experiment was the 606th used and we are thankful for that when we understand that it is to be the synonym for 'dimethyldioxiarsenobensoldichlorhydrat.'

Dr. Erlich has this to say about the discovery: "The most important point about this remedy is that one injection utterly destroys all spirochetes, but is harmless to the animal tissues. In the course of my investigation I have made hundreds of mixtures with which to accomplish this, but only after several years of experiments did I, in company with Dr. Hata, in November last, discover the present medicine * * * * and the cure 'sterilsatio manga,' so-called because of its great effect of killing all parasites at once. In March last being so satisfied with the results ot my trials on animals, I decided to apply the medicine to human beings, but having no hospital under my control, I asked my friend, Dr. Wechselmann, to undertake the conduct of the experiment." The report of Dr. Wechselmann and others verify the claim of Dr. Erlich. * * * *—Journal A. M. A.

This preparation will be ready for the market soon and it will be tried by the profession of the world practically at the same time. It is to be hoped that the claims are not extravagant and that it prove the success that is claimed for it.

DR. J. N. McCORMACK.

National Organizer for the American Medical Association, will spend the month of October in Oklahoma at the following places:

Vinita	October 3
Muskogee	October 4
Eufaula	October 5
McAlester	October 6
Atoka	October 7
Durant	October 8
Hugo	October 9
Ardmore	October 10
Pauls Valley	October 11
Norman	October 12
Oklahoma City	October 13
Chickasha	October 14
Duncan	October 15
Waurika	October 16
Lawton	October 17
Anadarko	October 18
Hobart	October 19
Clinton	October 20
El Reno	October 21
Watonga	October 22
Cherokee	October 23
Enid	October 24
Guthrie	October 25
Shawnee	October 26
Holdenville	October 27
Okmulgee	October 28
Sapulpa	October 29
Tulsa	October 30
Bartlesville	October 31

It should be borne in mind that some slight change may be necessary in the above program on account of delayed trains, etc.; and if for any reason, Dr. McCormack cannot reach a place on the date he is scheduled to appear in that place the meeting at that town will have to be cancelled and the regular meeting held in the next town on the fixed date.

PERSONAL

DR. BLESH'S LETTER.

Wien, Sept. 3, 1910.

Dear Dr. Thompson:

In accordance with my promise before leaving America I shall write you my impressions of matters medical in Vienna. However, as I have just arrived here I am not yet in possession of the facts necessary to do this with any degree of accuracy or authority. In these letters I shall endeavor to deal with the facts only and in such a manner that they will be of some little value, I hope, to those contemplating the luxury of a trip and course of study here.

So this letter will not deal with medical matters at all, but with your permission I will give you my impressions of the much advertised Passion Play at Obergammergau. To these simple minded, deeply religious mountain people the things they represent are real. Let this fact be ever in mind while reading these few comments of mine. Above all they are not dishonest people.

The drama has its foundation in the still deeps of human sorrow. It is said that in the 12th century a crude representation was made but this was interrupted by the wars of Gustavus Adolphus. The Bavarians have always adhered to the Catholic faith and for this were especially marked by the victorious Swedes who at this time were the champions of Protestantism. Following the devastation of war came that of pestilence which decimated all the villages round about with the exception of Oberammergau which, by the enforcement of a primitive but effective quarantine, escaped until Caspar Schuchler, who got caught on the outside, broke through carrying the death-dealing infection with him. In a short time many of the villagers were dead. These simple minded folks although wise enough to enforce a quarantine, looked upon this plague as the mark of the displeasure of an angry God to appease which they vowed hereafter to perform the Passion Play at least once every 10 years, provided these measures were effective. This is another way of applying the saying "Put your trust in God, but keep your powder dry." The Lord was to be given a fair trial but no effort was to be wasted. It is a matter of tradition (they say history) that the affection ended at once even to the recovery of those who were sick.

Since that time (about the time the Pilgrim fathers landed in America) the drama has been enacted every 10 years, as stated above it has been a mat-ter of religion with these people who are in many ways quite primitive indeed.

The play itself is enacted in an open air theater and requires about 8 hours in its performance. The personnel is composed entirely of villagers who earn their livelihood by other means. The plays with them is not a matter of finances but of devotion.

This statement will be criticised by visitors to Oberammergau and with apparently good reason. When one has paid five times the price he should pay for board and lodgings he has a right to assume that some one has a graft hid away somewhere. To illustrate, my family is composed of five members, two children and three adults. I was in Oberammergau one day and two nights. Our accomodations were most excellent and our hostess very attentive and pleasant. Below is a copy of my bill for same;

Oberammergau, den 31, Aug. 1910.
Reichnung
fur Mr. Dr. Blesh,
Zimmer No. 112.
Pension pro tag niel Zimmer M. 20.
2 tage (note that we were charged for two days) fur 5 personen M. 200.

One mark German money is about equal to 25c American, so you will see I paid $50.00 for 1 day and 2 nights accommodation. I was not especially "stung" for I found that the larger members had been similarily robbed. I also found upon further investigation that those who dealt directly with the citizen of Oberammergau were not held up in this manner, but got their accommodations extremely cheap while those who purchased through Thos. Cook and Son paid the high prices The reader may draw his own inferences from the above facts. I am quite clear that if I were to again arrange a visit to the Passion Play, it would not be through Thos. Cook and Son, but I would arrange the matter direct with Anton Lang or some one

170   JOURNAL OF THE OKLAHOMA STATE MEDICAL ASSOCIATION.

of the other players a few months in advance.

As to the play itself it altogether depends upon what one expects. This play is not strictly speaking a theatrical but is the expression of a profound and deeply rooted religious devotion, of a simple and child-like faith of a sincerely religious people.

Reverentialy considered (and it should be viewed in no other light) it has its deeply enduring lesson. For this simple faith however childish and immature it may seem finds its echo in all human hearts everywhere, so do we hark back to the time when our race was young. In this primitive village a century passes as a day. The child follows in the footsteps of the father.

As a play the hypercritical could find much to criticise in the way of stage settings and acting. Johann Zwink as Judas the betrayer would appear with credit on any stage, Andreas Lang as Peter was also good and the same may be said of Anton Lang the Christ. The vocal music was exceptionally good for untrained voices. Perhaps the most just criticism that might be offered is as to the length of it.

To sum up I would leave the play as it is, the people as they are, but if possible would un-syndicate it from the grasp of those who are debasing it by making money out of it.

Very truly,

A. L. BLESH.

DR. POSTELLE WRITES ON THE RECENT ELECTION.

Dr. Claude Thompson,

Muskogee, Okla.

Dear Doctor:

The recent election is suggestive of the following points:

1st. The total vote of Dr. Davis and myself will, in future elections, be reckoned by politicians and the public politic as the doctors' vote.

2nd. This vote will be estimated at not less than 35,000 in the Democratic primaries, and not less than 50,000 in a general election.

3rd. This large vote given to any candidate in a primary or general election, would elect likewise if against would insure his defeat.

4th. These facts taken together will hereafter make the doctors influence a potent factor in politics and insure recognition of any measures presented by our physicians to the law making bodies of the state.

I consider this test of the physicians' influence a great victory, although to secure the same I suffered defeat. I am optimistic, have no sore spots, no wounds to heal, and am ready at any time to take up a fight that promises in the least to gain a point that will add influence in promoting the welfare of my brother practitioners or to the general health laws of our state.

I would suggest that every physician interested in medical and health legislation study our present laws carefully and write their individual opinions on same making suggestions, additions, changes, etc., to suit their own individual ideas. Submit these briefs to the Legislative Committee of the Oklahoma State Medical Association for their consideration in the framing up of future legislative bills. The committee can glean from this multiplicity of ideas many golden thoughts that would otherwise never be put into action.

I want to thank my many friends in their untiring efforts to secure for me the nomination of Lieutenant Governor, and, also congratulate the physicians of Oklahoma on their victory, and urge the profession to make good use of the advantage so gained.

I would like to further suggest that each physician get away from the old idea that a physician "has no business in politics." The family physician has more influence than any other class of men, he has more to do in shaping the morals of the country; more to do in the education of the people; more to do with the upbuilding of public institutions; his money and work stands for more than all other professions combined and yet custom has caused him to relinquish that which justly belongs to him and he takes a back seat when it comes to the political affairs of his country.

Some of our physicians are now awakening to their duties to the body politic, and the sooner every physician keeps his finger on the public pulse and studies the political condition of the country just that soon a great intellectual influence will be felt in the management of affairs that has in the main, hitherto been left undeveloped.

Very truly yours,

J. M. POSTELLE.

Dr. H. T. Ballantine, of Muskogee, has returned from a vacation in Tennessee.

Dr. Claude Thompson, of Muskogee, will spend part of October and November, in Chicago, doing post-graduate work.

Drs. F. B. Fite and J. L. Blakemore, of Muskogee, have returned from their vacations spent in North Carolina and Colorado.

Dr. A. M. Young, Jr., who has completed an interneship in St Thomas Hospital, Nashville, Tenn., has returned to his home in Muskogee, and will locate there.

DRS. WEST AND NOBLE DISSOLVE.

The firm of Drs. West and Noble, of Guthrie, Surgeons, announce their dissolution. Dr. A. A. West announces that he will continue the practice of surgery in Guthrie, as heretofore.

ABSTRACTS AND EXCHANGES

THE TREATMENT OF ECLAMPSIA.

By Barton Cooke Hirst, M. D., Philadelphia Pa.

The Census Bureau states that on June 1, 1910, the estimated population of the United States is 89,599,209. Applying the birth-rate of England and Wales for last year 25.58 per thousand of the population, as our own figures are unobtainable, there were 1,291.922 labors at term in this country during the last twelve months.

It is generally admitted that eclampsia occurs once in 300 pregnancies. There

(*Reprinted frm the American Journal of Obstetrics and Diseases of Women and Children, September, 1910.*)

were, therefore, at least 4:306 cases in the United States last year. The mortality of eclampsia in general practice is about 33 per cent.; consequently, 1,435 of our country women lost their lives last year by this disease.

Those of us who have ample experience in the treatment of eclampsia, and who must keep informed upon the subject, know that the mortality can and ought to be kept below 10 per cent. It appears, therefore, that the lives of more than one thousand women are unnecessarily sacrificed in our country every year. These women, in the majority of cases, are primiparae, just entering upon wifehood and motherhood.

Mere words and figures convey no adequate idea of the irreparable loss to the family and to the community indicated by these statistics. Moreover, this irrefutable statement is a serious arraignment of our profession.

It would seem, therefore, that a national society such as ours could devote itself to no worthier object than an inquiry into the cause of an unnecessarily high mortality of a common disease, and suggestions to the profession at large for improvement in treatment that will insure better results.

What follows must be an expression of individual opinion, which I hope will be supplemented and corrected by the views of our members.

Time will be saved by a succinct statement of the writer's present routine treatment, preventive and curative, of eclampsia.

If the blood pressure is carefully observed and regarded as an invariable index of toxemia in the latter half of pregnancy when over 150, and if pregnancy, is interrupted if it is impossible to reduce the blood pressure below 180 by a rigid antitoxemic regimen, eclampsia can almost always be prevented.

In the treatment of the actual convulsions the following scheme can be depended upon to reduce the mortality under 10 per cent.

Lavage of the colon and stomach removes a possible additional intoxication from the alimentary tract. Purgation is a valuable means of elimination. The stomach-pump is utilized to introduce two ounces of caster oil with a drop or two of croton oil. The purgation is continued by concentrated Epsom salt solution in 2-dram doses if the patient can swallow. Sweating is the most valuable means of elimination. The patient is put in a sweat cabinet for thirty minutes every four hours, in steam heat. Every physician who may see such patients should be provided with a portable sweat cabinet.

Hypodermoclysis.—After the first sweat a quart of salt solution is injected under the breasts.

Subsequently at least a quart of the solution is injected between the sweats in the colon.

Vensection.—If the blood pressure is over 180, sixteen ounces of blood should be withdrawn.

Medication. Fifteen minims of veratrum viride fluid extract is given hypodermically. Subsequently 1-100 gr. of nitroglycerine is given every four hours. Chloral by the bowel and chloroform by inhalation during the convulsions may be administered, but they are unimportant. Parathyroid extract is of value. One grain is administered every four hours.

Obstetrical Treatment.—If the woman is pregnant or in labor, nothing should be done except to puncture the membrane, which more quickly and decidedly reduces blood pressure than anything else. Any form of accouchement force adds to the risk and increases the mortality. After puncture of the membrane and with the active eliminative treatment an easy spontaneous labor is the rule within eight hours.

I am aware that this statement will not pass unchallenged by some of my colleagues, and is not in accord with the views of many specialists in Europe, but it is based on a personal observation of more than two hundred and sixty cases in which both plans have been tried. I find that in reviewing these cases that I can obtain better results by non-intervention than by active interference. In spite, therefore, of some predilection in favor of operative treatment I am compelled to adopt the course that experience teaches me is safest for my patients.

Finally, treatment must be continued for at least a week after the cessation of convulsions. Naturally, the severity is reduced as the patient improves.

STRICTURE.

V. C. Pedersen, New York (*Journal A. M. A.*, January 1), discusses the treatment of stricture of the male urethra, the most dangerous after-complication of gonorrheal infection. Early diagnosis of incipient obstruction is the first step and no case of gonorrhea should be described as cured without gentle complete examination of the urethra for thickenings or infiltrations. This should be done about a month after the other treatment when presumably all inflammation has ceased in order not to set up any irritation by too early interference. He quotes at length White and Martin's summary of the treatment of stricture with comments and summarizes the operative indications according to the clinical feature as follows: "1. Narrowing at or near the meatus, if treated at all, are always cut. 2. Strictures of large caliber (greater than 15 F.) are treated by gradual dilatation. Cutting is almost never required when such a stricture is in the deep urethra; it is sometimes necessary when the stricture is anterior to the bulbomembranous juncture. 3. Strictures of small caliber are treated by gradual dilatation if possible; when in the deep urethra they often require external urethrotomy; when anterior to the bulbomembranous juncture they usually require internal urethrotomy. 4. Impermeable strictures are treated by perineal section, followed at times by excision and mucous membrane grafting. 5. Soft, recent, uncomplicated strictures are always dilated. 6. Fibrous, nodular, irritable strictures complicated by urinary fever, fistula, etc., are always cut." He next takes up the treatment of stricture by dilatation in detail under the heads of the armamentarium, the preliminary treatment, the actual treatment, and the after treatment. He mentions the importance of prevention of reflex anuria and has found a very reliable and rational means of prevention by a reflex vesical action at the end of each treatment caused by filling the bladder with a blood warm antiseptic solution. For this purpose he has employed the tunneled or grooved silver, or the standard catheter. Strict asepsis is essential. He finds rigid instruments preferable to flexible ones except in extensive tortuous strictures, besides being more aseptic. A very important detail is care of and relief from the pus organisms and chronic urethritis before the dilatation treatment begins. He specially mentions the use of the irrigating sounds devised by himself which enable the antiseptic solution already mentioned to be used as the last step in each treatment. These add greatly to the comfort of the patient at the end of each dilatation. The after treatment he says is more or less neglected by general practitioners. During active treatment the patient should always have a few moments rest in the office, and in the intervals between treatments should be told to observe sexual rest as far as possible, and urinary rest by the avoidance of alcohol, condiments, and by adherence to simple diet. Urinary antiseptics are wisely administered for at least the first 24 hours after each dilatation, and free drinking of water is to be encouraged. A little pain on urination is to be expected and the patient should be informed. As to the terminal after-treatment, the patient should be taught that, since stricture is fundamentally only scar tissue and liable to contract, he must watch for the first symptoms of recurrence and report once or twice a year for observation and for the early and necessary correction of any slight relapse which may occur.

DIGALEN.

Speaking first of the disadvantages of digitalis, on account of its secondary effect, Worth Hale, Washington, D. C. (*Journal A. M. A.*, January 1), takes up the claims of digalen, introduced by Cloetta in 1904, as doing away with these defects. He reviews the literature on the subject and gives the results of biologic experiments made by himself on frogs, which led him to the following conclusions: "Diagalen is not a uniformly stable preparation, as shown by the gross appearance of Sample 1 and by biologic tests of the five different samples. Biologic tests also indicate that digalen is relatively much less potent than corresponding amounts of crystalline digitoxin, but that it is of about the same activity as digitalein. The experience of clinicians indicates that digalen is much less effective than is claimed, and that the secondary action of the digitalis group appears equally often after its use as with the older and cheaper galenicals. Its use in cases of acute heart failure, whether by intramuscular or intravenous injection, seems open to serious objection on account of the pain, and danger of thrombosis, and it would apparently be better practice in such cases to use either strophanthin, given intramuscularly, or one of the preparations of the suprarenal glands by intravenous injection."

THE ANTITOXIN TREATMENT OF DIPHTHERIA.

Again are we nearing the season when the problem of diphtheria and its treatment must be met and solved. The writer of this paragraph is forcibly reminded of the fact by the receipt of a modest but important brochure of sixteen pages bearing the title "Antidiphtheric Serum and Antidiphtheric Globulins." A second thought is that here is a little work that every general practitioner ought to send for and read. Not that the booklet is in any sense an argument for serum therapy. It is nothing of the kind. Indeed, the efficacy of the antitoxin treatment of diphtheria is no longer a debatable question, that method of procedure having long since attained the position of an established therapeutic measure.

The pamphlet is noteworthy because of the timeliness of its appearance, the mass of useful information which it presents in comparatively limited compass, and the interest and freshness with which its author has been able to invest a subject that has been much written about in the past dozen or fifteen years. Its tendency, one may as well admit, is to foster a preference for a particular brand of serum, but that fact lessens not one whit its value and authoritativeness.

Here is a specimen paragraph, reprinted in this space not so much to show the scope and character of the offering as to emphasize its helpful tone and to point out the fact that its author was not actuated wholly by motives of commercialism:

"Medical practitioners have learned that, inasmuch as the main problem presented in the treatment of a case of diphtheria is the neutralization of a specific toxin, the true antitoxin cannot too soon be administered; moreover, that, antitoxin being a product of definite strength, a little too little of it may fail when a little more would have succeeded—hence larger or more frequently repeated doses are becoming more and more the rule. One more point: if the medical attendant is prompt, as he must be, and fearless, as he has a right to be, the full justification of his course will hinge upon the choice of the best and most reliable antidiphtheric serum to be had; for while there is little or no danger of harm ensuing from the use of any brand issued by a reputable house, the best results—which may mean recovery as the alternative of death —can only be hoped for from the use of the best serum."

The brochure is from the press of Parke, Davis & Co., who will doubtless be pleased to send a copy to any physician upon receipt of a request addressed to them at their main offices, Detroit, Mich.

ARSENIC TREATMENT OF SYPHILIS

J. B. Murphy, Chicago (Journal A. M. A., September 24), discusses the treatment of syphilis with the Ehrlich's new preparation "606," and states the results which he has obtained with sodium cacodylate. He asserts that after administration of this sodium salt the spirochetes disappear from the lesions and from the blood somewhat as they are reported to do after administration of Ehrlich's "606," and reports briefly one or two cases. He urges physicians throughout the country to try this remedy (concerning which we know something) while waiting for the Ehrlich preparation to be put on the market.

NEW ORLEANS POLYCLINIC,
Post Graduate Medical Department Tulane University of Louisiana, Twenty-fourth Annual Session opens October 31, 1910, and closes May 27, 1911.

Physicians will find the Polyclinic an excellent means for posting themselves upon modern progress in all branches of medicine and surgery. The specialties are fully taught, including laboratory and cadaveric work. For further information, address:

CHAS. CHASSAIGNAC, M. D., Dean.
New Orleans Polyclinic,
Postoffice Box 797　　　　New Orleans, La.

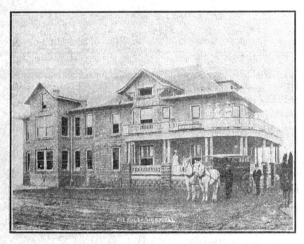

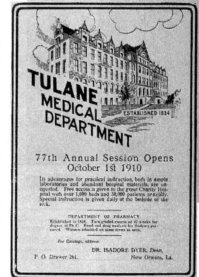

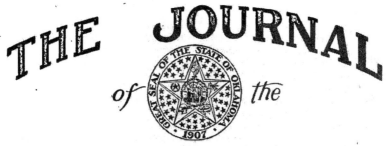

Oklahoma State Medical Association.

VOL. III.   MUSKOGEE, OKLAHOMA, NOVEMBER, 1910.   NO. 6

DR. CLAUDE A. THOMPSON, Editor-in-Chief.

ASSOCIATE EDITORS AND COUNCILLORS.

DR. J. A. WALKER, Shawnee.   DR. JOHN W. DUKE, Guthrie.
DR. CHARLES R. HUME, Anadarko.   DR. A. B. FAIR, Frederick.
DR. F. R. SUTTON, Bartlesville.   DR. W. G. BLAKE, Tahlequah.
DR. I. W. ROBERTSON, Dustin.   DR. H. P. WILSON, Wynnewood.
DR. J. S. FULTON, Atoka.   DR. J. H. BARNES, Enid.

Entered at the Postoffice at Muskogee, Oklahoma, as second class mail matter, July 28, 19109.

This is the Official Journal of the Oklahoma State Medical Association All communications should be addressed to the Journal of the Oklahoma State Medical Association, English Block, Muskogee, Oklahoma.

CARCINOMA OF THE SKIN

BY E. S. LAIN, M. D., OKLAHOMA CITY., PROFESSOR OF DERMATOLOGY, ELECTRO-THERAPY AND RADIOGRAPHY
STATE UNIVERSITY SCHOOL OF MEDICINE.

Cancer, as it is commonly called, is one of the most common of all the death-dealing diseases. We are almost appalled when we are reminded that statistics tell us that, of the total number of deaths after thirty-five years of age, cancer, or carcinoma, is the cause of from nine to twelve per cent. Only one other disease gives a higher death rate, and that at a different age, namely, tuberculosis, which has a mortality between the ages of twelve and thirty-five years of twelve to fifteen per cent. It is not so strange then that within recent years public opinion and municipalities have become so much aroused toward caring for the unfortunate victims of cancer. Several of our older states, also quite a number of our benefactors have begun to endow laboratories and institutions for the study of the cause and cure of this, one of our most rapidly increasing maladies.

It is our aim in this paper to discuss only one division or type of this disease, namely, carcinoma, which begins within the skin, or, the common term, which is more extensively used in America than elsewhere, epithelioma.

DEFINITION.

Dr. Pusey defines epithelioma as a "Carcinoma or malignant proliferation beginning in the epithelial structures of the skin." Dr. Stelwagon defines epithelioma as "an epithelial new growth with a destructive tendency having its origin in the epithelium of the epidermis or of the glands of the skin." A more explicit definition is given by Mac Cleod in his work on "Pathology of the Skin," namely, "a malignant proliferation of the epidermis which is capable of unlimited growth, has the power of invading the surrounding tissues and forming

mitotic power of every pathological cell produces a permanent cure.

PATHOLOGY.

Under pathology much has been written and demonstrated with the microscope of the character of the epithelial cells which are present in these lesions. Perhaps the most common pathological cells found are undeveloped columnar, cuboidal, and the so-

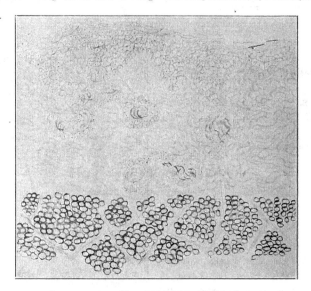

The proliferation downward through the germinal layer of the epithelial cells as seen in the common epithelioma, also, the epithelial pearls.

growths of a similiar nature in organs at a distance, and which cannot be checked except by complete eradication or extirpation."

Certainly no one who has been observing of these superficial malignancies for a number of years, or who has had occasion to treat a number of them, fails to appreciate the statement that nothing less than complete destruction or elimination of all the

called prickle cells. These cells, however, are nothing more than the undeveloped epithelial cell which has taken on an extensive proliferation, its growth extending in different directions, usually downward through the germinal layer into the connective tissue. It is in this tissue we so frequently find the so-called characteristic epithelial pearls. Much has been written concerning the formation of these so-called pearls, but suffice it to say, they have a central degeneration appearance or a collection of these undeveloped cells which are thinly surrounded by lines of connective tissue. No doubt these so-called pearls represent only nature's attempt to overcome this disease and foreign tissue.

ETIOLOGY.

Since the year 1904, when the State of New York, through its legislature, appro-

as the mouse, the guinea pig, or the dog. Since these investigations and observations the whole of our medical profession has been more thoroughly aroused until now practically all believe that individuals of susceptible age and skin, dwelling within the same house or in frequent contact with one who is infected with this disease, are most frequent victims of cancer. We recently heard a discussion by a number of leading surgeons and dermatologists from

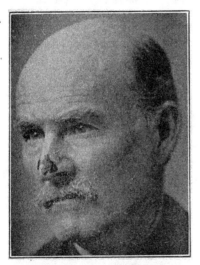

Rodent ulcer. 25 exposures, March, 1909, to April 25th.

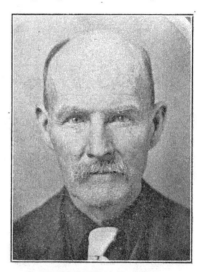

As appeared April, 1910, when he died from a brain lesion.

priated ten thousand dollars and provided for the appointment of a commission of permanent physicians and pathologists to experiment and study to try to learn the cause and a more successful cure of cancer a great deal of original research work has been done in many pathological laboratories. The investigations of this commission, as well as of many other pathologists, have clearly demonstrated that certain forms of cancer and sarcoma are transplantable or capable of being inoculated in animals, such

different sections of the United States relating cases of lip and other epitholioma which possibly had their etiology in a like lesion upon some other member of the family. The orders which have been issued from our State Commissioners of Health forbidding the use of the public drinking cup, etc., may not be fully appreciated by even the commissioner himself, unless he has been in touch with the vast amount of research work which is being done in demonstrating the inocubility of this disease.

Within our own observation we have seen some two or three cases which were, in our opinion, clearly traceable to some person or associate who was suffering from a like disease. In one case almost the day could be remembered by the patient. This patient, a lady, came to us with an epithelioma upon the end of the index finger which had resisted all ordinary methods of treatment. She remembered to have pricked this finger with a pin from the dressing of a cancer

is that of a man of about sixty years of age who was suffering with quite a large lesion upon the penis, extending to the left inguinal region, which had been diagnosed as carcinoma by his attending physician. His wife had died only a few years previous from carcinoma of the uterus.

With these facts before us, it would seem that it should be an easy matter to stain and demonstrate some particular micro-organism or parasite, or some particular cell

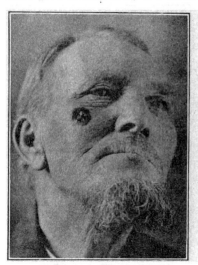

The common typical epithelioma 29 exposures
beginning October, 1909.

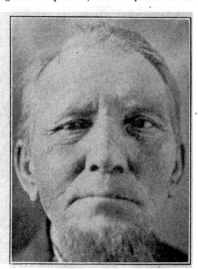

As appears today, more than 12 months
after healing.

upon the face of her father nine months previous.

Another case was that of an elderly man who was sent to us by a local physician. This man had a typical epithelioma upon the cheek. Not many months after its development his wife was a victim of carcinoma of the uterus. The lesion upon his cheek yielded to treatment nicely but even before his wife had died another like lesion had begun to develop upon his lower lip.

Another one of our cases of recent date,

as a specific cause for carcinoma. Such has been our most earnest anticipation for some months in the past, but as yet not realized. 'Tis true that in making a positive diagnosis the pathologist by careful cutting of perpendicular sections of the tissues, and with cautious staining and mounting, can clearly demonstrate the invasion of these characteristic undeveloped epithelial cells. Most generally they, too, are demonstrated to proliferate downward through the germinal layer into the corion, and thence to the lymph and other channels. By these aids we have learned to clearly recognize the pathological changes which take place in the tissue infected; but the distinct cell or parasite from which this growth takes its origin remains yet a mystery, which we trust shall be solved in the near future. Please pardon the trustful prophecy that within another decade we shall know the exact factor or distinct micro-organism of this disease which is now being so earnestly sought.

Certain factors or causes connected with

years of age. However, these, as we are aware, are the exceptions. Trauma, or exciting causes, may be many. All physicians have had acquaintance perhaps with one or more cases which have given a history of trauma. The mole, wart or nevus, located favorably on exposed parts which render them liable to friction and trauma, are the frequent beginnings of epithelioma.

Lupus, particularly the varicosus form, tubercular syphilides, and the well-known Padgett's disease, are also common sites for the development of malignancy. Just the

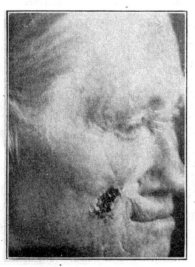

Epithelioma, a return from a former treatment by sloughing. Given 35 exposures from June, 1904, to October.

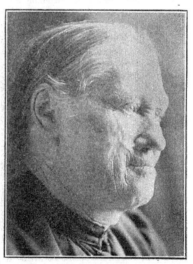

As appears today more than 6 years after treating by X ray

epitheliomas may be classified as: First, age; second, trauma; third, predisposing and heredity. *Age*: We have all learned that epitholiomas are rarely found under forty years of age, though quite a number of cases are reported at an earlier age. Dr. Pusey reports several cases between the ages of twenty-three and thirty years. Dr. Hartzell reports one case distinctly diagnosed as epithelioma in a patient fourteen

exact part which trauma plays in connection with these predisposing lesions in the development of epitheliomas is not definitely known. However, an injury to such a lesion is frequently the dating point for the beginning of a rapid proliferation of malignant cells. So many patients have come to us with this common story, "Doctor, I had a mole (or a wart, or a small rough place) on my face, and after picking it (or having a slight injury to this place) it began to grow and to give me slight tingling pains in that locality. I went to see my family physician. He examined the growth and told me that it was not cancer and to just let it alone, not to bother it and perhaps it would never give me any trouble." ·

One of our recent cases gave the history of having a small lesion located between the eyes, and in looking after her chickens she was pecked on this lesion by an old hen who objected to her meddling with the

years without any apparent growth, giving but slight discomfort to the patient, nevertheless they are a pathological lesion and should be guarded by the intelligent physician with the utmost care.

Of recent years I have been telling my patients that nearly all ordinary infected so-called sores, under antiseptic lotions or salves, should heal within a period of four or five weeks. If they did not heal within this time to submit at once to an investigation by their physician. Nine times in ten

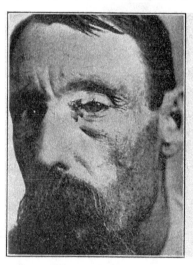 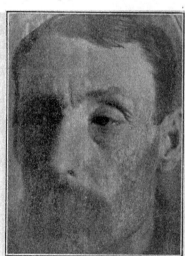

Cauliflower type of epithelioma after clipping off level with skin Given 37 exposures dating from February, 1904.

As appeared 3 years after treating. Recently learned that he is living and well, now 6 1-2 years later.

brood. This sore never healed but after a period of a few weeks began to spread, until, at the time she came to us, it was a typical crater-form epithelioma about the size of a twenty-five cent coin.

Another predisposing lesion which is the most frequent of any is the small scaly or senile lesion, termed by dermatologists "senile keratoma." The face and backs of the hands is a favorable location for this disease. These keratomas may remain for

such sores have proven to be either syphilitic, tubercular, or malignant.

Upon my attendance this summer at the "Skin and Cancer Hospital," New York, we heard practically the same advice given by the chief of the clinical-staff to many such patients. At the last meeting of the A. M. A., St. Louis, before the Dermatological Section, Dr. Bloodgood, a noted surgeon of Baltimore, made this assertion: "The majority of tumors and epitheliomas of the upper part of the body date their beginning to some trauma or constant irritation, especially is this true of the face and trunk." He added that, "After removal by excision, I am sorry to report, the greater number so removed have returned." Whether this return was due to the method of treatment or to the lateness of the period at which most patients submit to surgery, we have presumed to briefly discuss under treatment.

Regarding heredity, let us assert this as our belief, namely: Heredity plays only such part as is now attributed to the same cause for tuberculosis, namely, heredity is a factor only so far as association or contact is concerned. True, the factor of heredity has been handed down from age to age, and from text to text, yet the same has been true of tuberculosis until the past few years. Dr. Cullen, of Philadelphia, who has made as wide investigations of statistics upon the subject of heredity in cancer as perhaps any other man, tells us that statistics show a history of heredity in only about nineteen per cent. We believe we can safely assert that the time is now at hand when we shall claim for heredity only such part as the weakened body of infected parents thereby a frequent association. This is proven by pathologists who have found that by inoculating mice and dogs the offspring of the animals infected appear to be more susceptible to such inoculation, though such animals do not transmit such lesions to their progeny.

DIAGNOSIS.

As has been intimated in the former part of this paper, we consider the microscope one of the most valuable aids. However, certain signs or clinical manifestations are so obvious that they become, to the experienced, quite reliable. This history will in most cases differentiate syphilis or other destructive lesions. The early tubercle or roughened appearance, the degeneration in

the center of the lesion, or, perhaps, it may extend back under the edges of the epidermis, or, may be the opposite, an excessive proliferation of central tissue, presents to the trained eye immediately a suspicion of malignancy. The common rolled appearing edges of the epithelioma are not, in our experience, present in so great a number of cases as text books would imply. Nor do we have the described short or darting pains until after distinct evidence of lymphatic absorption has begun. The depth of the lesion, its tendency to bleed upon slight irritation, its continued invasion of surrounding tissue, in spite of the ordinary treatment which has been given, are, in our opinion, strong evidence upon which we may base a diagnosis.

From lupus it is more difficult to differentiate, perhaps, than from any of the common lesions, but if we consider that lupus is usually slower in growth, accompanied with slight, if any pain, its more superficial nature, the less tendency to bleed upon irritation, its frequent so-called apple jelly exudates, are points which should, if carefully considered, differentiate from epithelioma.

One other disease which seems to be rapidly increasing in the United States, in which country it was first discovered and described, is to be differentiated, namely, blasto-mycosis. If we remember that blasto-mycosis in its early stages is very superficial, extending only to the corion, and that it is also studded by many small or miliary pustules or openings from which pus may be made to exude on slight pressure, and the simplicity of a microscopic examination for blasto-mycetes, we should have no trouble in differentiating.

The initial lesion of epithelioma, as has been previously mentioned, is, in a large number of cases, the senile keratoma. It is this stage which is most difficult to diagnose. This, too, is the stage in which a more perfect and certain cure may be promised. Usually the family physician first sees the patient and if a request for a section of the lesion for microscopic examination is made in most cases it is refused by the patient, and yet the prognosis is almost entirely dependent upon the diagnosis of these malignancies at this stage, that is, before lymphatic dissemination and glandular involvement has begun. If we fail in this paper to impress you with any other thought, please let us repeat this one statement, do not, for the sake of your reputation in after years, and for the sake of the life and welfare of your patient who is looking to you for conscientious and intelligent advice, make the too often serious error of advising him to, "just let it alone, don't bother it, forget it and it will amount to nothing."

TREATMENT.

Were we to attempt to name all the remedies which have been tried upon cancers, or even to mention all the "sure cures" of the Cancer Quack, perhaps in no other disease would there be an equal number of remedies unless in the one previously mentioned, tuberculosis. Though all methods may be classed as either, (1) Internal; (2) Surgical; (3) Destructive, either by drugs or by mechanical means; (4) Radiation; and as a fifth, we might mention the probable future method which is at present only experimental, injection with different fluids, serums, etc.

Of internal treatment, let us dispose in short by saying none can be recognized by an intelligent observer.

SURGICAL.

Surgery has been for ages a method and is still the method of choice by all for certain localities upon the body or stages of the disease. But with due respect for this method and for the men who practice it. let us say that, according to statistics by

Bloodgood and others, even by this method the greater per cent have a recurrence within one to three years. This, however, may be due, as some surgeons are prone to imply, to the disposition of the patient to make surgery the last method tried.

With regard to drugs. This is the method practiced chiefly by quacks and cancer charlatans, thereby causing the regular profession to look upon this method with prejudiced eye, yet in spite of the very unsightly scars or contractures which so frequently follow the use of this method by the ignorant "Cancer Quack," we are compelled to confess that they have produced a complete cure in many cases of a true skin cancer.

Of the regular profession who have for so long a period advocated and practiced the caustic methods and who have so tenaciously improved and taught us this method, none deserve more credit than Dr. Robinson of New York.

The chief objection found to the caustic or sloughing processes, are, our inability to judge the depth of the slough we may get; the violent reaction and pain which usually follow the application; and the unsightly scars and contractures, especially if located upon the face. Even the Paquelin cautery or the red hot iron has been successful in many cases. We recently heard Dr. Pusey assert that if you gave him a red hot poker he could absolutely cure a great per cent of lipitheliomas in the primary or preglandular stage.

RADIATION.

With reference to radium, we pass it briefly by saying we have had experience with this agent; however, we believe its effects practically the same as X-Ray, but the expense is almost prohibitive.

Since a period of only a few months following the discovery of the X-Ray in November, 1895, it has been given a great ovation as a therapeutic agent. It soon became a favorite method by the advertising M. D. And so soon did the serious evils begin to be learned only by sad experience, by patient and operator alike. After which the pendulum of public opinion by the more conservative or the prejudiced M. D., then began to swing extremely to the reverse. Such was the status of the X-Ray. But thanks to the persistent and observing few, and all honor to the seventeen or more medical martyrs to this agent, the X-Ray has been clearly demonstrated to be a strong agent capable of good or evil just in proportion to the caution and intelligence of the operator.

You ask me in my enthusiasm would I assert that the X-Ray will cure all cases of epithelioma? Nay, indeed. No such agent as a specific is yet known. Then, what may we claim for this agent? It is this: That, according to statistics from skilful and intelligent medical operators of machines, the X-Ray has proven to be just as effective, when cases are treated for a sufficient length of time, and is followed with perhaps less returns in the primary or pre-glandular stage than any other method practiced today. It should be the method of choice for all accessible and exposed lesions, particularly those located upon the face, before glandular involvement has begun. After glandular involvement, first operate, then follow with X-Ray. This is the opinion not only of most dermatologists, but of our foremost surgeons as well.

Pathologists have clearly demonstrated to us from sections made from lesions before and after treatment by both the caustic and raying methods, that their effects are somewhat similar, namely, that the terminal blood vessels, lymph spaces and channels, are obliterated or blocked in such manner as to greatly hinder absorption and dissemination of the pathological cells or the infected material, whereas, in surgery, the clean-cut incisions, however wide they may be, leave open vessels where pathological

material may be taken up readily by the freely open spaces, channels and vessels, just back of the occluding clot.

Please do not misunderstand my statements, for surgery, even with its great percentage of returns, is the best known method today in any case where glandular involvement has already taken place. A custom practiced today by the largest number of our leading surgeons, is, that after a complete removal of all visible pathological tissue, to refer the patient immediately to X-Ray as a precaution against further malignant cells or infective material which so frequently remains. Such custom is also becoming more popular since time is differentiating the percentage of returns from the former methods of surgery alone. We heard Dr. Pusey recently assert that out of a series of about 500 cases of epithelioma treated by him with X-Rays since 1901, he had no cause as yet for regrets.

Regarding the recent experiments with injections or serum prepared from the acetic fluid of an individual suffering from cancer, also the somewhat similar experiment that has been carried on in the Rockefeller Institute for Medical Research in New York, let us still hope.

We have of recent months become quite optimistic in the faith that the dawn of the day which shall illumine the true etiology and a more perfect treatment of this, one of our most distressing and fatal maladies, is at hand.

In the meantime let each of us be more observing in regard to etiology, become more adept in making an early diagnosis, and cautiously select the best method of treatment for each particular case.

We append some photographs of cases before and after treatment by X-Ray, and only for the length of the paper do we refrain from narrating some interesting histories connected with same.

E. S. Lain, M. D.
Oklahoma City, September, 1910.

CRETINISM WITH REPORT OF CASE

BY DR. J. E. HUGHES, SHAWNEE, OKLAHOMA

Cretinism is a type of mental and physical degeneracy, due to an absence or diminution in the function of the thyroid gland. The disease is rarely congenital—developing, usually, the first year of extra-uterine life; occasionally not manifesting itself until the fourth or fifth year.

Sporadic cretins are found the world over. No race is known to be exempt. It is this type we have largely to deal with in this country. In certain shut in mountainous valleys of Switzerland, Italy Spain, Sweden and Brazil cretinism is an endemic disease, affecting a large per cent. of the inhabitants of those districts. No physical differences can be established between the sporadic and endemic forms, but an apparent difference as to cause is seen in the more frequent association of goitre with cretinism in the localities where both are endemic.

Just the relation between the thyroidal changes and the development of cretinism is not definitely understood, but the general accepted theory is—that the gland produces a substance which acts as an anti-body or antitoxin to certain toxic products of daily metabolism; and, if the toxic products are not antagonized, they remain in the body and exercise a deleterious influence principally on the nervous system, also on the skeletal and tegmental tissues of the body; and, if the individual is young, there will be an arrest of both mental and physical development and cretinism will ensue.

Several cases of cretinism have been reported following operation on children for the removal of the thyroid gland, the degree of cretinism depending on the age of the patient. The earlier the removal of the thyroid gland the more marked the cretonic state.

Myxedema, whether operative or a result of morbid changes in the thyroid itself, is essentially cretinism in the adult. The individual's mental and physical development well under way before the thyroid ceases to functionate. Experimentally, the removal of the thyroid gland in young-growing animals—if the animal survives—there is that same arrest of development analogous to cretinism in man.

Just what brings about these morbid changes in the thyroid our knowledge is quite lacking. In sporadic cretinism many theories have been advanced, foremost among which are consanguinity of parents, alchoholic intoxication at time of conception and thyroiditis as a sequela of infectious diseases, but the frequency of these conditions and the rarity of cretinism forces us to give little weight to these theories. In the endemic form of cretinism our attention is directed to the water supply as the probable etiological carrier of the disease; for in these cretin districts a change in the water supply is always followed by a marked decrease in the number of cretins. Even the boiling of the water renders it innocuous. This would suggest a bacterial cause for the disease. Much research has been done along these lines; and, like many other diseases of unknown origin, many bacteria have been isolated, but as yet none have fulfilled Koch's postulate, and we are still seeking for the true etiological cause.

The clinical picture of cretinism is very characteristic. There is a remarkable uniformity in the physiognomy of all cretins, so much so that the individuality of a normal human being is largely obliterated. Balzac, in his novel, "The Country Doctors," typifies the cretin as "a being without the physical beauties of an animal, or the mental endowments of a man." One of these creatures was brought to me for treatment about three years ago. The patient, a female, the fifth child of a family, to all appearances normal at birth, with a negative history as to gestation, porturition and heredity, continued to thrive until between the fifth and sixth month, when the mother noticed retrogressive changes in the physical and mental developments of the child. About the seventh month the child was first seen by me, and as I remember, this was the mother's statement: "Doctor, while our baby does not appear sick, she certainly does not look and act right." The child was rather short, the limbs stunted. The natural plumpness over the back and limbs was wanting, while there was an apparent over-deposit of adipose tissue about the face, neck and groins. Even the head appeared fleshy and rested directly on the shoulders, or rolled forward on the chest when unsupported. The hair was course and extended well down on the forehead. The face was stupid, expressionless and repulsive; the nose was broad, flat, with wide flaring nostrils. The mouth was large, lips fleshy and between them protruded a large swollen tongue. The skin was pale, thick and dry, and lay in folds or waddles. The abdomen was large and protruberent, presenting a large umbilical hernia. From the above picture, a diagnosis of sporadic cretinism was made and confirmed by one of my colleagues. Thyroid treatment was immediately instituted, and from the first there was a marked improvement in the child's general appearance. The fleshy face, the thick lips, the large drolling tongue and expressionless eyes, which had stamped the child an imbecile, gradually gave way to the features of a happy and

more nearly normal child; however, the body weight did not increase, in fact there was a slight loss of weight for the first two months, then a slight, but gradual, gain was observed. The child at one year of age passed from under my observation. In a recent communication from the mother, she writes: "We still continue the thyroid treatment—not continuously, but only when we are afraid she needs it." The child was able to sit alone when nineteen months old; walked at two years, and four months, and now at three and one-half years of age is regarded to be a healthy and normal child.

The thyroid treatment most probably will have to be continued throughout life, though a few cases of spontaneous cases have been reported. However, this is not to be expected, and can only be explained in that the administration of thyroid extract tides the patient over, until such a time when there may be a regeneration of new gland tissue, from some pre-existing or non-functioning thyroid cells. The grafting of normal thyroid tissue on to the peritoneum would seem a most rational procedure, and in a few cases improvement has been observed, but at the present time the daily administration of some of the thyroid preparations have proven the most satisfactory treatment.

DISCUSSION.

Dr. A. S. Hagood, Durant, Bryan County:

I enjoyed that paper very much. It shows that the Doctor has given it considerable study, and I think he has covered the ground entirely. I don't think anything could be added to the paper. There isn't much room for discussion.

Dr. Winnie M. Sanger, Oklahoma City:

I want to say that we have under treatment now our first case of sporadic cretinism. A child three months old who would answer the same description the doctor gave. We had the same experience that the doctor reports. The loss of flesh at first, but the child already looks more normal, and the rolling tongue very much less prominent.

Dr. R. L. Coons, Elk City:

1 enjoyed the paper very much. It was a very interesting, scientific paper, and all 1 wish to speak about is the heredity of cretinism. About fifteen years ago when I was studying medicine a young physician asked me to go with him back to Madison, Pa., to see a peculiar family. There were fifteen children in the family. The father had goiter, the mother had goiter, and every child in the family had some trouble with the thyroid gland. Three cretins in the family and the rest of the children had goiter. I don't remember of ever seeing another case of the kind.

Dr. Carl Puckett, Pryor:

I am about as well up on this subject as I might be on cholera or some of those diseases we don't have in this country. I could say but very little about this paper that would be of special interest, but I must say that I O. K. his treatment of thyroid extract. I haven't had any experience at all in cretinism, but other similar of mental troubles, sometimes epilepsy and other things which we find either from birth or from young childhood, or an arrest from physical development, I find that the thyroid treatment is the very best thing we can use.

Dr. D. E. Broderick, Kansas City Mo:

I was waiting for somebody to recite an experience like I had when I was in general practice a few years back, and I treated the child with thyroid for about three years. And on taking up the children's work in London I was acquainted with that class of idiocy known as the Mongola idiot. The difference between the Mongola idiot and the cretin depends on the shape of the palpebral fissure. And the other mental development is about the same as the cretin.

I wish to add that in treating cretinism small doses of thyroid are given. Large doses of thyroid extract are liable to produce a diarrhoea that is fatal.

I have seen between twenty and twenty-five cretin cases and all these cases were diagnosed in infancy during the first year. Unless the case is diagnosed in the first year thyroid extract does not improve the mental caliber. And as the doctor well brought out, the treatment has to be continued throughout the life.

FURTHER EXPERIENCE WITH INTERNAL SPLINT IN TREATMENT OF FRACTURES

BY HERMAN E. PEARSE, M. D., KANSAS CITY, MO.

Surgeon to St. Luke's Hospital; Surgeon to the General Hospital; Post Graduate Hospital; Acting Assistant Surgeon to United States Marine Hospital Service.

In May, 1909, I read a paper upon "The Use of Internal Or Direct Splint, in the Treatment of Bone." The matter had been called to my attention by the excellent work of the author of the method, Mr. Wm. Arbuthnot Lane, of the Guy's Hospital, London. At that time I stated as follows:

The revelations of the X-Ray have proven to us what post mortem findings had led us to suspect; we are never, al-most never, getting the ends of two bones in good apposition by extension, counter-extension and splint. The work of the masseur has proven that we kept the parts too long immobilized. We too often have had stiff members. These have been the heritage of the old system of "setting" fractures—pain, long loss of use, crooked parts, poor use of mended members, some-times loss of reputation and occasional damage suits, and the more the X-Ray is educating the public, the oftener comes the protest against the result.

A large number, perhaps a majority, of the suits filed against doctors are from results after fracture "setting."

The following are insurmountable ob-stacles to exactness and, hence, to perfec-tion of results under the external splint method;

1.—It is impossible to see the ends of bone, hence impossible to secure accurate apposition of ends.

2.—Breaks are never so exactly trans-verse as act to slip side-wise upon occasion.

3.—Portions of fascia and muscle will become misplaced and engage between the ends of the bone.

4.—The hemorrhage from broken bones does not stop until the parts are packed with a blood clot that must be absorbed and whose presence increases the stiffness, and uselessness of the mended member.

5.—External splints applied over the parts, separated from the actual bone by muscle, fat and skin cannot hold the parts in more than indifferent position, and then only by exerting undue pressure upon the soft parts.

6.—Too often one fragment of the brok-en bone is too short to afford proper bear-ing for the splint and thus maintain the axis of the bone in its proper position.

7.—Every factor of the external splint

process used to maintain apposition, splints, bandages, pressure, extension and rest, all these tell against nutrition.

8.—Early motion which is the panacea for stiffness and loss of function must be sacrificed to the need for bony apposition.

In view of these reasons for imperfect results, the external splint method has been recognized as faulty, and I am desirous of presenting to you a much better method, which is applicable to any recent fracture whenever perfect aseptic technique can be carried out, i. e.—The incision of the soft parts and the application of a steel splint or splice fastened with screws directly to the replaced fragments of the bone in such a manner as to maintain perfect apposi-tion. If the fragment is a condyle or other projection it can sometimes be simply fast-ened by screws, nails or steeples.

I have done this operation up to the present time upon twenty-three cases, the complete records of which were mostly de-stroyed in the fire which burned the Rialto Building, December 23rd, 1909. These splints open up a new and legitimate field of surgery that should not be abused by careless invasion but if properly approach-ed and cultivated will result in the saving of many limbs that would otherwise be amputated and in the very great lessening of time required in the repair of serious fractures. There will also be many straight strong, useful members where now are crooked and useless ones.

I employ the method:

1.—In single fractures where external splinting, plaster of paris or extension fails to retain the broken bones in fairly good apposition.

2.—In simple fractures very near a joint or involving a joint.

3.—In compound fractures where on ac-count of the location of the external wound or of damage to soft parts proper immobilization can be done.

4.—In ununited fractures where I formerly used silver wire.

The questions usually asked me are about the following:

1.—"Do you take out the splint after the fractures is united?"

No. The splint is left permanently in place if possible.

2.—"Does the splint ever come out?" Yes, nature will some times cause a splint to loosen and come away, months or even years after it is put in. Should it be seen to be causing trouble it is best to cut down and remove it. This is devoid of danger if aseptic technique is employed.

3.—"What about the splint in compound fractures?" Usually I pack down to the splint. I do not expect the splint to remain over eight to twenty weeks in a bad compound case—only long enough to secure solid bone union, then remove it.

4.—"Do you treat all fractures by this method?" No, the method is applicable to all classes of fractures, but in my practice there has been so far need of the splint only once in four or five cases of fractures. In my service at the Kansas City General Hospital, I think I operated about once in four cases.

5.—"What is the technique?" I feel bound to quote the exact language of the author in this matter. Here is the technique as told by Mr. Lane himself in "Operative Treatment of Fractures:"

"The operative treatment of simple fracture is compartively easy in the majority of cases, and if due care be taken and reasonable skill be exercised the risk is practically nil."

"In certain small proportion of cases, the bone may be too friable, too thin, or too much broken up, and the surgeon may therefore be unable to restore it completely to its original form. Even in these cir-

cumstances he can almost obtain a much better result by operating than by any other form of treatment."

"Age is no barrier to operation; indeed, in old people an operation is often more imperatively called for them in vigorous life for the reason that prolonged recumbency in old age is a very serious matter, often entailing of necessity a fatal result. The shock sustained from surgical interference is trivial, old people bearing operation well. Alcohol patients, in whom the soft parts about the fracture have been very severely damaged as a result of direct violence, incur more risk from the injury than healthy ones, so it follows that the additional risk consequent on operation in these cases is naturally greater than in the normal subject, not because of the operation but because of the conditions in which the operation is performed. In other words, alcoholism and direct injury to soft parts increase the danger of fractures and also add to the risk of their operative treatment. I have found the bones of chronic alcoholics to be frequently thin and friable."

"Many complaints have been made by surgeons who have failed to obtain good results by operation. For example, some have said their screws would not hold and others that they could not obtain union. These failures are due to the fact that the very moderate cleanliness necessary to obtain a good result in ordinary operations is quite insufficient to meet that required when a large piece of metal, whether steel or silver, is left buried in the wound."

"If the surgeon has not succeeded in such a simple operation as wiring fractures of the patella without killing or permanently disabling many of his patients, he had better bring himself to believe that the results of the generally accepted methods of treatment are excellent, and that any statements to the contrary are exaggerated or imaginary, and leave operations on recent fractures alone, since they may test the methods and skill of the operator to the utmost."

"In performing these operations, not only must you not touch the interior of the wound with your hands, nor permit the patients skin to do so either, but you must never let any portion of an instrument which has been in contact with your skin or with that of the patient touch the raw surface. All sponges must be held in forceps and applied to the wound in that manner. They should not be handled in any way previous to being used."

"After an instrument has been used for a length of time, or forcibly it should be reboiled or placed in a germicidal solution."

"I have occasionally seen beginners employ the handle of a knife or dissecting forceps to separate adherent parts, or to displace some structure instead of using the particular instrument made for that purpose. I need not remind you that this must not be done on any pretext whatever."

"It is probably unnecessary to say that no germicidal or other liquid should be introduced into the wound."

"The details of the operation are as follows:

"Get the skin thoroughly clean. This may sometimes take several days, as the thick indurated epidermis of the foot and knee is often difficult to remove. I find large moist compresses with careful scrapings most effective in enabling one to get rid of suspicious material. When this has been properly done a germicide should be applied to render the skin as clean as possible."

"Choose a situation for your incision which involves a minimum chance of damage to important structure and a maximum advantage from the point of view of accessibility. Do not hesitate to make the incision of a length sufficient to enable you to deal effectually with the fragments. There is no greater mistake than to exaggerate the difficulties of the operations by employing an incision which is not sufficiently long to permit of easy access to and ready manipulation of the fragments. Its length in no way increases the risk the patient runs, but usually adds to his safety, since it enables the surgeon to deal with the fragments more readily."

"Having made the incision, exclude the skin of the patient from contact with the wound. This can be done effectually by attaching sterile cloths to the cutaneous margins of the incisions by forceps. These are made in several sizes."

"The fragments are exposed and examined, and when all clot and material intervening between them have been removed they are brought into accurate apposition. To do this much traction may be necessary, combined with the leverage action of elevators and the approximating influence of powerful long-handled forceps. The long, forceps I employ are very powerful and are made with a limited grasp to facilitate their use."

"If there be any bleeding it is effectually dealt with by strong compression forceps long enough to allow that portion of the handles which have come into contact with the fingers to protude beyond the areas of the wound. Their grip is sufficiently firm to occlude the vessels if they are kept on for a short time, and so the necessity for a ligature is obviated."

There are certain points I wish to emphasize:

1.—The incision should be long and free; it is a great mistake to try to work through an insufficient incision.

2.—Make the incision at whatever location the bone can be approached with least damage to soft parts.

3.—Hold the bones in close apposition by heavy forceps while fitting the splints and drilling the holes. Have a sharp drill the exact size of the screw to be used. If larger the screw will not hold. If smaller you will have trouble in driving the screws home.

4.—Boil everything that is to touch the wound one hour except rubber gloves and cutting instruments. Boil former ten minutes; place the latter in 95 per cent. carbolic acid or 5 per cent. formalin for thirty minutes, then in alcohol thirty minutes.

5.—Pay particular attention to the periosteum. Get it closely laid on the bone. Splints go outside the periosteum. In bad, compound fractures one can depend on the periosteum to build in new bone if it is properly place.

The bone is seized by strong forceps, and the fragments are closely fitted together under the eye of the surgeon; every portion of the break is made to fit accurately. No further oozing occurs from broken bone ends. Blood clots in the soft parts are carefully wiped away. Any fragment of periosteum or fascia that may have been displaced is placed in its proper relation. From the supply at hand taken clean and boiled from the sterlizer, the surgeon selects one splice or internal splint that fits the parts and secures it firmly. More than one can be used if desired. These splints are from fine, malleable, steel strips, ground out, shaped, smoothed and polished by a machinist and screw holes made at convenient distances. They may be made of silver or other material if desired, but steel answers all purposes, and can be made by any one having some mechanical skill in a short time. After fitting the splint carefully the holes are drilled into the bone to receive the screws. These are short, and are intended to be received into the proximal bone only. The narrow splint and the short screws are recent modifications.

The splint may not be retained but it usually is. If not a sinus forms, or there is some irritation, and the surgeon cuts down and removes the splint through a small incision.

The case shown here received a gunshot wound of the arm, when the upper arm was lying over the muzzle of a shot gun. There was severe sepsis when he came to me for amputation. After making clean the wound which required much time and some further incision of soft parts, the ends of the shattered bone were brought in apposition and I decided to try to save the arm with some four or five inches of the bone gone. A metal splint with screws was applied and continuous irrigation used for seventy-two hours. The temperature dropped but suppuration continued intense. At the 10th day the splint broke during sleep. I supplied two others next day, each heavier than the first. One of these broke and the other loosened at the upper end at the end of four weeks and the bones separated about one and one-half inches. It then held and rendered the arm quite firm as the cross arms of the T splint had been bended around the upper fragment. The periosteum commenced building about the sixth to eighth week as I remember and finally has become quite firm. One splint has been removed. The other is still in place.

A complication of this case was an attack of tetanus occurring the nineteenth or twentieth day from which you will see he has recovered.

He has a shortened arm, but is pitching hay, plowing and doing farm work with the new bone formation and the iron splint in place.

Suite 618 Commerce Building.

DISCUSSION.

Dr. Berry:

The matter that the doctor calls attention to is a very radical procedure, and we have been seeing a great deal about it in the surgical journals, and I heard Prof. Matas about two months ago in New Orleans, discuss fractures and discussing re-uniting of these fractures by this and other methods along that line, and those who are present and are conversant with Prof. Matas' experience, know that there is no man who has had more experience, and he says it is best never to put a foreign body next to the bone. He never uses a screw, practically never. He says that he makes a rare exception, but his rule is never, because he almost invariably has to take it out. It may be that the doctor's method has something to do with making the condition tolerant, but it seems to me that that would be a very hazardous undertaking for the average surgeon over the country. However, I feel sure that there are cases where it might be a good practice to take those splints out. I believe that a damage suit would be likely to come up as a result of this operation because it is a radical operation. I see a decision rendered by justice Dunn in a fracture suit, in which he takes a very sensible view that the bad result is the inability of nature to respond to the conditions, and proved to be correct in this case. It is the duty of every physician to stand by those who are involved in damage suits. Any of you can be sued without any cause, and be caused a great deal of expense and trouble, no matter what method you try. And getting down to the last analysis, I believe that the simplest treatment is the best.

Dr. Pearse: I was glad to hear the doctor say it is dangerous. It is a good deal like the Irishman's whiskey. There isn't any danger in it if you just remember it's dangerous. And so if we can take care of it we will have very little trouble. There is no hurry in doing it; there is no necessity in doing it the day the patient is injured. Say at the end of a week, tell your patient, I have done everything that can be done to get these bones in apposition, and have not done so. Will you take the risk your self of having a crooked arm, or will you have the arm operated on? Then the patient takes the blame. My patients usually say, "I want a straight member." "Very well, I will operate and fix it for you." And I don't have much trouble. If we get these bones in a straight line and hold it there, the growth of the bone will be maintained, and will complete itself beyond what it will if the two ends are not in apposition. There is a limit to the amount of a foreign body which nature will tolerate but these splints are tolerated so nicely that you will be surprised to see the people going around and working with them without any trouble whatever. There are just two reasons for taking them out. The first is where they are close to the skin and hurt; and the second is where the uncontrollable curiosity of the surgeon is responsible for his cutting down and taking them out.

MEDICAL ETHICS

BY DR. L. S. WILLOUR, ATOKA, OKLAHOMA.

I feel greatly honored to be asked to present to this Society a paper on Medical Ethics, at the same time I feel considerable you, in that I am not an authority upon the subject, and in a great many ways I fall far short of maintaining the ethical position which goes so far toward making the perfect professional man.

At many times and upon many occasions, a doctor acts unethically without any intent whatever, this is due more or less to carelessness and many complications that arise from these inadvertant acts could be avoided by being a little more thoughtful and using greater care to think before we speak or act.

Some professional men I fear, think that nothing is unethical if it is not found out, the same opinion is held by some with regard to right and wrong, that a person only does wrong when they are caught with the goods, but this is a very low standard indeed, and I am sure that you will all agree with me that confidential reports should bear the same mark of a high ethical position as should be maintained in our open personal relations. As Secretary of the Atoka-Coal County Medical Society, which position the Society was unfortunate enough to have me fill for two years, I had a great many inquiries regarding the professional standing of many of the members and always the replies were to be held strictly confidential. I am glad to say that it never was necessary for me to make an unfavorable report and I would maintain the position that any doctor who can retain his membership in our County Medical Society is of a professional character that would entitle him to a very favorable consideration. If he is not worthy of your recommendation for an office of trust, don't be hypocritical enough to let him retain his membership and then condem him in some confidential report where you feel sure he will never know the origin of the knock he has received.

I have been fortunate enough during my professional life to live most of the time in communities where the relation existing between the members of the medical profession was the most pleasant, of course there have sometimes been misunderstandings, but I have a prescription for this trouble which works in most instances, bringing the best of results, it is always to go to the doctor whom you think has done you an injustice and then and there have an understanding, don't go to someone else and make bitter remarks, for your primary visit to the man you think has wronged you will, as a rule adjust the matter as a proper explanation of both sides of a question will usually do.

There is no use for me to attempt to lay down any fixed rules or regulations regarding the conduct of the doctor, who would be professional and ethical, but there is one great rule that covers the ground very thoroughly, that is, the Golden Rule, let the doctor abide by this and professional misunderstandings will be few and far between. Every thinking man despises a knocker, so remember that when a derogatory remark is made by one doctor about another, it is the remarkor rather than the remarked about who receives the damage.

Medical ethics does not stop merely with the relation which exists between the doctor and his colleague. We should above all things be honest and ethical with our patients, how many times is the physician tempted to give some treatment or do some operation, where the pay is good, when we are confident it will be of no advantage to the patient.

It may be hard for some of us to even confess this to ourselves, but we are all human and I know from personal experience that when the bank book looks as red as an autumn sunset, we may make the fatal mistake of taking advantage of some patient, who has placed in us implicit confidence.

There are, of course, times when it is

best to withhold the truth regarding the condition of a patient, but this is very infreqently the case, I am inclined to believe that we are apt to mislead ourselves regarding this matter, and will often withhold our true opinion when it would be far better to state the absolute facts. Of course, this is a matter for each man to decide for himself, but let us all use the greatest care and the very best judgment, when we make any statement to a patient.

Any profession will succeed just in direct proportion to the loyalty of its members, consequently, it stands the members of the medical fraternity in hand, to show and practice, the highest possible degree of medical fraternalism. At this time we are being imposed upon by "pathies" and "isms" that would fain displace us to make room for some "watch that the hand does not decieve the eye" cure, and it is only by a concerted effort upon the part of the doctors that we are able to show to the people the quackery that is about to be imposed upon them, therefore, let every member of the medical profession stand shoulder to shoulder with his brother practitioner, and help to maintain the dignity of the healing art and not allow it to fall to the level of a street faker as some of our friends who practice quackery are endeavoring to bring it.

I am confident that all I have said has been for naught as I am sure there are no men in this meeting who would conduct themselves in other than an ethical manner, and among ourselves I could only suggest that we be more thoughtful and try to preserve a professional balance that will be looked upon with envy by the medical profession in other localities.

It is occasions of this character that tend to develop medical fraternalism. What man can come here and after associating with his fellow practitioners for a day, and together enjoying such a sumptuous repast, and so excellent a brew go back to his practice and do otherwise than treat his neighbor doctor ethically. To develop the social relation among the profession has always been my remedy for the sore head; consequently, I would make a very favorable prognosis, of any case that may have started for Aylsworth with this trouble, if there be one, allow me to pronounce you cured. and if there is a relapse, the chances are that it will be your own fault, so, when you begin to see the prodromal symptoms either of a relapse or a new attack, call in the doctor whom you think has not treated you with the professional courtesy that is your due, and over two small bottles of "Bud" talk it over, the result will be very gratifying, not only the result of the talk, but also the "Bud."

A CASE REQUIRING HERNIOTOMY AND LIPECTOMY

BY DR. C. N. BALLARD, OKLAHOMA CITY, OKLAHOMA

Associate Professor of Gynecology and Clinical Gynecology at College of Physicians and Surgeons (Medical Department of the University of Illinois); Surgeon to Marion Sim's Sanitarium, Chicago; Attending Surgeon at West Side Hospital, Chicago; Attendant in Gynecology at the West Side Free Dispensary.

When asked to appear upon the program to read a paper before this audience of medical men, it seemed that it would be difficult to select a subject that could be of interest.

There is so much written that one feels that each subject had been exhausted, but like biblical literature, the more we think and investigate the more new means of discussing the same old subject, present themselves. New fields for discussion are noted daily.

New minds, researchful in tendency, unfold advanced ideas that enable us to understand, even our old hobbies, more thoroughly.

There is no man, who loves his profession, but has or should have some hobby, something he can do better than his colleague.

He may, in discussing his special work, seem to be an extremist, yet it is only through these extremists that we are to perfect a working mean. So let them work on and we will sift the chaff from the mixture and appropriate the real kernel.

The title of this paper is indefinite, it is not explanatory of the thought in mind.

It is such a common condition that most men have refrained from discussing. it, yet so new no one has satisfactorily explained why it exists. First, because it is as old as woman-kind; second, because it has been called "a freak of nature" and nature allowed to care for it.

Howard Kelly, in 1899, reported his first case, and that was for the removal of fat alone. Since that time he has operated on seven other cases, four for the cosmetic effect, and three complicated with umbilical hernia. There has been but one case reported, and that was by Wienhold, in 1909, a case complicated with umbilical hernia. The case which I shall report in this connection is my fourth, two for cosmetic effect and two complicated with umbilical hernia. The first three were clinical cases and not reported.

The technique in each writers report, has been independent and different, each one reporting success alike. This shows that it is not always the technique, but each surgeon to his perfected technique, that makes his work a success.

In considering fatty deposits, we are to distinguish between lipomata and pipo-matosis. The former is an encapsulated fatty accumulation, which may have a distribution as wide as adipose tissue.

It is the most generalized genus of tumor which occurs in man, except sarcomata. There is usually one to be found, but there may be many, varying in size.

The skin and peritoneum rests upon a cushion of fat, the thickness of which varies greatly in different individuals as well as in different locations in the same individuals. As examples, in the renal region, and in the mesentary and omentum, the deposit is abundant, while beneath the peritoneum covering the liver, uterus, Fallopian tubes and ovaries, but little is found. Encapsulated collections of fat are to be found, variously distributed in the subserous tissue.

They obtain a large size in the mesentery, in the fat at the base of the broad ligament, and in relation to the peritoneal fat.

Their size makes them difficult to diagnose from many other abdominal tumors. The lobulated collections of subserous fat found in the region of the inguinal and femoral ring may simulate hernia by protruding into the sac and drawing a small pouch of peritoneum with it. This same linea alba, this so called, fatty hernia of the peritoneal pouch is sometimes found in the linea alba may be later accompanied by a loop of bowel, and complete a true hernial sac.

Encapsulated subserous fatty accumulations have been found in the lumen of the bowel, having protruded through the muscular coat of the gut and caused obstruction. In these cases a dimpled appearance can be noticed on the serous side of the bowel. Virchow has found this condition in the stomach.

Deposits of this nature have been found in the joints, most frequent in the knee. Very large tumors of this kind are often found between the muscles of the abdominal wall, of less size in the periosteum of bones, as the scapula femur and ischeum.

They are to be found in the trunks of nerves, as in the mediam at the wrist, and the great sciatic in the ham.

A case is reported of a growth the size of a child's fist, growing from the sella turcica, extending into the middle fossa of the skull, causing periodic pains in the head and finally ptosis.

The lipoma proper is usually easily diagnosed, yet it is found in some locations, where to diagnose it is difficult, as examples, when found connected with the periosteum of the long bones it may be mistaken for sarcoma, or when imbedded in muscle tissue, or the tongue.

Large lipomata in the subperintoneal tissue mimic most acurately an ovarian tumor. A deposit of fat over the sac of spina bifida, may be mistaken for a fatty tumor and the sac be opened in consequence. These tumors proper, are very closely connected to the skin, they have a definite outline, and a doughey feel. This will in ordinary locations enable us to make a diagnosis.

Fat presents two opposing conditions, fatty infiltration and fatty degeneration. The former, with which this paper has to deal principally, is storage fat, accumulated in the cells, either as the result of an intake of food material, affording neutral fats over and above the capacity of the tissue to organize, or of oxidative capacities of the tissues below the normal, so that food-stuffs reach the stage of neutral fat, but do not, forth-with pass beyond that. Neutral fat is found in most of the tissues of the body, but this, in a state in which it is not recognizable in the cells, either by simple microscopic or microchemical means.

Adami states, "that the kidney tissue may, by all the usual microscopic methods, or by osmic acid, show not a trace of fat, yet by appropriate chemical means as much as 23 per cent of the total solids of the kidney may be demonstrated to consist of fats.

Properly speaking, fatty infiltration is more accurately defined and demonstrated when it accumulates between the fibers that constitute the bulk of the organ, as fatty deposits among the fibers of the heart muscle.

During pregnancy we find the liver cell the seat of the accumulation of fat, as another example of fatty infiltration. This accumulation is sometimes extreme, even 4-5 of the solids of the organ being fatty tissue and 41 per cent of the total cell substance, might be fat. In the liver, the liver cell proper is affected, while in other parts of the body the connective tissue cells are involved.

This accumulation of visible neutral fat in the otherwise normal cells of connective tissues, and the liver, occurs in various conditions. Seemingly fore-stalling its necessity during pregnancy and lactation, we find it heaping up in various places, especially in the liver. In the performance of our various functions of life, more fatty matters may be taken in or elaborated than can be burnt up. The "Aldermanic" type of individual, and the over-fed "Strassburg goose" are familiar examples of this form of fatty infiltration.

We find a substitution form of fat accumulation in the liver of those addicted to the use of alcohol, notwithstanding they are usually small eaters. Two factors are operating in these cases.

Alcohol acting on the nerve centers, or directly on the cells of the body, lowers functional activity and oxidation, and so the fats absorbed are not burnt up; again, alcohol is in itself a food-stuff capable of easy oxidation, and that it replaces the fats, so that these not being oxidized remain and accumulate.

The obese are unable to oxidize the fat acids reaching the intermediate metabolism with the same intensity as do healthy persons, and that the defective transformation of the fatty acids leads to the accumulation of neutral fat in the cells.

So much for the general consideration of the different parts of the body.

The history of the patient follows:—

Mrs. E., Age, 39; Married—10 years, widow 6 years. Menstrutation began at 13 years, always regular and profuse. She has had no children and two miscarriages. The miscarriages were early in her married life and were produced at about six weeks. The first child is now 15 years of age and in good health. The second, died at four months. Both deliveries were instrumental and tedious. Soon after the recovery from the last delivery she felt a tearing pain occasionally in the region of the umbilicus, This symptom grew worse and was aggravated by standing or straining.

In a few months she noticed a lump in this region; it was hard and tender. These symptoms continued, accompanied by a rapid increase of fat, especially in the abdominal wall.

For the last year or more she was often compelled to lie on her stomach to relieve the pain and neusea after meals.

Even standing for some time, loosely clad would bring on these symptoms and necessitate the prone position for relief.

Her digestion was poor and hemicrania frequent.

In the family history it might be interesting to state, that the father and mother and two brothers all had hernia.

Fat is usually destributed uniformly over the body acting as cushions and fillings were needed to give shapely form to the body. If the pigment of the body be properly distributed it gives to the skin its uniform color, but if not so arranged, there are spots too deeply colored, and others correspondingly too lightly pigmented.

So with the fatty deposits, if evenly distributed, symmetry and plumpness of the body, the delight of women-kind, is the result but if not so distributed, then we have that burdensome, unsightly form of body. Women would lose any other visible feature than part with this. One may be a little too thin, another harbor a little too much adipose tissue, and yet as long as symmetry of form, exists, no embarrassment attends it, but let it become asymmetrical, then all hope of beauty of form and activity of body is gone.

Uniform accumulation on either side of the ligamentum nuchea, and under the chin, are well known. These fatty lumps are in no wise to be considered as tumors, but only as diffuse lipomata.

She has an unnecessary burden which she carries without her consent. It is unsightly and can not be hidden. It can not be left home to be cared for by the domestic. It is obnoxious to her while mixing with her society folks. Its room would be more welcome than its company. It is a filled hammock without a welcome hanging. It cannot be given away in whole or in part, but must be cared for by its possessor even though an unsolicited ownership.

She is unwieldy in appearance, waddling in gait, awkwardly balanced, and usually short of breath. The care of her person is difficult, especially the toilet of the lower part of the body.

The patient is practically incapacitated for work or even for recreation. She is not sick, but not well. She is disabled yet not injured. It is not produced by the disease of the organ, then what is it? Is it a pathological condition, or is it a physiological one?

Why has there not been more said about

it, because this, like many other neglected conditions, has been lookel upon as natural, as well as inevitable, and irremediable?

Fat shows strange freaks, for which physiology, as yet, offers no adequate explanation.

The intaking of more food or drink than is necessary to supply the wants of the body, we call intemperance, so when a seemingly physiological process continues beyond the limit of the necessities of the body why should we not call it a pathological condition.

The line of demarkation where a physiological process becomes a pathological one is impossible to define, hence the different opinion of authors as to this being a disease.

After a thorough examination of this patient, in different postures, I was unable to say for certain, as to the existence of a hernia. The patients history and symptoms given, lead me to believe in the certainty of an existing hernia. However I was called in to decide what was best to do to relieve her of the distress produced by the immense deposit of fat in the abdominal wall.

Abdominal supports had been tried and all other known means but no direct pressure over the most prominent point could be used on account of the pain being aggravated.

She was unable to support this mass of fat in any other way, other than by having a specially improvised corset made which would allow her to raise the mass into the upped or breast supporting portion of the instrument, so it would rest here and thus remove the direct pressure and prevent the dragging.

The skin was stretched transversely, as well as vertically, hence it was necessary to remove fat and skin from above downward as well as from side to side. I removed an eliptiform piece of tissue down to the fascia extending from within three

inches of the symphysis pubes and eight inches of its greatest width. I then removed two large V-shaped strips transversely from about the center of the perpendicular incisions.

When the stitches were in place the incisions described a cross, the center of which was a little below the point of the umbilicus. In about all 15 pounds of tissue were removed.

The vertical incision made the hernia was plainly seen. It was about the size of a six months old babe's head.

A closer examination showed it to be irregular or saculated, adherent and irreducible. A portion of the sac being found that was not adherent, an incision was made and this proved it to be an omental hernia, with many small sacs, each of which were filled with omentum adherent to its walls. In each small sac was an opening through which a small strand of omentum extended, connecting that within the small sacs to that occupying the main sac. This was the condition throughout.

The omentum was adherent to the walls of the main sac down to the abdominal opening, to which lower portion was attached a knuckle of bowel.

This protrusion, in umbilical hernias, is usually composed of bowel principally, accompanied by some omentum, but in this case it was omentum principally, containing only a loop of bowel.

The coverings of these are usually thinned, unhealthy, and somewhat discolored, but this one was covered with so much fat that is could not be outlined. The saculation could not be determined, until the incision was made.

Adherent, irreducible hernias can not be well treated with mechanical appliances.

Umbilical hernias are frequent in children, easily diagnosed, and easily treated, but when found in women past middle life, it is more difficult. They are usually corpulent patients, some excessively so. Their tissues do not have the firmness necessary to retain their normal form; they have a feeble muscular development; their digestion is not good and constipation is the rule.

Their excess of fat makes them bad subjects for operation.

Free hernias of this form strangulate easily, and are not safe if left unprotected.

Practically every case of irreducible umbilical hernia should be operated upon. Reports are many, of unsuccessful attempts at radical cure. If proper care is taken the results are usually satisfactory.

The structures about the opening are not as firm as would be desired. The recti muscles are of little use, as they are thin and flabby at this point. They are not sufficiently strong to afford a hold secure enough for the sutures. We can rely only upon the sheaths of these muscles, which are arranged in two layers. These layers are to be coaptated by sutures of strong kangaroo tendon, which should be placed through both layers as close as possible. This tendon suture becomes organized into fibrous tissue, and remains as such for an indefinite time. I have used as many as 20 sutures to close an opening three inches long.

Because of the many unsuccessful attempts to close the opening in these cases, requiring repeated operations, surgeons are at varience as to the best technique.

Mayos advises a transverse incision with verticle suturing, while Treves, the English surgeon, differs, and says that the opening is greatest vertically, hence there is less tension when the sutures are placed transversly. Metal plates and silver filigree have been used, but cnly in extreme cases, where suturing in impracticable.

This case presented those symptoms so characteristic in a true fatty hernia; namely, radiating pain and nausea both of which were aggravated by pressure.

An omental hernia will elicit neither resonance on percussion nor gurgling on manipulation and reduction.

If it be irreducible it will not show any change in size by different positions of the body, nor show enlargement by the strain incident to coughing. If the abdomen be one of extreme fatty deposit, a hernia of this kind may be easily overlooked.

The nausea and pain especially the nausea, was aggravated when the patient was in the erect posture. This latter symptom constantly annoyed her, as the hernia increased in size, and especially when it was not held up by the sling-like support.

Nausea is a symptom invariably present in large omental hernias, and is due to the traction on the stomach by the adherent omentum. In practically all hernias of this form we would advise the radical operation. If there existed an excess of fat in the abdominal wall, we would consider it our duty to remove that portion which seemed to be in excess at the same time we were doing the operation for the hernia. But if a case came to us with the excess of fat alone we might hesitate to operate. We would more likely advise that it was only natural, and the patient, treating it as a matter of fact, would continue to eke out their miserable existence. We might attempt relief by the use of some clumsy mechanical appliance and thus add to instead of relieving the condition.

By a little surgical ingenuity we are able to eliminate natures excess and utilize that which is necessary to make a natural support for that which should exist as a normal body.

After this simple surgical procedure our patient will show a better paise in standing and a better poise in walking. The movements once awkward will now be graceful.

She will be able to dress with convenience and comfort.

She can make the toilet of her body complete. Her figure is changed from unsightly and awkward to that of symmetry and gracefulness. This once over-sensitive patient, now occupies a more normal and natural relation to society. We not only note a great benefit in a physical way, but the physical effect is marked.

Were there no other reason for the operation than the cosmetic effect, I should recommend it for that alone.

POLIOMYELITIS ANTERIOR

BY J. DONOHOO, AFTON, OKLAHOMA.

In presenting the subject of Poliomyelitis to this Association we feel that it would be better taken in the section on pediatrics as it is essentially a disease of infants, and children, seventy five per cent of all cases occurring before the fourth year, the last half of the first, and the second years, being the age at which it most commonly occurs, however young adults are not immune.

The etiology of this disease has been studied by many high authorities with quite different findings and conclusions. Flexner's recent researches has convinced him that the diplococus intercellularis is the specific virus causing this disease and reaches the spinal cord through lymphatic connections existing between it and the nasopharynx, he also claims that cultures made from the secretions of the masopharynx of those suffering the disease, when injected into the lumber spinal canal of monkeys, will shortly produce paralysis. As to the pathology all agree that atrophy of the anterior of motor horns of the spinal cord is the chief pathological lesion.

The symptoms seen in the initial stage, or before paralysis is noted, are very similar to other infectious disease, the child usually has fever reaching 101 or 102, F. and occasionally higher, it sometimes vomits, and rarely has convulsions.

Poliomyelitis anterior is most apt to be mistaken for cerebral paralysis or the mild-er form of cerebro spinal meningitis, but we do not have the well marked meningeal congestion, tenderness on pressure over the spinal column, headache, and rigid muscles as in the latter disease.

We know of no other disease where the diagnosis and prognosis should be more scrupulously withheld, especially in its early stages as what would appear today, to be a trifling disturbence of digestion or a mild form of many other diseases. A few hours or at least a few days delay in making a positive diagnosis, is very often very essential, as our present knowledge of the etiology does not warrant an early diagnosis without paralysis has taken place in certain groups of musles.

I differ from some who have written on this subject as to the relative time of recovery, my experience has led me to believe that once a group of muscles are paralyzed from this disease, they seldom fully recover, so far as a fatal issue is concerned if the child survives the first week or ten days its

c__ are good for a partial recovery, however when the respiratory muscles are involved death often takes place in a few hours.

During the summer of 1902 I had the misfortune to treat sixteen cases of these little patients, with results that were not at all incouraging, one died the first day due to failure of the respiratory muscles, the other fifteen had permanent paralysis in the extensor muscles—in one or both lower extremities. Three had one, and two had both arms paralyzed.

The subsequent history of these cases showed them to have been physically wrecked during the acute stage, as only three of the remaining fifteen were living in 1905 three years after the original attack, and some of them were not able to survive even a moderate attack of malaria, or a trifling burn; hence their early demise.

The treatment by drug means, I consider has about an equal value as the pfenig or German half penny.

The faradic current possibly prevents atrophy and should, in the absence of nothing better, be applied.

Gentle massage is indicated and should be persistently done for years, and I would add by the child's nurse or parents.

The orthopedic surgeon has a fertile field in this malady. Tenotomy for the various forms of talipes is often of great value, and ankle braces should be applied, for the relief of flail feet.

It would seem from the vast number rendered helpless and physically disabled for life each year, that infantile paralysis has been to a degree neglected, and it is hoped that modern scientific laboratory investigations will reveal the true cause, and produce a remedy for its prevention and cure.

EDITORIAL

THE MEDICAL ASSOCIATION OF THE SOUTHWEST, MEETING IN WICHITA, KANSAS, OCT. 11, 12, 1910.

General Session, October 11, 9 a. m.

The Fifth Annual Meeting of the Medical Association of the Southwest was called to order at 9 a. m., in the Scottish Rites Temple by Dr. Chas. E. Bowers, Chairman of the Committee of Arrangements. After the invocation, Dr. Bowers introduced Hon. C. L. Davidson, Mayor of the City of Wichita, who welcomed the delegation on behalf of the citizens of Wichita. Dr. O. P. Davis, President of the Kansas State Medical Association, then welcomed those present in behalf of the State Association, and Dr. J. E. Oldham in behalf of the local profession, after which Dr. Bowers introduced Dr. G. H. Moody who in turn called Dr. Joe Becton of Texas, to respond to the word of welcome, after which Dr.

Bowers as Chairman of the Committee of Arrangements, reported upon the program with especial reference to the social features which were to take place.

The President then appointed as a Committee on Resolutions: Drs. Jabez N. Jackson, E. H. Martin and W. L. Allison.

Dr. Jabez N. Jackson then moved, which was duly seconded and carried that as many of the Physicians had not yet arrived, we spend the remainder of the morning session in General Scientific Session, each Chairman presiding in turn.

Dr. H. F. Lyle, Chairman of the Section on General Medicine, called upon Dr. E. H. Thrailkill of Kansas City, who read a paper upon "Colica Mucosa" with report of cases. This paper was freely discussed by Dr. Hertzler and Robinson of Kansas City and the discussion closed by the Essayists.

In the absence of Dr. Wm. Keiler, Chairman of the Section on Surgery, Dr. D. A. Myers as Vice-Chairman called upon Dr. D. W. Basham who read a paper upon "The Post Operative Care and Treatment of Supra Public Prostatectomy," with especial reference to the method of drainage and the treatment of shock and hemorrhage. This was discussed by Drs. Jackson, Bransford, Lewis, Mark, Griffith, Becton, Hill, and Norberg, and closed by the Essayists.

At the Caucus of the various State Delegations the following were nominated as members of the Nominating Committee:

From Texas, Drs. St. Cloud Cooper, E. H. Martin, J. M. Griffin and C. H. Cargile.

From Oklahoma, Drs. C. Thompson, E. S. Lain, J. H. Scott, D. A. Myers, and J. H. Barnes.

From Missouri, Drs. G. W. Robinson, E. H. Thrailkill, Jno. Punton, A. W. McAlester and Bransford Lewis.

From Kansas, Drs. C. C. Goddard, J. W. May, S. E. Sawtelle, E. E. Liggett and R. Claude Young.

Tuesday, October 11, 1910. 7 p. m.

General Session called to order after a delightful informal Musical and Scenic Program, furnished by the Committee of Arrangements, after which Dr. D. A. Myers, Vice-President, introduced Dr. G. H. Moody, who delivered the Annual President's Address, which was very timley, he using as his subject "Fatigue."

Dr. Edward H. Ochsner was then introduced and delivered a masterly address upon the "Prevention and Treatment of Septic Infection of the Extremeties."

Among the many social Programs provided by the Physicians of Wichita, especial mention should be made of the Programs of musical numbers and the beautiful scenery of the Scottish Rites Temple. All enjoyed very greatly the splendid voice and musical numbers rendered by Mrs. Campbell as well as the scenic effects produced through the kindness of the Superintendent of the Temple. Of course no one missed the banquet tendered the Physicians and their wives and which took place immediately after Dr. Ochsner closed his oration.

The speakers for the evening were:

Dr. J. M. Griffin, of Sulphur Springs, Arkansas, whose subject was "The Arkansas Traveler."

Dr. A. K. West, of Oklahoma City, Okla., who told all about "The Sooner."

Dr. Bransford Lewis, of St. Louis, Mo., who "Show'd Me."

Dr. S. S. Glasscock, of Kansas City, Kans., on "The Sunflower" and last but not least,

Dr. Joe Becton, of Greenville, Texas, who handled "The Lone Star" in his usual "Becton Manner."

All joined in saying that the Profession of Wichita had "done themselves proud" and had provided an evenings entertainment long to be remembred.

The following were selected as officers:

President, Dr. M. L. Perry, Parsons, Kansas.

Vice-President, Dr. J. M. Griffin, Sulphur Springs, Kansas.

Vice-President, Dr. W. H. Stauffer, St. Louis, Mo.

Vice-President, Dr. E. S. Lain, Oklahoma City, Okla.

Vice-President, Dr. W. L. Allison, Ft. Worth, Texas.

Secy.-Treasurer, Dr. F. H. Clark, El Reno, Okla.

Section Officers, 1911.

Executive Committee to serve 3 years:
Dr. W. A. Wood, Hubbard, Texas.
Dr. S. S. Glasscock, Kansas City, Kans.
Dr. J. H. Scott, Shawnee, Okla.
Dr. St. Cloud Cooper, Ft. Smith, Ark.
Dr. J. D. Griffith, Kansas City, Mo.

For place of meeting, 1911, Oklahoma City, Oklahoma.

Dr. S. G. Burnett gave notice that at

the next Annual Meeting he would move to amend Act 6 and Act 1.

Dr. Claude Thompson gave notice that at the next Annual Meeting he would move to amend the by-laws so that the Publica-tino Committee shall be instructed to divide the papers among the various Medical Jour-nals of this organization.

Section Officers 1911.

Surgery: Chairman, Dr. J. F. Kuhn, Oklahoma City, Okla.

Vice-Chairman, Dr. Spitler, Wellington Kans.

Secretary, Dr. Howard Hill, Kansas City, Mo.

General Medicine: Chairman, Dr. C. C. Conover, Kansas City, Mo.

Vice-Chairman, Dr. A. D. Young, Ok-lahoma City, Okla.

Secretary, Dr. G. W. Robinson, Kansas City, Mo.

Eye, Ear, Nose and Throat: Chairman, Dr. H. C. Todd, Oklahoma City, Okla.

Vice-Chairman, Dr. J. H. Barnes, Enid, Okla.

Secretary, Dr. J. W. Hay, Kansas City, Kans.

The President appointed as a Publish-ing Committee for the coming year:

Dr. Claude Thompson, Muskogee, Okla.

Dr. Morgan Smith, Little Rock, Ark.

Dr. J. W. May, Kansas City, Kans.

Dr. Ho'man Taylor, Ft. Worth, Tex.

Dr. E. J. Goodwin, St. Louis, Mo.

ERLICH'S 606.

More recent contributions to the reports on Erlich's 606 would indicate that it is be-ing most favorably received by the profes-sion, who have had an opportunity to give the preparation a test.

At a symposium recently held in Chi-cago, more than twenty patients were pre-sented on whom the drug had been used

and no untoward results had been noted. It was the unanimous opinion that the ef-fect of a single injection was most remark-able. The spirochaeta were not to be demonstrated after a lapse of from twelve to twenty-four hours after the injection and the intractable chancre was reduced to a simple sore; all other conditions accom-panying syphilis were ameliorated, with the exception of iritis and brain gum-mata. In this connection it is well to men-tion that a note of warning has come from the occulist that in some cases blindness has been produced by its use; a partial report of its use in seven cases of tabes, by Dr. Frank Billings, indicated that no special changes had been noted, but Dr. Billings believed or hoped that more time might change the re-sult. Another investigator present had seen considerable sloughing follow the injection; sloughing to the extent that required com-plete excision of the parts.

Dr. J. B. Murphy insists that sodium coccodylate gave the same initial results in those of his surgical cases requiring pre-paratory anti-sylphilitic treatment, but ad-vanced no opinion as to the permanency of the results.

To those inclined to use either of these treatments their arsenic constituents should be remembered as most of the bad reports are believed traceable to the arsenic or the idiosyncrasy of the patient to that drug. A summing up of obtainable data leads one to the belief that in the treatment by 606 a great advance has been made.

THE RE-ELECTION OF DR. F. H. CLARK.

The action of the Wichita meeting of the Medical Association of the Southwest in re-electing Dr. F. H. Clark, of El Reno, as Secretary will be most gratifying to mem-bers of the organization and especially to those in Oklahoma who know him.

Dr. Clark has been secretary since the inception of the Association and his activity in organization is evidenced by the growth of the body which in a few years has spread over the five great states of its territory.

This efficient work will be more appreciated when one understands that other similar organizations having larger cities and more populous communities to draw from do not excel it in attendance or interest, notwithstanding they are much older.

This honor coming each year as it has done, and without solicitation on the part of Dr. Clark, is a high token of the appreciation in which he is held by the medical profession of the Southwest.

ABSTRACTS AND EXCHANGES

TREATMENT OF SYPHIILIS WITH DIOXYDIAMIDOARSENO - BENZOL.

So far, Wechselmann has treated over 600 cases of syphilis with this remedy. He says that the erosive chancres become clean after from 12 to 24 hours and heal rapidly; in pronounced sclerosis the cleaning process is of the same rapidity, but absorption takes longer. In 4 cases there appeared after the healing of the prisary lesion an exanthem which healed spontaneously in 2 cases in which it appeared on the first and seventh day after the injection; the 2 other patients received a second injection. Mucous patches of the mouth heal in from 24 to 48 hours, even if the patient is an inveterate smoker. The roseola disappears in a few days, as do also the malign ulcerous syphilis, the rupia, the watery papules, the small papulous syphilides, which are otherwise so pertinaceous, and the gummata. Slower is the disappearance of the large papulous syphilides, and for these a second injection becom sometimes necessary. Favorable are the effects on syphilis of the bones; especially the night pains of the bones disappear as by magic. In view of experience with other arsenical preparations Wechselmann sees that every patient has his eyes examined by a specialist before giving the injection. In cases in which there are changes in the optic nerve— a circumstance which frequently occurs— he has not given an injection. Visceral lues also show quick recovery, especially syphilis of the testicles and of the brain (epileptoid attacks). Icterus which has existed for a considerable time disappears in 10 days. Syphilitic growths of the larynx which has produced such severe dyspnea and stridor that the case was received as one for tracheotomy disappeared quickly and remained only as solid infiltrations, which were treated 4 weeks later with a second injection; and edema of the larynx, of which he was very much afraid at first, did not occur. Two patients with tumors from cerebral lues stood the injections well, although the symptoms were very severe. The same was the case with 2 patients who had only lately suffered a luetic apoplexy and a patient with a luetic apoplexy a few weeks old; these 3 patients plainly showed improvement. As to the parasyphilitic diseases, Wechselmann has not observed clear results in cases of progressive paralysis, although he is of the opinion of Alt, that a trial should be made in early cases. At all events a favorable influence will be produced on the symptoms of lassitude, depression, and abnormal irritability which occur early and quite threateningly. In tabes also a quick improvement has been plainly noticeable. Altogether, the tabetics are very well satisfied. Some symptoms seems to improve in some cases; for example, the girdle sensation; the dull headache which had existed for years; very severe intercostal neuralgios; in one case weakness of the muscles of deglutition. which had existed for a number of years and which produced difficulty in swallowing dry nourishment. Diminished potentia cæundia was in one case so improved that daily intercourses was accomplished. A debility of the sphincter vesicæ which had existed for 8 years, and on account of which diurnal incontinuence occurred, while on a sudden impulse immediately evacuation of the bladder took place, disappeared a few days after the injection. In 2 cases an improvement of the rigor pupillæ was shown, also an improvement of the disturbances of sensibility. Furthermore, some patients state that the gait is improved. In advanced cases, Wechselmann says that one cannot hope for success, but we must not forget that there exist in partlysis and especially in tabes, besides the process which cannot be repaired, such as scleroses of certain systems. syphilitic lesions, especially of single vessels, gummata, meningitic growths, particularly in the atypical forms of tabes, pseudotabes, in which an improvement is possible It is evident that such an improvement is of the greatest import for the patient even if the improvement occurs in small, circumscribed locations in an organ, as, for example, the spinal column, which so many important nerve courses are crowded together in the smallest space. Several observers, such as Truffi, Pazini, and especially Wechselmann's assistant, Dr. Siesskin, have proved that the spirochetes disappear from papules and primary lesions, in some

cases after 24 hours, while in other cases they still exist after days, even if they are swollen and very little movable. Iversen has lately made similar observations in preparations of glands.

The Wassermann reaction usually disappears, as has been stated by Alt, and Lange has found that a time from 8 to 40 days is necessary to prove this effect, according to the primary severity of the reaction.

Wechselmann has not observed bad after effects of importance, but it has found that otherwise light infections, such as those with coryza or angina, even if they appear on the ninth day, are accompanied with very high fever, with a temperature from 104 to 105.8 F. A patient with a weak heart should therefore be carefully guarded; besides, in such cases the injection seems not to be without danger. Otherwise, the influence of the remedy appears generally to be of an exciting and invigorating nature. It can therefore be given with benefit to very miserable patients, as, for example, to the tuberculouse, in contradistinction to mercury. Nor has he observed widespread and severe recurrences, such as occur after mercurial treatment. Isolated cases have remained refractory and made a second injection necessary, which was then successful as in cases of recurrence. Although, naturally, it cannot be positively stated whether it will be possible to cure syphilis permanently, Wechselmann hopes that we shall be able to do this in certain cases.

Review, New York Medical Journal, September 3, 1910. *Journal A. M. O.*

THE MANUFACTURE OF ANTITOXIN.

In the treatment of diphtheria the physician of today uses antitoxin, as a matter of course. It is his first expedient and his last resort. He believes implicity in its efficacy. But does he understand and appreciate all that is involved in the production of that antitoxin—the scientific knowledge, the skill, the caution, the minutiae of detail? This thought is forced upon the writer through the perusal of a recent publication of Parke, Davis & Co., which deals in part with the subject of antitoxin manufacture. Here is a specimen chapter:

"In the selection of the horses which are to act as the living laboratories for the production of the antitoxin, we apply not commercial or academic knowledge merely, but, what is more to the point, veterinary skill. The animals must be vigorous and healthy. They are carefully examined, their temperature noted for several days, and the presence of glanders excluded by the delicate mallein test. It is the blood-serum of these animals that is to be injected into the patient later on, and no precaution can be regarded as extreme which contributes the slightest positive assurance of its purity.

"Not only must the horses be in good general condition when inoculated; they must be kept so. They are fed, stalled, groomed and exercised for no other purpose than to maintain to the full their self-protective, antitoxin—producing powers. Thirty miles removed from the noise, smoke and dust of the city is our stock farm, equipped with model stables and supervised by expert veterinarians. Here, at Parkedale, on more than three hundred acres of sunny slopes, at an altitude of six hundred feet above the level of the Great Lakes, live the horses which we employ in serum-production. Amid these favorable surroundings they maintain the physical condition so essential to satisfactory service as serum-producers.

"These are preliminary considerations. Young, healthy, well-kept horses, indispensable as they are, would be of little use in the elaboration of a reliable antitoxin unless the work of injecting them with toxin were conducted accurately, aseptically, systematically, and throughout a period long enough to allow physiological reaction up to the limit of attainable immunization. We have horses enough, so that there is no occasion to be in a hurrry with any of them; the exact length of time required for complete reaction is determined in each individual instance by carefully scheduled observations.

"It goes without saying that in the preparation of the toxin and its injection into the horses, as well as in obtaining the blood serum, the most rigid bacteriological technique is maintained. The methods we employ agree substantially with those of Roux, Aronson, and Behring, and are from first to last in charge of experts. The varying susceptibility of different animals, whether guinea-pigs or horses, to the diphtheria poison; the more or less rapid physiological reaction; the variation in strength of the antitoxic serum from different horses; the absolute purity of the finished product—these are all important and delicate questions demanding for their determination a high degree of skill and scientific accuracy of observation. These qualifications, in our judgment, outrank all other considerations in the work of producing a reliable antidiphtheric serum."

The foregoing has reference to but a single step in the process of serum production, and affords but a hint of the safeguards with which Antidiphtheric Serum (P. D. & Co.) is hedged about at every stage of its manufacture—conditions which enable the company to guarantee the purity and potency of its antitoxin.

BOOK REVIEWS.

Surgical After Treatment. By L. R. G.

Crandon, A. M., M. D., Assistant in Surgery at Harvard Medical School. Octavo of 803 pages, with 265 original illustrations. Philadelphia and London. W. B. Saunders Company, 1910. Cloth, $6.00 net; Half Morocco, $7.50 net.

This splendid work contains fifty-three chapters and an appendix devoted to "Some Invalid and Convalescent Food Receipts."

Nothing in the practice of surgery troubles the profession as much as the after care of operative cases, and until recently the writings have been meagre on the subject, but this work goes most thoroughly into the different phases of surgical treatment encountered after operation, not neglecting the preparatory care of cases. The work is decidedly more expensive than such works usually are, but contains no immaterial matter.

Aside from the minute directions for after treatment the volume contains chapters on Immunization and Vaccine Therapy which are most valuable on account of their completeness as to detail, application and technique.

The work is worthy a place in the library and should be cultivated by all who have to contend with the questions and problems confronting the operator or physicians left in charge of a case.

DISLOCATIONS AND JOINT FRACTURES.

Dislocations and Joint Fractures. By Frederic Jay Cotton, A. M., M. D., First Assistant Surgeon, Boston City Hospital. Octavo of 654 pages, 1,201 original illustrations. Philadelphia and London: W. B. Saunders company, 1910. Cloth, $6.00 net; Half Morocco, $7.50 net.

This is a splendidly prepared work of thirty-five chapters and as indicated above is most profusely illustrated, the illustrations being to a great extent from both photographic reproductions verified by good accompanying X-Ray pictures.

Great stress is laid upon the radiograph as the most useful solution of many of the difficulties met with by all who treat fractures and injuries about the joints. When it is remembered that most of the troubles of the surgeon anent fractures and dislocations come from those at or near the joints the coming of this work will be well received.

A great deal of space is given the operative treatment of fractures as might be expected where there are injuries near a joint and union is sometimes so difficult to attain without deformity or injury of function.

The illustrations closely accompany the text and in this way the reader is enabled to judge of the effects of various forms of treatment of the injury and select the best applicable to the trouble.

We feel that a few lines under the head of "Generalities" should be quoted. "Accurate reposition is almost never attained, except by open operation, but it will be years before the laity, including the courts will appreciate this. What is important is the obtaining of good functional results— an entirely different matter."

BOOKS RECEIVED.

The Practical Medicine series. Volume V, obstetrics.

Edited by Joseph B. De Lee, A. M., M. D. Professor of Obstetrics, Northwestern University Medical School, with the collaboration of Herbert M. Stowe, M. D. Series 1910. Cloth, $1.25. Chicago. The Year Book Publishers, 40 Dearborn Street.

General Medicine, Volume VI.

Edited by Frank Billings, M. S., M. D., Head of the Medical Department and Dean of the Faculty of Rush Medical College, Chicago.

And J. H. Salisbury, A. M., M. D. Professor of Medicine, Chicago Clinical School. Cloth, $1.50, Chicago. The Year Book Publishers, 40 Dearborn Street.

INTERNATIONAL CLINICS.

Volume III, Twentieth Series.

Edited by Henry W. Cattell, A. M., M. D., Philadelphia, U. S. A. With the collaboration of many other writers.

Volume Three, Twentieth Series, 1910. Philadelphia and London.

J. B. LIPPINCOTT COMPANY.

Practical Medicine Series, Volume Seven.

Pediatrics and Orthopedic Surgery.

Pediatrics Edited by Isaac A. Abt, M. D., Clinical Professor of Pediatrics, Northwestern University Medical School, with the collaboration of May Mitchell, M. D.

ORTHOPEDIC SURGERY.

Edited by John Ridlon, A. M., M. D., Professor of Orthopedic Surgery, Rush Medical College. With the collaboration of Charles A. Parker, M. D.

Series 1910.

Chicago, The Year Book Publishers, 40 Dearborn St.

PROGRAM.

1 "The Obliterated Appendix and its Clinical Manifestations,"
——————— Horace Reed, Okla. City
2 "The Trend of Modern Obstetrics," ——— A. B. Leeds, Chickasha
3 "Injuries During Chilbirth and Their Care," J. S. Hartford, Okla. City.
4 "Eclampsia," Lee Watson, Ok. Cy.

5 "The Importance of Differentiating Between Blastomycotic and Other Skin Lesions,"
——————— Clarence E. Lee, Okla. City
6 "Skin Cancers," E. S. Lain, Okla. City
7 "Fractures,"
———————G. H. Thrailkill, Chickasha
8 "Paper," subject to be announced
——————— E. S. Ferguson, Okla. City
9 "The Tonsils," J. H. Barnes, Enid
10 "Cholecystitis,"
——— J. F. Messenbaugh, Okla. City
11 "Pellagara; with Report of Case,"
———————J. R. Phelan, Okla. City
12 "Incapacity, without Local Disease," ——B. W. Russell, Chickasha
13 "Paper," subject to be announced
———————Dr. Cook, Chickasha
14 "Tuberculosis of the Kidney, with Report of a Case,"
———————S. N. Mayberry, Enid.

PERSONAL

DR. BLESH'S LETTER

In describing medical matters here I shall simply describe what I see as accurately as I know how.

To the student upon his first visit to this city it will be of great advantage to speak and understand the German tongue. While this is not indispensible since some of the courses are given in English, yet it must not be forgotten that the German when endeavoring to give expression to his thoughts in English is laboring under the same handicap that the English speaking person is who is attempting the use of the German tongue. Also it should be remembered that a good understanding of a spoken language can be acquired much sooner than a fluent speaking command if it can be. This is clearly demonstrated in the English courses put on, while the language is excellent it requires evident effort on the part of the speaker and requires much time in delivery. Time, however, does not mean as much to the German as it does to the American.

Again not the least valuable requisition to the professional man is the mastery of the German tongue, for today the real science of medicine is being worked out by our patient neighbors, the Germans, and the ability to read this at first hand is a great satisfaction. Language loses in translation.

The clinics are, at the present time being run by the first assistants mostly for the reason that the professors have not returned from their summer vacations.

A first assistant here, unlike with us, is quite usually a man of large experience who has served in that capacity for many years, frequently his chief when the latter is called to larger and more lucrative fields. He has worked up from the bottom passing through the successive stages of fourth, third and second to his present enviable position. He hopes ultimately to fill his chief's place and as a rule does do so. He operates in the absence of his senior and quite usually as skilfully; thus it will be seen that the first assistant is a man of ripe experience and liberal education.

More often than his senior he is able to use the English language, an accomplishment of which he is evidently quite proud. His course not infrequently is really better than that of the professor since he has his professional following to make and his spurs to win.

The wealth of material is great and it used to the best possible advantage. An American clientele, even though a charitable one, will not stand the manipulation necessary for demonstrations that these people will. To illustrate, I was the sixth to pass the ureteral catheter in the ureter of one patient today and by the time my turn came there was considerable bleeding provoked by the previous manipulations not all of which were the most gentle.

The subject of cystoscopy and ureteral catheterzations should not be passed without noting the fact the course given in this subject by Dr. Blum in Prof. Von Fritsch's clinic in the Poliklinik is a revelation to those accustomed to the American method. The latter is usually done by the *direct* method. This method requires a much larger calibered instrument as well as more side to side movement both of which cause most of the pain incident to the maneuvar in the male. Here the *indirect* method is used altogether and the field magnified by means of lenses, a smaller instrument can be used and by means of a director (Hobler) the catheter is guided directly to the opening which owing to the magnification, is plainly to be seen. By the assistance of the director but little lateral movement of the instrument is necessary, and hence but little if any more pain is experienced by the patient than is provoked by the passage of an ordinary sound. As with us the ureteral catheter is used for both treatment and diagnosis. It purifies its principle function in the latter. It is really wonderful the refinement of diagnosis in all the courses that have been participated in by the writer. The poorest patient receives the most painstaking examination with the object in view of making a correct diagnosis before operation. With respect to advising operation our German colleagues are indeed most conservative, but when he does operate he is most truly radical.

In my next letter I shall speak more directly relative to the work in these clinics as well as to the American Medical Association of America.

A. L. BLESH.

Dr. J. W. Riely, city health officer of Oklahoma City, attended the meeting of the American Public Health Association, in Milwaukee.

Dr. C. J. Fishman, of Chicago, has located in Oklahoma City, limiting his practice to internal medicine and diagnosis.

Dr. G. T. Tyler, of Owensboro, Kentucky, 1st Lietutenant M. R. C. U. S. A., has located in Oklahoma City.

Dr. D. D. McHenry, of Cushing, has removed to Oklahoma City, and has offices in the Colcord building.

Dr. E. J. Sapper, of Warner, Oklahoma, has been attending the New York Polyclinic Medical School.

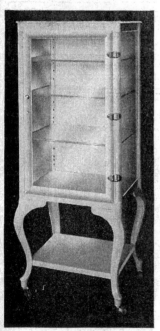

DR. W. E. WRIGHT, OF TULSA, MARRIES.

Dr. Walter E. Wright, of Tulsa, and Miss Katherine Grigsby, of Bardstown, Ky., were recently married in Memphis, Tenn.

The Journal and a host of friends in Oklahoma congratulate Dr. Wright and wish for he and Mrs. Wright many years of happiness and prosperity.

FOR SALE.

$3,000.00 annual practice, fine country location, 11 miles from railroad, nearest opposition 8 miles and 12 miles, good people, good fees and good colelctions. 'All I ask is for man to buy small stock of drugs and driving outfit. $700..00 will handle the deal. Don't write unless you mean business.

Adress:

DR. W. R. LEVERTON,
Cloud Chief, Okla.

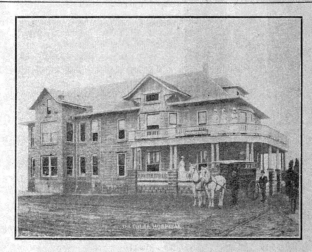

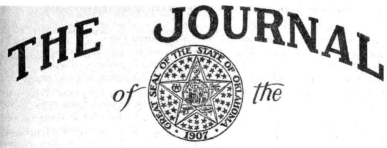

THE JOURNAL

of the Oklahoma State Medical Association.

VOL. III.   MUSKOGEE, OKLAHOMA, DECEMBER, 1910.   NO. 7

DR. CLAUDE A. THOMPSON, Editor-in-Chief.

ASSOCIATE EDITORS AND COUNCILLORS.

DR. J. A. WALKER, Shawnee.	DR. JOHN W. DUKE, Guthrie.
DR. CHARLES R. HUME, Anadarko.	DR. A. B. FAIR, Frederick.
DR. F. R. SUTTON, Bartlesville.	DR. W. G. BLAKE, Tahlequah.
DR. I. W. ROBERTSON, Dustin.	DR. H. P. WILSON, Wynnewood.
DR. J. S. FULTON, Atoka.	DR. J. H. BARNES, Enid.

Entered at the Postoffice at Muskogee, Oklahoma, as second class mail matter, July 28, 1910

This is the Official Journal of the Oklahoma State Medical Association All communications should be addressed to the Journal of the Oklahoma State Medical Association, English Block, Muskogee, Oklahoma.

THE GENERAL PRACTITIONER—(Esau Despised His Birthright)

BY DR. CHARLES W. FISK, KINGFISHER, OKLAHOMA.

Jacob and Esau were twin brothers. Esau was entitled to inherit all the honors that belonged to the chieftain of the clan. A man of energy and restless activity. A man of the fields and woods. This nomadic life, providing his daily sustenance from the uncertainties of the chase, gave him little time to dream and in his dreams to see himself the honored progenitor of a great nation. So in an evil hour, because of the very limitations of his horizon due in a measure to the character of his daily toil, he sold his birthright to his ambitious brother for a mess of pottage.

Read before the Annual Meeting of the Oklahoma State Medical Association, Tulsa, Oklahoma, May, 1910.

Esau despised his birthright and recovered it not though he sought for it with tears.

Much of life consists in the airy substance dreams are made of. The vision of today may be the reality of tomorrow. Our ideals shape our destiny.

The life of Esau is a type which we may apply to the general practitioner. He labors without cessation at his monotonous daily toil. He sees no vision, he meets many discouragements, and in the hour of his despondency he feels that the glory of his calling has departed.

At our state associations a few of us meet in this section on general medicine.

At the meeting of the South Western Association in Kansas City, an enthusiastic surgeon made the statement on the floor that in ten years the section on general medicine in our associations would be abandoned. So we are told we see the passing of the general practitioner.

The men who turn their energies toward surgery display a commendable zeal in perfecting themselves in their chosen field. They see in surgery the highest perfection in the art of healing. They feel in their hour of exaltation that the general practitioner has lost his birthright and that they themselves have fallen heir to all that is worth saving of our art.

The student in medical college gives careful attention to the surgical clinic. There is the spectacular array of uniformed surgeons and assistants, the flash of steel, the rapid and skilful execution of intricate details. All this appeals in an irresistable manner. The call to the ambitious young man is to become a surgeon. The medical clinic is sufficiently prosaic with its routine examination and the prescribing of formulae by number. Materia Medica, the foundation of medicine, has no charm for the average student. Pharmaceutical incompatibles and physiological incompatibles and a thousand other things come before him in inextricable confusion. He starts in bravely at absinthium and finds himself thoroughly mystified long before he reaches zingiber. He comes out of college with insufficient training in the art of prescribing and falls an easy prey to the promoter of the latest patent medicine. He practices his profession following carefully the treatment recommended in the last pamphlet that has fallen into his hands. It would be better not to know so many things than to know so many things that are not so. He carelessly drifts along and allows himself to be classed with the proprietor of the country store who prescribes Peruna and Hosteters bitters.

So we are told today that there is no real science of medicine. There is no really dependable treatment for disease except in the exactness of our modern surgery. It matters little to the surgeon if the operative procedure of today is abandoned tomorrow. He is not discouraged or disheartened. Perhaps he may have misgivings that in the progress of his art lives have been sacrificed, which could just as well have been saved. It must be so if there is real progress in his work. He sees the unbounded horizon, he believes in his ultimate success in his chosen field of activity. This is the spirit of optimism that wins.

This criticism is not aimed at the surgeon, who lifts his eyes to the limitless expanse, but to the general practitioner who casts his vision at his feet, who dispises his birthright. The world is not yet ready to dispense with his services. he is the most important factor in the field of medicine in its all inclusive application. He is to be reckoned with in life saving surgery. He must be so thoroughly expert in surgical diagnosis that he can give his patients the benefit of surgical treatment at the opportune time. It has been well said that there is no need for the term surgical diagnosis. What would the surgeon do with his statistics and percentages, if the general practitioner were unable to diagnose a case of appendicitis or cholecystitis until general peritonitis supervenes and death is imminent? If this responsibility rests upon us it is our duty to meet it squarely by perfecting ourselves in diagnosis.

We too frequently underestimate the general practitioner. One of our great surgeons once said that he always did a Caesarian section for placenta praevia because, having no experience with the method, he lacked the requisite skill to turn and deliver.

A prominent instructor in medicine once said that it would be necessary to appeal to the general practitioner to learn how to treat pneumonia. If diphtheria antitoxine is to be tried out, the court of last resort is the general practitioner.

It is first of all necessary for us to more correctly estimate the importance of our calling, to lift up our eyes and see the boundless opportunity that lies before us. General medicine is only now beginning to come into its own. Ten years will see marvels in this field. What has been accomplished in the last twenty years? An up to date work on physical diagnosis is a sealed book in many of its pages, to the man who graduated in medicine twenty years ago, unless he has kept step with the ownward march of progress. The demand today is for men who will keep pace with this onward march. The practice of medicine is no longer purely empirical but is rapidly developing into an exact science. Rational therepeutics is one of the demands of our time. No longer can the physician treat all manner of disease with the shotgun prescription and trust to some over ruling providence to cause this heterogeneous mixture to produce only beneficial results. If a drug has a potency to do good it must have a possibility of doing harm. Simplicity in prescribing with an accurate knowledge of the action of drugs is necessary for the successful treatment of disease. Simplicity should not consist in the employment of one drug for fever, another for every bladder symptom and so on throughout the whole range of symptomatology. An artist was once asked what he used in mixing his colors. He replied that he mixed them with brains. This ingredient is quite as necessary in mixing medicine as in mixing paint.

With the advantage we possess, having standardized drugs and alkaloids of very nearly uniform activity, we should be much more successful in the treatment of disease than were the physicians of a generation ago. I believe we are more successful.

The Council on Pharmacy and Chemistry of our National Association are doing invaluable service for the cause of scientific medicine. This is one of the most important movements of our time and marks an epoch in the history of medicine. They demand the support of every progressive general practitioner. The Committee is being assailed by medical journals and by circulars that are being sent to every physician whose name is on the directory. It is very important that we be very careful in our judgment. We have too much at stake to allow ourselves to be influenced by those who are not our friends, who have not the interests of the profession at heart, but are looking only for dividends.

We are facing conditions such as never before confronted the general practitioner. There is a feeling, which is daily growing stronger, that the general practitioner in some particular manner is a public servant. He is the guardian of the public health, whether he is an officer or not. He is to a very large extent the guardian of the public morals. This proposition probably does not appeal to all physicians, but today the burden of the fight for the purity of manhood is placed directly upon us as an organized profession. While we spare no effort to reach the highest proficiency in our art, the public has a right to demand a reasonable service. We as good citizens are in duty bound to respond to the call. President Schurman of Cornell University says: "Physicians and surgeons are not mere practitioners, they are also human beings. A university must think of training them for manhood and citizenship as well as for the practice of medicine and surgery."

The campaign of education is on, the martial call has already sounded. The call is to the general practitioners. The surgeon, the specialist must meet with us on a common plane if they enlist for this campaign. Education is necessary on the folly of promiscuous dosing by the use of patent medicines. The newest fake that appears is the home made prescription with such simple ingredients as cardiol and cadomene. The fact that they are used is an index that the public is trying to get away from the ready made prescription. Newspapers cannot be depended on to give the needed information. It must be done by the open meeting and by the personal efforts of the general practitioner.

The habit forming drugs are getting in their deadly work. Morphia, cocaine and chloral are too well known to call for comment. The coal tar derivatives have their slaves. Some of our number may have fallen into the trap which was skilfully laid by some of the headache remedy promoters. While negative evidence is very poor evidence it was indeed surprising to read this pamphlet that has been sent to all physicians and to the laity. You will look in vain for my name with the illustrious throng. It adds nothing to the dignity of our profession for so many of our number to write endorsements and testimonials with so little deliberation. The Department of Agriculture wrote letters to 925 physicians of whom 400 responded giving 813 cases of poisoning, 28 deaths, and 136 instances of habitual use of the coal tar derivatives.

The general practitioner is too busy to write any endorsements for heart tonics of this kind.

Instruction in the nature of disease and the means of prophylaxis is necessary. We do not need to confine our efforts at enlightenment to the submerged tenth. Only by a little missionary work can one realize how little the average citizen, whether educated or untutored, knows about the laws of health and disease.

Every time a hue and cry is raised against vaccination we are astonished to find among the rabble men of education and intelligence. It is a disgrace to our profession that we are compelled to fight against chiropractors and osteopaths and all others of the kind in a vain attempt to protect the public. Every generous unselfish effort of the general practitioner is misconstrued and the health officers are maligned. London has more inhabitants today, who are susceptible to small pox, than at any time since the deadly epidemics of the past. The protection of the so called liberties of the people have rendered the health officers powerless. Who can tell how soon a dreadful penalty will be executed for such shortsighted legislation. Why should our own Association be compelled to address the legislature of our state to keep them from passing an anti-vaccination measure? It would increase our self respect and educate the public thoroughly, quickly and permanently should we abandon all quarantine measures against small pox. The system is inefficient. It is expensive and it places the burden upon the educated, law abiding citizen.

Many of our county societies have already held open meetings to instruct the public on tuberculosis. In this work the general practitioner is doing effective service. Much good is being accomplished but it will take patient, persistent effort to reach all classes of people, which is absolutely essential. The first effect of education the ill defined sense of danger, will soon be forgotten unless it is stimulated from time to time. If we can fully inform the public of the contagiousness and curability of this disease and the means of prophylaxis we shall have less difficulty in enforcing proper regulations.

There is a need of a campaign of education on the social evil. This has been avoided and shunned until today it is a virulent cancer that threatens the very existence of our nation. Tuberculosis exacts its annual deadly toll of our brightest and most promising. We part from them with aching hearts and cherish the memory of their brief lives as a sacred treasure. The social diseases exact their deadly toll. The farewell is spoken with words of anguish, often with hearts broken by the shame, the memory of blasted lives, of dishonor and despair. Men are stricken down in the prime of manhood as a result of a disease contracted in the ignorance of youth. Too long we have delegated this matter to the ministry and to the churches. We can no longer wash our hands and shake off our responsibility. It is not simply a question of morals it is a grave question of political economy.

This need of education must be supplied. This field of enlightenment has been preempted by the confidential quickly cured vultures. We as a profession have not realized what an influence has been wielded by this class of people. It is often a tragedy when one of their books falls into the hands of the boy. When we can so easily place sane and helpful literature into their hands, have we done our duty if we have made no effort in this direction? It is argued that nothing can be accomplished in a campaign of education. It is admitted that every other system has been ineffective and this has never been tested. The various societies of Social and Moral Prophylaxis of our land are backed by the best men in our profession. Our own National Association has taken a prominent part in the crusade against the social evil. Now that we hope for a National Department of Public Health our responsibilities in this direction will be greatly increased.

The general practitioner can do a work that no one else can accomplish. He is in a position to instruct parents and to place suitable literature into their hands. They must be made to realize the necessity of a careful supervision of their children in infancy and during the time of their development. How many parents have been informed that the rubber pacifier used to quiet the fretful infant, may lead to habits that will cast a shadow over the whole life. Parents do not know that dangerous tendencies may originate in infancy. Fathers should give early instruction to their sons and mothers to their daughters. If they do this it will be very largely through the influence of the general practitioner.

When an opportunity offers it is our duty to do work in a more public manner for the promotion of a pure manhood and womanhood. There is no class of citizens in our new state, which can wield so large an influence for good or harm as the medical profession.

In general education the general practitioner compares favorably with any of the professions. As regards special training and the exact knowledge which is necessary to make a man master of his profession, and the ability to make application of that knowledge immediately in time of urgent need, the practice of medicine is the most exacting of them all.

The command was given by the Master to his disciples to go into the world, to heal the sick and to cast out demons. We are the accredited bearers of this commission. Christian Science and the Emanual Movement are not seeking to do this work in the Master's way. God's method has always been to raise up men for service, who use their God given powers to carry out the divine command not without great toil and danger. The command to subdue the earth was not given alone to the man who tills the soil, but also to him who eliminates the once impassable barriers of the mighty ocean, to him who with bands of steel makes the most distant cities of a great continent to join hands, to him who flies the air on the wings of the eagle, and to us who wage a ceaseless warfare upon the tiny disease microbe.

"Ye shall not be afraid of the pestilence that walketh in darkness nor of the destruction that wasteth at noon-day." It is for us to claim this promise. We shall conquer by the natural forces that are placed within our hands, just as we have brought the earth, the sea and the air under our dominion. The general practitioner has no need to be ashamed of his calling. If we have despised our birthright, if we have considered ourselves as merely hewers of wood and drawers of water, let us take a broader view of our duties and of our privileges. Then will we come into a full measure of our inheritance.

CEREBRAL MENINGITIS.

BY F. B. ERWIN, M. D., NORMAN, OKLAHOMA.

This is one of the diseases which we, as physicians, dread to meet because of being unable to successfully treat it. We meet with it most frequently in children under five years of age. In fact, it may well be called a disease of childhood. The nervous system is the highest organized portion of the human body. Being the most delicately and intricately constructed it is thereby the most easily torn down and the hardest to repair of any portion of the body. When it is irritated from any source an inflammation is soon set up. Cerebral-meningitis comprehends a much broader field than I shall attempt to treat in this short paper. It may mean an inflammation of either the dura-mater or outer covering of the brain, or the pia-mater or inner covering. In general, when we speak of meningitis, we mean an inflammation of the pia-mater or lepto-meningitis. Therefore, this paper will deal with lepto-meningitis. As we have said, it is distinctly a disease of childhood and more often attacks males than females.

Etiologically, it is either primary or secondary. The primary is a simple purulent, tubercular or syphilitic. Secondary when due to other diseases such as: Pneumonia, scarlet fever, typhoid fever, ulcerated endocarditis, measles, variola, septicemia, rheumatism, toxic, trumatic or idopathic.

As to location, it is found either on the convexity of the brain or the base. Metastatic meningitis is most frequently found at the base.

It occurs epidemically or sporadically. The cause of this disease is due to a micro-organism. This organism can reach the meninges in but two ways; either through traumatic or destructive lesions of the bony and fibrous coverings of the brain or through the vascular supply on the other hand. This micro-organism is found in the primary form of the disease as the causative factor. In the secondary form there are many different forms of micro-organisms, such as: Pneumococcus, streptococcus pyogenes, intra-cellular diplococcus, and pneumo-bacillus. The conditions which prepare the field for the invasion of this disease are: Ill-health, mental overwork, early childhood and male sex. Leyden discovered the intra-cellular diplococcus in 1883. Frequently a history of phthisis, tubercular milk and unhygienic surroundings are found in these cases.

It is either a fibro-purulent or purulent

Read before the Annual Meeting of the Oklahoma State Medical Association, Tulsa, Oklahoma, May, 1910.

disease. The base of the brain is more often affected than the convexity. The inflammatory deposits are more conspicuous along the Sylvian fissure and vessels branching form it; the optic chiasm; posterior and under surfaces of the cerebellum and the sides of the Pons. There is an increase of fluid in the ventricles and arachnoid cavity. This fluid may be turbid. We find that the brain substance is oedematous so that it fills the skull closely and the convolutions appear flattened. There are also small hemorrhages noticeable.

The symptoms of the disease depend upon the location and causative agents. If located on the convexity, we find covulsions and other general symptoms of the disease more conspicuous or pronounced. While if located at the base, the special sense symptoms are very pronounced, owing to the fact that the special sense nerves rise mainly from the base of the brain. The symptoms of tubercular meningitis are quite distinctive from the other forms. The symptoms, as a rule, during the whole course of the disease are of longer duration and not so pronounced as in other forms of the disease.

The disease may be classed as having four well defined stages: Prodromal, irritative, depressant and comatose. Detailed symptoms depend considerably upon location of the lesion, as before stated.

The disease, especially in children, is frequently ushered in by a convulsion or a severe chill. When not beginning this way about the first thing noticeable, in the prodromal stage is that the patient is easily irritated; general malaise; headache; loss of appetite; some constipation. Gradually this passes into the irritative stage in which we find the symptoms much more pronounced; delirium; beginning rigidity of neck; hyperesthesia of the skin; retraction of the head; vomiting; irregular fever; contracted and often unequal pupils; sometimes optic neuritis or retinitis; incoherent muttering; opisthotonos and *tache-cerebrale;* sometimes suppression of the urine. Pulse is high and full; temperature irregular; purpuric spots may appear; respiration frequently irregular; patellar reflexes increased.

This stage of excitement gradually passes into a stage of depression. The patient becomes dull and hard to arouse; vomiting checks and the fever is lower. The hyperesthesia of the skin is less; pulse irregular and intermittent; respiration irregular and slower; bowels constipated; urine small in amount and sometimes albuminous; patellar reflexes diminished; boat-shaped abdomen; Cheynes-Stoke respiration. Sometimes sugar or casts are found in the urine. The spleen is enlarged.

When the comatose or paralytic stage is reached the patient can hardly be aroused to be given his medicine. There is some rigidity except in the last stage; abdomen is greatly retracted; pupils dilated; skin moist; bowels and bladder move involuntarily. The patient gradually passes to his death.

These are the symptoms, in general, of a case of lepto-meningitis. When the tubercle bacillus is the causative factor, the tubercles are found along the course of the veins, the Fissue of Sylvius and the floor of the ventricles. Acute mania frequently develops in the course of tubercular meningitis, especially in adults. In general, a few of the diagnostic symptoms of meningitis are: Constant and severe headache; persistent constipation; explosive vomiting; inequality of the pupillary reflexes and *tache-cerebrale.*

The prognosis of all cases of meningitis is bad, but should be guarded as some few cases recover. Also, unless there is absolutely no doubt as to the diagnosis, there is a possibility of a mistake along that line.

As to the treatment of these cases, we have nothing definite to offer, therefore we treat the cases symptomatically. There are several general lines of treatment, a few of which I will designate. The one which is probably used the most is that one in which the eliminative organs are increased. For the bowels the drugs most generally used are, calomel, podophyllin, and the salines. For the kidneys, spirits of nitrous ether, potassium acetate, milk and water. The skin is kept active by different drugs and bathing. Depressants are given to quiet and ease the patient. Sometimes morphine is the only agent whereby this may be obtained. Heart stimulants should be given —digitalis. Nourishment should be given frequently, per rectum if necessary.

The serum treatment is in its infancy and we hope to see it soon be made practical in the hands of the general practitioner. Some good results have been reported from its use, thus far, and I think where indicated might be well used in many cases possibly with good results.

The hot water treatment has given some good results as reported by some. This consists in placing the patient in water at a moderate temperature and gradually increasing the temperature till it reaches about 104 degrees Fahrenheit. After which the patient is thoroughly sponged dry. This treatment is continued every day for two or three weeks. In some well selected cases good results have been reported.

The treatment by lumber puncture seems to give some good results in those cases where the collection of fluid in the ventricles produce great pressure symptoms. As in most cases of diseases of whatever kind, prophylaxis is the most important item.

I wish to give a brief history of three cases which I saw with another physician. The first child was a child of about five years of age. It took sick one evening with vomiting and the family, thinking it was possibly a "bilious attack," sent for something for vomiting. The child continued to get worse and the next morning we saw the child. There was great prostration and the child was in somewhat of a stupor but not vomiting so much. The bowels had been moving freely; pulse rapid and weak; urine scanty. There was no retraction of the head to speak of but the family said that it had been at times. Respirations were rather weak and somewhat irregular. While there another child vomited some but nothing much was said about it. The first child continued to get worse and died that night. The second child continued to get worse and the next day we were called again. When we got there two instead of one were in bed. The second child was about seven or eight years old and the third was about fifteen. All had begun with vomiting. The fever of either of the last two was not at that time nor had been, thus far, very high. We noticed the patients for a time and saw the purpuric spots so frequently found in those cases. The pulse was irregular; temperature irregular; easily irritated; respiration somewhat irregular; bowels constipated; urine scanty; pupils somewhat contracted. We gave medicine to purge the bowels and for the kidneys; also supporting medicine and to ease the patient. Before the next morning the second child was dead. The remaining one gradually got worse. The fever got higher and very irregular; very restless; opisthotonos marked; bowels continued constipated; urine scanty; pulse irregular; sometimes weak and sometimes strong; respiration irregular. It required morphine to ease the patient. Nothing else would do the work. Regardless of treatment, the patient continued to waver between life and death for ten days or two weeks. We kept the bowels thoroughly purged out all the time. The kidneys were kept active; the heart was supported by digitalis; heat and plasters were applied to the spine as was also ice-packs; ice was applied to the head as much as the patient would stand but it seemed to irritate her at times and had to be removed; supportive medicines were given for the system.

We used ergot for the contractile power it is supposed to have on the arterioles of the brain and spinal cord; nourishment was given at regular intervals as well as could be given per mouth and also per' rectum; the pupils at first contracted became irregularly dilated; the patient was isolated as well as was possible in a country home. She lay in a stuporous condition for several days but' gradually regained consciousness. It was several weeks before she recovered and when she did she was absolutely deaf and remains so till the present day, I think. The mortality of this disease is very great and the most of the recoveries might be better off had they not recovered for they are generally severely afflicted, frequently one of the special senses lost.

Thus we see that this disease, located as it is in the vital centers, and unless we can get a more satisfactory treatment than we now have, it means either death or to pass the remainder of his life maimed in a very serious way.

DISCUSSION.

Dr. A. S. Riser, Blackwell:

There isn't anything I can add much in the discussion, but I would like to give you a case I had of meningitis, secondary to pneumonia. The patient was about two years old. I had her three days under treatment and she seemed to be doing very well, and the third day her people called me up and said she wasn't doing so well. I called to see the girl and found a well developed pneumonia on the left side posterior. She proceeded for ten days, apparently getting along well, temperature going down and she seemed to be on the high road to recovery, when on about the eleventh day her mother reported she wasn't so well. I called to see her and found a slightly higher pulse, she wasn't quite so bright and hadn't taken so much nourishment. The day following there was no change, but early on the morning of the third day I called to see the little girl and found nothing but a ptosis of the right eye lid, and the other symptoms were about the same. On the following day the condition continued. The ptosis was very marked, the right pupil dilated, the left pupil normal, but the stupor increased and the temperature in the right axilla about two degrees higher than the left. The pulse gradually increased and grew more irregular and slightly higher in rate, and then a very few hours after that she died.

This was a very sad case from the fact that this was the only child of her parents and there came to me the thought if we could only avoid that complication following pneumonia and if there is not any way of avoiding it and if there is any way of treating it, and I must confess that I know of no satisfactory way of treating it, and I should be glad to hear from any of the gentlemen present.

APPENDICITIS.

BY DR. W. T. TILLY, PRESIDENT STATE BOARD OF MEDICAL EXAMINERS MUSKOGEE, OKLAHOMA.

Mr. President and Fellow Members of Muskogee County Medical Society:

I consider that I have been assigned one

Read before the Muskogee County Medical Society, September, 1910.

of the most important subjects that your committee could have assigned me, for appendicitis has come to stay. It is one disease that will never be of less interest to physicians and surgeons than it is today, unless every child both male and female, should be operated on in its infancy and have its appendix removed and do away with appendicitis by breeding it out as they breed stump tail dogs—a theory which I believe is possible but however, not practicable.

Etiology: One of the most frequent causes, I think, is constipation and in my experience I have found that almost invariably patients suffering with appendicitis, give a history of constipation. Other causes are foreign bodies entering the canal of the appendix and remaining until irritation is produced followed by inflammation. Ad hesions of the abdominal viscera play an important part in producing appendicitis by extending and involving the appendix. Personally, I have found but few cases that I operated on containing seed or foreign bodies, but as a rule my cases have contained fecal concretions. We also have a constricted appendix produced by adhesions.

Symptoms: The symptoms of appendicitis vary in different cases and are sometimes very deceptive. There is no one symptom pathognomonic of it. I do not believe that there is any disease to which the human being is heir in which we are so liable to be mistaken in our diagnosis as in appendicitis. Ordinarily, however, attacks of appendicitis come on, in typical cases, by what is known to the laity as cramp colic, beginning in the region of the umbilicus and radiating over the entire abdomen in the acute stage, centralizing, after a few hours, at McBurney's point. Pain though, is not always a leading symptom in appendicitis. Vomiting occurs in the majority of cases, but is not always present. Constipation, as I have before stated, usually exists. In typical cases, we usually have a wiry, high tension pulse and we may or may not, have any elevation of temperature. But usually

within forty-eight hours of the onset, we have an elevation of from one to three degrees. Very often we only have tenderness and soreness in the abdomen which may not be confined to any particular place. The patient may linger for days or even weeks, without showing any leading symptoms of appendicitis. We very often have symptoms of ovarian or, tubal troubles which are very easily mistaken for appendicitis, vice versa. I have operated on a number of cases where the leading symptoms were those of salpingitis or ovaritis, and upon opening the abdomen, find that I had a typical case of appendicitis. We often find the appendix and tube united which condition produce more leading symptoms of tubal or, ovarian trouble than that of appendicitis. I have recently operated on one case at least, where the appendix and left tube were united. A case in which it would have been impossible to diagnose appendicitis by the leading symptoms as are usually laid down in our text books. In other words, I consider each case a law unto itself and it must be treated accordingly. Like all other diseases with which we come in contact, it is impossible to make a diagnosis from our text books only. The greatest assets a physician possesses in the diagnosis of appendicitis, as well as in other diseases, are experience and common sense, of which any successful physician or surgeon must possess at least a reasonable amount of each. I want here to add, that there are two classes of physicians whom I wish to class as extremists and very dangerous to deal with as far as the patient is concerned. One is the physician who makes a diagnosis of appendicitis of each and every ache and pain that may be in the abdominal region. The other, who never makes a diagnosis of appendicitis, it matters not what the symptoms may be. The latter, I would consider the more dangerous of the two as far as the patient is concerned. I will give here two cases that have occurred in my practice which will illustrate the foregoing: Case No. 1. Was called in consultation to see Miss A, and found her suffering intensely with a typical tumor in the region of the appendix as large as a common saucer, a sausage shaped indurated mass, very sensitive and painful to touch, temperature of 104, anxious expression, pulse thready—120, constipated, vomiting and in fact, every leading symptom of appendicitis. A case in which no one should have made a mistake in his diagnosis. The abdomen was covered with an ointment of ichthyol and vaseline and on top of this was an antiphlogistine poultice. This patient had been suffering for two weeks with all the leading symptoms present. I immediately ordered that the patient be prepared for operation and operated within the next three hours. Upon making my incision, I found a sack of pus, the like of which I had never smelled before, and after a thorough cleansing, drained the cavity. The end of the caecum together with the appendix had sloughed off leaving an opening through which fecal matter has passed ever since. This patient is able to go around wherever she pleases, but there still remains a slight fistula which may close of itself by and by, or will require a secondary operation. Case No. 2. Was called in consultation to see a woman who had been suffering intensely for four or five days with pain in the abdomen. The physician had diagnosed appendicitis, but on examination, I found that she was suffering with gall stones and advised an operation. She was brought to Muskogee and I removed at least one-half a pint of gall stones from the size of a quail egg to black sand, the patient making an uneventful recovery and has enjoyed fine health ever since. These two cases illustrate to my mind very clearly the importance of making a correct diagnosis and the liability of making an incorrect

one. It is plain that neither case would have recovered without the proper diagnosis and treatment.

Treatment: As you all know the treatment varies with different men as much as the diagnosis. But to my mind, after having made a diagnosis of appendicitis I wish to go on record now as saying that there is only one method of treatment which is safe and sane and that is an appendectomy. And I do not agree with a great many men who are, owing to their advantages and experience, a great deal better qualified to judge than I, who advocate that after 24 or 48 hours we should wait 10 or 12 days before operating. I have never been able to make myself believe that a patient is safer waiting and allowing a large pus cavity to form and taking the chances of perforation followed by peritonitis and death, than they are to operate at any stage from the hour of attack on. There is just as much reason to my mind in a theory of that kind as in the old theory that physicians as well as the laity, advanced that a wound was not doing well unless it discharged pus.

As to the medicinal treatment, I consider the morphine splint the best of all and keep it applied all the time. I do not believe in giving cathartics in appendicitis unless you are prepared for an immediate operation. I consider it both useless and dangerous but think that the peristalsis should be absolutely controlled. Quiet, rest in bed, and take nothing into the stomach if we are compelled to treat on the expectant plan. As to the operation, it is not necessary to take up your time with a detailed description of it as it is fully understood by each and every physician present and the technique is about the same with all.

Hoping that the ideas advanced here and the discussion of the same will be beneficial to each of us, I thank you.

INTESTINAL OBSTRUCTION.

BY DR. J. C. WATKINS, HALLETT, OKLAHOMA.

Ileus or intestinal obstruction is an abnormal condition of the intestinal portion of the alimentary canal in which the feces is prevented from passing on.

There are three principle types of Ileus; Vis. *Adynamic, Dynamic,* and *Mechanical.* In the adynamic form we find the condition due to an absence of the power of propulsion or a paralyzed condition due to the interference with the mesenteric nerve supply. The dynamic form is one in which the contracting power of the intestinal wall is in excess of normal, the peristalsis being produced by some pathological stimulus. The mechanical form, the most common of all, is one in which the fecal stream is blocked by some mechanical · device such as, strangulated hernia, foreign bodies, (worms, empacted feces, gall-stones, etc.). bands, congenital and acquired; peritonitus from acute appendicitis; volculus, and intussusception.

The diagnosis of ileus is made upon the following general or cardinal symptoms: *pain, corpostasis, vomiting, meteorism, shock* and *collopse.*

The treatment of ileus is premeninently a surgical one. Valuable time is often lost in the use of drugs, injections, etc. Celiotomy is the only procedure.

I wish to go more specifically into that special form of ileus, the result of intussusception.

Intussusception is that form of intestinal obstruction where one part of the intestine is prolapsed or invaginated into the lumen of an immediately adjoining part. The condition may be acute, sub-acute or chronic. The intestine is not always obstructed at first, but soon becomes so, due to the adhesions formed, and the rapid swelling which soon takes place. The circulation is soon interfered with, the blood supply being shut off from the teloscoped portion of the gut, it soon becomes gangrene.

The aetialogy of intussusception is rather obscure, but is generally conceded to be due to some irregular peristalsis induced by the presence of some foreign material, undigested food worms, impacted feces, or polypoid-tumors, etc. A portion of the gut may become paralyzed, thereby causing the adjacent portion to telescope.

The condition is usually found in children, seventy per cent. of the cases before the third year. Males seem to be more predisposed than females, when a record of sex has been observed.

In addition to the cardinal symptoms of ileus, the diagnosis of intussusception is made by considering the age, the more abrupt onset, severe colicky pains of paroxysmal nature, vomiting, first the contents of the stomach and later becoming stercoral. It has been suggested that vomiting whether early or late suggests the location of the obstruction, whether high or low. At first there are a few diarrhoeal stools, followed by bloody musous discharge, then constipation becomes complete, not even the passage of gas. Can usually make out a tumor mass in abdomen, before the distension becomes too great. The temperature soon becomes sub-normal, pulse weak, fast, thready, cold clammy skin.

In making a diagnosis it is not wise, as a rule, to wait till one is sure of an intussusception, but all that is necessary is to make a positive diagnosis of acute obstruc-

Read before the Annual Meeting of the Oklahoma State Medical Association, Tulsa, Oklahoma, May, 1910.

tion and proceed to the treatment at once. The treatment of intussusception and obstruction in general is a surgical one.

Holt, recommends, to first attempt reduction by inflation or injection, the procedure to be done under an anesthetic, and if unsuccessful to proceed at once to do a celiotomy.

Clubbe, (Brit. Jour. Child. Dis. July, '99) insists that the treatment of ileus and especially intussusception is celiotomy. He states that out of 173 cases of intussusception under his care, that sixteen were reduced by injection method, 157 celiotomies with a mortality of about twenty per cent.

Dr. John Young Brown of St. Louis, (American Jour. Obstetrics, Nov., '09.) reports a case of intussusception in which an artificial anus was produced by sticking a trocar into the abdomen. This condition was of three and one-half years standing, the large bowel being out of commission all this time. He did a celiotomy with a resection of the occluded bowel, thereby establishing continuity. I mention this case to show that if a patient is in too profound a shock, to go through the operation, that one may quickly form a fecal fistula above the obstruction, and later doing a secondary operation.

The above is only a digest of the literature on the subject.

I wish now to report briefly a case that came under my own care hoping it may be of some interest to some one.

On Monday, July 26, '09. I was called to see Lizzie P., a girl of 8 years of age.

The history and physical examination revealed the following facts; was just recovering from a two weeks attack of malaria, was very anaemic. On Saturday before she had eaten five or six large pickled peppers, some green apples, candy, nuts, etc. She took sick Saturday night, with severe cramps in the stomach, nausea and vomiting, constipation since Saturday. The abdominal pain was general over the abdomen, very slightly localized at umbilicus. The abdomen was slightly tender to touch. There was no rigidity of muscles, no tympanitis and no tumefication either by abdominal palpation or per rectum. Temperature 98 3-5, pulse 84.

I prescribed the usual treatment for acute indigestion.

On Wednesday, July 28, I was called again. Patient had not been able to retain any food or medicine, no action of any kind of the bowels; temperature now 98, pulse 100. Pain about the same, still no tympanitis, nor tumefication. I then made a diagnosis of intestinal obstruction, and insisted upon an operation but was refused. I then tried reduction (for suspected intussusception) by enema of hot water with oil, in knee-chest position.

On Thursday, July 29, the vomiting became stercoral with a very offensive odor, temperature now 97, pulse 130, still no tumefication, tenderness slightly increased. Tympanitis, becoming very marked could outline coils of small intestines, vomiting still increasing. Pain now so severe that had to give hypo 1-8 gr. morphia, 1-150 gr. strychnine.

An operation was still refused. On Friday morning, July 30, vomiting much worse. temperature had gone down to 94, (rectal temperature) pulse 160 and barely perceptible, skin cold and clammy, in fact was in state of profound shock, a semicomatose condition. Now got consent to an operation, and started at once for Oklahoma City, reaching the hospital about 7 o'clock p. m. Patient seemed to rally some, while making the trip of 85 miles to the hospital, as her pulse was now 106, temperature 96. We decided to watch the case that night and next morning it was decided by the consulting surgeons that it would be unwise to operate as it was thought she would die upon the table.

We started at once for home hoping to get there with her before she died. She stood the trip fairly well, much better than we expected.

She lingered along until Aug. 16, when she died, just twenty-four (24) days after taking sick.

During all this time her temperature ran from 84-96, pulse 140-160. Constipation was absolute the entire time, at times she would go five or six hours without vomiting, towards the last the vomit was nearly pure bile, abdominal tenderness was not very marked at any time, there was slight rigidity of muscles all along.

Tympanitis was very marked at times only, would be much worse just before vomiting, when she would go a few hours without vomiting. The last fifteen days, she would take orange juice with a little whisky and a little iced butter-milk, and retain it two or three hours.

We kept ice bags on her abdomen most all the time and let her eat small pieces of ice every little while.

The injections were kept up two or three times every day. Would make the irrigations high with rectal tube, could retain from two or three quarts of water in knee-chest position.

I was permitted to do an autopsy, and I found upon opening the abdomen, all the abdominal organs in a normal condition except the lower portion of the ileum. The appendix was in a normal healthy condition. There was not a trace of peritonitis. No adhesions except in the telescoped portion of the Ileum.

About ten inches above the Ileo-caecal valve there was an intussusception of the Ileum, about fourteen inches of the gut was telescoped into the portion just beyond. There was a small rim of the gut glued together, at margins of the intussusception, forming a blind sack, which contained about one pint of thick yellowish fluid. The entire large bowel was collapsed. No trace of fecal matter. The small intestine was very much distended with gas, above the obstruction.

I have gone into details in reporting this case, hoping it may be of interest to some one.

This case shows that however small the chance for recovery may seem, there is yet hope, for "While there is life there is hope" and the effort should be made.

I wish again to call attention to the importance of an early diagnosis in cases of acute intestinal obstruction, of whatever nature; and the still greater importance of an early operation as valuable time is lost in delaying.

DISCUSSION.

Dr. Noble, of Guthrie: This case strikes me because it is only about eight weeks since I had a case, and it also shows that one cannot get a typical case. This little boy, four years old, was taken ill with severe headache and vomiting, with pain in his muscles and bones. He did not complain of any abdominal pain; his abdomen was flat and he was passing some gas and a very little fecal matter. The diagnosis of the attending physician was La Grippe. Saturday night I was called on the phone, and Sunday I saw the boy. He then had a temperature of 100 and the pulse was about 110. The abdomen was flat. He was not complaining of any pain in the abdomen. He did not look very sick. I advised operation, and although this was a week after the start it was surprising to see how little trouble there was. The boy made an uninterrupted recovery and was out to Sunday-school four weeks later.

Dr. Berry, of Okmulgee: The point that strikes me in this case is the fact that the doctor impress the patient with the importance of an operation. That fact ought to be a lesson to every man who is not doing surgery, because every man who practices medicine ought to be able to diagnose a case of intestinal obstruction. I saw a case that had been under the care of the family physician for five days, last year, and I was asked to operate. I said, "Doctor, we are operating on a dead boy." When a patient goes three days with a complete intestinal obstruction, you have got a dead patient.

I had another case similar to the one that the doctor just now reports. A physician called me from a neighboring town, and he had made a diagnosis. We immediately placed the child in the hospital, operated in less than twenty-five minutes, never had a bit of trouble, and the child was well in less than three weeks.

___

Dr. Mayberry, Enid: Just one little point about the ileus that I had some personal experience recently; that is the danger of allowing the backed up fecal matter to pass down into the bowel after relieving your obstruction. Often times you operate and find a full bowel above the obstruction and find a full bowel above the obstruction and an empty bowel below. Your obstruction is sometimes easily removed. But allowing that accumulated fecal matter ripe in bacterial poison to pass down into the bowel below is something you should always bear in mind in intestinal obstruction. I had a case of strangulated hernia and very nearly lost the case, and I am satisfied that it was due to the accumulated fecal matter passing into the part below the obstruction. I would like to have some instructions on the point of when to drain that off.

___

Dr. White, Muskogee: Sometime ago I heard Dr. T., of Australia. He said he had had 125 cases of in-

tussusception. And he laid great stress on the early diagnosis, and also to importance of a bloody stool. He relied more on the bloody stool symptom than any other one symptom. Sometime ago I had a case and I am satisfied that that is what produced death in the child. It was a young baby, about three years old, stood the operation very well, and about 25 hours afterwards she began to have convulsions and died.

___

Dr. Fortner, of Vinita: We have been discussing the diagnosis. I want to ask, what is there serious about cutting a hole in a baby's belly? What is there about it that we should postpone so long and be so afraid of it?

___

Dr. Grossheart, of Tulsa: The paper in my estimation only should educate the man that is in the general practice that where he is refused by the family, after he has made the diagnosis, he should absolutely refuse to go further with the case. If every honest practitioner would do that, where he has asked for a consultation first, and if you and your counsel see the case alike, and your judgment is that it is a surgical case, and needs surgical interference, then if your family refuse and will not give their consent, or the patient will not give his consent to surgical interference, step down and out and quit it honorably. It is a fact that there are always in a community a few that will keep holding on to run a bill, etc., and that is not the proper way to educate your people. In regard to diagnosis of intussusception, I have had no great sight of experience. I have seen a few cases and operated a few for bowel obstruction.

It is very easy to make an artificial anus and drain the bowel, and in a good many cases that is better than to operate.

___

Dr. Blesh, of Oklahoma City: I was

interested in the report of this case, but unfortunately I did not get here in time to hear the paper. However, I believe I was the surgeon consulted in regard to this little patient, and I will state that it seemed absolutely in an unoperable condition. It did not look like it could survive an anesthetic, and operative deaths must be recognized as unfortunate always in their effect upon the public. That is to say that one operative death, while it has accomplished nothing with respect to that individual case, has barred many cases, or frightened many cases from that vicinity whom the surgeon might have benefited. I am not afraid to take long risks where I think there is some good to be accomplished and a chance to save the patient's life. But where it seems likely to terminate with death on the table I am very cautious for the reasons stated. The greatest good to the greatest number must to a large extent guide us in deciding upon an operation. My judgment, as a matter of fact was in error in the matter. Since then I have operated several cases of intestinal obstruction, and several before, and have made nice recoveries. I regret very much in view of the subsequent history of the case that I did not operate.

Dr. Rector, of Hennessey: I have had very good results with treating the bowel with normal salt solution. I have got one of those patients here with me now. I think it is a good idea to do that before you resort to surgery.

Dr. Pearse, Kansas City: I will speak only about the operation. Make the incision at the point where you have the best reason to believe you can find the obstruction.

Do not handle the bowel.

Use a munyon tube. Slip this into the bowels, and it will empty itself of gas for a space of four or five inches. Slip that part over and it will empty another six or eight inches up to the next kink.

Dr. Watkins: All I wish to add is that in the rural districts where I live, especially where you have to deal with religous fanatics as this case was, the parents being opposed to any form of medicine, and especially surgery, it is very hard to obtain consent to an operation. I insisted very strongly on an operation but they held off. They thought the child was dying. Its mother did. But we made even that last desperate effort, and as far as diagnosis is concerned, when I first saw the child, with the history of what she had been eating—those large pickled peppers, green apples, candy, nuts, etc., I thought it was just acute indigestion. It did not seem very sick, temperature normal, pulse normal, only about ten hours since it has had an operation, so at the start I merely diagnosed the case acute indigestion, but later about thirty-six hours I made the diagnosis intussusception, and suggested operation but was refused.

MANAGEMENT OF FRACTURES OF THE EXTREMITIES.

BY DR. JAS. A. FOLTZ, FORT SMITH, ARKANSAS.

I am here in response to the very kind

Read before the Annual Meeting of the Oklahoma State Medical Association, Tulsa, Oklahoma, May, 1910.

and much appreciated invitation of your distinguished chairman, to read a paper before your society. In trying to select a subject, I was much puzzled. I was ashamed of the fact that I had not invented an improvement in the technic of the shortening of round ligaments. I was forced to confess I had developed no original technic in abdominal surgery, and found that I had been amputating breasts very much along the same lines laid out by Halstead and Jabez N. Jackson.

My perineorrhaphys and trachelorrhaphys had been done along lines familiar to you all. I could not even offer an improvement on the Mayo Method of removing goiters.

While thinking along these lines, it occurred to me that, as I had been doing quite a little fracture work in my railroad surgery, I might find something here that would interest you and be of practical importance, and, when I considered further that the records of the great hospitals in this county and in England show that from one-seventh to one-fifth of all accidental injuries treated in these institutions are fractures, and that court records show that about seventy-five per cent of all suits for damages against physicians and surgeons, as well as against railroad companies and other corporations, is for poor functional results following the treatment of fractures, I thought a few remarks along the management of fractures might not prove uninteresting.

I want to say in the beginning, there is no claim made for originality. I have only endeavored to touch some of the points frequently overlooked in the management of fractures.

About the poorest advertisement a doctor can have in a neighborhood is a crooked and powerless limb. No argument can offset this damaging evidence. Thus we see an error in diagnosis or a failure to apply proper remedial measures at the proper time, may end disastrously not only for the patient, but for the doctor as well.

Duncan Eve has said, "a thorough knowledge of the anatomical relations of structures, a wide experience, practical common sense, calm judgment, and constant vigilance are the characteristics a surgeon who is called upon to treat fractures, stands most in need of."

The most important of these points, to my mind, is constant vigilance. There should be in every case of fracture, or suspected fracture, a careful and frequent inspection of parts. In order that this may be carried out, I invariably use some form of a splint which may be easily and frequently removed with but little disturbance of parts.

Of late years, I have been using the wood fiber splints. They are light, can be easily molded by placing in warm water, and are very strong. They are made to fit almost any kind of a fracture.

In this connection, there is one point I want to urge. It will always stand one in good play. I make it a rule in the management of fractures of the extremities, when seen early before we have a great amount of swelling, to make a careful comparison with the opposite member. In this, we have nature's most perfect guide. Never be satisfied to leave a broken arm or leg until its contour exactly corresponds with its fellow on the opposite side. Always have both injured and uninjured limbs fully exposed. Always do your work under an anesthetic.

In my judgment, whenever a surgeon allows himself to attempt the reduction and subsequent immobilization of a broken limb with the patient's muscles stiff and rigid, and the patient himself probably writhing with pain, he is doing himself and his patient an unnecessary injustice.

Remember that in setting a broken bone, celerity, so much praised by our chairman, is of little value. Here, you may take your time. With your patient anesthetized, carefully and thoroughly make your reduction, compare parts, and use constant care and vigilance that the bones do not become misplaced while applying your splints.

I think it is an excellent rule, and one which we follow in our railroad hospitals, to remove splints and inspect all fractures at least once every week. One exception to this rule we sometimes make, in case of a simple fracture to the tibia or fibula, in the middle or upper third, which may be safely treated after the first week, by using the plaster cast which need not be removed for three or four weeks.

I feel sure that this custom has saved both myself and the railroad company considerable trouble.

Before submitting for your consideration a few cases illustrating the points I have endeavored to bring out, I want to say a few words in regard to the value of the X-Ray in the management of fractures.

That the X-Ray has been of very great value in assisting us in our diagnosis of fractures and other injuries to the long bones, there can be no doubt; but that it is infallible, is not true.

One thing particularly the X-Ray has proven to us, is the fact that excellent functional results may be obtained in almost any kind of an injury, even though the apposition of the bones is far from perfect; and that perfect apposition and alignment is a condition, which far from being ordinary, is, indeed, an exception even in the work of our most experienced and competent surgeons. This point has its value particularly in those cases where a doctor will be sued for malpractice on account of a crooked arm or leg.

First: J. S. A compound comminuted fracture of both condyles of humerus.

The shaft of humerus projected out through tissues and skin about one and one-half inches above external condyle. At the time this case was seen, which was

within thirty minutes after the accident occurred, there was very little swelling, and diagnosis was easily made. Some small nutrient artery had been cut by jagged end of bone, and bleeding was profusely. This artery was caught and tied under anesthesia, and reduction made.

The arm was at first put up in a small posterior long splint, extending from just below the shoulder to just above wrist, completely immobilizing the elbow extension.

This splint was left on for ten days, and the wound which had been packed with iodoform gauze, was dressed every other day without disturbing the splint until it healed, which was about the seventh day.

On the tenth day this form of splint was exchanged for a right angle splint which I had constructed by a tinsmith for this fracture. The arm was allowed to remain in this for ten days more, when a Plaster of Paris cast was applied, and an X-Ray taken through cast.

The X-Ray showed I had very poor apposition of the bones. Though everything felt all right, the X-Ray showed that humerus was not in proper place and projected markedly to one side, while a small piece of external condyle was pushed outward by shaft of humerus.

The cast was removed, and under an anesthesia, I attempted to correct this error, after which the arm was again put in a right angle plaster of Paris cast, and another X-Ray taken, which, while showing an improvement, still showed far from perfect apposition.

I decided that this was the best I could do and that it must be that the arm slipped within the cast.

I pursued the plan of allowing this cast to remain on for ten days, at which time same was removed and upon inspection the wound appeared all right, and the cast was again put on for ten days more, after which time I cut the case so as to make two distinct parts, one posterior and one anterior. These parts I kept together by adhesive strips, and began examining the arm every other day.

Finding that the union was fairly good, I begun passive motion. For three months active and passive motion was persisted in so that today Mr. S. has an arm which has yielded nearly three-fourths its original functions.

This was a type of injury which I think I am safe in saying, would ordinarily have resulted in a stiff elbow, with the loss of probably seventy-five per cent. of motion. This, I am sure would have been the result had the cast been put on permanently instead of any form of splint.

I may say here that I have since examined this by X-Ray, and it looks anything but pl-asing. However, functional results are good.

Second: T. J. S. A compound comminuted fracture of both bones of both legs, caused by patient falling twenty-six feet from top of coal chute and having a railing with about a ton and a half of coal fall on his lower extremities.

The fibula of the right leg was sticking out about two and one-half inches through patient's underclothes, pants and overalls, when I first saw him in the ambulance en route to the hospital.

Further examination under anesthesia, showed tibia to be broken in four places, the middle third for about two inches, being literally crushed.

The fibula of the right leg was broken in two places, once in the middle third, and the other about one-half inch above malleolus.

I decided that it would be worth while temporizing with this leg in order to save it if possible. To do this, I made an incision above anterior surface of tibia about fourteen inches long, fully exposing the bone, and removed some twelve or fourteen small fragments, and with no other splint save a pillow, protected by sterile gauze, and strapped with ordinary canvas strips to leg of patient, he was put to b.d. The wound, after controlling hemorrhage, was packed with iodoform gauze soaked in a mixture of ichthyol, castor oil and balsam peru.

This open and expectant plan of treatment was continued for about three weeks, after which time the sloughing, of which there was considerable, had ceased, and the wound found to be granulating nicely.

I then had a fracture box made at a local machine shop, and continued same plan of treatment, except using the fracture box instead of the pillow. In seven months from date of accident, Mr. S. was able to leave hospital on crutches. The wound inflicted by right fibula was still open and discharging some pus. Several spicula of bone worked out through this wound during the next six months, but at the end of one year and six months from the date of the injury, Mr. S. resumed his occupation as railroad conductor, and has continued to work steadily up to this time. He walks with a slight limp, but is active and capable.

I have not mentioned the treatment of the left leg because no complications worthy of mention developed in the treatment of same.

These two cases will suffice to show that one has plenty of latitude for originality, and one's ingenuity is often taxed to the limit in the treatment of fractures.

It also shows that only by constant personal care can we hope to obtain good results in the more complicated forms of fractures.

The two cases illustrate the point that it is very very rare, indeed, that a fracture, or a complication of fractures, will require the amputation of the limb.

THE COUNTY MEDICAL SOCIETY.

BY DR. D. ARMSTRONG, MEAD, OKLAHOMA.

In attempting to write a paper on the subject, The County Medical Society, I do so in the hope, that it will invite a discussion of medical organization, it's purpose, advantage and possibilities, with the results that we all will be supplied with that vigor and enthusiasm so essential to any prosperous medical society. We are living in an age of organization where most every line of human activity is organized, with the followers of each looking after the interest peculiar to their line of work, therefore, all must admit that medical organization is a necessity as well as a benefit.

The first and noblest object for which a medical society is created, is the education of its members in that which relates to their work, there is no profession in which it is so necessary to constantly study as that of medicine, for while medicine is not an exact science, yet it is progressive and until perfection is obtained and all of natures secrets revealed, it will continue a progressive one, making new discoveries every day, which requires, that to keep up to date we must constantly study and investigate. The man who starts out from medical school with his degree is laboring under a most serious mistake if he thinks he is educated, for if he has mastered the knowledge of the day, which is improbable, he has entered a profession which is moving forward and onward and if he would keep in the front ranks he must associate with those in the front and be spurred on by their enthusiasm and assistance, he who does not is bound to be left behind.

By reading the best medical journals a fair knowledge of the progress being made

Read before the Bryan, County Medical Society, September, 1910.

in medicine can be obtained, but with difficulty, and I am sure but few doctors keep up to date by reading alone.

By meeting together in medical societies every statement. is discussed by those best able to pass judgment and every member gets the benefit of the accumulated knowledge of the whole. The meeting together makes physicians broad minded and liberal towards the views of others and makes the average doctor recognize his short comings and the ability of others, thus stimulating study and investigation for the greatest stimulus to study and investigation comes from association with students and investigators.

The physician, especially the general practitioner of the country works under peculiar and in some respects unfortunate conditions as he works alone, men in other callings either work together or meet each other to exchange views regarding their labor, even the farmer manages to meet his neighbor at the store or elsewhere and discuss crop conditions and exchange experiences. A lonely worker in any pursuit is liable to become self-reliant in what he does, too much so for his own good and those whom he serves and especially does this apply to the physician for his is a progressive work, in which practice does not make perfect, and if he will not associate with fellow workers he certainly should be classed with the mossbacks. The doctor who works alone day after day will in spite of himself become narrow, fall into a rut and his ability to relieve the suffering, will soon be confined to his own narrow views and experiences; he is convinced that he is doing his work better than others, he is not stimulated with the ambition to progress, because he does not know, and will not believe that others are progressing. Nothing will prevent this deplorable condition better than an occasional attendance at the County Society, where we come together to discuss scientific questions which vitally affect our reputation and work, and the physician who attends the meetings will become broad minded, liberal to the views of others, and treat his professional brother in an ethical and professional way.

The second and very important object for which a medical society is created is the social side. One of the greatest curses of our profession is the existence of petty jealousies among those practicing in the same locality, and it is not necessary for me at this time to say why these jealousies exist, suffice to say, that it can be summed up in the one word "misunderstanding." Too often enmity is created between doctors living in the same town through the tattle of idlers, prejudice founded on imaginary insults or wrongs are allowed to grow into deadly animosities, and one of the best preventatives as well as the best remedies for this bickering and enmity is the coming together of the supposed enemies and face to face talking the matter over. An active medical society is a good place to keep down these troubles, especially if a little time be given to sociability, an occasional smoker, or banquet, the results in this regard will be surprising, for bickering and enmity can not long endure the mellow sunshine of the social hour. If a medical society had no other value than that of a social club it would be well worth all it cost. Another need for medical organization, and especially in Oklahoma is for active work in enforcing medical laws, to simply put laws on the statute book, and do nothing else is only accomplishing half the good that is sought to be obtained. We may theorize as long as we please about it being the duty of the County Attorney to attend to this matter,

but the fact remains that those politically elected officers will not do their duty only in rare instances, because a united profession does not demand it, and the individual member of the profession who takes upon himself this task will generally live to regret it, hence it is imperative that a united profession assert their rights and demand the enforcement of proper laws.

A fourth and essential need for the medical organization is the proper looking after the business side of the practice of medicine. High ideas, noble motives, and self-sacrificing work, are the characteristics of the average doctor and his daily work, is proof of this but there is a business side to the practice of medicine and the majority of us are sadly liking in this matter, although it is hard to say why. It is not my purpose to discuss this very important question, but only suggest that a mutual exchange of views in regard to the business side of our work, would result in much good. A mutual understanding of physicians living in the same town, (such as that agreed on by the physicians of Durant) as to fees, collections, etc., could not but result in many instances in a much better provided home for the doctors family, and a great deal for the comfort and enjoyment to himself. If one doctor persists in placing a low price on his work or services in opposition to the wishes and practice of the other physician of his country, I say, gentlemen, he should be ostracised both professionally and socially by his fellow practitioners. Such a physician will soon learn that no man ever made a reputation by placing his services lower than those of his neighbors, and that he who places a low estimate on his ability will find that his patients will generally judge him by his own standard. A good county medical society will be of great value in bringing about a mutual understanding among physicians, which will redound to their mutual good welfare.

EDITORIAL

THE HYGIENIC EDUCATION OF HIGH-SCHOOL STUDENTS.

A perusal of literature, medical and lay, indicates that there is a vast movement on foot throughout the country looking to the sane investigations of the cause of disease and its prevention along sane lines.

One is struck by the fact that there seems to be so little cohesion of forces and endeavor in this direction; one state having splendid laws, so far as their constitutional limits permit, and the neighboring state by dissimilar laws and regulations does much to undo the work done across the border.

It is noticeable that all meetings and discussions of public health matters ends with the understanding that some move will be undertaken to make the people acquainted with the principles of the spread of disease and the principles underlying its prevention.

By reason of the fact that many of our contagious diseases are little understood and their control, even to a small degree, a matter of knowledge of the past few years only, many erroneous opinions prevail among the profession and certainly to a greater degree among the people, as to the simpler means of preventing disease. This lack of information or the knowledge as to how the different situations should be handled necessarily means inadequate and poor handling.

Years of time and patient endeavor are necessary to accomplish any great good and no reform can be inaugurated and put into force until the people affected by the proposed reform understand the underlying principles. When this is understood educators and reformers will begin at the proper age in life to inculcate the proper knowledge.

Our high schools should have a department of hygiene and properly qualified lecturers should be employed to educate the growing mind in the fixed and undisputed points of disease prevention.

A department in the state with this in view could be economically organized and maintained. That Federal control of all public health matters would be theoretically ideal cannot be disputed; for the protection and conserving of the public health is certainly a matter of most vital importance to the National existence, but to reach this ideal condition the people must know the reason for the changes and the breaking down and invasion of what they consider their greatest heritage, their constitutional rights, as they are now in force and interpreted, must be preceded by a wide education of the people and when they are shown the importance of the eradication of state lines so far as public health is concerned no objection will be raised by sensible people.

When the states are educated in this respect there will no longer be raised the objections that one now hears on every side that Federal control of state health matters is unconstitutional and an infringement of the rights of the people. If necessary that part of the constitution written years ago and applicable to then existing condition can be rewritten by order of the people to conform to the modern knowledge of today, but before this can be done the people must know the reason for it and to know this they must be taught the principles involved, just as they are today taught the principles of electricity, engineering and agriculture in a way absolutely unknown when our present binding constitution was written.

INFANTILE PARALYSIS.

Recent reports to the State Commissioner of Health indicate the presence in the eastern portion of the state of infantile paralysis. While isolated cases have appeared from time to time in the western portion of the state no cases have been reported in the eastern half until now.

It is well to remember that this disease is of an infectious or contagious nature so far as we know and that its control rests on the same rules that the control of other infectious diseases do. Unfortunately no known treatment affects the result so far as the paralysis is concerned, but the total results are probably influenced by an eliminative treatment, as are many other infectious diseases, a liquid diet, quiet and thorough isolation.

The ultimate control of this affection will probably be found in serum therapy or along these lines, but as an early diagnosis is impossible according to our present limited information of the disease we should bend every endeavor to have those cases we do find placed under a strict quarantine and the case more closely isolated than we now isolate diphtheria.

A BLOW AT MISBRANDING.

The National Association of Pure Food, Drugs and Dairy Departments, meeting in New Orleans, November 28-December 3rd, adopted a resolution demanding that all patent medicines be truthfully and legibly labelled.

This resolution should in reality be unnecessary, but it is notorious that many of the patent medicines sold are brazenly labelled in violation, of at least, the intent of the law governing such matters.

Many of them have dropped the word "cure" but replace it with evasive claims and elusive statements, which are more potent to the uneducated reader, the reader who is the usual victim of their cheap and unreasonable claims.

DIRECTORY OF OFFICERS AND SECTION CHAIRMAN OF THE OKLAHOMA STATE MEDICAL ASSOCIATION.

President—Dr. D. A. MYERS, Lawton.

Vice-Presidents—*First*, Dr. C. L. REEDER, Tulsa; *Second*, Dr. H. M. WILLIAMS, Wellston; *Third*, Dr. JAMES L. SHULER, Durant.

Secretary-Treasurer—Dr. CLAUDE A. THOMPSON, Muskogee.

Delegates to American Medical Association, 1911-1912—Dr. CHAS. R. HUME, Anadarko; Dr. WALTER E. WRIGHT, Tulsa.

SECTION CHAIRMEN.

Surgery—Dr. ROSS GROSSHART, Tulsa.

Medicine—Dr. J. H. SCOTT, Shawnee.

Mental and Nervous Diseases—Dr. F. B. ERWIN, Norman.

Ediatrics—Dr. W. G. LITTLE, Okmulgee.

Eye, Ear, Nose and Throat—Dr. MILTON K. THOMPSON, Muskogee.

Gynecology and Obstetrics—Dr. B. W. FREER, Nowata.

Section on Pathology—Dr. ELIZABETH MELVIN, Guthrie.

For Councillors see first page.

Place of meeting, Muskogee, May 9, 10 and 11, 1911.

卐 | COUNTY SOCIETIES | 卐

ADAIR COUNTY.

Meeting at Stilwell, December 3rd.
Diphtheria: Its Diagnosis and Treatment—Dr. D. A. Beard, Westville.
La Grippe and Its Sequellae—Dr. C. C. Barnes, Westville.
Tuberculosis: How Shall We Handle It?—Dr. P. C. Woodruff, Stilwell.
Surgery—Dr. T. W. Blackburne, Cane Hill, Ark.
Sanitation and Prophylaxis—J. A. Patton, Stilwell.

OKLAHOMA COUNTY.

October Meeting:
Subject—Acute Gastro-Enteritis in Children.
Etiology and Pathology—Dr. W. M. Taylor, Oklahoma City.
Symptomatology and Diagnosis—Dr. J. A. Coley, Oklahoma City.
Treatment—Dr. John S. Pine, Oklahoma City.

TILLMAN COUNTY.

The Tillman County Medical Society will have a Post-Graduate course for the remainder of the year and will carry out the following program which was arranged by a committee consisting of:
Drs. A. J. Hays, L. A. Mitchell, J. Angus Gillis.

PROGRAM.

Diseases of the Lungs and Pleura.

Oct. 28.—Dr. A. B. Fair, Anatomy of the Lungs.
Nov. 4.—Dr. L. A. Mitchell, Histology,

of the Lungs; Dr. J. D. Osborne, Physiology of the Lungs.
Nov. 11.—Dr. A. J. Hays, Anatomy, Histology, and Physiology of the Pleura; Dr. A. M. Boyd, Pleurisy.
Nov. 18.—Dr. F. G. Priestley, Topography of the Chest; Dr. T. E. Spurgeon, Anatelectasis.

Lobar Pneumonia.

Nov. 25.—Dr. J. N. Ryan, History, Etiology and Pathology: Dr. H. C. McGee, Symptomatology Diagnosis and Prognosis; Dr. H. L. Roberts, Treatment.
Dec. 2.—Dr. J. Angus Gillis, Lobular Pneumonia; Dr. R. L. Wilson, Other forms of Pneumonia.
Dec. 9.—Dr. J. P. Van Allen, Bronchial Asthma; Dr. M. F. Patterson, Other forms of Asthma; Dr. O. G. Bacon, Emphysema.
Dec. 16.—Dr. A. B. Fair, Empyemia, Hydro and Pneumothorax; Dr. W. W. Beach, Abscess and Gangrene of the Lungs; Dr. A. J. Hays, Traumatism of Lungs and Pleura.
Dec. 23.—Dr. J. W. Collier, Acute Miliary Tuberculosis; Dr. J. H. Hanson, History and Etiology of Chronic "T. B."; Dr. F. G. Preistley, Pathology and Symptomatology.
Dec. 30.—Dr. J. W. Comb, Diagnosis and Prognosis of Chronic "T. B."; Dr. J. Angus Gillis, Climate; F. C. Rosenberger, Treatment.

A. B. FAIR, Secretary.

CLEVELAND COUNTY.

The Cleveland County Medical Society have outlined their work for the years and will follow the following subjects on the dates indicated. All meetings will be held in Norman.

PROGRAM.

November Seventeenth—
Erysipelas:
Diagnosis and Treatment.

November 24th—
Annual Meeting Oklahoma Academy of Science.

December—
General Topic:
Respiratory Diseases.

December 1st—
Anatomy of the Respiratory Tract.
Physiology of the Respiratory Tract.

December 8th—
Acute Bronchitis.
Chronic Bronchitis.
Discussants.

December 15th—
Lobar Pneumonia:
Etiology, Pathology and Symptomatology.
Diagnosis and Treatment.

December 22nd—
Lobular Pneumonia:
Etiology, Pathology and Symptomatology.
Diagnosis and Treatment.

Decemebr 29th—
Etiology, pathology and Symptomatology.
Diagnosis and Treatment.

January—
General Topic:
Anaesthesia and Surgical Shock.

January 5th—
Local Anaesthesia.
Minor General Anaesthesia.

January 12th—
General Anaesthesia:
Chloroform.
Ether.

January 19th—
Surgical Shock:
Physiology and Etiology.
Diagnosis and Treatment.

January 26th—
Annual Election of Officers and Smoker.

February—
General Topic:
Diseases of Children.

February 2nd—
Rubella.
Discussant.
Rubeola.
Discussant.

February 9th—
Scarlatina:
Etiology, Pathology and Symptomatology.
Diagnosis and Treatment.

February 16th—
Pertussis.
Varicella.
Spasmodic Croup.

February 23rd—
Acute Anterior Poliomyellitis.
Etiology, Pathology and Symptomatology.
Diagnosis and Treatment.

March—

General Topic:
Syphilis.

March 2nd—
Primary Syphilis:
History and Etiology.
Diagnosis and Treatment.

March 9th—
Secondary Syphilis:
Pathology.
Symptomatology.
Diagnosis and Treatment.

March 16th—
Tertiary Syphilis:
Pathology and Symptomatology.
Diagnosis and Treatment.

March 23rd—
Hereditary Syphilis:
Theories of Transmission.
Diagnosis and Treatment.

March 30th—
Clinical Meeting:
At this meeting all members are requested to exhibit clinical cases or present case reports, especially of Syphilis.

April—
General Topic:
Obstetrics.

April 1st—
Physiology and Management of Pregnancy.
Management of Normal Labor.

April 13th—
Complications of Pregnancy.
Management of Abnormal Labor.

April 20th—
Management of the Puerperium.

Complications of the Puerperium.

April 27th—
Plastic Surgery of the Cervix and Perineum.

May 4th—
Entero-colitis:
Etiology and Pathology.
Symptomatology.

May 11th—
Diagnosis and Treatment of Entero-colitis:
Acute Entero-colitis.
Chronic Entero-colitis.

May 18th—
General Diseases of the Heart.

May 25th—
Diseases of the Blood Vessels.

June 1st—
Parasitic Diseases of the Skin:
Scabies.
Pediculosis.
Tinea Trichophytina.

June 8th—
Non Parasitic Diseases of the Skin:
Eczema.
Seborrhea.
Dermatitis.

LOCATION WANTED.

A graduate, fifteen years' experience and well equipped, wants a good location for general practice. Partnership in general practice will be considered.

Address "DOCTOR," Care this Journal.

BOOKS RECEIVED

Transactions of the Fourth International Sanitary Conference of the American Republics. San Jose, Costa Rica, December 25, 1909, to January 23, 1910.

Published under the auspices of the Pan-American Union, John Barrett, Director General, Washington, D. C.

A COMPEND OF THE ACTIVE PRINCIPLES.

(With Symptomatic Indications for their Therapeutic Use.)

By Harold Hamilton Redfield, A. B., M. D., Associate Professor of Therapeutics, Bennett Medical College, Chicago; Professor of Therapeutics and Physiology, Reliance Medical College, Chicago.

Cloth, price $1.00, post paid.

The Clinic Publishing Company, Chicago, Ill., 1910.

THE PRACTICAL MEDICINE SERIES, VOLUME EIGHT.

Contents, Materia Medica and Therapeutics, Preventive Medicine and Climatology, Edited by George F. Butler, PH. G., M. D.; Henry B. Favill, A. B., M. D., Norman Bridge, A. M., M. D.

Series 1910.

Chicago.

The Year Book Publishers, 40 Dearborn Street.

THE PHYSICIAN'S POCKET ACCOUNT BOOK, by J. J. Taylor, M. D., 212 pages. Leather. Price $1.00 postpaid. J. J. Taylor, Jublisher, 4105 Walnut St., Philadelphia, Pa.

The especial feature of this book is a system of accounts whereby each transaction can be recorded in a moment's time in plain language, so that it is strictly legal as evidence in court without personal explanation, and so arranged that any patron's account can be ascertained on demand without any posting. There is only one entry of each transaction, and this in such a form that no posting is ever required. It saves time, labor and worry, and insures that your accounts are always up to date, so that you can send statements out every month without any delay and can inform any patron, wherever you may meet him, of the exact state of his account. This feature alone in the course of a year will secure payments for you— that would otherwise be missed—sufficient to buy your account books for a whole lifetime. It is the simplest, quickest and easiest legal account system on the market.

The book also has some easy and practical directions for billing and collecting, some excellent business and legal hints, some valuable forms for emergency use, such as "dying declarations," "form for wills," etc., an average medical and surgical fee bill, besides miscellaneous tables, clinical directions, etc. Having a good cash account department and various clinical records—vaccinations, deaths and confinements—it forms a complete year book for the physician's pocket.

For those who prefer to keep their accounts at the desk, the same system has been enlarged into a desk size book of 400 large sized pages, the price of which is only $5.00 per copy.

THE PRACTITIONER'S VISITING LIST FOR 1911:

An invaluable pocket-sized book containing memoranda and data important for every physician, and ruled blanks for recording every detail of practice. The Weekly, Monthly and 30-Patient Perpetual contain-

32 pages of data and 160 pages of classified blanks. The 60-Patient Perpetual consists of 256 pages of blanks alone. Each in one wallet-shaped book, bound in flexible leather, with flap and pocket, pencil with rubber, and calendar for two years: Price by mail, postpaid, to any address, $1.25. Thumb-letter index, 25 cents extra. Descriptive circular showing the several styles sent on request. Lea & Febiger, Publishers, Philadelphia and New York.

DISEASES OF THE SKIN.
New (6th) Edition, Revised.

A Treatise on Diseases of the Skin. For the use of advanced Students and Practitioners. By Henry W. Stelwagon, M. D., Ph. D., Professor of Dermatology, Jefferson Medical College, Philadelphia. Sixth edition, revised. Handsome octavo of 1195 pages, with 289 text-illustrations, and 34 full-page colored and half-tone plates. Philadelphia and London: W. B. Saunders Company, 1910. Cloth, $6.00 net; Half Morocco, $7.50 net.

A MANUAL OF DISEASES OF THE NOSE, THROAT, AND EAR.
New Second Edition.

A Manual of Diseases of the Nose, Throat, and Ear. By E. Baldwin Gleason, M. D., Professor of Otology at the Medico-Chirurgical College, Philadelphia. Second revised edition. 12mo of 563 pages, profusely illustrated. Philadelphia and London, W. B. Saunders Company, 1910. Flexible leather, $2.50 net.

THE PRACTICE OF SURGERY.

The Practice of Surgery. By James G. Mumford, M. D., Instructor in Surgery in the Harvard Medical School. Octavo of 1015 pages, with 682 illustrations. Philadelphia and London, W. B. Saunders Company, 1910. Cloth, $7.00 net; Half Morocco, $8.50 net.

HYDROTHERAPY.

Hydrotherapy: A Treatise on Hydrotherapy in general. Its application to special affections; the Technic or Processes Employed; and use of Waters Internally. By Guy Hinsdale, A. M., M. D., Lecturer on Climatology, Medico-Chirurgical College of Philadelphia. Octavo of 466 pages, illustrated. Philadelphia and London, W. B. Saunders Company, 1910. Cloth, $3.50 net.

THE HYPODERMATIC TABLET AS AN EMERGENCY AGENT.

If there is one class of therapeutic agents which more than another should be chosen with discretion and judgment, the hypodermatic tablet represents that class. When he administers a preparation hypodermatically the physician wants prompt action, and he wants to be certain that he is going to get it. To have that assurance he must use a tablet that is active, that has definite strength that dissolves promptly and wholly. Cheap tablets poorly made tablets, tablets concerning which there is the slightest doubt as to medicinal quality, may well be left alone. And there is no need to err in the matter of selection. Hypodermatic tablets of the better sort are easily obtainable. Perhaps the brand which comes most readily to mind is the brand which is exploited so extensively to physicians under the familiar caption of "Five Seconds by the Watch." The makers, it is hardly necessary to add, are Messrs. Parke Davis & Co., who guarantee their hypodermatic tablets unequivocally as to purity, solubility, activity and stability.

AN UNCONVENTIONAL COUGH SYRUP.

There are "cough syrups" without end. Some of them, it is needless to say, have little or no therapeutic value. Conversely, there are some that no physician need heitate to prescribe. One of these—Syrup Cocillana Compound (P. D. & Co.)—is so exceptional in many particulars as to be worthy of special mention just now, when coughs are so plentifully in evidence. By its name no one would recognize it as a preparation for "cougs" and "colds," and this, in connection with its general efficiency, constitutes one of its chief claims to distinction. It is a product which the layman knows nothing about. It does not encourage counter-prescription or self-medication. It was designed especially with reference to the needs of the prescriptionist.

The formula of Syrup Cocillana Compound which of course is plainly printed on the label, is quite unusual. Let us briefly consider its components: Euphorbia pilulifera—serviceable in the treatment of chronic bronchitis and emphysema; wild lettuce—a mild and harmless narcotic, useful in spasmodic and irritable coughs; cocillana—valuable expectorant, tonic and laxative, exerts an influence on the respiratory organs similar to that of ipecac; syrup squill compound—serivceable in subacute or chronic bronchitis, as an expectorant, and as an emetic in croup; cascarin—the bitter glucoside of cascara sagrada, useful for its laxative action; heroin hydrochloride—a derivative of morphine and extensively prescribed in the treatment of cough, especially of bronchial origin; menthol—

THE NEW HYPNOTIC CALMINE.

It is safe to say that every doctor in practice has sometime wished for a better hypnotic than the materia medica afforded. None of those available quite "filled the bill" but they have been prescribed out of necessity because that better one was not yet evolved.

Now, apparently it has appeared. Calmine is its trade name; in chemical parlance it is sodium diethylbarbiturate—a fine, white-water-soluble powder with an alkaline taste. THE ABBOTT ALKALOIDAL CO. of Chicago supply it in the form of 2 1-2 grain tablets—twenty-five in a package.

Calmine has been thoroughly tried out by leading clinicians in this country and abroad, all of whom pronounce it an entirely satisfactory hypnotic, sleep inducer and nerve-calmative. It acts promptly. It is followed by no bad after-effects, no "head," no nausea, no tremulousness the next day. It seems to be absolutely harmless. It may be dissolved in water and given per rectum if desired. And, last of all but not by any means least, it is reasonable in price.

A well-known physician who used it in insomnia following worry said it: "An average dose afforded me a calm and restful sleep from which I awoke without the headache, nausea and tremulousness that succeed the ordinary hypnotic."

Calmine should prove very useful in the treatment of insomnia, nervous irritability, delirium tremens, sea-sickness, hysteria, mania, and every type of nerve-storm. It certainly acts ideally in the wakefulness that follows worry, mental overstrain, excitement and too free indulgence in coffee and tobacco.

THE ABBOTT ALKALOIDAL CO., of Chicago are sending samples on request and circular matter describing the agent in full. Every doctor should certainly send for this package.

stimulant, refrigerant, carminative and antiseptic, serviceable in coughs of pharyngeal origin.

Syrup Cocillana Compound would seem
to be worthy of extensive prescription.

FOR SALE.

One Sixteen plate static machine, with
X-Ray attachment. Will trade for good
microscope or sell at a bargain for cash.

Address Dr. C. B. TAYLOR, Spencer,
Oklahoma.

LOCATION WANTED.

WANTED—Small town location pay-
ing $2,500, or more annually, will purchase
office equipment. Give full particulars first
letter.

DR. HARWOOD,
Milton, Ky.

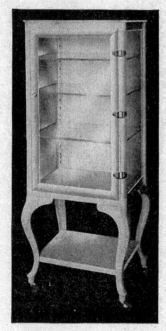

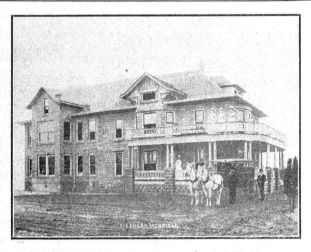

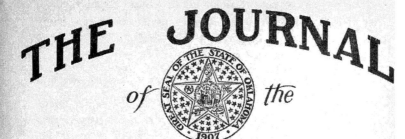

Oklahoma State Medical Association.

VOL. III.   MUSKOGEE, OKLAHOMA, JANUARY, 1911.   NO 8

DR. CLAUDE A. THOMPSON, Editor-in-Chief.

ASSOCIATE EDITORS AND COUNCILLORS.

DR. J. A. WALKER, Shawnee.	DR. JOHN W. DUKE, Guthrie.
DR. CHARLES R. HUME, Anadarko.	DR. A. B. FAIR, Frederick.
DR. F. R. SUTTON, Bartlesville.	DR. W. G. BLAKE, Tahlequah.
DR. I. W. ROBERTSON, Dustin.	DR. H. P. WILSON, Wynnewood.
DR. J. S. FULTON, Atoka.	DR. J. H. BARNES, Enid.

Entered at the Postoffice at Muskogee, Oklahoma, as second class mail matter, July 28, 1910

This is the Official Journal of the Oklahoma State Medical Association All communications should be addressed to the Journal of the Oklahoma State Medical Association, English Block, Muskogee, Oklahoma.

THE PREVENTION AND TREATMENT OF SEPTIC INFECTIONS OF THE EXTREMITIES

BY EDWARD H. OCHSNER, B. S, M. D., CHICAGO, ILLS.

If we could secure accurate statistics of the havoc caused by seemingly insignificant injuries of the extremities, I am sure most of us would be appalled by the large number of people who annually lose the full use of one or more of their extremities, or who lose one of their members, or who succumb to these infections. Besides the loss of time caused by these infections there is a very considerable economic loss to the body politic. I dare say every physician of a few years practical experience can recall some patient who has lost his life or his limb, or has been left with contractures as

Address Before Surgical Section, Medical Association of the Southwest, Wichita, Kansas, Oct. 10, 12, 1910.

the result of a septic infection consequent upon what seemed at first a trivial injury. It is for this reason that every abrasion of the skin, every pin prick, thorn prick, cut, etc., should receive the proper treatment as soon as possible after the injury occurs. I do not want to seem to be an alarmist and be understood to say that every time a farmer or mechanic gets a small cut or abrasion or a seamstress pricks her finger she must hasten to the doctor and undergo elaborate treatment, because such a contention would be ridiculous, but if every layman were taught simply how to care for the slighter injuries and if physicians and surgeons were more careful in treating the severer ones, the working and earning capacity of our people as a whole would be greatly enhanced, for we must not forget that the young vigorous productive portion of our population is the portion that suffers most from these infections and their consequences. The layman should know two things: first, how to care for the simple injuries and, second, that in all extensive superficial wounds no time should be lost in consulting a thoroughly competent, conscientious and painstaking physician. The layman can take care of the minor injuries satisfactorily by gently squeezing or sucking the wound so as to draw outward with some fresh blood any particle of septic material that may have gained entrance. Besides fresh blood is the best germicide we have and if the vigorous, active leucotyes can get at the few bacteria that may have gained entrance they will usually quickly destroy them. If in addition to the above the layman will wash the member carefully with clean soap and water and will apply a freshly laundered cloth over the wound and keep the wound clean for a few days these smaller wounds will scarcely ever cause any trouble. Should the part become tender a wet dressing consisting of one-half alcohol and one-half boiled water applied over night will usually relieve the trouble permanently. Witch hazel and a great number of similar remedies had real virtue, but it was all dependent upon the alcohol in them and people have been exploited and overcharged for decades because we have not informed them that half alcohol and half water would be just as effective and only one-tenth as expensive and besides they would then have been disillusioned as to the supposed almost miraculous potency of these advertised remedies and would not have had undue confidence in them.

I make these preliminary remarks because if we will perform our duty to the people and if we wish to rob the patent medicine quack and other quacks of their power we must become more and more active and efficient in teaching prophylaxis and personal hygiene to all of our patients.

The severer wounds that naturally come to the physician from the very first we must divide into two classes, the more superficial wounds that are likely to be infected with ordinary pyogenic micro-organisms only, and those which are likely to be infected with the tetanus bacillus in addition.

In the latter the same method of disinfection is used as in the former with the addition that we always give a prophylactic dose of antitetanus serum and if the wound is deep or likely to contain foreign material we lay it wide open, remove the foreign material and leave the wound gaping and to heal by granulation subsequently. In some parts of Chicago tetanus is quite prevalent, and up to seven years ago we had quite a number of cases, but since we have followed the above routine we have had only one case of tetanus develop and that in a case of severely infected compound fracture who came to us on the sixth day after the injury. All fresh wounds are treated in the following manner when they first come in: If the laceration is very extensive the patient is given a general anesthetic, if less severe the extremity is immersed in a two per cent. carbolic acid solution in tepid water, from five to ten minutes. This is an excellant local anesthetic and makes it possible to thoroughly scrub the parts without causing undue pain. We now scrub the extremity thoroughly with soap and sterile water by the aid of a brush or pieces of sterile gauze; then wash it off with ether, scrub it well with turpentine, swab it with tincture of iodine, rinse it with alcohol and finally put on a sterile dressing. I go thus into details for four reasons: First, because when I was a medical student and even now the learned professors seem to consider it beneath their dignity to give the students detailed instructions about these matters. They were and are much more likely to go into great detail about some rare abdominal operation that possibly not five per cent. of their students will ever do than to give them accurate instructions how to treat cases of which they will treat dozens, yes, hundreds, during their professional career. Second, because I have noticed many a medical man go at these cases in a mighty bungling manner. Third, because I have had to treat many of these cases subsequently, a large number of which could have been saved the infection if the above routine had been followed, and finally by scrupulously adhering to the method just described I have not seen a case of alarming septic infection develop in a large number and great variety of traumatic injuries.

If in spite of the above precaution or because of their neglect septic infection does develop, by instituting and rigidly adhering to a definite rational plan of treatment we can secure healing with practically no mortality, rarely, if ever, lose a member and usually without permanent impairment of function. Thus in a period of over fifteen years I have not lost a case, amputated even a finger or toe and have not one single claw-hand to my discredit in cases which came to me before incision had been made.

As most of these infections occur in young vigorous persons at the height of the economic productiveness, the prognosis must be viewed from four angles, namely, mortality, loss of member, permanent disability, and period of convalesence. The last three may be classed under the general term morbidity. While it is of the utmost importance to save the life and limb of such a patient it is almost as important to prevent permanent contractures, such as claw-hand, etc.; and to shorten the period

of illness and convalescence as much as possible. When the pathology of septic infections is once fully comprehended the treatment becomes easy and satisfactory. Whatever the exact species of micro-organism may be the pathologic process and the principles involved are fundamentally the same. It is a warfare between the bacteria and the defensive powers of the body. We must try to destroy the former, the bacteria, with something which does not weaken the latter, the defensive powers, and to strengthen the latter by means which do not favor the former.

In practice these things can actually be done quite readily. We know that healthy leucocytes in the presence of opsonized blood serum will destroy innumerable bacteria. We have learned that the blood of a vigorous healthy individual that is well aerated has serum of high opsonic power and leucocytes of great vigor. For these reasons we place the individual under the best possible hygienic conditions and provide good arterial blood for the involved extremity. The patient is placed in the best possible hygienic conditions, plenty of fresh air and sunlight because we have learned that oxygen and sunlight greatly increase the opsonic index of the blood. The patient is put on a restricted diet, first, because most persons consume from two to four times as much food per day as they really require and, second, because a febrile patient cannot assimilate properly even the normal ration; the patient is given a moderate dose of saline cathartic to remove any residue that is left in the bowels because a patient with fever will because of faulty metabolism generate a variety of toxin which, if absorbed, will reduce his resistance; in addition the patient should be given a glass of hot or cold water every hour to secure better elmination. We have long been talking about elmination, but most of us have failed to realize that in addition to excreting chemic poisons the kidneys, liver and skin will excrete millions of bacteria. Only recently I was able to collect pneumococci in pure culture from the gallbladder in a patient who recently had had a pneumonia and about two years ago we had a young woman suffering from colon bacillus septicemia who eliminated millions of colon bacilli with her urine and from whose blood we obtained a pure culture of colon bacilli.

How can we provide the affected part with arterial blood? This can be easily accomplished by securing full unobstructed circulation and preventing stasis. As soon as the infection takes place edema and swelling develops and if special attention is not paid to this matter the edema will soon make pressure on the thinner-walled vessels, the lymphatics and veins, and stasis will result. This can be avoided by elevating the extremity and applying a loose hygroscopic elastic dressing. In applying the bandage we must avoid extending the bandaging proximally beyond the gauze and cotton and thus causing the constriction. If these directions are followed the edema will soon subside, the circulation become full and unincumbered, and sufficient arterial blood will bathe the tissues.

In this relation permit me to make a passing remark about the Bier passive hyperemia: From the first it did not appeal to us as rational and we have never employed it. I have, however, seen some cases where it was used and I am sure better results could have been obtained by other methods. The great trouble with it is that it actually causes venous congestion instead of arterial hyperemia. In actual experience we have a beautiful illustration of Bier's hyperemia in the case of a washerwoman with varicose ulcers wearing an elastic garter. After reading Bier's article one would expect such an ulcer so treated to heal rapidly and spontaneously but the

thousands of women who walk around with such ulcers prove the contrary. Bier's passive congestion is theoretically untentable and practically worse than useless.

In addition to the elevation of the affected extremity rest not only of the extremity but of the whole patient is very essential.

A patient with septic infection with pyrexia be it ever so slight should be kept in bed with the extremity elevated in a comfortable relaxed position. This last point is of considerable importance. If the muscles are not relaxed they make pressure on the lymphatics and veins and hinder return circulation and the tenseness of the muscles tires the patient unnecessarily and reduces his resistance. The two factors which lower resistance almost more than any other two are pain and fatigue and by observing the rules here laid down these can be reduced to the minimum.

We have now briefly considered the factors that support the defensive powers and raised the opsonic index of the patient How can we destroy the bacteria, or at least, materially reduce the virulence without at the same time injuring the tissues or impairing the resistance of the individual? Such remedies we have in carbolic acid, boric acid, alcohol, and tincture of iodine, and by their proper combination and judicious application one can practically always obtain the desired results.

Ninety-five per cent. carbolic acid is a very powerful germicide and can be safely applied with a cotton swab over the reddened, inflamed area until the area turns white, if it is then quickly washed off with strong alcohol. It has often surprised me how much 95 per cent. carbolic inflamed skin will tolerate. It will tolerate an amount that would destroy normal healthy skin. It will instantly destroy innumerable pathogenic 'micro-organisms, almost instantly relieve the pain without injuring the skin in the slightest, providing, of course, that it be properly applied. After this preliminary application the extremity is encased in a large hygroscopic elastic wet dressing. For wet dressing we use a saturated solution of boric acid in water, to which 1-6 to 1-2 of 95 per cent. alcohol is added. Saturated solution of boric acid is, in my judgment, the best non-toxic antiseptic we have, and alcohol is a powerful dehydrant and in addition keeps the part warm and comfortable, preventing that cold, clammy feeling which a wet dressing is so apt to cause. Boric acid does not seem to have much power in inhibiting the growth of pathogenic bacteria, but I am fully convinced it has great power in reducing their virulence. I have repeatedly withdrawn a 30 m. syringe full of a pure culture of streptococci from a septic patient that had this dressing on for several days, then injected into the peritoneal cavity of a guinea pig and even a mouse without causing the death of these test animals. You know that ordinarily these animals are very susceptible to virulent strains of streptococci.

For a number of years the ultra-scientific have been trying to tell us that the application of an aqueous solution of any remedy to the skin was old-womanish and useless.

In making these statements they have often assumed the superior, supercilious, obnoxious air of the pseudo-scientific.

At my suggestion, Professor Louis Kahlenburg, of the University of Wisconsin, has made a series of chemical investigations, which has scientifically proven beyond possible contradiction and doubt that not only aqueous solution of boric acid, but also various other chemical substances when dissolved in water and applied as a wet dressing to the skin will be absorbed in very appreciable quantities. Thus for a time when a patient with a septic infection of an extremity would come to the hospital, I would apply a large wet dressing consisting of a saturated solution of boric acid in water and 95 per cent. alcohol in the proportions above mentioned, collect the urine every two hours, put each specimen thus obtained in a separate bottle and ship them all to Professor Kohlenberg. He found that easily detectible quantities of boric acid would be present in the urine one hour after the application of the dressing, to continue present constantly during the application of the wet dressing, and remain present several days after the wet dressing was discontinued.

Permit me here to emphasize the importance of having the boric acid in a saturated aqueous solution. Some fifteen years ago I found that in order to be effective it must be saturated; and almost twelve years ago I published these findings in the transactions of the Illinois State Medical Society.

The saturated solution is much more agreeable—immeasurably more effective than either the super-saturated or the unsaturated solution. The super-saturated solution causes a deposit of fine boric acid crystals on the skin which is both uncomfortable to the patient and seems to interfere with the rapid absorption, while the unsaturated solution is uncomfortable, macerates the skin and is absorbed in much smaller quantities than the saturated solution. Thus one patient being treated with a saturated solution, showed 0.001 per cent. of boric acid in the urine within an hour after the application, increased to .05 per cent. Another patient treated with the saturated solution showed from .002 to .1 per cent. Again, another varied between .02 per cent. and .2 per cent. while another patient treated with a .2 per cent. solution of boric acid never showed more than .001 per cent. of boric acid in the urine, and this not until the dressing had been in place continuously for 46 hours.

These experiments explain satisfactorily for the first time, I believe, why the saturated solution is absolutely essential to the success of the method.

You may recall that about 20 years ago boric acid had quite a reputation which subsequently declined considerably, and I believe this decline was due to the fact that it was not always used in saturated solution. In my study of the literature, Sir Frederick Treves is the only one I have found who advises always employing a saturated solution, but he simply makes the statement, without giving any reason for it, or without emphasizing it.

We now come logically to the discussion of the question of drainage. In the great majority of cases, the veins and lymphatics can be drained by simply elevating the affected extremity, and this can be done so effectually that incision rarely becomes necessary. This drainage by elevation is assisted by the dehydrating power of the alcohol.

There is an old rule in surgery, so old that I have not been able to trace its origin, which says: *"Ubi pus, ibi evacuo,"* or in English, "Where these is pus, there evacuate." This rule with certain modifications, is still a good one, but in recent times it has too often been exceeded. Many surgeons seem to have construed it to read: "Before there is pus, evacuate," which of course is an absurdity. To many of you the above statement may seem like an exaggeration, but in reality it is not. Sometimes these too-early incisions are due to excessive zeal, and again they are prompted by fear of criticisim on the part of one's fellow practitioners.

I have no doubt but that every one of you can recall one or more cases either in his own practice or that of a colleague when this early incision was actually practiced. I can recall many such cases, of which the following is a fair example: On May 27th, 1910, a colleague 38 years of age, was brought to the Augustana Hospital. Five days before admission he operated upon a very septic patient, and while scrubbing up after the operation he pricked himself with one of the bristles of the scrubbing brush, under the thumb nail. He thought nothing further about it until the following day, when he noticed a small infection under the thumb nail. The swelling, pain and redness increased so that the day before entering the hospital he cocainized the thumb himself, made two spival incisions around the thumb, and removed the nail. The infection spread rapidly, and on admission the whole left arm was swollen, red, hot, painful and tender. The lymphatic glands in the axilla were enlarged and painful. The thumb was greatly swollen and portions of the skin necrotic, the raw surfaces covered with white septic membranes, and the systemic disturbance was expressed in pyrexia and intermittent delirium.

One would think he had had enough energetic treatment, but instead he clammered for more cutting, and we had some difficulty in persuading him that it would not be wise to make more extensive incisions. Above all, he insisted on having axillary glands removed. We finally persuaded him to let us try the treatment above outlined, and in eight days he left the hospital with all active manifestations completely under control. There was no pain, no redness, no pyrexia, no delirium. All that remained was the granulating surface which he had himself caused by his incisions. Now, what this physician had tried to do was not to evacuate pus before it was present, but to secure drainage. One should always secure drainage just as soon as an infection occurs, but until macroscopic pus develops, this can be done much more safely and effectually without incision. If pus has formed before the patient applies for

- treatment, or as will sometimes, though rarely, be the case, in spite of the treatment, and a localized abcess develops, as manifested by fluctuation, the proper thing to do is to secure reasonably free drainage by incision, and the old rule finds its proper application. There are, however, several points about the incision that are of the utmost importance. First of all, before the part is incised, it is always well, whenever possible, to apply an Esmarch constrictor proximally to the proper point of the incision, and after the incision is made, pack the wound with a strip of gauze which has been soaked in tincture of iodine. The Esmarch will block the veins and lymphatics until the tincture of iodine can secure the closure of the cut ends, when the Esmarch can safely be removed. If these precautions are not observed, it often happens that the incision and necessary manipulation forces virulent septic material into the general circulation which may cause pyemic abscess or general septicemia, as manifested by severe chills, marked pyrexia, and delirium a few hours after the operation. The part should be manipulated as little as possible in order to avoid these undesirable consequences, and especially is this last precuation to be observed if the incision is in the same part of the body where an Esmarch cannot be applied. One more precaution in reference to the incision should always be within the line of demarkation or distal to it. An ordinary boil is always surrounded on all sides, except the skin covering it, by a wall of leucocytes. It can practically always be incised without getting through this line of defense. An infected finger is elmininated from the rest of the body by an infiltration of the tissues with innumerable leucocytes standing guard and ready to destroy any bacteria that come their way. The ridge can always be seen and felt, and

it is just as easy to make the incision distal to this wall as to break down this barrier. I could cite many cases where this little rule was not observed, and almost always the convalescence was unnecessarily prolonged. One case in particular do I remember where extensive incisions were made without an Esmarch and no attention was paid to the line of demarkation. The patient developed a chill within a few hours. The temperature rose to 106 degrees F. and he died within two days from septicemia.

Even if the patient is not thus overwhelmed with the septic posion, the wrongly executed incisions always inflict new areas which take much time and vitality to heal, and sometimes the convalescence is thus unnecessarily prolonged for weeks and even months.

For a long time it was the practice of many surgeons to excise all accessible, enlarged lymph glands. I believe this is a grave error. When a lymph gland has broken down, is suppurating, drainage is, of course, necessary but so long as it is simply inflamed, it shows that it is doing its duty, and it would be just as wise to withdraw an active fighting garrison from the last fort as it would be to excise an active lymph gland, even though it be inflamed. So long as it is not suppurating, it is waging a winning battle and demands our support. It is sometimes the only barrier left, and its removal may lead to general sepsis.

Vaccine therapy has its field of usefulness in the septic infections, but in my opinion only in the later stages, and then only autogenous vaccines.

There are so many species and strains of streptococci, staphylocci that stock vaccines may do more harm than good, and it always takes several days to prepare autogenous vaccine. In the neglected cases, when the resistance has been greatly reduced, and who are sluggish and do not respond properly after the acute symptoms have subsided, the judicious use of vaccine will sometimes greatly hasten the recovery. But let me repeat two cautions: the vaccine must be autogenous vaccine, and it must be given in doses much smaller than are ordinarily recommended in the literature.

In conclusion, permit me to briefly recapitulate: I. Absolute rest and proper elevation of the affected extermity. Recumbency in bed of the patient if there is the slightest pyrexia.

Do not incise until there is unmistakable evidence of pus, and do not remove the lymph glands unless they are necrotic and suppurating. If incision becomes necessary, it should be within the line of demarcation, and, if possible, distal to it and to an Esmarch constrictor. Swab the incision with tincture iodin before releasing the constrictor so as to close the cut veins and lymphatics.

Manipulate, knead, and squeeze the inflamed part as little as possible. Attend to general hygiene and elimination. If very red and inflamed, paint the skin with ninety-five per cent. carbolic acid until it turns white, and then wash it off with strong alcohol, and apply a copious wet dressing, consisting of from one to five parts of saturated solution of boric acid, and one part of ninety-five per cent. alcohol.

If these directions are carefully followed, healing can be secured in a relatively short time, with almost no morbidity and practically no mortality.

2038 Lane Court, Chicago.

OBSTETRICAL SURGERY AND SECONDARY REPAIR OF LACERATED PERINEUM

BY J. M. TRIGG, M. D., SHAWNEE, OKLA.

The present may be designated as the age of specialism in medicine. The human body has been divided and sub-divided and the ills peculiar to its different parts have been carefully studied by man whose superior knowledge derived from such study, has made them known as specialists. Time was when it was not considered derogatory to the surgical specialist to have a family practice as well. Nowadays, and probably rightly, the surgeon is compelled by the sentiments of the laity and his colleagues to be a specialist in every sense of the word.

Now all this specialism has had its effect upon the general practitioner. If he be conscientious, he wants his patient to receive the best treatment and the cure of his patient. Yet if he refers every patient for every ailment to the specialist, he will soon have no patients or practice, and only be acting the part of an umpire whose business it will be to decide which specialist his patient must employ, and occasionally throw in an anti-constipation pill. Yet in the midst of all this specialism, has it ever occurred to you that there is one department of medicine quite free from specialism? That is the obstetric specialist.

One reason is the fees received, and the physician teaching the public that it is a physiological act, and that every woman is destined to get through her pregnancy and confinement without mishap. As a consequence they resent a larger fee for such work. Secondly, the general practitioner has always striven to retain his obstetric practice,—he may refer any other case to the specialist, but he draws the line when it comes to obstetric work. That is his peculiar province, and has been for centuries, and he proposes that it shall be his forever. For he knows, as his competitors know, that the doctor who brings the baby into the world and administers to the mother in her convalescence, will be the family physician in the majority of cases. So the general practitioner is the obstetrician of the country. Being the obstetrician, is it any wonder that he desires to do the surgery connected with his midwifery cases? —in fact, insists upon doing it. Are there any reasons why he should not do it? and do it well, if he be properly trained and studies his cases as he should.

Now, in order to be a good obstetrician means much, both to the physician and patient, for he should be able to handle all the graver conditions met with in obstetric practice, such as vaginal cesarean section, and if needed, abdominal cesarean section, or podalic versian, for the value of any obstetric operation must depend, after all, upon whether it can be performed by the general practitioner, for he has a hundred cases of confinement to the specialist's one. And the practitioner has proved his ability to successfully perform difficult obstetric operations, specialists' opinion to the contrary.

At one time or another the practitioner has been warned against attempting the operations of obstetric surgery, for fear he has not the necessary skill. But did you notice that the warning came from men who hold themselves a little above the average as regards their operative skill? However, they forget that, taken as a class, there is nothing in their mental make up which warrants their high opinion of themselves. The human brain is of about the same caliber, when everything is taken into consideration. Intelligence, industry and opportunity are all that are necessary to make one proficient in any line of work. Why then, should not the general practitioner possessing these, perform any and all the necessary obstetric operations and

do them well? There is absolutely no reason, and for the benefit of those who shake their heads and cite the bad obstetric surgery they have seen by general practitioners, it may be said that just as bad surgery has been performed by those who consider themselves in a different class. To my mind, the American physician is naturally a skillful and successful surgeon. I mean that, as a man, he is quick to see, thinks for himself, and above all is resourceful and able to work himself out of a tight place.

Yet while the specialists sympathize with us general practitioners in our efforts to retain our field of surgery ourselves, it cannot be gainsaid that there is vast room for improvement in obstetric surgery as it is practiced today. If they concede to the general practitioner the right to this province, they have the same right to demand that in a way we shall be a specialist in this department. It is not even sufficient that he acquire and put into practice a high degree of operative skill. Like any other surgeon we are supposed to possess this, or we are not fit to practice this art. Above all, we should be a good diagnostician and have an intimate knowledge of indications for or against an operative procedure. We should prepare for such work as a general surgeon does, work out our technic and all necessary asepsis. In many cases a little boiled water and a few bichloride tablets are all that are employed in even a major operation. Why should obstetric surgery be more slovenly performed than any other kind of surgery? It cannot be denied that this is true.

It is dangerous to undertake a serious operation alone when aid can be procured. So let the general practitioner cling to his heritage if he will, and do all the obstetric surgery his practice necessitates, but let him have a just appreciation of his responsibilities in this matter. Let him realize that faults of omission are just as reprehensible as faults of commission, and let him make of himself the kind of obstetric surgeon he would call in for one of his own family.

Now, how is this reformation going to be brought about? The oldest offenders probably will never change. Habits of cleanliness and mastery of efficient technic are not learned late in life. The practitioner over forty with slovenly habits will carry them with him to the grave, in the meantime hastening many a poor woman toward hers, and leaving many a woman for the operative gynecologist to repair her lacerated perineum, and this is no small operation if done properly.

The operation as it is usually done suggests more of a mathematical than an anatomic basis for its existence. They have generally consisted of excisions of mucous membrannes from the posterior vaginal wall, having geometric patterns, that vary as do the fancies of the different operators.

In repairing a lacerated perineum, the following principles should be followed:

First: No tissue is removed or extensive denudation made.

Second: Buried, absorbable, layer sutures are used exclusively, none of which penetrates the skin or mucous membrane.

Third: The operation is done from the outside of the vagina, rendering the introduction of sutures easier, and the exposure of tissues better than with those operations done from within the vagina.

Fourth: Each structure is sutured with precision under the guidance of the eye; there is no blind groping with the needle for tissues not seen and perhaps not felt.

Fifth: Each of the layers of the perineal floor wall, submucosa, muscular supports, fascial planes, and skin are united seriatem in layers, after the better types of herinotomy.

Sixth: The vagina is not separated

from the rectum, and therefore there is no danger of wounding the bowel.

The operation has the following advantages:

It restores and increases the length of the vagina instead of shortening the posterior wall of the vagina, as occurs with many of the operations. There is the added advantage that no sutures require removal that no foreign bodies in the shape of shot, suture ends, or the like, are left in the vagina to promote and hold secretions and that the seaton action of through and through sutures is avoided. And there is less danger of infection and suppuration by doing the submucous perineorrhaphy.

In doing this operation, one should realize the vagina runs nearly parallel with the skin perineum. Lateral to the vagina one may nearly always distinguish the thick broad bands of the anterior levator ani muscle. By placing a finger against the anterior edge of this muscle, on either side, and comparing the relative depths of the muscle from the surface, one may acquire an idea as to the relative injury to the muscles.

TECHNIC OF THE OPERATION.

First, the parts are carefully asepticized in the usual manner, and the anus covered by a sterile towel or gauze pad held to the skin by clips. The labia separated. the sharp point of a pair of scissors is introduced into the subcutaneous cel'ular tissue, just external to the orfice of Bartholins gland. The incision is carried around the posterior margin of the introitus, just external to the carunculae until a point external to the orifice of the opposite Batholin's gland is reached. A pair of tenaculem forceps is fastened in posterior median line of the wound to serve as retractors No separation of *vagina from rectum is necessary.*

The second step consists in the exposure of the lavator ani. The edge of the muscle is located between one finger placed against the lateral wall of the vagina, and a second finger or thumb placed in one side of the wound. Having located the muscle in the wound, a pair of sharp pointed scissors is thrust through the depths of the wound to the situation of the anterior edge of muscle, then opened and withdrawn. The opening is enlarged by stretching with the fingers, or if necessary, by a few touches of the knife. The muscle is freed on its inner and outer sides by the finger, grasped with a pair of tenaculum forceps or hooks, and pulled into the wound. The isolation and exposure of the muscle is usually easy and requires but a few seconds of time.

The third step of the operation consists in the repair of the vaginal mucous membrane. With a curved needle and No. 1 plain catgut, the mucous membrane is united, beginning near what was the posterior commission. A continuous suture is used, engaging the submucous cellular tissue, a short distance from the wound edges and uniting the upper border of what was a transverse incision in a vertical manner. In doing this, the part of the vagina that was near the posterior commissure comes to occupy a point some distance above the introitus, and the length of the vagina is restored. Suture No. one, which has thus made a partial submucous closure of the vaginal wall, is then temporarily laid to one side to be finished later.

The fourth step of the operation consists in uniting in the median line the edges of the levator-ani muscle, which are located by the attached tenaculum forceps or hook. Continuous sutures of chromic or iodized catgut may be employed, but the muscle must not be united so far anteriorly as to unduly constrict the vaginal orifice. Some of these sutures catch the underlying submucous tissues to prevent the formation of a dead space. Posteriorly, a simple, or figure-of-eight suture is employed to bind together the various structures that meet here, and if necessary, to give support to the sphincter ani. With the union of the levator muscles, the rectum, anus and vagina, will be found to ascend to a higher position in the pelvis, and to be carried forward toward the pelvis.

The fifth step of the operation consists in the suturing of the inferior fascial plane to reinforce the muscular support. The outer edges of the incision which the levator ani muscles have been brought, are united in the median line by continuous sutures of No. 1 Chromic catgut. This support, which includes the posterior part of the urogenital trigone, affects the layers of the triangular ligament and the deep transverse perinei muscles, and posteriorly serves to increase the tension on the transverse perinei muscle.

The sixth and final step of the operation consist in completing suture No. 1, which after completing the submucous union of the vagina, is continued posteriorly under the skin, uniting the subcutaneous and callous fascia, until the posterior portion of the incision is reached. The two ends of the suture Number One are then tied, binding together the various structures that have been united; the knot is permitted to sink under the skin, the ends being cut short.

Thus there has been built up in the layers of a perineum consisting of united mucosa, muscle, fascia, and skin. All the sutures being buried and the layers bound together compactly there are practically no dead spaces, then the usual dressing is applied and after two or three days begin vaginal douche, patient is up in a few days, and able to resume her work in two weeks.

OPHTHALMIA NEONATORUM

BY DR. MILTON K. THOMPSON, MUSKOGEE, OKLAHOMA.

I have undertaken to write upon this subject by special request. It is one of the most important subjects under discussion today; one that is attracting much attention, and one which cannot be brought before the public too often.

It is such a pitiful sight to enter a home or school and see these little helpless blind children compelled to grope their way through life, dependent in every respect upon the charity of others, and it is appalling when we stop to think how many of these are in this condition by carelessness, and we might further say needlessly blind. Think of it a moment, about 30 per cent. of all the children admitted to our blind schools today are blinded by this disease. Nearly 25 per cent. of all the blind in the world are victims of this unnecessary disease, the education of whom cost the states from 10 to 15 times as much as it does to educate the ordinary child, which has to be appropriated by the state. Therefore, we expect the legislature to help us in this fight, and thus save money for the state, as well as do good in saving the hundreds of babies yet to be born, from their certain suffering and ultimate misfortune unless something be done to prevent infection, as a cure after infection is too uncertain as to results.

Opthalmia Neonatorum is an inflammation of the conjunctiva characterized usually by great swelling of the lids with an abundant secretion of a contagious pus.

The causes—are infection in the genito urinary track, or soon thereafter. The majority of cases, and especially the severer ones are caused by the gonococcus

of Neiser but many other micro organisms may appear in conjunction with, or alone. Viz: Pneumococcus, Streptococcus, Diplococcus and Staphylococcus and Bacterium coli, the latter infections are of a milder type with a tendency to recover without any serious damage being done—any of these micro-organisms may get into the eyes during birth from a muco-purulent discharge of an infectious nature in the vagina or elsewhere along the track of delivery—or after birth by soiled cloths or fingers carrying infection during bathing. The time of infection matters little the symptoms and results are the same. Beginning in one eye in from 12 hours to a few days as a slight congestion; usually shortly afterward the second eye becomes likewise involved, the congestion rapidly increases until it is intense with cushion like swelling of the conjunctiva—severe pain and photophobia, the discharge which was at first watery changing to a dirty color and at this stage to a thick yellow or greenish yellow pus in great quantities running out from under the lids onto the face or pent up in the culdesac to pour out on opening the lids. The lids are much swollen, the upper one overhanging the lower, at first are tense and hard to evert, are velvety flecked with lymph, shortly becoming dark red with rough elevations and bleeding cracks. The ocular conjunctiva is chemotic and infiltrated with a hard tense rim, endangering the vitality of the cornea. The cornea appears sunken and dull ulcers due to strangulated vessels or the active infection may form anywhere on the cornea, but more especially near the limbus, breaking down and spreading rapidly with much destruction of tissue with a tendency to perforation and all the evil consequences of a perforation, depending upon the ex-

Read Before the Annual Meeting of the Oklahoma State Medical Association, Tulsa, Okla., May, 1910.

tent and location of the perforation and the amount of the tissue involved. The next stage the lids become flabby, puckered with elevated papillae, are easily averted and bleed freely. Pus is still abundant mixed with blood and serum, however the disease begins gradually to improve, and in about six or eight weeks the discharge stops though the palpebral conjunctiva remains thickened with elevated papillae for some time and perhaps cicatricial changes may remain permanent with deformity of the lids. There is an acute simple conjuncti-vitis of the new born which, as any other inflammation of the eyes, should be attended to promptly, though it will not run such a disasterous and destructive course. The prognosis in this variety is not unfavorable, but may continue for several weeks. Pro gnosis is always grave in the gonorrheal types. If seen before the cornea becomes dull, there is some chance of good results. After the disease has been acquired the treatment is symptomatic. The mild variety is treated as a simple conjunctivitis. The more severe types as the stage demands. In the early part or tense stage cold or hot applications are made, some prefer cold, cotton plegets or cloths from ice, others the hot formentative with equal regularity, but above all, cleanliness. It is generally conceded that cold may be used when desired from any reason only as long as there is no haziness of the cornea, otherwise the hot applications. Irrigation and treatments with mild astringents, and as the discharge increases a constant removal of the same. In the first stage the stronger salts of silver are contraindicated, but as the pus becomes free and lids puckered, then is time to apply silver from 10 to 20 grains to the ounce, or I have found in some instances, carefully applied as strong as 10 per cent. acts like magic when the weaker ones do not seem to check the disease.. Other preparations are Protargol,

10 to 40 per cent. Argyrol 10 to 25 per cent., these salts are the most frequently used and next to nitrate silver are in my judgment best.

I've obtained the best results by application of nitrate silver in strong solution from 2 to 10 per cent. once a day, and Argyrol 10 to 20 per cent. every 2 or 3 hours between applications of the nitrate, keeping pus cleaned away with a boric solution. If only one is affected, the other eye is protected by a shield. Atropine or Eserine only used when needed and carefully. The time to treat the disease with the best results is before it develops. With our knowledge of antisepsis and careful midwifery and an understanding public, the percentage of blindness by this disease should diminish, and I am delighted to see not only the wives of the profession, but other women so interested in our meetings and proceedings and know that it will help in this one of our gravest curses of today. It is impossible to measure by any standard we know the individual injury done one of these poor unfortunate innocent babes by the carelessness, and neglect of the person attending the mother at the time of the childs birth that this horrible disease is allowed to develop, one that could be prevented by just a little knowledge, a moments time, and a very little expense, and yet regardless of the fact that nearly 30 years ago the prevention was pointed out to the profession. I repeat 30 per cent. of all the children entering the schools for the blind today are there from this unnecessary disease.

In 1881, Prof. Crede, of the University of Leipsic announced that a 2 per cent. nitrate of silver solution dropped into the new born infants eyes would prevent this disease where infection was present and do no harm to a sound eye, showing that previous to the use of this method where one case in 10 was affected there was a reduction of 1 in 500 by employing the method. In our medical colleges this method and other preventative treatments are taught, and there is no reason why the medical profession of today should not have a minimum per cent. of infection by only being careful as routine practice to use silver in some of its forms in all cases, especially when there may be reason to believe that there was a chance of infection. Of course the vaginal tract should be rendered as thoroughly aseptic as possible previous to the birth, but immediately after the child is born, this treatment should be used. For routine work, one of the milder salts may be used, argyrol or protargol. Of course an indiscriminate use of drugs may do a great deal of harm to the cornea, or cause a conjunctivitis.

There has been brought to us from Germany, Austria and other foreign countries, who regulate by rigid laws the practice and registration of midwifery a system of uneducated midwifery in our midst, with no laws to govern them, or if laws exist, they are not enforced with reference to qualifications and reporting births. Especially in cities, so many babes are brought into the filthiest kind of surroundings by the filthiest kind of a person posing as a competent midwife. These people do not know anything about anti-sepsis or prophylaxis and care less. Is it any wonder that the percent of blind children remains so high? It is a common practice among a certain class of midwives, if the childs eyes appear weak, to put any filthy concoction at hand in the eyes, and thus perhaps make a simple case more complicated. A sterile solution of silver or anything else would be entirely out of place in such hands. That which we need in this particular branch of our profession are laws governing the practice of midwifery, requiring education, competency, registration and prompt reports of all births. These laws must be enforced. Some states have good laws, but they are not being enforced. In many states there is now being waged a fight for the childs eyes and appropriations have been gotten. The public is being educated with reference to this particular treatment and prevention. Until we can make some progress along these lines the fight is going to be an up hill one, and every physician must resolve to do his best—not only to use the preventative treatment at all times himself, but must use all his influence toward getting legislation and enlightening the public with reference to the dangers of incompetent and filthy midwifery, not only to the child but to the mother.

REPORT OF SOME CASES FOUND AMONG THE DEPENDENT CHILDREN OF OKLA.

BY CARL PUCKETT, M. D., PRYOR, OKLA.

In writing a paper on this subject I will give experiences with the wards of the state in the Oklahoma State Home for Dependent Children.

Most of you may imagine what kind of physical weaknesses we would expect to find in this class of children, but if you have not thought of it I will say that among those that are orphans, about 75 per cent. are the children of tubercular parents and usually have the consequent weaknesses; which lead to catarrhal troubles, enlarged tonsils, scrofulosis and diseases of this kind, during the winter months, and these extending deeper to bronchial affections. It requires constant vigilance to prevent sickness of this kind that may be paving the way for the future dread disease, tuberculosis. If by proper care of these children we can develop strong, robust bodies, that can ward off disease and teach these children how to care for themselves, we have done a great work for the anti-tuberculosis movement and also will have done a great deal toward lessening other kinds of diseases that are brought on by violation of natural laws of health.

A great many of our children come to the institution, infected with the malarial parasite which is very hard to remove because of the deep seated hold it has on the individual and we have to treat this disease along with other troubles that for the time being have the upper hand.

I will give a report of some cases of Broncho-pneumonia, the first two of which are associated with malarial infection. These two are brother and sister, their father dying one day with pulmonary tuberculosis, and mother the next day with a conjestive chill, and children were a short time afterward brought to the institution.

Case 1. D. C. Girl—Age 8:

Admitted to institution about 6 months previous with two brothers and one sister, all infected with malaria in latent form having the swarthy, sallow skin, tired appearance, and enlarged spleen, in fact the general characteristics that are present in those that live in malarial countries and put up with "Fever and Ague" as a necessary evil. This girl at intervals was in the hospital with acute attacks of malaria that would readily respond to treatment of calomel purge and quinine. For six or eight weeks previous to this time she was in a fair condition of health due to a course of quinine, iron, strychnine and arsenic of about three weeks.

She was admitted to the hospital on December 20th, with a chill and severe cold. On first examination it seemed to be nothing more serious than the usual attack of malarial intermittent or remittent fever.

The bronchial symptoms increased and the high fever persisted till on the 25th I was convinced of Broncho-pneumonia. It probably was present sooner but the symptoms were masked by the malaria present, which no doubt was indirectly the cause of this attack of bronchial trouble.

Malaria is not ordinarily classed as one of the causes of broncho-pneumonia but it is my experience that it acts as a predisposing cause in many cases, by weakening the resistive power of the individual and is frequently associated with it in malarial districts.

Another predisposing cause in this case was the weak lungs inherited from the tubercular father. The symptoms were those usually found in these cases; cough, dyspnea, restlessness, and fever, the latter, unchecked, running from 103 to 105.5, higher than usually found, which no doubt was due to the presence of the malarial parasite. All symptoms were severe from the start; Cyanosis was extreme; chest expansion was small, but respiration was moderate, running from 40 to 48. Percussion note was dull over both lungs. On auscultation subcrepitant rales were heard over the greater part of both lungs and there was present the inspiratory retraction of the lower ribs.

In the early treatment I had given her a malarial prescription of quinine 1 1-3 grains, carbonate of iron 3-5 grains, and strychnine sulphate 1-130 grain, every 5 hours. At the positive diagnosis of broncho-pneumonia, I placed her also on a prescription of potassium citrate 4 1-2 grains, aromatic spirits of ammonia five, glycerine one, and nitrous spirits of ether nine minims, with Liquor Ammonium Acetate q. s. to make one dram, every 4 hours; as a cough medicine and expectorant on ammonium chloride 1 1-2 grains, spirits of chloroform 4, Syrup of squills compound 12 and Syrup of wild cherry 20 minims with syrup of lemon q. s. to make one dram. I used cold sponging for high fever and nervous symptoms and kept the room thoroughly ventilated. I kept her on this treatment until symptoms began to abate and before convalescence was well established I began to reduce other treatment and increase the malarial prescription. With convalescence I placed her on cod liver oil tonics and later on quinine, iron, strychnine and arsenic, followed by complete recovery. In this case fever was continually present for 5 weeks with occasional recurrences for two weeks longer.

Case 2. E. C. Boy—Age 10:

This boy had more trouble with attacks of malarial fever than any of his brothers and sisters with spleen much larger. He was admitted to the hospital on February 28th with measles. From the first he seemed to have aggravations of all symptoms. Respiration was short and rapid yet the other pulmonary symptoms seemed about the same as usually found in measles, but before two days were up I knew that I had a tussle on hands with broncho-pneumonia. His temperature ran as high as 105.5 but was kept down most of the time with cold sponging to from 101 to 103. Respiration ran as high as 65 and pulse to 150. In this case the greater part of lower left lobe was consolidated and gave a great deal of pain. I kept him on practically the same treatment as Case 1, but added some things for severe symptoms. I gave aromatic spirits of ammonia and tincture digitalis separate to what I was already giving for respiratory and heart effect with excellent results. This case ran a course of four weeks and at beginning of convalescence was placed on quinine, iron, strychnine and arsenic, for two weeks with rapid improvement. After that I gave him potassium iodide for four weeks to reduce tonsillar and splenic enlargement, with good results.

Case 3. R. W.—Boy—Age 10. No history of parents:

The boy went to bed with measles on same day as case 2, with almost the same symptoms but lesser severity. He had some consolidation of right lower lobe. I placed him on the same treatment except the malarial prescription. He ran a course of three weeks and got up with both ears suppurating and hearing very poor. His tonsils were enlarged and follicular. I used hot saline irrigations daily with potassium iodide three times daily as internal treatment. Suppuration ceased in ten days when irrigations were discontinued, but the potassium iodide was kept up for four weeks when the hearing was almost normal.

At the time of these last two cases I had two other, following measles, one with malaria present, the other not, the one running a course of 2 1-2 the other 4 weeks.

In these cases we may see the difference in simple broncho-pneumonia and malarial.

Case 4. E. B.—Boy—Age 12. Report of accident:

This boy came to the institution with trachoma in latent form with contracted lids and other evils caused by this. On treatment he was greatly improved and had been in school a short time. On November 27th, I was hurriedly called to the home. I found this boy in great pain from a burn of face and eyes caused by an explosion of melted lead that the boys were playing with and had poured on a wet board. I found the face and forehead badly burned, eyelashes full of hardened lead and partially burned away, with epidermis of eyelids destroyed. I immediately dropped a 2 per cent. solution of cocaine over lids and in eyes. On opening the lids I found a small strip of lead molded back under right upper lid about 1-4 inch wide and 1-3 inch long; a small round piece about the size of a B. B. shot imbedded in the sclerotic coat of left eye, to left of cornea. I also found numerous small particles in eyes and had to cut the remaining lashes off to remove the lead from them. There were several burns on the cornea but nothing deeply imbedded. Lime water and linseed oil had been applied to the flesh wounds before my arrival and the pain was reduced to some extent. I washed out eyes thoroughly with saturated solution of boracic acid, then dropped 2 drops of 1 per cent. Atropine solution in each eye. I then sponged and cleansed the other wounds antiseptically and applied a moist bichloride dressing. Then as daily treatment I used saturated solution of boracic acid, atropine 1 per cent. and Argyrol 10 per cent. as eye treatment. I used moist bichloride dressings for the flesh wounds. On account of the destruction of epidermis of eyelids and the necessity of handling them in the dressings I used cocaine solution as local anesthetic. I kept this treatment up for two weeks when bandages were left off. His eyelids were treated till January 1st, when he was dismissed and started to school.

DISCUSSION.

Dr. R. H. Harper, Afton:

I enjoyed the paper and description of the conditions found and approve of his treatment. It seems there is very little left for discussion. We sometimes try to find some place to disagree with a man with some of his ideas, but I fail to find anything in the paper except to commend.

Dr. J. H. Scott, Shawnee:

Mr. Chairman: Just a question of diagnosis. I don't wish to assume the attitude of disagreeing with the Doctor's diagnosis. I just want to suggest that we frequently diagnose a condition from the symptoms that we might diagnose from positive findings and I believe in an institution that these positive findings ought to be made. I really don't believe for

certain that this malarial condition he speaks of was responsible for the aggravated condition he found in the case described. I would just as much feel justified in assuming from the history that it was a tubercular condition that was responsible for the condition as a malarial condition.

Therefore, I say that when the opportunity exists to make positive findings by microscope or otherwise, I believe it ought to be done.

Dr. G. R. Gordon, Wagoner:

I certainly enjoyed the paper of the Doctor very much, and agree with him almost unanimously, while I agree with Dr. Scott also. I believe that the more positive we can be in our research along the line of science the better. I certainly agree with him about the malaria and in a new country like this a diagnosis is almost always right for we certainly have an unusual amount of malaria. And I think we should treat thoroughly with calomel and quinine and then follow with the iron and arsenic.

Dr. Carl Puckett, Pryor:

I have but very little to say on the subject, but it seems to me that a very large part of our cases come from the southern part of Oklahoma and up and down the rivers where we have so much malaria. I myself am a crank with calomel and quinine and I have never had any trouble yet with any cases of tuberculosis, with the exception of one, and it died with a sudden hemorrhage. That is the only one we have had in about three years. Of course we can't say in so many children, and I find that this giving of quinine and calomel is one of the best things we can do. Of course, we usualy include a great deal of iron, arsenic and strychnine.

Dr. Harper, Afton:

What condition do you find, fever or absence of fever or enlarged spleen, or, on what do you base your assumption that these cases have malaria in general?

Dr. Puckett, Pryor:

We all learn when we see malaria once and can look at any patient and pretty nearly tell. I base my opinions generally on the enlarged spleen and the history, and a great many of them will give history of having had chills, and usually if they have had trouble of that kind they are not so very long until they develop trouble with malaria.

Chairman: It seems the Doctor has lived in a malarial district and they all have some malaria, and it seems to me his position is well taken.

Dr. Harper, Afton:

It may be an indiosyncrosy of mine, but I don't believe in giving medicine unless there is some definite reason for it, and I don't exactly believe in saying any one has malaria unless there is some reason for it. I think Dr. Scott's suggestion is a good one that in a State Institution we should unite in urging the legislature to provide means to furnish necessary apparatus and microscopes and fluids in order to make scientific diagnoses in the State Institutions. The State takes care of these children, the taxes care for them, and we are entitled to some benefit in the way of returns by scientific apparatus with which to make diagnoses.

Dr. J. H. Scott, Shawnee:

I don't want to assume the attitude of criticizing any one, I believe we are all liable to come to the old style of diagnosis. I believe the conditions the Doctor describes can be present for no reason except malaria and some of these children he has down there he could do nothing to them but the administering of supporting, building and nourishing treatment and he would get exactly the same results. I am satisfied from the description that a certain per cent. of the children there are syphilitic and on nourishing treatment he would get the same results.

Dr. Davis, Enid:

It seems to me that the criticism would be proper if these patients would die, but the Doctor's report shows that his patients recover, and results are what count in any case. I am satisfied that Dr. Puckett is right in his treatment because his people have recovered.

Dr. F. R. Wheeler, Mangum.

Perhaps there is not a person here who is in a malarial district where the malaria is so heavy as I have. I am most pleased with the Doctor's paper and his treatment and as Dr. Davis said, they didn't die and wouldn't you rather be cured by an Arkansas Doctor's treatment of calomel and quinine than die scientifically.

THE MODERN TREND OF OBSTETRICS

BY A. B. LEEDS, M. D., CHICKASHA, OKLA.

The medical profession, today, in spite of the great advancements made in the

Read Before the Annual Meeting of the Oklahoma State Medical Association, Tulsa, Okla., May, 1910.

science and practice of medicine, stands self-accused and convicted of palpable neglect of one of its most important branches, that of obstetrics.

The realization of this fact, by the profession, is emphasized by the discussions, to a great length, in the medical journals, and association meetings, big and small, of the latest methods for applying the forceps, the most correct Ceasarian section, operative interference, of every description, and the befuddling views, of individual operators, for the correction of abnormal conditions.

In the mad race for surgical and gynecological fame and the springing up, like mushrooms, during the last decade, of embryonic surgeons, we have entirely forgotten, neglected and overlooked the greatest need, along his line, that of the prevention of these abnormal conditions.

We have been tugging at the wrong end, we have had the cart before the horse, we have waited until the barn was all ablaze before we attempted to clean out the stable to prevent the fire.

From a careful and exhaustive study of the papers, discussions, etc., which could be found along this subject, it appears that, like the social evil, these are considered necessary evils and that all of our efforts must be directed along the lines of operative interference and herculean means exerted, at the time of confinement, to remedy these conditions.

Having considered, for some time, that this view of the matter was erroneous and false and there was great need of an awakening, on the part of the profession, to some vital facts, concerning this subject, the author was persuaded, when invited by the chairman, of this section, to contribute a paper at this meeting, to accept the invitation and to select the discussion of this subject as his theme.

To point to a few causes, their reasons and remedies, and attempt to show that, in the great majority of cases, patience and intelligent instruction, on the part of the medical profession, in the early months of pregnancy, will obviate and prevent the most of these abnormal conditions and hasten a return to the good old days, of our grandmothers, when the use of forceps, the bottle-fed baby, ceasarian sections, extra-uterine pregnancies etc., were, if not practically unheard of, at least, a rare complication, will be the purpose of this paper.

When the position is taken, by the author, that the medical profession are responsible, in the vast majority of cases, for the deplorable physical wrecks, resulting from the complications of modern pregnancies, he anticipates a storm of protest.

Yet, the hollow-eyed and pinched face, with the freshness and bloom of youth forever gone; aged, as it were, in a day or night, are walking accusers of our palpable neglect of this subject.

The girl, of today, not only in the cities but also in the rural districts, in the majority of cases, are ill-prepared to undergo the physical demands of a normal pregnancy, much less an abnormal one, with its usual serious complications.

The practice, so prevalent, of mothers not preparing and educating the girl for the advent of the menstrual flow and through this ignorance, the health of the girl often neglected, at this time, with frequent serious consequences; allowing the girls to have company before they are hardly able to add and subtract, much less being prepared, physically, for irregular hours and the consequent exposure; the wonderful corset, in its shapes and latest cuts, varied as the legs of a dragon; the modern plays, shows, magazines and novels, with their usual perverted sexual suggestions; rapid, irregular, irrational and indiscreet eating, as practiced by the American people; nick-nacks, candies, ice-cream, low-necked and thinly arranged clothing; early marriages, with no knowledge of the sexual side of married life; the horrible effects of gonorrhea and venereal disease, contracted, previously, by the husband and disseminated through the system of the young wife, during the usually active sexual habits of the newly-weds; the practice of the old women and especially, the average physician, for that matter, of telling the recent pregnant woman that, no matter how varied the aches and pains, there is nothing to be feared or peculiar and by this method and their attitude of jest and lack of interest and attention, lull the fears and anxieties with a false sense of security, all contribute their part to the overburdening and poisoning of the ill-prepared systems and are responsible, to a great extent, for the results obtained, in modern pregnancies and so often vividly and horribly depicted.

The old adage and saying "that the only service to be rendered, by a physician, during confinement, is to prevent hemorrhage, turn the child or use the forceps," not only does this apply to modern pregnancies, but it is this view of the matter promulgated, so assiduously, by the old women and the attitude of the average physician, that is the curse of obstetrics, today.

This case will illustrate; in 1903, Mrs. T., age 22, wife of a stockman, the family history negative during the early months of pregnancy, the husband consulted the author, and at this visit, was told of the necessity of reporting, frequently, the condition of his wife, also the dangers, etc., resulting from neglect. The husband was assured that it was so much better to be looking for trouble and not to find it than to allow trouble to steal upon you and overwhelm, before we realized that that there was any. About a month later, after the return, of the husband, from his ranch, he reported that while his wife was visiting a neighbor, some days before, she had been introduced to another physician and in the course of the conversation, his wife had been told that it was no more

than natural for Dr. Leeds to make a big fuss, over his confinement cases, as he charged $25.00, also this physician had noticed that Dr. Leeds always did put his pregnant patients to a lot of unnecessary trouble and that his wife need not anticipate any trouble, as long as her mother had not had any, with any of her children. One examination, of the urine, a day or two before confinement, was mentioned as being sufficient, also the charges would be $12.50, instead of $25.00. The lady being naturally thrifty, this conversation appealed to her. The sample of urine, at the time suggested, was taken to the $12.50 physician, who, holding the urine up to the light, remarked that it was the best looking sample observed, in a long time. The fact had never been considered that the mother of this patient had never had on a corset and during her child-bearing period, as the wife of a farmer, had led an unusually active out-door life, further, that this mother had always tried to shield her daughter from every kind of hard work. About midnight, a few days later, the author was called, with the admonition to come as quickly as possible as this patient was having convulsions. The other physician and the author had a blood-sweating time, the patient not only had a very close call but a very tedious convalesence. Forceps and heroic efforts for very active elimination of all of the emunctories was the treatment necessitated. An examination of the blood and urine revealed an overburdened and poisoned system.

It is needless to say that, the family and patient are not only thoroughly convinced of the necessity of the proper preparation of the patient, during pregnancy, but they do not allow an opportunity to pass, without making a comparison between the methods of the two physicians.

Which doctor had you rather be?

A cursory and occasional examination of the urine, during pregnancy, does not suffice; nor will it give a true picture of the patient, because the symptom-complex, characterized by nausea, vomiting, headache, visual disturbances, delirium, coma, with or without albuminuria, casts or edema, hyperermesis gravidarum and eclampsia does not mean so much a crippling of the kidneys as it does that there is too great a burden on all the emunctories.

Instead of being lulled by a false sense of security, when we find that the urine is free from albumin, in a patient, complaining of some of the symptom-complex, though these may be slight, we ought to realize that the liver is an organ barely capable of performing normal function, in normal health, and that, when you add the natural toxins of pregnancy to its burden of every-day metabolism, it is but logical that the liver should undergo some degree of deterioration, also that the kidney trouble and edema, if present, are secondary and that it is the clogged emunctories which need our immediate and urgent attention.

Why can not we realize that the modern woman is an uncertain quantity, nervously, though she may be, apparently, well prepared physically?

Also, why can not we try to appreciate that the nervous organization, of our modern women, has been undergoing a gradual change, since the time of our grandmothers?

Do we consider that our civilization has made such persistent and exacting drains on the organization, that not only has the physical development been dwarfed but there has been developed a highly strung bundle of nerves, poorly nourished and sadly out of tune, hardly able to stand the little jars, of every-day life, much less the depressing effects, of pregnancies, without

very material aid at the hands of an intelligent and careful medical adviser?

If we expected a horse to come anywhere near winning a race, we would hardly fail to give him the benefit of thorough, careful and intelligent training?

Do we use this same common sense, which the Maker is supposed to have given us, when we allow our pregnant patients to go along, in a hapazard manner, during pregnancy, without any intelligent instruction and preparation?

Are we treating them as we should, when we do not do all we can to place them in the best condition, possible, for the great demand which is made on both the physical and nervous systems, at the time of confinement?

Can we anticipate anything but hapazard results, with our usual treatment of these cases, previous to confinement?

Can we conscientiously be surprised and wonder when, with the treatment usually accorded these cases, we have the accidents and complications, so common, in modern pregnancies?

Does it not appear somewhat sneaking and comtemptible, after obtaining these hapazard results, for us to flounder around, in our endeavor, to not only satisfy the family and clear our own skirts, of any blame, but also attempt to shift the responsibility to other shoulders than our own?

The author was advised, by one of his professors, to consider every patient tainted with venereal disease, until a careful and exhaustive examination proved otherwise.

If this same advice was applied to our pregnant cases, so far as being normal or abnormal was concerned, we would surely obtain better results if we proved by careful and exhaustive examinations that there was no abnormality present.

Then, again, instead of lulling our

ly establishes our diagnosis. We must not lose sight of the fact however that a similar nodular salpingitis of the insthmus of the tube is found in chronic gonorrhoea. These nodules are due, it is thought, in both conditions, to a swollen, thickened mucus membrane encroaching upon the muscularis and thus producing the characteristic nodular feeling.

Early the mucosa of the tube may become infiltrated with round cells, vascular, and thickened, containing many giant cells. At this stage, in these cases, the muscularis is unchanged. Later the epithelium degenerates and disappears. Necrotic changes follow, affecting the tubercle first and then the muscle tissue is encroached upon. If the necrosis affects all the coats or coverings of the tube, rupture and escape of the contents occur. This is rather rare unless it be mixed infection.

Secondary tuberculosis of the tubes may occur by extension from the peritoneum, ovaries and uterus. The disease is usually bilateral, yet both tubes may not be affected to the same degree. In our observation of many cases, we are convinced that the tube presents fertile soil for the production of the tubercle bacillus. We can assign no definite reason for this unles it be due to the previously existing inflammatory or circulatory disturbance, and disorders arising during menstruation and the puerperium.

If the infection is of the descending type it generally begins in the mucus membrane of the ampeulla. The affected tube is thickened, more or less tortuous. The muscular coat is hypertrophied and the fimbria are thick, firm and shortened. Many adhesions are found about it, binding it firmly to adjacent tissue. On incising the tube in the earlier stages the mucosa is found swollen and reddened and the folds are adherent. It has the appearance of chronic productive salpingitis. As it becomes more advanced, greyish points show themselves in

the mucosa, or caseous nodules or streaks are seen.

Microscopically in the secondary form, the mucus membrane is swollen and infiltrated with round and epithelioid cells. Tubercles are to be seen near the lumen, with central caseation. As the disease advances the mucosa becomes largely caseous, with the progress noticeable in the muscular and serous coats. In the earlier stages the lesions produced are not unlike those of lesions produced are not unlike those of chronic salpingitis from any other cause. Microscopically the resemblance is close in both forms there being added, in the primary form, giant cells in the neighborhood of the cellular infiltration. Caseation soon sets in and the tubercles are recognized as greyish elevations. The epithlium of the crypts show evidence of cloudiness and degeneration. The crypts disappear in the course of the coalescence of the caseous masses and the formation of tuberculous granulation tissue. The lumen of the tube becomes filled and distended with a cascopurulent detritus. The process of destruction extends into the muscularis. The walls become greatly thickened, adhesions form and the tube becomes tortuous. Small caseous foci may be formed or simply areas of cellular infiltration with giant cells.

The caseous detritus retained in the lumen may undergo degeneration, becoming liquified and puriform. This often results in sacculation causing tuberculous pyosalpinx.

Ulceration and perforation in purely tubercular cases are rare, as the abscess is usually walled off by adhesions, attaching it to the uterus, appendix or other adjacent tissue.

Pus infection may occur in tubercular disease, or it may be a mixed inftction from the beginning, both forms taking place from the one foci. When the primary focus is a mixed infection, its extension is by ulceration, coagulation necrosis and other than extension by continuity of surface, or through the lymphatics.

If the primary focus of mixed infection is the tube, the end of the tube becomes sealed, and a pyo-tubercular salpingitis is established. The extension may be by ulceration through the fimbriated end, and the formation of an abscess in the Cul-de-sac, ovary or anywhere the end of the tube may become attached. Extension from a mixed infection salpingitis is by ulceration through its walls to the adjacent tissue. If it becomes attached to the ovary, the result is a tubercular abscess in one of the graffian follicles.

If it become adherent to the intestines, perforation most likely will take place and a tubo-intestinal sinus result.

This is one of the conditions to be apprehended in operating for tuberculosis of the tube or peritoneum, and is one of the most serious conditions with which we have to contend. Fistulas of the bowel, of tubercular origin, are difficult to suture on account of the infiltrations of the wall of the intestine and the adjacent tissue.

Resection is difficult and should seldom be undertaken on account of the extensive adhesions.

The rapid healing tendency of the peritoneum, which is so all important, has been destroyed by the tuberculous process, and therefore it is difficult to get primary peritoneal union sufficient to support the walls. If repair is inevetable, several rows of sutures must be inserted to approximate enough surface that apposition may be insured during the process of tissue regeneration.

The fundus of the uterus has been utilized, by suturing it to the opening in the bowel, so as to secure enough normal peritoneal surface to repair the opening.

Many cases might be mentioned where the fimbriated end of the tube is united to the bowel and the disease transmitted to the bowel in this way, the disease being primary in the tube.

There being no pathognomic symptom of genital tuberculosis, we find it necessary to make a systematic microscopic examination of the scrapings, and discharges for the bacilli.

We must remember, however, that the bacilli may not be found on every slide, for as an average, it exists only in one out of every 47 slides examined. Hence it requires a careful examination of many specimens to make a positive diagnosis. The smegma bacillus is so very similar to that of tuberculosis that much pains is required to differentiate them. The inoculation method is sometimes a useful adjunct to the microscope. In doubtful cases, a general systemic examination is necessary. The thermometer is of great help in tubal tuberculosis. A constant slight rise in the evening temperature, and a normal or slightly subnormal morning temperature, are very suggestive of the tubercular nature of the tubal affection. Our attention is often directed to the frequent coincident of tubal pregnancy and tubal tuberculosis. This is of much interest from a diagnostic standpoint. When we are confronted with a tubal pregnancy we are to take into consideration the possibility of tubal tuberculosis.

Sterility is the rule in tubal tuberculosis. Early, the menstrual disturbance is slight. Later, there may be either amenorrhoea or menorrhagia. Menorrhagia in young girls should arouse our suspicion, as to there being tuberculosis. Many times will our efforts be rewarded by finding the bacilli, while it would have otherwise remained undetected. Caseous mases may be found in the discharge and yet not especially significant unless the bacilli be found. Pain is not common unless it be confined principally to the tube and salpingitis exists.

The tubes are predisposed to tuberculosis because of their spiral form and the irregular mucosa which tends to stagnate pregnancy successfully.

Bear in mind, that there are many wo- men who can not accomodate themselves to the changed conditions, of pregnancy, and with them, there is need of an ever- lasting intelligent advice and instruction as to the dangers, etc., of neglecting them- selves and the wonderful benefits to be de- rived in assisting nature.

Study carefully each patient so that you will be able to intelligently advise her, as to her individual needs, for in individual- izing your obstetrical cases, you are laying a firm foundation for success.· in these cases.

Be firm with your pregnant cases and when you find that they antagonize your efforts or fail to follow your advice. it will be to your interest to insist upon them getting some one else.

A case will illustrate; Mrs. W., age 24, history of fall, with permanent injury to · spine and hip, also deformed pelvis. De- livery at 7 months advised, but patient overpersuaded the author to wait until full term. Results, an 18 lb., still-born child, patient living a week and death from shock.

Another case; Mrs. D.. age 25, history of husband having had syphilis, 10 years before, but no signs in past 5 years. Anti- syphilitic treatment for wife was advised, by author, but as husband insisted that if this treatment was given, that he would be compelled to explain his previous condi- tion, the author was overpersuaded. The result was a still-born, syphilitic child and a serious and tedious convalescence, for wife. The husband refused to make a clean breast of the trouble so that his wife could have the proper treatment and· as the re- sult of another pregnancy, occurring very shortly, after this, there was a miscarriage, at 3 months, of a syphilitic child, and as this occured when the author was out of the city, another physician was called who explained to the wife, the cause of the

trouble. The husband confessed his part, but denied the advice and previous sug- gestions of the· author. You can imagine the present standing, of the author, with that family.

Another case; Mrs. *, age 23, husband gave history of case of gonorrhea, ap- parently cured. Anti-gonorrheal serum treatment, for wife, suggested to husband, but refused owing to the necessity of an explanation having to be given to wife. Another physician was secured; for the case, and after delivery, an infection de- veloped, which a third physician pro- nounced due to the carelessness of the 2nd physician, though the patient was treated for a gonorrheal infection.

Use your abdominal binders and sup- porters, during convalescence and for sometime afterwards, as they will give much needed assistance to the weakened abdominal muscles and internal organs of generation, also assisting, materially, to preserve the previous symmetry of the mother's figure.

In case of fever, following confinement, be sure to examine the blood for malaria, for, often, a latent malarial infection will demonstrate itself, after the depressing effects of confinement, and, too, in this way. you can often explain and treat intelligent- ly an infection which might otherwise be a source of embarassment and censure to the attending physician.

Make repeated examinations, during pregnancy, of the blood and urine, for a clogged condition of the system will of- ten be shown, which when taken in time, is easily corrected, but if allowed to persist may become of a serious nature.

The use of normal salt enemata, fre- quently, during pregnancy, especially, when any symptoms of toxemia are present, is a valuable aid.

The routine use of lithiated sorgum

comp. or liq. ferri. et. ammon. acetate gives excellent results.

The early and persistent massage of the breasts, with olive oil, together with alcohol or similar preparations applied to the nipples, will prevent many bottle-fed babies.

Persistent and regular massage, of the abdominal muscles, with olive oil, increases the muscular tonicity, and in this way, often obviates instrumental interference.

A heart to heart talk, with the husband and wife, as soon as convenient, after you have been consulted, will give you their confidence and also establish a hearty co operation.

A lack of an ever-watchful eye, on your pregnant cases, sooner or later, will develop, for you, a horde of obstetrical wrecks, with tongues never stilled, waxing eloquent in every listening and sympathetic ear, as they depict the suffering and agony, which they will have to endure, always, as a result of the services rendered by you. and this never ceasing tale of woe will surely and persistently limit and eventually terminate a physician's usefulness, in a community.

Be serious and earnest, with your recent pregnant woman, do not treat her aches and pains, in a light or frivolous manner, because, to her, it is a serious strange, wonderful and oftimes fearful experience.

Encourage her confidence and discourage her seeking or accepting advice from the neighbors or meddling old women.

Tell her that instead' of a bother or trouble, that it will be a pleasure, for you, to give her a common-sense reason for every phase of her condition.

If you will explain these things, to her, in a language which she can understand, and are kind and patient, she will appreciate the treatment received, at your hands, and you will steadily establish an obstetri-

cal practice, like unto those things described, in the Good Book as "Treasures laid up, which thieves can not take nor rust or moths destroy."

It is needless to more than mention that, especially, in obstetrics, "Cleanliness is next to Godliness."

Adopt a rule and adhere to it, strictly and religiously, that you will not accept an obstetrical case, unless you are permitted to watch and care for it, at least, three months before confinement.

Tell them that the ultimate successful termination of pregnancy depends upon a thorough preparation, and that the more common sense used and the more rational assistance rendered nature; the less medicine will have to be taken and the less serious trouble and complications will have to be overcome.

Give them a good sensible reason for everything that you ask and tell them to do.

One of the most important things to do, is to charge $25.00 for your uncomplicated cases, then do good work and make your patients pay.

No one will value your services any higher than the estimate you place upon them, yourself.

Does a $7.50, $10.00, $12.50 or $15.00 suit of clothes receive the same respect and treatment that a $25.00 suit does?

Whenever you find people that consider themselves, wives and physician, like unto a $7.50, $10.00, $12.50 or $15.00 suit of clothes, you had better advise them to employ someone else; in that confinement case, for your financial and professional reward, from such cases, will be of little value to you.

A thing or service cheaply obtained has little value, no matter what it may be or from whom it may be obtained.

When you insist upon your confinement cases being given to you, at least three months beforehand, it is much easier, then, to arrange for the amount of the fee and the manner of its payment, than to attempt to quibble over the fee, at the time of the call for your services.

The author had found that the husband or other members of the family, for that matter, under the strain and excitement of the impending confinement, are very prone to be very prolific and rash, in their promises and even more dilatory in their efforts to fulfill them.

My obstetrical cases understand that this work is C. O. D. "Cash on delivery" and wherever, beforehand, it seems expedient the full fee or the greater part has been in the hands of the author, before the services have been rendered, sometimes being collected, in amounts of $1.00 or $2.00, at a time.

With this fee, for your services, and its payment practically assured, you can afford and ought to have an obstetrical grip, which you use for no other purpose and which is equipped for any emergency, which might arise, in these cases.

Have it like unto the Virgin's lamp, in Biblical verse, "Always ready, filled, trimmed and burning, so that when the baby. instead of the bridegroom, cometh," you can grab your grip and run, satisfied that nothing can arise which will necessitate a serious delay, while you, or someone else, runs, rides or walks back after something forgotten.

Thus can we, as members of the noblest profession, on earth add our mite to the dignity of the craft and help to place the branch of medicine on the high and important plane, to which it is entitled.

BRONCHO-PNEUMONIA

BY DR. LEONARD S. WILLOUR, ATOKA, OKLA.

In preparing a paper on Broncho-pneumonia I cannot help but feel that the subject has been very thoroughly threshed out in many medical society meetings, and that perhaps it will be hard for me to inject enough new material into this paper to elicit the discussion of the members of this section. I am aware of the many times in our practice we meet this disease either as a primary condition or complication, and how grave the symptoms appear to the friends of our patient as well as the attending physician and will consequently try to the best of my ability to bring to your attention some points that may have been overlooked by you in your study of this disease.

Broncho-pneumonia is a disease of infancy and early childhood, it is very uncommon in children after the sixth year.

It is a disease of such character that it is hard to classify clinically as there is a complexity of symptoms which indicate rather a combination of diseases, but there is always present the one common factor capillary-bronchitis.

Primary broncho-pneumonia rarely exists, I have never seen a case myself, and from the best authority I can obtain, it occurs in about one per cent. of all cases.

Of its etiology it is safe to say that it appears as a complication of most all of the diseases to which our baby patients are heir, its most virulent forms complicating measles and diphtheria. The frequency of the complication depends upon the nutrition and age of the child, it being more common in infancy and in the poorly nourished chronic and debilitating diseases such as scrofula, marasmus or syphilis are predisposing factors, as when a child is in the necessarily debilitated condition that one of the above mentioned diseases would cause its resisting powers are very much lowered and it is impossible to cope with the ravages of infectious organisms so constantly present in the upper respiratory system.

With regard to symptoms, it is necessary for me to say but little as we are all so familliar with the characteristic breathing, dyspnea, which is aggravated by the very least exertion or excitement, the constant cough terminating in a sharp cry which indicates pain, the dilated nostrils, sinking in of the soft tissues of the chest which of course, shows the extreme effort nature is putting forth to supply sufficient oxygen for our little sufferer. The one symptom which is not at all characteristic is the temperature. When broncho-pneumonia presents itself as a complication. we find a rapid rise of temperature to a 104° to 105° F, and while it remains high it is subject to fluctuations and often shows in twenty-four hours a variation of three to five degrees. This is, no doubt, the most common character of the temperature, but the fact never-the-less exists that the temperature is sometimes of a constant variety. When the child is suffering from extreme malnutrition a much less elevation of the temperature is present.

I will not take any of your valuable time with physical signs, but go on at once with the treatment.

In the debilitated condition in which we usually find these patients it is of paramount importance that we preserve each and every unit of vitality, this may be accomplished somewhat by arranging the medication, local treatment and nourishment to come at the same time, and this at intervals of sufficient length to give the patient ample time for rest and sleep, as the reconstructive and recuperative powers of rest, cannot be overestimated.

The arrangement of the sick-room should not be left to the family without several important suggestions from the attending physician. There should be plenty of fresh, pure air which can be arranged by the adjustment of a window board, and with the necessary thermometer to be religiously watched to see that the temperature of the room does not exceed 70° F. or fall below 65° F. we have an arrangement which will give us a change of air and that not superheated.

With regard to medication the first suggestion I would make is, that many of the ordinarily used cough syrups be set aside and that the already weakened digestive aparatus should not be taxed with these heavy mixtures. Expectorants must be handled with the utmost care and in my opinion, are much better given in powder or tablet form. For a child one year of age I would recommend 1-100 gr. of tarter emetic and 1-40 gr. of ipecac, where it is necessary to add a sedative to the combination 1-4 gr. of Dovers powder is of value.

It is always of great importance to have the digestive organs in the best possible condition, and to attain this end a few small doses of calomel followed with two or three drams of caster oil at the onset of the disease will accomplish much. It is necessary to keep the bowels open and this can be done with castor oil or glycerine suppositories.

It is most always necessary during an attack of broncho-pneumonia to administer heart stimulants, and the indication for their use should be carefully considered. I have accepted as a rule the suggestion of Chas. G. Kerley, of New York, and find it to be of great value. It is to the effect that when the pulse is 150 per minute or of a slow, soft, irregular character and not favorably influenced by sponging, it is time to begin medical stimulation. At this time it has been my practice recently to use tincture of strophanthus, using in a child one year old one drop in a little water every three hours. Sometimes when proper results cannot be obtained by the use of this agent I use 1-300 gr. strychnine increasing to 1-100 gr. making the intervals in proportion to the indications, watching carefully for symptoms of strychnine poisoning. In a pulse of the soft, irregular character strychnine is always the preferable remedy.

Our guide in dealing with the temperature should not be the registration of the thermometer as much as the effect the amount of fever present is having on the patient. If a child has high fever and by reducing it we can make it more restful or improve its digestive power it is our duty to bring into play our antipyretics. Of course by reducing the temperature we can reduce the heart action, which no doubt will be of great value as every pulsation saved may be of decided advantage later in the attack.

Hydro-therapy is the method par excellence in reducing temperature and plays the double role of lowering the fever and acting as sedative. In the cold spongings which I start at a temperature of 95° F. and gradually cool to 70° F. to 75° F. I sometimes use either salt or alcohol using two teaspoonfuls of salt to a quart of water, or one part of alcohol to three parts of water.

I do not often use the cold pack as it is not safe in unskilled hands and it is often impossible for the physician to be present during this procedure. Of course if I have a trained nurse on the case it removes this objection and then I use this valuable agent.

When it is necessary to use drugs to reduce the temperature the following combination is of value, caffein citrate gr. 1-3 Dovers powder gr. 1-2 aspirin gr. 2 at four hour intervals. Guiacol carbonate in 1 gr. doses appears to have a favorable influence upon the temperature as well as possessing some curatave properties.

One of my objects in presenting this paper is to describe a method of applying counter-irritation which has been very satisfactory in my hands and which I have never seen mentioned in the literature on this subject. It is a mustard pack prepared and applied as follows: One pint each of alcohol and water are placed in a large bowl, to this is added one to three ounces (according to the severity of the case) of spirits of mustard. A large piece of flannel is moistened in the mixture and wrapped around the child from his neck to his knees, he is then enveloped in a dry sheet and the pack is left on until the skin is a bright red, usually fifteen to thirty minutes. The child is then taken out and wrapped and left for one-half hour in a pack wet with one part of alcohol and two parts of water. At the end of this time the child is wrapped in a dry sheet.

Usually one pack causes marked improvement but relapses are frequent and it may need renewal, once in twenty-four hours being often enough in all but the most urgent cases.

The physician should apply the first pack to determine the necessary strength and instruct the parent or nurse.

The advantages of this form of counter-irritation are first; its surprisingly rapid effect, second, its light weight does not materially embarrass respiration, third, it can be applied without removing the enfeebled patient from the bed, fourth, it is inexpensive, fifth, it is clean.

In cases where there is a large lung area involved oxygen given for one or two minutes out of every seven to ten gives gratifying results, if given for less time or at much longer intervals I have failed to see equally good results.

———

DISCUSSION.

Dr. Winnie Sanger, Oklahoma City:

I enjoyed the paper very much. Of course, we disagree very much about treatment on some lines. The principal difference is the use of opiates. I think we should be very careful in the use of opiates.

Dr. Leonard S. Willour, Atoka:

I wish to say in closing, that I am not in favor of the universal use of opiates and only use them when their sedative action is absolutely necessary as when it is impossible to get satisfactory rest and quiet for the patient by the use of hydro-therapy and every other method that can be used. When the cough can not be cured without a sedative, I think the best sedative is Dovers powders. I rarely have to use them and there is hardly enough opiates in the mixture prescribed to have any constipating effects, and this can be readily controlled by an occasional dose of castor oil.

EDITORIAL

THE ANNUAL MEETING, MUSKOGEE, MAY 9, 10 AND 11TH, 1911.

Once again it becomes the duty of the Secretary to urge all concerned to prepare early for this meeting.

Chairman of Sections should begin at once to prepare their programs for the meeting in order to not delay the program and leave off any who wish to offer papers, as was inadvertantly done last year in a few instances, which was not necessarily the fault of the Chairman concerned so much so as the contributor waiting until the last moment to send in the title of his paper.

If you have a paper for this meeting consult the directory at once, locate the name and address of the Chairman of the Section to which your paper properly belongs and write him at once. Do not make the mistake of waiting for him to write you, he might be very busy and forget it or not know that you have the paper.

While on the subject it is not out of place to remind all members that their dues as members of the State Association are paid for the year 1910 only, and that now

is the time to remit them to your county secretary. Do not wait for him to hunt you up, for his time is valuable as well as yours and the salary attached to his office is not sufficient for him to give the office all his time in making collections, so just help him out and set a good example by mailing him a check and stating in your letter that the amount is for membership dues and subscription to the JOURNAL.

———

FEEDING IN TYPHOID.

Considerable attention is being paid at present to the increase in the diet list of typhoid patients comparatively speaking.

There seems to be no happy medium in medicine, the pendulum is given to swinging too far one way or the other and this fact prompts the expression of this note.

The writer personally knows of typhoid patients eating most anything that struck their fancy, patients who neither knew nor observed any rule ordinarily accepted as proper for a typhoid and yet the course was not disturbed so far as could be seen by this grave departure from the teachings and advice of the physician. I also recall cases in which the slightest deviation from an extremely weak fluid diet caused grave symptoms such as tympanites and rising temperature and which symptoms abated promptly on the withdrawal of the offending food.

Obviously it follows that every case is a law to its self and must be treated and fed on its individual merits. A liberal diet would certainly not affect the first-class of patients mentioned while the same diet used with the second-class would result in disaster to the patient and unlike many other conditions the trouble is so easily encountered and so difficult to get rid of that it is well to consider carefully any departure from those rules that the general practitioner has had the best results with.

Aside from the general rule to keep the temperature down by approved methods, water, ice and alcohol, keeping the bowel empty with oil or salines, using some of the so-called intestinal antiseptics and a food that agrees with the individual patient in hand any other marked change is likely to result in trouble for both patient and physician. We should not too quickly desert those remedies and habits that have served us fairly well.

THE RESULTS OF DR. McCOR-MACK'S VISIT.

From the different sections of the state gratifying reports are being received of the organization of various working bodies within the county society membership for the purpose of either following out the post-graduate work as detailed by the Journal of the American Medical Association, or following an original plan of work and study as agreed upon.

This feature was one strongly urged upon the profession by Dr. McCormack and one that is found to be effective of more general good to the entire profession than any plan heretofore adopted. The medical profession is composed of many diverse

characters; some are indefatigable workers; constantly posting themselves and leaving nothing undone to keep abreast and in many cases, ahead of the times, in their communities; others are content to rely on the knowledge they obtained in college, backed up by experience and rarely a trip of a short time to some medical center, while others are totally negative as to efforts of self improvement and simply content themselves by getting by the State Board requirements. It is needless to say that this class bring the profession into disrepute with the people who they come in contact with, and fortunately they are becoming so well known to the general public that their opportunity for doing damage is daily growing less.

A small body of earnest investigators who have regular meetings and follow out a general plan of work, will surprise themselves with the information gained, they will soon attract their more careless brother physician and the public will soon have them stamped as men worthy of respect and trust and as men as to call on when in trouble. The day is past when one or two abdominal operations or difficult cases brought to a successful conclusion will establish a lasting reputation for the man doing them. The medical profession is nothing of not progressive and the man who today stands still will soon find himself too far behind to ever recover his lost prestige.

We should try by faithful effort to prepare ourselves to properly repay the trust of the people reposed in us, the result will not be noticed in a day but soon it will be noticed and we have the added satisfaction of knowing that we are doing something all the time for our mental advancement. The lowliest and poorest prepared physician in the state need not despair if he is honest with himself, becomes acquainted with his limitations and deficiencies and starts about finding a remedy, and the remedy will be found in the motto "work."

REPORT OF THE STATE COMMISSIONER OF HEALTH.

The First Biennial Report of The State Commissioner of Health, Dr. J. C. Mahr, is just completed and has been transmitted to the Governor.

The report is an interesting document of 349 pages and contains many interesting photographs depicting public health conditions in the state and is valuable from a statistical standpoint.

It shows that the state has gained in population during the time up to and including September 30th, 17,082, there having been deaths to the 9,692 with a birth record of 26,774 and it is estimated that the figures cover 60% of births and 80% of deaths.

The report recommends that a stringent law be passed requiring reporting of marriages and divorces and that they be made a part of the vital statistics of the state; concludes the cause of typhoid in the state to be due to carelessness in handling garbage, non-protected water supplies and fly infection of food stuffs. Of the deaths recorded the Commissioner concludes that 3,406 were due to preventable disesase, and enumerates them as follows:

Typhoid	.699
Measles	159
Tuberculosis	645
Diphtheria	187
Smallpox	97
Scarlet Fever	77
Whooping Cough	61
Pneumonia	1,384
Hydrophobia	3
Puerperal Sepsis	94
Total	3,406

Taking this summary into consideration it is recommended that there should be rigid and continued medical inspection of schools.

One phase of this report will meet with the hearty approval of every physician in the state who has the state's welfare at heart. Under the head of Indigent and County Farm Inmates the Commissioner has this to say: "The prevailing policy pursued is to award the medical care and treatment of these people to the lowest bidder, giving little or no thought to the class of supplies furnished, or the character of scientific treatment secured or the nature of environments. All of these are important features in health work. When these are furnished as a result of competitive bidding, inferior service is to be expected.

Probably the greatest crime being perpetrated in Oklahoma is that of letting to the lowest bidder the contract to care for our sick and indigent."

PERSONAL

Drs. P. P. Nesbitt, and Sessler Hoss, of Muskogee, will spend February in Chicago, doing Post-graduate work.

Dr. W. L. Kendall, of Durant, will move to Oklahoma City, in the near future. Dr. Kendall carries with him the best wishes of the local profession in Durant, where he has lived for several years.

Dr. Frank Jackman, of Cumberland, has moved from that place to Mead, and President Evans of the State University has appointed Dr. Gayfree Ellison, of Oklahoma City, Assistant in the Department of Bacteriology. He will have charge of the Public Health Laboratories at Norman, the appointment taking effect at once.

Dr. J. L. Blakemore, of Muskogee, spent the holidays in Virginia, with his son.

Dr. W. K. Callahan, has returned from Chicago, where he has been doing post-graduate work and will locate in Muskogee.

Professor John Dice MacLaren, of the State University School of Medicine is offered the Professorship of Physiology in the Oregon State University Medical School at Portland. More time for research in a better laboratory at an increased salary has caused him to tender his resignation to President Evans and the Board of Regents at their regular meeting on Monday, December 12th. In 1908 Dr. MacLaren began work in the State University of Oklahoma with 20 students in 6 classes. He now teaches 108 students in 5 classes. This is sixteen college credit-hours a week which requires the Professor to be at least thirty hours a week with the students.

Dr. John Dice MacLaren won his degrees of A. B., M. S., and B. D., by completing the Biology course and the Philosophy course in Kansas State University.

Then the pre-medical course in John Hopkins University and the Clinical Courses in John Hopkins Hospital were completed. His successful experience as Professor of Biology in the State University of Wyoming and Director of the U. S. Experiment Station, and as acting President of the South Dakota College, was followed by the degree of M. D., from Columbia University and the practice of medicine in New York, to 1908. In 1909 Tulane University Medical School offered him an assistant Professorship and in 1910 the Mississippi State University Medical School offered him a Professorship but he preferred to stay in Oklahoma.

Professor MacLaren is a member of both the American and British Association for the Advancement of Science; of the American Medical Association; the Sigma XI scientific fraternity; the Society of Medical Jurisprudence; the Oklahoma State Medical Society, and the University Club of Oklahoma City. He was recently elected a Fellow of the Oklahoma Academy of Science, and is President of the Cleveland County Medical Society. He now holds the Professorship of Physiology and Experimental Medicine in the State University of Oklahoma, and is Secretary of the Medical School.

COUNTY SOCIETIES

TILLMAN COUNTY.

The annual meeting of the Tillman County Medical Society held in Frederick, Okla., December 27th, selected officers as noted below:

President—Dr. A. B. Fair, Frederick.

Vice-Pres.—Dr. F. E. Rosenberger, Grandfield.

Secy.-Treas.—Dr. J. P. Van Allen, Frederick.

Delegate—Dr. H. L. Roberts, Frederick.

Alternate—Dr. J. D. Osborn, Jr., Frederick.

Censor—Dr. J. H. Hansen, Grandfield.

Dr. A. B. Fair, President of the society, who is also Councillor for his District is making an attempt to greatly increase the membership during the early months of the year.

TULSA COUNTY.

Held its annual election for officers for the ensuing year with the following results:

President, Ross Grossheart.

Vice-President, P. R. Brown.

Secretary, W. E. Wright.

Treasurer, Dr. S. D. Hawley.

Censors, Dr. F. S. Clinton, Dr. J. C. W. Bland, Dr. N. W. Mayginnis.

Delegates, Dr. G. H. Butler, Jr. and Dr. M. L. Garvin.

Alternate, Dr. W. E. Wright and Dr. J. C. W. Bland.

BRYAN COUNTY.

Bryan County held its annual election of officers in Durant, December 13th, and elected the following officers:

President, Dr. J. F. Park, Durant.

Vice-President, J. H. Durham, Durant.

Secretary-Treasurer, D. Armstrong, Mead.

Delegate, Dr. A. S. Hagood.

Alternate, Dr. J. H. Kay and J. L. Austin, Durant.

STEPHENS COUNTY.

The annual meeting of this society was held in Duncan, December 21st, with the following results:

President, Dr. P. M. Haraway, Marlow.

Vice-President, D. Long, Duncan.

Second Vice-President, Dr. H. A. Conger, Duncan.

Censor, Dr. H. C. Frie.

Committee on Public Health, Dr. C. M. Harrison, Comanche; Dr. C. E. Frost, Duncan; R. L. Montgomery, Marlow.

ATOKA-COAL COUNTIES.

The Joint County Societies of Atoka and Coal, elected officers in Coalgate, December 14th, and selected:

President, Dr. J. S. Fulton, Atoka.

Vice-President, Dr. W. A. Logan, Lehigh.

Secretary-Treasurer, L. S. Willour, Atoka.

This society expects to increase its membership greatly before the annual meeting in May.

MAJOR COUNTY.

Held its annual meeting at Fairview, December 13th, and after reading and discussing the following papers, Adenoids, by Dr. J. H. Barnes, Enid and Surgical Appendicitis, by Dr. S. N. Mayberry, of Enid, elected the folowing officers:

President, Dr. W. L. Gleason, Fairview.

Vice-President, Dr. J. S. Lindley, Fairview.

Secretary-Treasurer, Dr. Elsie L. Specht, Rusk.

Delegate, Dr. B. I. Townsend, Fairview.

Censors, Dr. P. C. McCall and Dr. B. I. Townsend, Fairview.

MUSKOGEE COUNTY.

The annual election of officers in this county resulted as follows:

President, Dr. W. S. Aiken, Muskogee.

Vice-President, Dr. G. A. McBride, Ft Gibson.

Secretary- Dr. H. T. Ballantine, Muskogee.

Treasurer, Dr. S. M. Fryer, Muskogee.

Delegates, Drs. P. P. Nesbit and Dr. W. T. Tilly, Muskogee.

Censor, Dr. J. T. Nichols, Muskogee.

After the meeting was over a smoker was indulged in and the plans for the annual meeting discussed, the President being empowered to appoint an executive committee of five members who were authorized to nominate the various committees necessary to arrange the annual meeting.

GALL-BLADDER DISEASE.

J. P. Runyan, Little Rock, Ark., (*Journal A. M. A.*, December 31), reviews the pathology and diagnosis of morbid conditions in the gall-bladder and bile ducts. He accepts the evidence that infection frequently occurs by the route of the portal vein. The history is of great importance and we should not regard the statement that gall-stones may produce no symptoms, and also remember that they may occur before middle age. The most prominent symptoms of gall-stone disease is a history of long-standing dyspepsia and digestive disturbances, usually independent of ingestion of food and frequently relieved by it. In gall-stone disease we have often at the beginning a sense of constriction rather than actual pain and accompanied with a sort of characteristic chilliness, jaundice, hematemesis, etc., are later symptoms after complications have occurred. From a surgical standpoint it makes no difference whether we have gall-stones, gastric or duodenal ulcers, pericholecystic or perigastric adhesions; the same incision will do for all. The consequences of gall-stones and inflammatory diseases of the gall-bladder are noticed in order. Whenever there is obstruction and the bile is absorbed into the blood we have jaundice The toxic biliary salts are responsible for some of the consequent toxemia and the exclusion of the bile from the intestines interferes with the absorption of fats which undergo excessive cleavage from the action of intestinal bacteria and ferments and give rise to irritating decomposition products and produce diarrhea. Fats should therefore be excluded from the diet in these cases, as the pancreas has the unfortunate defect of sharing its outlet with the bile it often becomes involved, probably in close to 50 per cent. of the cases, and gall-stone

disesase may therefore be considered as the cause of a very large proportion of cases of pancreatitis. Complete exclusion of the pancreas secretion is rare without coexisting exclusion of bile. The cleavage of fats in the intestines is considerably diminished and some claim its absorption is also lessened. There is much fat in the stools, which are large and the muscle nuclei pass through the intestine undigested, as shown in Schmidt's test. In addition, lipase may appear in the urine (Hewiett's test) and pentose (the Cammidge reaction) and much dextrose. The nature and extent of the operation for gall-bladder and gall-stone disease must depend on the condition of the pancreas. In biliary disease with chronic pancreatitis, the removal of the stone with temporary free drainage is generally sufficient. The removal of the gall-bladder is not advisable unless there is malignant disease. The keeping of the gall-bladder intact allows of a secondary cholecystenterostomy if necessary and we must keep in mind that the mucus of the gall-bladder has a function and protects the pancreas as well as relieves the tension in the common duct at the head of the pancreas. Runyan has always been impressed with the importance of chronic pancreatitis and has always advocated a cholecystenterostomy in all cases of distended gall-bladder and dilated common duct, with or without stones. In performing this operation we should always bear in mind the function of the bile in the intestines and never make an anastomosis between the gall-bladder and the colon unless the conditions demand it. The most logical place for such union is between the gall-bladder and the duodenum as near the opening of the common duct as possible, though this may not always be practicable. In acute pancreatitis complicating gall-stones or gall-bladder disease the pancreas should be incised and free drainage established; the anterior abdomnial incision is better than the posterior. If the patient's condition admits it and there are stones in the gall-bladder or ducts or an acute infection of the bile passages, the stone should be removed and drainage of bile established through a right lateral incision. If jaundice is present drainage is imperative. In all diseases of the gall-bladder and ducts we can prevent complications only by an early diagnosis. There is danger in waiting for an attack of biliary colic, vomiting, hematemesis or pancreatitis to make the diagnosis before operating.

VACCINES IN TYPHOID FEVER.

J. M. Anders, Philadelphia (*Journal A. M. A.*, December 10), says that certain accepted facts and principles should be understood by the clinician who attempts to use vaccine in the treatment of typhoid and other diseases. Among these are the following: 1. The object of vaccine therapy is to induce an active immunity by introducing an added amount of morbific materials so that by increasing the amount of protective bodies in the body, the growth of the invading organism can be inhibited. The *Bacillus typhosus* undergoing solution in the human body sets free an endotoxin which is the cause of its pathogenic action. In the process of immunization both bacteriolysis and phagocytosis come into play. Emery rightly says that phagocytosis is of chief importance in typhoid, since the typhoid bacilli liberate their endotoxins when dissolved by means of bacteriolvtic serum. In serious cases of typhoid, when the system is overwhelmed with the toxins, the vaccine treatment may therefore be a source of fresh danger and aggravate the symptoms. The determination of the opsonic index is too time-consuming to be practicable in general practice; fortunately, it is not generally considered necessary. Ty-

phoid is an acute bacteremia plus toxemia, often fulminating in character, and not a localized infection. Hence brilliant results from vaccine treatment can hardly be looked for. It is doubtful whether it is safe to use typhoid vaccines in severe cases. It is in chronic infections, in which the specific organism is walled off from the general circulation with slow absorptions of toxins into the blood, that vaccine therapy is most useful. The reports of those who have used tphyoid vaccine are somewhat varied. In 8 cases Anders himself used small doses, 25,000,000 in the beginning and subsequent ones of 50,000,000 each, repeated as a rule at intervals of 75 hours. For the reasons already given, he does not believe in massive doses of from 300,000,000 to 350,000,000. In his series, except in one case, there was no febrile reaction from the use of the vaccine, but in 2 cases the nocturnal remissions became distinctly greater and in one case of protracted subfebrile temperature in typhoid they seemed to bring the temperature down to the normal in a few days. His observations do not show that small doses stimulated phagocytosis very much, but he thinks the effects of the vaccines on the leukocyte count should be carefully investigated. If, however, the process of immunization is dependent chiefly on phagocytosis, and it can be shown that the bone marrow can be thus stimulated then vaccine therapy is advisable. The routine use of vaccines is not to be encouraged, but an antiendotoxic serum would, by neutralizing the endotoxin, be an ideal treatment. Before rejecting vaccine therapy, it should be thoroughly investigated, especially in mild cases. Finally, he says, in the present state of our knowledge the value of vaccines for the following purposes must be conceded: "(1) As a means of prophylaxis; (2) in suitable cases when continued during convalescence, to prevent relapses; (3) to combat local infections with the tyhpoid bacillus, as, for example. bone suppurations which arise in the period of convalescence; and (4) for the removal of the typhoid bacilli from the feces and urine in the case of typhoid-carriers." An endotoxic serum has been prepared by MacFayden and favorable results have already been reported from its use when administered early in typhoid cases. Anders thinks it not improbable, that serum treatment in typhoid, except as indicated above, will be by the method of establishing passive immunity by means of antiendotoxin. In view of the discrepancy among clinical observers as to the size and repetitions of doses, there seems to be a great necessity for the consideration of these aspects of the question of therapeutic inoculations in the future.

TREATMENT OF WOUNDS.

The reparative processes in wounds are described by A. Carrel, New York (*Journal A. M. A.*, December 17), who says that with asepsis we have not the right to believe that we have reached the last step in the treatment of wounds. He asks if it would not be feasible to act on the processes or repair themselves and expedite them We might thus greatly improve the therapeutics of wounds and fractures, and we must therefore analyze the mechanisms which are instrumental in cicatrization of wounds, the factors which modify their functions, the stimuli by which they are started, and the causes of their reciprocal action in the common work. The anatomic processes of cicatrization have long been known. These phenomena can be divided into four periods: quiescent period, period of granulous retraction, period of epidermization, and cicatricial period. The experiments on which he bases his article were performed on dogs. The cicatrization of a resected flap of skin, rectangular, trapezoidal or circular, was observed. In order to locate the edges of the old epidermis, black

animals were used or the edges of the wound were stained with India ink. The quiescent period lasts until granulation begins; during the first one to three days the dimensions of the wound do not vary. At the end of this period the edges of the wound inclines downward, sometimes suddenly, and begin to approach each other, thus beginning the period of granulous retraction. This reduction in size is very marked for the first days of this period. Then it gradually becomes slower and comes to a standstill, when the dimensions of the wound are only 20 mm. and is zero when the edges have reached a distance of from 10 to 15 mm. from each other. The larger the wound the greater the speed of retraction, and the rate of reparation is directly proportional to the size of the wound. It thus becomes important in the healing of middle-sized and large wounds. The end of the granulous period corresponds to the beginning of the epithelial wandering from the edges of the wound, which seems to stop immediately their retraction. It can be easily observed on a wound the edges of which are stained with India ink. The new epithelium spreads very slowly on the surface of the granulations, and it is difficult to locate its free edge accurately. It is exceedingly delicate and many factors interfere with its development. Its time and rate of growth depend on the dimensions of the wound. The rate is inversely proportional to the dimensions of the wound. It is very slow when the distance between the edges is more than 10 mm., and its maximal activity seems to be when the cicatrization is nearly complete. The cicatrical period is very long, the evolution of the scar being slow. There is a progressive enlargement of the scar after the epidermization is completed, the edges of the wound having a tendency to go back to their former position. The progressive enlargement of the scar lasts for a long time. While the processes of repair are continuous and progressive, they have their periods, of minimum and maximum activity. During the quiescent period, the end of the period of granulous retraction and the beginning of the period of epidermization the rate is slow. It is maximum at the beginning of the period of granulous retraction and at the end of the period of epidermization. The two mechanisms are adapted to the healing of small and middle-sized wounds, the width of which is not over 45 mm., but if the wound is larger—60 or 70 mm.—the retraction of the granulations cannot bring the edges to the minimum distance. They remain at a distance of about 20 mm. The mechanisms are efficient for the healing of the common injuries incurred in fighting of the animals, but they do not work as well for the larger wounds. The article is the first of a series on the subject.

BOOKS RECEIVED

INTERNATIONAL CLINICS, (VOLUME FOUR).

International Clinics, Volume Four, 1910, Twentieth Series. J. B. Lippincott Company, Philadelphia and London.

This volume is richer in material than any of its predecessors for the year 1910, containing the report of operations for July, 1910, at St. Mary's Hospital, Rochester, by the Mayo brothers and their assistants, by E. H. Beckman, M. D. Erlichs 606, by Henry W. Cattell, M. D., Philadelphia. The Technic, Aims and Limitations of Spinal Anaesthesia in the Young, by H. Tyrrell Gray, London, and many other good and useful contributions. The book is especially rich in contributions on nervous subjects Epilepsy, Hysteria and Traumatic Neuroses being given notice by various writers, and contains an exhaustive article on the Psychological Interpretation and Practical use of Hypnosis in the Diagnosis and treatment of Disease.

THE PRACTICAL MEDICINE SERIES (Volume IX, 1910.)

Skin and Venereal Diseases, by William L. Baum, M. D., Professor of Skin and Venereal Diseases, Chicago Post-Graduate Medical School and Harold N. Moyer, M. D., Chicago, Ill. Cloth, $1.25.

The Year Book Publishers, 40 Dearborn Street, Chicago.

REPRINTS.

The Journal desires to acknowledge receipt of reprints of articles of Drs. W. J. and C. H. Mayo, E. S. Judd, M. S. Henderson, Christopher Graham, Louis B. Wilson, Wm. Carpenter MacCarty, W. F. Braasch, Byrd C. Willis, H. S. Plummer, E. H. Beckham, Dudley W. Palmer, Justus Matthews, Donald C. Balfour, H. Z. Giffin and Donald Guthrie, of the staff of St. Mary's Hospital, Rochester, Minn. These reprints reflect the great amount of good work being done in Rochester and cover a large field of subjects.

DA COSTA'S MODERN SURGERY.

The New (6th) Edition, Greatly Enlarged.

Modern Surgery, General and Operative. By J. Chalmers DaCosta, M. D., Professor of Surgery and Clinical Surgery in the Jefferson Medical College, Philadelphia. Sixth Edition Greatly Enlarged, Octavo of 1502 pages, with 966 illustrations, some in colors. Philadelphia and London, W. B. Saunders Company, 1910. Cloth, $5.50 net; Half Morocco, $7.00 net.

This is one of the most complete works

on surgery in one volume published today and its contents are brought up to the present time in a thorough manner. The recent advancements in surgery of the blood vessels, brain and thoracic surgery are given attention and much of the brilliant work of the Mayo's, Murphy, Halstead, Cushing, Crile, Bier and Wright is incorporated in its pages.

The chapters on nerve and brain surgery and exophthalmic goiter are splendid and while the work abounds with descriptions of operations of various authorities, the author has given his views and reasons in a clear and convincing manner, on the same operations. He has also gone at length into the diagnosis of surgical affections making the work a text-book as well as clinical work.

Taking the work in its entirety it may be said to be one of the criterions among surgical works and as such will be welcomed by the student, general practitioner and surgeon.

PULMONARY TUBERCULOSIS AND ITS COMPLICATIONS.

By Sherman G. Bonney, M. D., Professor of Medicine, Denver and Gross Medical College, Denver, Colorado. Octavo of 955 pages, with 243 original illustrations, including 31 in colors and 73 X-Ray photographs.

Philadelphia and London. W. B. Saunders Company, 1910. Cloth, $7.00 net; Half Morocco, $8.50 net.

We have in this admirable work the last and best word as to Tuberculosis in its varied forms and manifestations. The author modestly disclaims intention to make the work "encyclopedic" in scope or of use to any but the general practitioner, but he has exceeded his intentions for he has presented a most thorough work on this great subject, a subject that is engaging the attention of the thinking people of the world whether engaged in medical pursuits or in other affairs.

With the subject completely in hand the author takes up its consideration from a practical standpoint; an enormous amount of space is devoted to the sanitary aspects, to climatic considerations and to the open air treatment.

The deductions in the volume are those of intelligent effort from the pen of one who lives in the tubercular center of the United States and its immensity testifies to the abundant material for observation in the locality in which he lives. There are many cuts and illustrations of sanitariums and open air institutions in the vicinity of Denver. The work devotes much attention to the causes of the spread of contagion in tenements and unsanitary surroundings and suggests means of prevention and treatment. The details as to treatment are highly valuable. This book should be read by every physician in the country and an intelligent following of its teachings will be of inestimable benefit to mankind.

MISCELLANEOUS

SPECIAL SYPHILIS NUMBER.

The Editors of the INTERSTATE MEDICAL JOURNAL, St. Louis, announce the publication of a symposium number on Syphilis for January.

The list of articles reads as follows:

The Influence of Syphilis on Civilization—*Wm. Osler, M. D., Oxford University.*

Present Status of the "Noguchi Test"—*Hidego Noguchi, M. D., New York.*

On the Means of Finding the Spirochaeta Pallida, with Special Reference to the India Ink Method. (From the Laboratory of the Michael Reese Hospital)—

J. S. Cohn, M. D., Chicago.

The History and Methods of Application of Ehrlich's Dioxydiamido-arseno-benzol. (From the Royal Institute for Experimental Therapeutics)—*Lewis Hart Marks, M. D., Frankfort, a. m.*

Recent Progress in the Treatment of Syphilis—*H. Hallopeau, M. D., Paris.*

Treatment of Syphilis with Ehrlich-Hata "606"—*Abr. L. Wolbarst, M. D., N. Y.*

Syphilis of the Nervous System—*Ernest Jones, M. D., Toronto.*

Syphilis and Pulmonary Tuberculosis—*Robert H. Babcock, M. D., Chicago.*

Syphilis as a Cause of Pauperism—*A. Ravogli, M. D., Cincinnati.*

Giant Cells in Syphilis—*John A. Fordyce, M. D., New York.*

Personal Observations with the Ehrlich-Hata Remedy "606"—*B. C. Corbus, M. D., Chicago.*

Syphilis and the Public—*Isadore Dyer, M. D., New Orleans.*

Sanitary Regulation of Prostitutes—*Prince A. Morrow, M. D., New York.*

In addition to the above, there will be four "Collective Abstracts" (critical reviews of recent literature in collective form) on (1) Ehrlich Hata "606", (2) the Cerebrospinal Fluid in Syphilis and Parasyphilitic Diseases. (3) Serum Diagnosis of Syphilis, (4) Diagnosis of the Osseous Lesions of Syphilis by the X-Ray.

A NEW LINE OF PARKE, DAVIS & COMPANY.

"Everything under the sun for physicians" might be suggested as a motto not inappropriate for Parke, Davis & Co. The thought is prompted by the recent incursion of the company into the field of surgical dressings. It was something like a year ago, if we mistake not, that Chloretone Gauze and Formidine Gauze were launched in modest fashion, the purpose evidently being to let them find their way into the medical armamentarium in the natural order of events rather than by artificial fostering. Their reception by the profession must have been gratifying, for the line soon began to expand. Now it numbers six gauzes and tapes, and we note a disposition on the part of the company to bring them more prominently to the attention of physicians. For this reason a word or two in explanation of them may not be out of place.

The line includes Chloretone Gauze, Formidine Gauze, Formidine Tape, Adrenalin Tape, Plain Tape, and Anesthone Tape. What has been said of the therapeutic properties of Chloretone, Formidine, Adrenalin and Anesthone (and most physicians are well acquainted with these products) is applicable to the surgical dressings. Chloretone Gauze applied to raw surfaces exerts an anesthetic and antiseptic action, promoting the comfort of the patient. It is markedly useful in extensive burns. Formidine Gauze takes the place of iodoform gauze. It is more actively antiseptic, does not stain the clothing, is non-toxic, and is practically odorless. Formidine Tape, which comes in two widths (1-2 inch and 1 1-2 inches) is used for packing cavities antiseptically. Adrenalin Tape, supplied in 1-2 and 1 1-2 inch widths, is serviceable in tamponing cavities to check hemorrhage. Plain Tape, which also comes in the two widths above mentioned, is used for packing and draining small wounds and cavities. Anesthone Tape is serviceable in the various forms of nasal hyperesthesia. All of the tapes are double selvaged and when removed from wounds do not leave short threads to cause irritation.

Parke, Davis & Co., issue a small pamphlet descriptive of their medicated gauzes and tapes. Physicians who have not received a copy are advised to write for one. The dressings are pretty generally carried in well-stocked pharmacies.

THE AMERICAN PROCTOLOGIC SOCIETY'S PRIZE FOR THE BEST ORIGINAL ESSAY ON ANY DISEASE OF THE COLON BY A GRADUATE OF (NOT A FELLOW OF THE SOCIETY) OR A SENIOR STUDENT IN ANY MEDICAL COLLEGE OF THE UNITED STATES OR CANADA.

The American Proctologic Society announces through its committee that the cash sum of $100.00 will be awarded, as soon as possible in 1901, to the author of the best original essay on any disease of the colon in competition for the above prize.

Essays must be submitted, to the Secretary of the committee, on or before May 10, 1911. The address of the Secretary is given below, to whom all communications should be addressed.

Each essay must be typewritten, *designated by a motto or device, and without signature or any other indication of its authorship, and be accompanied by a separate sealed envelope, having on its outside only the motto or device contained on the essay, and within the name, the motto or device used on the essay, and, the address of the author.* No envelope will be opened except that which accompanies the successful essay.

The committee will return the unsuccessful essays, if reclaimed by their writers within six months, provided return postage accompanies the application.

The committee reserves the right not to make an award if no essay submitted is considered worthy of the prize.

The competition is open to graduates of medicine, (not fellows of the Society) and to members of the senior classes of all colleges in the United States or Canada.

The object of the prize and competition is to stimulate an increased interest in, and knowledge of Proctology.

The committee shall have full control of awarding the prize and the publication of the prize essay, and it shall be the property of the American Proctologic Society. It may be published in the Transactions of the Society and also as a separate issue if deemed expedient. The committee may increase its membership if deemed advisable.

DR. DWIGHT H. MURRAY, Chairman,

DR. SAMUEL T. EARLE,

DR. JEROME M. LYNCH,

DR. ALOIS B. GRAHAM,

DR. LEWIS, H. ADLER, Jr., Secretary.

1610 Arch St., Philadelphia, Pa.

FOR SALE.

$2,500.00 practice free to purchaser of four room residence, town of 200 on the Rock Island Railway, good country and roads, no opposition, nearest competition is 7 and 12 miles.

M. SHADID, M. D., Stecker Okla.

A·TRIUMPH IN PILL-MAKING.

Parke, Davis & Co. confess that their soft-mass pill, which is now receiving so much favorable attention from the medical world, was for a long time a "hard nut" to crack. They had set out to produce by the soft-mass process a pill that should be a credit to their house and to manufacturing pharmacy. The task at first seemed simple enough. Here, as elsewhere, theory and practice were at variance. As a matter of fact, a good deal of experimentation had to be done. Time was consumed. Money was expended. In the end, of course, ingenuity triumphed.

In structure the soft-mass pill, as manufactured by Parke, Davis & Co., consists of a plastic mass encompassed by a thin, soluble chocolate coating. It may be flattened between the thumb and finger like a piece of putty. An important advantage of the soft-mass pill is the readiness with which it dissolves or disintegrates in the digestive

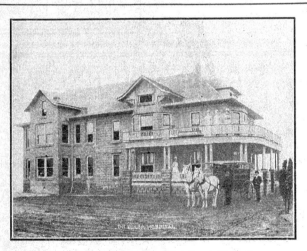

tract. Another commendable feature is that, no heat being applied in the process, such volatile substances as camphor, the valerianates, the essential oils, etc., are not dissipated, so that any pill embodying one or more of these substances may be depended upon to contain just what the label says it contains.

Parke, Davis & Co., are putting out close to thirty formulas by the soft-mass process —all of them listed, we believe, in advertisements now appearing in the medical press. Practitioners under whose eyes these announcements do not happen to fall may profitably write the company, at its home offices in Detroit, for a copy of a recently issued folder on "Soft-Mass Pills," which contains titles and complete formulas of all the pills now manufactured by Parke, Davis & Co. under the process referred to, together with some other important information.

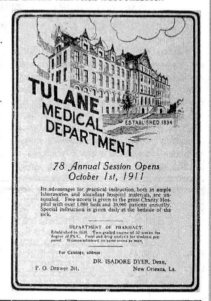
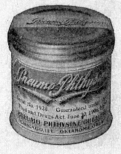

DIRECTORY OF OFFICERS AND SECTION CHAIRMAN OF THE OKLAHOMA STATE MEDICAL ASSOCIATION.

President—Dr. D. A. Myers, Lawton.

Vice-Presidents—First, Dr. C. L. Reeder, Tulsa; Second, Dr. H. M. Williams, Wellston; Third, Dr. James L. Shuler, Durant.

Secretary - Treasurer — Dr. Claude A. Thompson, Muskogee.

Delegates to American Medical Association, 1911-1912—Dr. Chas. R. Hume, Anadarko; Dr. Walter E. Wright, Tulsa.

Section Chairman.

Surgery—Dr. Ross Grosshart, Tulsa.

Medicine—Dr. J. H. Scott, Shawnee.

Mental and Nervous Diseases—Dr. F. B. Erwin, Norman.

Ediatrics—Dr. W. G. Little, Okmulgee.

Eye, Ear, Nose and Throat—Dr. Milton K. Thompson, Muskogee.

Gynecology and Obstetrics—Dr. B. W. Freer, Nowata.

Section on Pathology—Dr. Elizabeth Melvin, Guthrie.

For Councillors see first page.

Place of meeting, Muskogee, May 9, 10 and 11, 1911.

STANDING COMMITTEES OKLAHOMA STATE MEDICAL ASSOCIATION.

On Public Policy and Legislation.

Dr. J. C. Mahr, Oklahoma City.

Dr. C. S. Bobo, Norman.

Dr. D. A. Myers, Lawton.

Dr. C. A. Thompson, Muskogee.

MEMBER OF THE NATIONAL LEGISLATIVE COUNCIL OF THE AMERICAN MEDICAL ASSOCIATION.

Dr. J. M. Byrum, Shawnee, Oklahoma.

COMMITTEE ON NECROLOGY.

Dr. E. S. Ferguson, Oklahoma City.

Dr. L. T. Gooch, Lawton.

Dr. Chas. Blickensderfer, Shawnee.

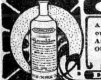

OFFICERS OF COUNTY SOCIETIES

COUNTY	PRESIDENT	SECRETARY
Atoka	J. B. Clark, Coalgate	T. H. Briggs, Atoka
Alfalfa	Z. J. Clark, Cherokee	G. A. Nylund, Helena
Adair	T. S. Williams, Stilwell	C. M. Robinson, Stilwell
Bryan	J. L. Shuler, Durant	D. Armstrong, Mead
Blaine	D. F. Stough, Geary	J. L. Campbell, Watonga
Beckham	J. M. McComas, Elk City	G. Pinnell, Erick
Coal	J. B. Clark, Coalgate	T. H. Briggs, Atoka
Choctaw	E. B. Askew, Hugo	J. C. Ellis, Hugo
Custer	J. Matt Gordon, Weatherford	O. H. Parker, Custer
Caddo	W. W. Gill, Gracemont	Chas. R. Hume, Anadarko
Cleveland	John D. McLaren, Norman	A. C. Hirschfield, Norman
Commanche	T. L. Gooch, Lawton	D. A. Myers, Lawton
Carter	E. A. Ballard, Lone Grove	C. B. Clark, Ardmore
Craig	C. P. Bell, Welch	Louis Bagby, Vinita
Creek	O. C. Coppedge, Bristow	C. L. McCallum, Sapulpa
Canadian	D. P. Richardson, Union City	Jas. T. Riley, El Reno
Cherokee	W. G. Blake, Tahlequah	C. A. Peterson, Tahlequah
Ellis	H. W. Hubbell, Arnett	John F. Sturdivant, Arnett
Garfield	J. H. Barnes, Enid	Julian Field, Enid
Grady	Walter Penquite, Chickasha	Martha Bledsoe, Chickasha
Garvin	W. C. High, Maysville	N. H. Lindsey, Pauls Valley
Greer	M. M. DeArman, Mangum	T. J. Dodson, Mangum
Haskell	S. E. Mitchell, Stigler	F. A. Fannin, Stigler
Hughes	A. L. Davenport, Holdenville	A. M. Butts, Holdenville
Jackson	J. W. Echols, Altus	L. A. Hankins, Altus
Jefferson	F. W. Ewing, Terrall	T. E. Ashinhurst, Waurika
Kay	W. A. T. Robinson, Ponca City	A. S. Risser, Blackwell
Kingfisher	C. W. Fiske, Kingfisher	C. O. Gose, Hennessey
Kiowa	G. W. Stewart, Hobart	J. M. Bonham, Hobart
Logan	E. O. Barker, Guthrie	R. V. Smith, Guthrie
Lincoln	C. M. Morgan, Chandler	E. F. Hurlburt, Chandler
Love	B. D. Woodson, Monroe	R. L. Morrison, Poteau
LeFlore	T. J. Jackson, Marsden	B. S. Gardner, Marietta
Mayes	E. L. Pierce, Salina	F. S. King, Pryor
Major	B. F. Johnson, Fairview	Elsie L. Specht, Rusk
Muskogee	H. C. Rogers, Muskogee	H. T. Ballantine, Muskogee
McIntosh	W. A. Tolleson, Eufaula	M. R. Nowlin, Eufaula
McLain	G. S. Barger, Wayne	G. M. Tralle, Purcell
Murray	W. H. Powell, Palmer	J. A. Adams, Sulphur
Marshall	W. L. Davis, Kingston	John A. Haynie, Aylesworth
McCurtain	A. S. Grayden, Idabell	W. B. McCaskill, Idabell
Nowata	L. T. Stother, Nowata	J. R. Collins, Nowata
Okmulgee	Wm. Cott, Okmulgee	W. G. Little, Okmulgee
Okfuskee	G. A. Reber, Okemah	Benton Lovelady, Okemah
Oklahoma	A. A. Will, Oklahoma City	W. R. Bevan, Oklahoma City
Payne	C. H. Beach, Glencoe	D. F. Janeway, Stillwater
Pottawatomie	T. D. Rowland, Shawnee	G. S. Baxter, Shawnee
Pittsburg	R. I. Bond, Hartshorne	H. E. Williams, McAlester
Pontotoc		
Pushmataha		
Rogers	W. F. Hays, Claremore	A. Lerskov, Claremore
Seminole	W. L. Knight, Wewoka	M. M. Turlington, Seminole
Roger Mills		
Sequoyah	A. A. Hicks, Muldrow	M. D. Carnell, Sallisaw
Stephens	R. L. Montgomery, Marlow	D. Long, Duncan
Texas	Jas. M. McMillan, Goodwell	R. B. Hayes, Guymon
Tulsa	G. H. Butler, Tulsa	W. E. Wright, Tulsa
Tillman	F. G. Priestly, Frederick	A. B. Fair, Frederick
Washington	G. F. Woodring, Bartlesville	W. E. Rammell, Bartlesville
Washita	J. W. Kerly, Cordell	A. H. Bungardt, Cordell
Wagoner	F. W. Smith, Wagoner	J. L. Reich, Wagoner

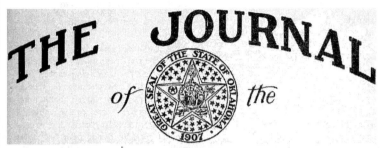

Oklahoma State Medical Association.

| VOL III. | MUSKOGEE, OKLAHOMA, FEBRUARY, 1911. | NO 9 |

DR. CLAUDE A. THOMPSON, Editor-in-Chief.

ASSOCIATE EDITORS AND COUNCILLORS.

DR. J. A. WALKER, Shawnee.
DR. CHARLES R. HUME, Anadarko.
DR. F. R. SUTTON, Bartlesville.
DR. I. W. ROBERTSON, Dustin.
DR. J. S. FULTON, Atoka.

DR. JOHN W. DUKE, Guthrie.
DR. A. B. FAIR, Frederick.
DR. W. G. BLAKE, Tahlequah.
DR. H. P. WILSON, Wynnewood.
DR. J. H. BARNES, Enid.

Entered at the Postoffice at Muskogee, Oklahoma, as second class mail matter, July 28, 1910.

This is the Official Journal of the Oklahoma State Medical Association All communications should be addressed to the Journal of the Oklahoma State Medical Association, English Block, Muskogee, Oklahoma.

SOME DISORDERS OF SLEEP.

BY DR. A. D. YOUNG, PROFESSOR NERVOUS AND MENTAL DISEASES, MEDICAL DEPARTMENT
UNIVERSITY OF OKLAHOMA, OKLAHOMA CITY, OKLA.

The disturbances of sleep are mainly symptomatic; but they frequently reach such proportions as to attain almost the dignity of a disease and it is then that the services of a physician are required.

Of the physiology of sleep, though it is more necessary to life than food, little is known. During sleep there is muscular relaxtion, the respiration is superficial, the lids are closed over the upturned eyeballs and the appearance is one of repose. None of the mental or physical functions are in complete abeyance. It is believed by many, myself included, that dreamless sleep never occurs, but only such dreams as are vividly impressed upon the mind of the individual, or such that occur during light slumber, are remembered. About one-seventh as much air is inspired during sleep as during wakefulness. Breathing is superficial, the diaphragm acting but slightly and the respiratory pause is absent. There are marked changes in the circulatory system. The superficial circulation is increased often producing a flushed condition of the skin. The brain in a measure is anaemic. The circulatory changes occur in a precise manner, reaching their maximum in a hour or two then gradually subsiding until the waking moment. Thus it is that the first few hours of sleep are the profoundest and therefore the most restful. The tendency to night-sweats and the ease with which one becomes chilled attest the increased activity of the skin. Just before and during the first moments of sleep, the reflexes are exagerated thus accounting for the sudden movements when one is dropping off to sleep. The pupils of the eyes are contracted according to the depth of slumber.

Infants should sleep most of the twenty-four hours—adults eight or ten. Old people seldom enjoy continuous sleep, but maintain a fair average by means of frequent naps during both night and day. The peculiarities of the individual, his environments and mode of living must determine the required amount of sleep every case.

The foregoing remarks pertain to persons in health and any considerable departure from these conditions require the advice of a physician. The most frequent disorder of sleep is called insomnia, which is the inability to obtain the requisite amount of sleep and is a symptomatic condition. The causes of insomnia are numerous. In fact any deviation from health may cause disturbances of sleep; but a bad sleep habit once established tends to persist notwithstanding the corrections of the conditions from which it had its rise. Many persons are naturally light sleepers and any slight jar or noise may be sufficient to awake them. Hunger over eating tea, coffee, tobacco, alcohol, lead-poisining malaria, syphilis, fevers, cardiac disease, physical disturbance, neurasthenia, worry, grief, old age and over study, are among the principle causes of sleeplessness.

Some persons readily fall asleep but awake soon after midnight and lie awake until morning. Others complain of not being able to sleep the first part of the night, while another class cannot obtain continous rest but sleep or lie awake at intervals throughout the night. Patients of this kind are prone to exagerate the amount of sleeplessness and if watch is kept are found to rest very well. Much loss of sleep is manifested by a weary look, loss of courage, and an irritable mental state. The appetite is poor, bowels constipated,

tongue coated and the secretions are sluggish.

Since insomnia is merely a symptomatic condition, the treatment must be directed to the removal of the underlying cause. The examination of the patient must omit nothing, heridity, personal history, habits, enviroment, occupation, and present physical condition must be investigated. A cure cannot be expected by means of a few doses of medicine and treatment will avail nothing without the co-operation of the patient. Any heriditory stigma so far as possible must be removed. If insomnia is the result of a previous sickness the removal of the obstacle will bring about the desired result. Likewise if it is the continuance of a bad sleep habit the treatment is obvious. Should the surroundings or occupation of the individual be at fault they must be modified and the physical condition be put in order. Among the general means to be employed is a warm bath taken quietly at bed time and alcohol sponge, cold pack or hot lemonade. The hot bath flushes the skin and produces the circulatory changes necessary for sleep. Large doses of whiskey are not advisable, although efficient for a night or two. The stomach should be neither empty nor over loaded. The bladder should be evacuated just before retiring. A preliminary feeling of drowsiness is physiological and should be cultivated. Any drug that sufficiently masters the organism is pernicious, but hypnotics are sometimes necessary.

They do good principally by re-establishing the sleep habit. My asylum experience has convinced me that chloral is the most reliable. Its effects are quickly obtained; it should be given one-half hour before retiring. Trional is slower in its action, Bartholow to the contrary not withstanding and is best exhibited in those cases characterized by restlessness in the latter part of the night. It should be given at bed time and then reaches its maximum at the proper period. I do not believe it dangerous to life, even in large doses. One of my patients, at the Illinois Central Insane Hospital, a physician by the way, saved his nightly dose of trinol until he had sixty grains and took it all at one dose with suicidal intent. He obtained a good night's rest, and except a feeling of drowsiness the next day was as well as usual. Some patients improve after a change of scene and are most benefited by a lake or sea voyage as it is devoid of sight seeing and the excitement incident to travel by rail. It is well to bear in mind that insomnia is often the initial symptom of approaching insanity.

In somnambulisam the person acts his part of a dream. It may be partial or complete by which is meant talking or walking during sleep. The motor apparatus is awake and responsive to the mind and there is a peculiar increase in the subjective powers of the sleep walker. Often there is great sensitiveness and analgesia combined The patient takes notice of only those things that pertain to his dream story and when awakening has no recollection of his acts although he may repeat the same performance on several successive nights. The feeling of double consciousness is nothing more than the misty remembrance of a previous attack of somnambulism and gives rise to the belief in a few weak minds of supposed scanty recollections of a previous incarnation. Sleep walking is a neurotic stigma and makes its appearance usually about puberty. The individual attack is sometimes traceable to a preceding mental state. The mere suggestion of sleep walking in the discussion of the subject has been followed by the act. Often the patient continues the occupation in which he was engaged just before retiring. I remember one young man who having taken a bath just before retiring no sooner fell asleep than he arose and insisted on repeating the act. It is needless to say the cold water soon restored him to a knowledge of his surround-

ings. The treatment of this condition should be broad enough to cover the neuropathic make-up of the patient and should be directed principally to the mental element. In these with a minor degree of self control a strong suggestion is often sufficient to prevent the attack. In children a cold spinal sponge accompanied by the announcement that it is to prevent walking in the sleep or a promise of reward will be sufficient. A dash of cold water or a breath of fresh air is generally effective in arousing the patient but in highly nervous children some milder method should be employed. Adult cases often resist all treatment and precautions must be taken each night to prevent accidents.

Dreams are perfectly physiological, but are frequently of special medical significance. Persons affected with hysteria neutashenia or melancholia seldom have pleasant dreams such as are enjoyed by well and contented persons. The former complain constantly of dreams of distressful incidents, a fact that is due to their light slumber, dreams being then more readily remembered. Many persons with a lowered physical and mental state are tormented by some particular dreams occurring several times the same night or on different nights. Janel says. "The influence of a terrifying dream in hysteria may equal a severe mental shock in the waking moments and may be the basis of a hysterical idea leading to paralysis, anaestheia, contractures or assertions of attempts upon chastity." In hysteria also the features of a dream may be prospected for an hour or more after the person becomes awake, thus constituting a delirious accident.

Night terrors is confined to children. The little patient suddenly starts from a sound sleep, screams and clings to its mother, uttering terrified cries and endeavoring to escape from wild animals or some disagreeable person. They may even go so far as to run about the room, climb on the furniture, etc. After a few moments the excitement subsides and the child, returning to sleep awakes the next morning without any knowledge of what has occurred. Night mare is not true pavor nocturnus. True night terror is of serious import, often fortelling apelipsy. Some investigations regard it as a true neurosis. Indigestion, over eating and an excessively tired body give rise to night mare. The patient has a feeling of suffication as if some great weight were on the chest. At such moments he suspends respiration and awakes with a start.

Nocturnal enuresis has aptly been termed somnambulism of the cord. This statement refers to that class of patients who dreaming that they are in a convenient place to urinate proceed to do so. Frequently if aroused and made to urinate, the child immediately, probably though suggestion repeats the act upon returning to bed. In the treatment of this most troublesome condition the first thing in order is attention to the general health and the quieting of nervous excitability. The urine should be frequently voided and what is more important of all a definite suggestion of self control should be installed into the mind of the patient. Elevation of the foot of the bed does good by gravitating the urine from the neck of the bladder. Belladonna should be given to reduce vesical irritability and the urine should be rendered unirritating by the use of proper remedies. A strong mental impression is of value. In the New York Medical Journal, of July 11, '96. Pendergast mentions the fact that he cured seventy out of 80 cases in a boys orphanage by a cold spinal sponge and a brisk rubbing down just before going to bed. I secured perfect results by similar treatment in a case during the past winter.

Narcolepsy is the condition in which the patient repeatedly goes to sleep during the day. It is caused by syphilis, diabetes, obesity, brain disease and is one of the accidents of hysteria. It may be an epileptic equivalent and several members of the same family may be thus affected. Treatment is removal of the cause if possible and the breaking up of the habit. Caffiene and nitro glycerine are useful in controlling the cerebral circulation. I have at present under treatment a patient who presents this symptom due to cerebral syphilis.

Hypnotisim is mentioned only to condemn it. As to the different methods of bringing it about. I shall have to refer you to books upon that subject. I do not care to discuss it at this time. Suffice it to say that dispite the extravagant claims made for it, it is yet of little service to the physician. In hysteria it is a two edged sword, one delusion may be removed only to be replaced by another such a one as needed ready. In general the number of susceptibles is so small that its general use is impossible.

A fair understanding of the part suggestion plays in therapeutics is one of the recent achievements of the most progressive medical needs.

DIFFICULT SURGICAL CASES.

BY V. BERRY, M. D., OKMULGEE, OKLAHOMA

There is perhaps no surgeon who does not feel grateful at the fortunate outcome of his difficult cases. I deem two of mine of sufficient interest to report in a general way.

The first patient was a negro woman, about 46 years old, from whom I removed a small dermoid tumor by abdominal section in October, 1908. She was rather hysterical and failing to recover her general health came to my office during the spring of 1909, asking the removal of the uterus.

After an examination which revealed a small, rather fixed uterus, general pelvic tenderness, which I believed partly hysterical as no marked pathological lesion was distinguishable, I advised against an operation. I might here mention the cessation of menstruation, of over two years previous. She left the office rather dissatisfied, and in two months was called to see her again and found she had been in bed for several weeks, and claimed to be unable to get up or walk without assistance.

She begged for an operation and I finally consented, to satisfy her mind more than any thing else for she seemed to have an insane delusion that she would never get up again unless the operation was performed. In July, 1909, I did a rapid vaginal hysterectomy by Pryors hemisection, completing the operation in about twenty-four minutes, and either incised, or tore a small opening in the posterior bladder wall. I immediately closed it with fine, parafined silk thread. Her progress was without event, except on the fifth day the bladder opening gave way. She was out of bed in ten days, and in four weeks I made an effort to close the fistula in the bladder. On introducing a broad, short bladed vaginal retractor I found a small fistulous sinus leading through dense sar tissue, which on separation revealed an opening rather high up on the posterior bladder wall, rather elongated transversely, about one fourth inch in its longest diameter. It was extremely difficult to pare the edges, in fact almost impossible, and even more difficult to pass sutures properly. As in the former closure I used fine silk, boiled in parafine, which makes a most excellent non-absorbable suture material. It took about fifty minutes to complete the operation, including the placing of a soft rubber catheter in the bladder for continuous drainage. To make a long story short the opening failed to heal, and began leaking on the third day.

I now had her get out of bed in a few days, and endeavored to get her in the best condition possible as to general health, and in October, following, made another effort at closure of the fistula. In addition to my former technique I made a button-hole opening into the bladder through the vesico-vaginal septum about two inches below the fistula. After paring and closing the fistula which was even more difficult than the former effort, I stitched a soft rubber drain tube into the button-hole opening to get free urinary drainage, and awaited results, and I only had four days to wait, for the whole thing gave way again; and I must confess to great mortification. From the repeated parings of the wound edges the hole was now very large, probably one fourth by one half inch. I decided to drop all efforts for several months, and then try again. In December she went to one of the larger cities of the state and was admitted into a hospital. The attending surgeon assured her he could close the fistula, and proceeded to do so after she had spent several days recuperating, but like Bangno's ghost, that fistula "would not down." She became thoroughly discouraged, and says the doctor did too. Any how she "came home to die," to use her own expression. On my return from post graduate studies in New Orleans, I received a note telling of her pitiable condition, and asking me to see her at once. On receipt of the message I arranged with Dr. Artz, of Beggs, in the vicinity of which the patient lived to meet me April 3rd, 1910, with the intention of closing the fistula through an abdominal opening, which we did as follows:

Patient was placed under ether, and after opening the abdomen under the strictest aseptic precautions, I had Dr. Artz place his left index finger in the vagina, and I then proceeded to dissect loose the bladder with Mayo's blunt scissors, and by brushing away the tissues with gauze stretched over my fingers. After tedious, and cautious maneouvers the bladder was finally released and brought forward as far as possible, which was not very far, and the edges of the bladder wound thoroughly pared. I then carefully, and accurately placed running suture of fine parafined silk along the full length of the wound, going about three sixteenths of an inch beyond the angles, and then doubled back and run another row to the point of beginning, continuous lembert-cozerney. I now placed a sheet of omentum over the wound and stitched it in three or four places, placed a loose gauze vaginal drain which came barely through the *cul de sac,* but did not touch the bladder wound, closed the abdomen by tier sutures, placed a Pezzer catheter in the bladder and put to bed. The bladder was washed daily under very low pressure with boric acid solution through the catheter, and on the eighth day the catheter was removed, the vaginal gauze drain having been removed the third day and I am gratified to say the result was perfect closure. I can say without boasting that from the standpoint of manual dextrity such a case as this requires a high degree of skill, and he who gets results is, I think, entitled to some self congratulation. Absolute asepsis, accurate, skillfully placed sutures after properly denuding the tissue, which can only be done by the aid of an efficient assistant are the keys to success. I do not believe it possible to have successfully closed this wound through the vagina.

My second case is one of compound, comminuted fracture of the tibia, and simple fracture of the fibula in the left leg of a woman 35 years old, which occurred M ay 24th, 1910. She was riding on the running gear of a farm wagon when her leg was caught on a stump by the break beam and both the tibia and fibula broken at about the juncture of the lower and middle third, the sharp, jagged end of the tibia protruding through the skin. Her husband pulled on the foot, pulling the bone back into the soft tissues without any preliminary cleansing of the wound, and several hours later called a physician to set the limb. I might here add that her physician is a thoroughly posted, and completent man, and that after cleansing the limb it was dressed in the usual manner. For several weeks it seemed union, and recovery would result. However infection, with necrosis finally eliminated all prospects of success, and the case was referred to myself for amputation, or an effort at union as seemed most feasable. I placed her in the hospital, and on the 24th day of July, one of the hottest days of the year, cut down to the seat of fracture over the anterior tibial border and found necrosis of both the upper and lower fragments, the lower one involved almost to the joint, the rapidity of the process being one to the soft, spongy bone near the joint. There was no union at all of the fibula, though I did not open the soft process being due to the soft, spongy bone tissues to it. After peeling the periosteum well away from the bone, I sawed off the upper fragment of the tibia well above necrosed tissue. Then with Farabeauf's curved bone curette cut away all necrosed bone to sound bone. Oozing both from soft tissues and the bone canal was profuse, and required firm packing for its arrest. The wound was filled with Claudiu's solution of iodine before packing, and after packing was firmly bandaged and put in flexible splints and fracture box. Forty-eight hours later all packing was removed, blood clots and debris thoroughly removed by irrigation with saline solution, and the wound repeatedly swabbed out with Claudiu's iodine solution, packed lightly and dressed. I now dressed every other day as follows, for two weeks:

Removed packing, poured wound full of

50 per cent. alcohol two or three times and mopped dry, then filled with 50 per cent. Claudiu's solution and mopped dry again, packed lightly with gauze wet with iodine solution and dressed with plain sterile gauze. In addition the limb was thoroughly cleansed with alcohol over a wide area from the wound, and changed in a few days from the fracture box to a long perforated posterior tin splint, which included the foot and thigh, there being a hinge joint at the knee. August 7th, the wound was thoroughly cleansed and dried out as above outlined, and the following preparation known as Mosetig's bone filling, introduced by Mosetig-Moorhoaf, of Vienna, poured in the cavity: iodoform 60 grains, spermaceti wax 40 grains, and oil of sesame 40 grains, all by weight. Place all in a small glass, or large test tube and sterilize for ten, or fifteen minutes. Then let stand twelve hours or more and resterilize for ten minutes again, and when just warm enough to pour—not hot—fill the cavity after preparing as above directed. Be sure the cavity is well dried out. In my case I had firm traction made on the foot and after filling the cavity let the limb relax which allowed a very firm filling between the ends of the bones. I now dressed the wound every day, smearing the gauze next the wound with oxide of zinc ointment to prevent the granulations growing into the meshes. I might here say I know of no method by which we can get an aseptic wound so quickly, together with such an abundance of healthy granulation tissue as by this method of swabbing with weak alcohol and iodine solutions.

With correct surgical application you can expect a healthy, aseptic wound in two weeks or less. The results in this case are little short of marvelous. There has never been a particle of discharge from the day the "bone filling" was applied except the discharge from the graulations of the soft tissues. All bone is completely covered, and the cavity is entirely obliterated (Aug. 17th,) with embryonic cells, and the only thing necessary to discharge the case with a sound limb is sufficient time for ossification, and perhaps a few skin grafts to cover the skin wound. When we consider the unhappy results of older methods of treating such cases in which, if the limb was not amputated a fistula persisted for years, with an almost useless limb, we can begin to appreciate the marvelous advance made by surgery in our own time. However there is an absolute and fixed price to be paid for such a result: Absolute sterilization of everything that comes in contact with the wound—dressings, instruments, hands. I doubt if success could be attained without the use of rubber gloves. All dressings and mops should be handled with sterile forceps where possible. The naked hands must never come in contact with the wound at any time. To facilitate dressing after putting in the "bone filling" I bandaged as follows: the foot was bandaged separately allowing the bandage to come within one inch of the wound. I then applied a bandage to the thigh, letting it come below the knee to within one inch of the upper end of the wound. That gave a firmly fixed limb with the wound entirely uncovered. Over this I placed a copious dressing of gauze which easily takes up all the discharge of twenty-four hours without soiling the permanent dressings above and below the wound. By this means I have been enabled to continuously change the dressings without removing the limb from the splint, or disturbing the dressings in any way whatever.

In conclusion I would say: given a patient with power of resistence near normal, with a compound fracture as here described, I believe any physician who would amputate without first making an effort to save the limb should be subject to severe censure. I now recall amputating just such a limb sixteen years ago. Patience is one of the prime requisites, but the results are well worth the price.

The tin splint was an ordinary trough shaped affair, perforated for ventilation, made by the local tinner at a cost of fifty cents, and is fully the equal in efficiency to an elaborate affair costing ten dollars at the instrument stores. It is applied well padded with cotton, and causes no discomfort whatever. There is a wooden foot piece by means of which the foot is rendered immovable. Feb., 1911, this patient is enjoying a useful limb as regenaration of excised bone is perfect.

THRUSH

BY DR. W. L. DAVIS, KINGSTON, OKLAHOMA

Gentlemen· In writing an article on this symptom which is ordinarily considered a harmless disorder, I hardly know how to proceed in a manner that will impress upon you the importance of giving due attention to the underlying conditions of which thrush is, with few exceptions, a symptom. Later on in this paper we shall discuss thrush as a primary disease. It is as ordinarily supposed an innocent disease of infancy, but sometimes ordinary types of the affection becomes difficult and dangerous, and generally because of some dangerous underlying pathological condition which, if we are careless in our examination, we may fail to detect. Hence we have that serious condition which sometimes make us careless general practitioners sit up and take notice. It is too often the case that after we are forced to recognize the seriousness of the situation, we are so far out at sea and in such deep water that we hardly know which way to turn to reach the land. Consequently we flounder about in our unpleasant situation and by and by our little patient dies and the mother says, "Dr. So-And-So is no good, he can't even kuore the thrash for he let it go plum through my baby and it died."

Now the idea I wish to convey is this— that any ailment however trivial it may seem if called to the attention of the physician should be considered important enough by him to be thoroughly investigated, a proper diagnosis made, and the underlying conditions carefully considered and prompt and proper line of treatment instituted and energetically carried out until the trouble is over. If we will take the time to make a painstaking and careful examination and look carefully after the little details of the case and carefully consider and plan the treatment (preventive, hyegeinic, dietetic, and medicinal), we shall oftimes or at least sometimes be spared the chagrin of loosing a patient with what is considered by the laity and general public to be a disease that is very amenable to treatment.

The duration of thrush varies according to the nature of the primary disease which it complicates. In young infants that have indigestion or slight gastro-intestinal catarrh, it is quickly cured by proper local treatment if the nutriment given be of the proper kind and the stomach and intestines be restored to their normal condition, however this advice is easier given than carried out. Our success in treatment will depend on our being able to determine the causitive factors in each case· These will often be found somewhere besides in the mouth. Hence we must not fall into the bad habit of making a careless and hurried examination, prescribing a little mouthwash, passing the patient by, and giving no thought to the underlying conditions which may later on make for us a serious and difficult case to treat. Thrush is a bad omen if the tongue and buccal surfaces be dry, red, and highly injected; the coating of the tongue be brownish in color, the infant fretful with the appearance of suffering on its face and a progressive loss of flesh. Such symptoms indicate in most cases a fatal form of gastro-intestinal catarrh. I wish again to impress upon you that it is not the common or ordinary forms of most diseases that tax our skill and give us trouble, but the severe and difficult ones that sometimes develops from the ordinary and harmless ones. This is especially unpleasant to the physician when he has been prescribing a mouthwash for a case of thrush, and is ultimately brought up against a fatal case of gastro-intestinal catarrh. We should always keep our eyes open and be thorough and careful in our examination and madication. This holds good with all patients but more so with infants, as it is almost as important for us to know what not to give as well as what to give. Each one of our cases is a case unto itself and demands our serious consideration. We must not make our examinations and write our prescriptions in a careless, half-hearted manner, but go into every little detail of each case and write our prescriptions according to the results of a thorough examination. If we will adopt this rule in each and every case, our results and our own personal satisfaction will amply repay us for the extra trouble. The laity is not slow to catch on, if we are thorough in our work.

Definition—Thrush is a specific infectious fungus disease of the oral mucus membranes. It is associated with or caused by the odium albicans. Some authorities say that it is due to the manilia candida. This last fungus grows upon mouldy wood, sweet fruits, lives in the air of rooms, clings to dirty rubber nipples and to the nipples of the breast, and in this way reach the mouth of infants who are otherwise healthy thus constituting the exceptions in which thrush is a primary disease.

Causes—The development of the thrush fungus is promoted and favored by all those conditions which are designed as unhygeinic, debilitated conditions of the general system, by neglecting to rinse and cleanse the mouth after nursing or bottle-feeding.

Age—Infancy with its concommittent gastro-intestinal disorders and catarrhal or acid condition of the oral gastric or intestinal mucosa   Even slight gastro-intestinal disturbances favor the growth of the fungus and it spreads very rapidly in debilitated or atrophic children. Diarrhoea, vomiting, and prostration which so often go hand-in-hand are probably not sequelae but are the active underlying causes of the disease. The cachectic states such as the last stages of consumption, cancer, diabetes, brights disease, and the late stages of low typhoid fevers. These are about the only conditions in which thrush will attack adults and when it makes its appearance in any of the above mentioned states, it usually means the beginning of the end.

Forms—Henoch recognizes two forms of the affection. First: isolated, white slightly elevated firmly adherent deposits in the form of dots and maculae which are situated upon the unaltered mucus membrane of the lips, tongue and cheeks and particularly in the folds between the lips and gums and between the cheeks and the alveolar borders. They differ from particles of coagulated milk, as they are easily removed while the apthous deposits are difficult to remove and often followed by bleeding. This the form usually seen in otherwise healthy children who are not kept very clean. Second: The whole mucus membrane of the mouth down to the pharynx is dark red, very dry, and covered with numerous white round or irregular shaped puncta or maculae which here and there are confluent and very painful during the act of nursing. Later on large white membranes may form covering the tongue, cheeks, and hard palate. This is especially liable to occur in debilitated conditions from gastro-intestinal or other diseases. The spots may be dirty, gray or yellowish instead of white and adhere more and more firmly the longer they persist. This form is more serious than the first mentioned.

Diagnosis—Milk curds, apthous stomatitis and diptheritic stomatitis only are to be considered. The child's grandmother will often have the diagnosis made for us by the time we arrive and will proceed to tell us in about the following language: "Doctor the baby has a bad case of the thrash, we have done every thing we knowed to do for it, we have been using honey and borax in its mouth and ever thing the neighbors told us to do, we got Timothy Ticklebritches who never saw his daddy to come and blow in the baby's mouth, they say he has never been knowed to fail to kuore the thrash, but this baby seems to be getting worser all the time, so we decided to send for you" The physician will note that the grandmother is correct in regard to the diagnosis and has recognized the danger signals but utterly failed to recognize from whence they came. Right here and now is a beautiful place for him to deliver to the kind-hearted old lady a short lecture in regard to superstitious remedies to which many lives have been sacrificed.

Prognosis—Good if promptly and properly treated and not accompanying some serious constitutional disturbance

Treatment—Here preventive measures assume a very important role. The very best plan of treatment is to prevent it if possible, though this is often out of the question. The time to begin preventive measures is when the baby is born. The following is a good form of instructions to give the mother: A large handful of boric acid is sewed up in a bag of cheese-cloth and placed in a clean fruit jar filled with boiling water and thoroughly shaken, after standing for a while a clear saturated solution of boric acid results. Some of this may be poured out in a clean glass and used

to cleanse the baby's mouth and the mother's nipples both before and after nursing. The following is the plan which I use: Some absorbant cotton is wrapped about the fore finger, lay the child across the lap face downward and thoroughly cleanse his mouth with the cotton dipped in the solution of boric acid. By placing him face downward, none of the solution is swallowed, however if it is no harm is done. This position is the one or similar to the one recommended by Kerley in performing the oral toilet of a child suffering with diphtheria. The mother's nipples are also cleansed with the same solution, and dried. Another good cleansing solution for the mother's nipples is equal parts of the boric acid solution and alcohol giving time for the alcohol to evaporate before allowing the child to nurse. This cleansing process may be gone through with both before and after nursing or as the attending physician sees fit. If nursing bottles are used, the nipples should be habitually kept in a covered glass of the boric acid solution. The bottles should receive the same scrupulous care also. If the family can be made to see the importance of these preventive measures, much good will have been done.

Treatment of a mild case—If thrush has already been developed and preventive measures have been neglected, the above routine should be resorted to immediately. It is my custom to give a few doses of mild chloride of mercury combined with a suitable amount of bicarbonate of soda, following the last dose in a few hours with a dose of castor oil. This usually clears away all offending substances from the intestinal canal. The nursing or feeding is regulated, ventilation, clothing, and bathing is looked after; gastro-intestinal disturbances or other abnormal conditions are looked for and corrected when possible.

Local Treatment—A piece of cotton is covered with boric acid and enclosed in a piece of sterilized gauze or cheese cloth and dipped in a one per cent. solution of saccharin and given to the child to suck and chew. Ordinarily this is all that is required in a mild case. If the fungus has already colonized, and the case does not respond to the above plan, we must combat it by the use of alkalies or alkaline antiseptics internally and applied locally by means of cotton on the fingers, or what I like better is to have these agents used with an atomizer. This fungus does not do well in an alkaline medium. The following formulae I have used personally and have all given more or less good results: five to ten per cent. solution of sodium bicarbonate used locally and internally, borax or sodium benzoate one-half to one drachm to two ounces of distilled water or salt water to be used locally. Also five to ten drops of a saturated solution of sodium hyposulphitr given internally every three hours and the same applied locally. The following is a good formula for a mouthwash:

Ac. boric, 12 drams.
Sodium borate, 1 dram.
Glycerine, 4 drams.
Hydrogen diox., a. a.
Aqua rosae q. s. ad., 4 ounces.

I wish to call attention to one drug which I have found very effective in nearly all forms of infantile sore mouth viz: infus. coptis (goldthread.) It may be used as a vehice for any of the above remedies. It is used both locally and internally. In obstinate cases a ten per cent. solution of iodine in glycerine applied once daily may be of service. In the more serious cases various antiseptics have been used. A one per cent. solution of formalin or a four per cent. solution of potas. permang. are mentioned. In the still more serious cases hourly painting with a 1-20 to 1-50 solution of argentum nitrate may be used if other means fail.

Syrup vehicles, honey or sugar are to be avoided for obvious reasons. A one per cent. solution of resorcine may be given in teaspoonful doses t. i. d. If a green or fetid diarrhoea is present, the following formula will do good service:

Bis. sub nit., 1-2 dram.
Resorcine, grs. v.
Glycerine, 2 drams.
Aqua dest. q. s. ad., 2 ounces.
M. Sig-Teaspoonful every two hours.

As a general rule all sugars and starches should be cut out of the dietary. If the growth of the fungus threatens to obstruct the oesoohagus, emetics should be used, but if these measures must be resorted to, the end is usually not far off. To sum up my plan of treatment is about as follows: Preventive measures, good diet and hygeine, correction present abnormal conditions.

Drugs—Saturated solution of boric acid, saturated solution of sodium hyposulphite, one per cent. solution of resorcine, infusion of coptis a two per cent. solution of pot. chlor. This last named drug is eliminated in the saliva and exercises a continuous effect. Some authorities caution us against its use if inflamtory conditions of the kidneys are present. Personally I have never had any trouble with it.

Read before the Marshall County Medicad Society, July 5th, 1910, at Aylesworth, Okla.

NEPHRECTOMY FOR INFECTED CYSTIC KIDNEY, RECOVERY

BY J. HUTCHINGS WHITE, M. D., MUSKOGEE, OKLAHOMA

Cystic Kidneys are rare affections and cystic kidneys with infection are still more difficult to find. This fact prompts me to report one of these cases which recently came under my care. Sieber found two hundred cases of cystic kidney on record and infection mentioned in about ten per cent. of these cases. Borelius found one of infection in his four cases. There seems to be very little information in the up to date surgerys on this subject, and while my article will not appreciably add to the literature it will increase the case reports.

These kidneys are converted into cystic masses and on cross section have a sponge like appearance. The cysts vary in size from a grape seed to a small apricot. Some of the cysts project from the surface of the kidney giving the organ the appearance of being made up of small round masses; or the surface of the kidney may be comparatively smooth, the cysts not projecting. The boundary between the cortical and medullary portion is not distinguishable. The ureter is small but pervious. The kidney sometimes attains enormous proportions and may seriously interfere with labor. Shattuck thinks it probable that these kidneys consist of a combination of mesonephros and metanephros; while Virchow regards the cysts as dilatations of the uriniferous tubules in consequence of the absence of the kidney pelvis. These kidneys are more often encountered in childhood and when present, at birth, Sutton claims they are incompatable with life. They are frequently associated with similar conditions in the other kidney and liver, and even though they may not apparently be present they are said to develop within two or three years. It is wise to realize this fact and avoid the error of removing a cystic kidney when a similar condition exists in the other kidney and liver. While these kidneys secrete for a time eventually the functionating power is lost and patient slowly dies from uraemia. These kidneys are often mistaken for other conditions owing to the fact that they are rarely encountered.

The following is the history of the case I recently operated upon. Mrs. A. P., age 28: Seen by Dr. A. B. Montgomery in consultation with Dr. J. H. McCulloch, of Checotah, Okla., and by these gentlemen referred to me. These gentlemen made a diagnosis of pelvic trouble in which diagnosis I concurred. Mother died of Typhoid fever and heart trouble, father living but health poor, has kidney trouble and piles. Patient had whooping cough and measles when a small child. Chills at the age of fourteen and fifteen. At about eighteen had a severe cold early in the spring and from then until the following winter had a great deal of throat and bronchial trouble, lost a great deal of flesh but at no time confined to bed. During the winter however her condition improved and she gained in flesh and strength. There is no history of tuberculosis in the family. Her periods began at fourteen, regular, lasting from four to five days, no dysmenorrhoea. Had one miscarriage after skipping two periods, from which was confined to bed three days. Had no children and gives no history of any kidney trouble until a few days after her miscarriage, when she had a burning, straining and inclination to continue urinating. This condition lasted about ten days or two weeks. About the tenth of February last she felt a pain and soreness in her bowels on the left side and low down. This lasted for a few days. After three or four days of comfort the pain returned and was worse than the first time. These attacks continued the pain becoming more severe and with less intermission until the pain was continuous. A mass appeared in the left inguinal region, which was very tender. She complained of pain across her back, nausea and vomiting. Hot applications were used with little effect. A brownish discharge appeared in the vagina, continuing for three days. In about a week her condition improved so that she was able to sit up in bed. Later she had another attack of this kind and the mass in her left side extended as high up as the ribs, difficult breathing and pain more extensive over the back. Perspired freely and hot and cold sensations. A diagnosis of tubo-ovarian pregnancy and peritonitis was made by her doctor at this time. Pain developed in the right inguinal region. This condition continued, first in bed a day or two and then out of bed a day or two, all the while running a fever. While in bed she was comfortable, having a good appetite but very constipated. On June 21st while under anesthetic and just before operation I again made a pelvic examination. A soft fluctuating mass, palpable through the vagina, was found to the left of the medium line of pelvis extending upward toward the left kidney. This mass was adherent. Still thinking I was dealing with a pelvic trouble I made a left rectus incision just above the pubes and found on entering the abdomen slight amount of cystic degeneration of one ovary, a purulent appendicitis and that the mass before referred to involved the kidney. Up-

on closer inspection I decided that it was an infected cystic degeneration. I then removed the cystic ovary and the appendix, shortened the round ligaments and after a careful examination of the right kidney and liver closed the abdomen. The patient was now turned on her right side and an oblique left lumbar incision made and the kidney which was attached up under the costal arch, extending to the pelvis was removed in toto. The wound was closed with the exception of small opening for drainage. Recovery was uncomplicated, the patient returning to her home July 27th. Since her return home her condition has materially improved, she has gained in flesh, looks and feels better than she has in a long time. Her urine however on last examination still shows pus corpuscles. These may be from the ureter which was not removed. The urine previous to operation was clear and free from pus.

DIAGNOSTIC RELATIONSHIP BETWEEN INTERNAL MEDICINE AND SPECIAL SURGERY

BY DR. J. BLOCK, KANSAS CITY, MISSOURI

Read before Annual Meeting of Oklahoma State Medical Association, Tulsa, Oklahoma, May, 1910.

Though the material for this paper was employed elsewhere and under a somewhat different caption, it was thought equally apropos to illustrate the relationship spoken of or mentioned in the title

A resume of the data about to be furnished will show that no argument is required to demonstrate its fitness.

Urinary bleeding attending the incipiency and development of every surgical urinary entity and, for that matter, not infrequently the genitary as well, to say nothing of those coming only within the purview of the internist occasionally, still remain the most attractive symptom in the search for cause and location to answer the pathologic

inquiry. Thus the frequency, amount, sequence, color and fluidity of the haemorrhages, the size, form and color of the clots, the initial or terminal association of either with the act of micturation are data of the utmost importance. And when considered with proper attention to the silent interval— a most important detail—the story becomes more convincing. The exact position and duration of this negative period applies to both macroscopic and microscopic haematurias.

The precise array of these qualifying factors, apart from the assistance derived from the collateral phenomena of pain, appreciable swelling, fever, pyuria or bacterial findings, etc. that may, and often do, develop during the course of the maladies under consideration, furnishes a better means ior a presumptive diagnosis than any other now at hand.

The brilliant results attending the employment of our modern instruments of precision taken alone are not as valuable. Their well known limitations and, at times, prohibitive precautionary restrictions render them valueless as a diagnostic asset. As a corroborative, their use is, however, at times indispensable.

In the light of this knowledge, we should be careful, now that we have passed the threshold of the mechanical era in diagnostic research, not to entirely ignore the painstaking clinical data gathered by our forbears. No better attests to their patience, persistance and power of analysis could be furnished than their studies of haematuria.

To awaken an interest in those unusual instances, however, where this sign is altogether absent, or appears so late in the history that it becomes a supernumerary, mocking the hopes of the surgeon, is the object of today's illustrations.

A very distinguished French genito-urinary surgeon created a clinical picture disclosing the presence of vesical tumors with such fidelity to detail that it still remains a masterpiece substituting the cystoscope at times where the well known limitations of this instrument become apparent.

Summarized, it presents the following characteristics: An unprovoked and painless urinary haemorrhage, lasting from a few hours to a few days, uninfluenced by rest or therapy and ceasing spontaneously. The succeeding bleeding follows after an interval varying from a number of months to many years. I had a case where the period of quiescence was as much as six years. After the second haemorrhage, the time intervening between the subsequent bleedings gradually shortens until it finally becomes practically continuous. As a rule, the latter part of the act of micturation expels the greater quantity of blood because of the de-

trusor's direct pressure upon the growth.

Until the bladder becomes infected, or the growth falls upon the internal urinary meatus during its expulsive contractions, there is neither pain nor cystospasm. This syndrome has repeatedly enabled me to make a diagnosis verified later by palpation, cystoscopy or incision and removal.

This is a faithful grouping of events alike applicable to benign or malignant growths.

But there are exceptions to all rules—even where this syndrome is accepted as pathognomonic. A brief resume of the following case will suffice to show an unusual exception.

A lady about 35 or 40 years of age, a patient of some fifteen years acquaintance and whose previous history has no bearing upon the details of the present narrative, had been treated for an alleged grippe during one of my vacations, about two years ago. Consulting me, on my return, regarding a number of vague neurotic symptoms, to which she was subject, I requested a specimen of urine, as a usual routine for examination, and found it to contain a few red corpuscles and a faint trace of albumin. Repeated examination at short intervals during about ten days always disclosed the same adventitious elements. Repeated inquiry always elicited the same negative answer—blood had never been seen in the urine nor had there been vesical pain or tenesmus, though she voided large amounts of hysterical urine at times and had a mobile right kidney. The cystoscope disclosed a papilloma the size of a hickory nut covering the right ureteral ostium. The base was of sufficient size to describe the neoplasm as sessile, and it was recognizable upon a vaginal bimanual.

The intact growth was removed through a supra-pubic incision and proved to be benign from apex to base. A cystoscopic revision of the case at intervals for eight months failed to disclose a recurrence. An attack of suppurative appendicitis requiring incision and drainage at the usual site, followed by another opening through the vaginal cul de sas a few days subsequently, invalided the patient for a number of months.

After this further search was discontinued; some two years after the urinary operation, the patient returned claiming to have seen blood in the urine. The cystoscope showed a recurrence of the growth at the same site about the size of the terminal phalanx of the little finger, and another on the left of the trigone. They were removed through an endoscope by the snare and cauterized.

Careful cross examination of this lady, after the fact permitted her to recall an instance of a possible haematuria some five years before the first operation, but she could not positively say whether it was an irregular menstrual flow to which she was at times subject or a urinary bleeding.

It is quite evident that since males, so to speak, urinate au jour they more readily observe a bloody urinary admixture than women. This usually excites suspicion, if not alarm, and the physician is at once consulted. Women, on the contrary, owing to the character of their garments, are not permitted this convenient form of aisance and they may remain ignorant of an haematuria for a long time. Again, where irregularities of menstruation obtain errors are quite common.

Practically, the case just reported was an accidental discovery, thanks to the routine microscopic examination of urines. The diagnosis was possible without the cystoscope, the palpating finger substituting the eye.

The report is of interest since it is at variance with the history so common to all forms of vesical neoplasms. Here it is very probable, however, that a microscopic siuntement obtained for some time before the observation.

Pursuing the subject further, we will report the next case of even greater interest.

Toward the end of January of this year, I was called to see a small frail woman of about 37, the mother of three young children and one prematurely still born. Nothing of importance in her previous or remote history bearing upon her present condition elicited, save that she was of a very nervous temperament and had in recent years lacked in endurance. Two of her deliveries were followed by postpartum haemorrhages. Following the modern vogue, after listening to the diluted strains emanating from the Concord siren, she enrolled herself under the banner of the latter's deluded followers, claiming a soothing effect upon her shattered nerves during the past four or five years. In April of last year, feeling more than usually run down, she consulted a charlatan for the cure of alleged haemorrhoids. The treatment was conducted under local anaesthesia, and was so severe that she went to bed for a month, a nurse constantly applying cocaine solution to obtain relief. As understood, there was but one operation and therefore incomplete. Though she steadily maintained there must have been exacerbations of the bodily temperature before the operation, judging from her feelings, its determination by theometric measurements compelled the quack to desist from further interference. His fears were further accentuated by a persistent cough that then appeared. Added to this, there was more or less nausea and almost daily vomiting of food—sometimes as often as thrice in one day. Under the advice of another physician, she went to Colorado for relief without, however, securing any definite benefits. She returned late in October and since then has had a daily intermittent fever, sweats, cough and vomiting, gradually losing flesh and strength. Some soreness of an indefinite and indescribable character situated in the abdomen, particularly to- ward the left, now extended the list of symptoms, and a gnawing hungry feeling was at times referred to the region of the stomach. A soreness and tenderness, some- times very severe, declared itself along the lower left intercostals from the sternum to the spine. About Chistmas time, she had the only acute attack which was at all comparable to a renal colic and it lasted but one day never to again return.

Upon examination I found a dark com- plexioned and very anaemic woman with flabby muscles and pale mucosae; a pulse of 120 and very weak; temperature, as measured by the nurse, subnormal in the morning and from 101 to 101·5 at night.

Heart and lungs negative; abnormal wall flabby though tympanitic; in the left hyperchondrium a mass, slightly movable upon respiration. At its summit, immedi- ately under the costal arch, it was limited anteriorly by the mammary line. From thence, it tapered downward, its tip cor- responding to an angle where the anterior axillary line crossed one drawn through the mid-costal iliac space. It was soft and smooth and somewhat elastic. No projec- tions or bosses could be demonstrated, and it was quite tender at its anterior border, near the costal arch, where the impression of a splenic notch was readily obtained.

In the right lateral decubitus, taking advantage of the relaxation following the end of expiration, just before the beginning of the next inspiration, I was enabled to in- sinuate my fingers between the upper end of the mass and the inner surface of the costal arch, but could not reach the summit of the former. Yet enough information was obtained to assume that this was a cap- ping to the lower half of the swelling, and more than twice its size. That it did not encroach on the pulmonary space, however, was evidenced by the maintenance of good pulmonary resonance and breath sounds in the lower shelving border of the corres-

ponding lung, and more importance still, that there was a well marked tympany over the tumor on its anterior aspect, and a corresponding dullness over its posterior surface, thus showing its retroperitoneal position.

The blood count by myself showed 4,000,000 reds and 60 per cent. haemoglob- in. A more careful examination by Dr. Brewster showed the following:

"Haemoglobin, 60 per cent.
Leukocytes, 16,000.
Erythrocytes, 3,880,000.
Malarial search negative.
Differential count:
Polymorphonuclears, 71 per cent.
Large lymphocytes, 21 per cent.
Small lymphocytes, 4 per cent.
Eosinophiles, 2 per cent.
Transitionals, 2 per cent.
Myelocytes, none.
Nucleated reds, none."

The small amount of frothy thin sput- um reacted negatively to the t. b. stain. Several urinalyses showed slight traces of albumen, hyaline casts and a few leucocytes, quantity above normal and gravity good· Urates in abundance but no blood cells. Several days later they appeared, however, following the cystoscopy then made, evi- dently due to the traumatism. Macroscop- ic bleedings positively denied. The cysto- scopy was done to secure information as to the presence of two functionating kidneys and to exclude vesical metastasis.

Ureteral papillae identical and normal, the alternating intermittent jets being equal, mucosae very pale. General exploration failed to show glandular or bony metastas- is.

Diagnosis: Neoplasm of left kidney, probably malignant; operation February 7th under gas-ether anaesthesia; oblique lumbo-abdominal incision, revealing an en- larged kidney with atrophied fat capsule, in which enormously enlarged serpentine veins were coursing; kidney slightly adhered above and toward the hilum. Nephrectomy closure by catgut tier suture. Small cigarette drain at upper angle of wound.

No shock, vomiting or nausea followed the intervention. Amount of secretion in the first twenty-four hours about twelve ounces, then gradually rising to normal or above.

Save for a few hours, the temperature never again rose above the normal. Nausea, vomiting and cough at once ceased as though by magic, appetite splendid, stools regular following enemas and sometimes without. Sat up on the third day, and out of bed on the fifth. Superficially applied Michaelis skin clamps were removed on the fourth, the wound having healed per prinum; a cystitis induced by catheter infection the only remaining annoyance, and pulse gradually going to normal.

A review of the literature shows that renal tumors without haematuria somewhere in the course of the development are among the clinical rarities. Indeed, in over 90 per cent, of the cases, it is the first of all symptoms, arousing the patient's suspicions. It appears long before an enlargement is observed, proceeding painlessly or with an accompanying colic, often defying the examiner to ascertain its cause, especially if the tumor is situated at the upper pole, and deeply buried within a largely domed costal arch and covered by a fatty abdomen.

It is a fallacy to assume, though a very popular one, that malignant renal tumors are painful. As a rule, they are not. Clot colics during the bleedings give rise to the pain. Circulatory disturbances, due to a fresh invasion of an infarct, may suddenly raise the intra-renal tension, because of an unaccommodating capsule, thus giving rise to a true renal pain. This happened but once in our case, near Christmas time.

The beginning of the necrosis at the upper pole may have been co-incident with an infarcation occurring at that date, or a sudden encroachment of one of the hypernephromatous plaques shown in the specimen may have been accountable.

We have most excellent authority showing that an absence of haematuria in the presence of renal neoplasms occurs in less than one case in twenty.

Our case is rendered doubly interesting when its clinical story and findings are taken collectively or in detail, each and all of which were veritable snares and pitfalls for the unwary.

A tumor in the left hypochondrium with a notched edge and this blood picture might suggest a so-called splenetic anaemia. The same growth, with a long continued pyrexia, a leukemia or even a possible protracted malarial intermittent. Then there was the cough, the nausea and vomiting in the absence of physical findings directly related to the symptoms, and yet the stomach had been gone over repeatedly, after the customary fashion, by a specialist by inflation, gastric test meals, etc. When its enlarged neighbor was pregnant with faults and suggestions. Pressure by encroaching upon the stomach or pulmonary area would hardly explain the symptoms. The physical findings negative this view, nor is it probable that an appeal to the subtle inter-relationship existing between the solar and renal plexuses and the pneumogastrics sufficiently explain.

If abundant evidence were not at hand showing that large necrotic tumor masses in the kidney do not affect the temperature, we might readily lend ourselves to this supposition.

My own notion is that the cough, nausea, vomiting and fever, each and all were due to the absorption of toxic elements. The immediate cessation of these symptoms on removal of the kidney certainly favor this argument. In a previous paragraph it was intimated that owing to the location and shape of the mass, one might mistake it for the spleen. Antrrior tympany and posterior dullness over the tumor on percussion soon dispelled this illusion.

Does the absence of palpable metastasis in the presence of this blood picture and peculiar color of the patient favor the view of present cacrexia and thus contra-indicate operation?

This was a most difficult and perplexing question to answer. Judging, however, from the results, I am inclined to favor the negative view, but it is too early to answer definitely. The estimate of the haemoglobin two weeks after operation shows but a five per cent. gain, too little to be certain when considering the personal equation, and the sweats that still continue. Cough, vomiting, nausea and fever having ceased perhaps may not be adequate to sustain this contention.

The absence of urinary bleeding in this case furnishes a most valuable instance of the occasional absence of haematuria in the presence of renal neoplasm. It again emphatically calls attention, which, however, must be impressed upon us again and again, that in the majority of instances where the somach is accused of being fault we find other viscera at the bottom of the trouble. To succssfully specialize this organ, one must needs be a master of internal medicine cr he is sure to go astray. Like a two edged sword, specialism is at once the blessing and the curse of medicine, and in seeking infinitessimal refinements, one loses sight of the woods because of the trees, as the Germans would say.

Like syphilis and hysteria, the stomach is fond of playing pranks, and they might aptly be termed the three disgraces in masquerade.

Here is the opportunity for the internist, —indulging in pessimistic fears lest the specialists appropriate his field,—to rise above being a mere assorter for these monopolists and instead further the interest of medicine, as well as his patients, by promptly urging needful surgery, as well as discouraging and condemning much that is needless and harmful.

"606" TREATMENT FOR SYPHILIS

BY EVERETT S. LAIN, PROF. OF DERMATOLOGY, RADIOGRAPHY AND ELECTROTHERAPY, STATE SCHOOL OF MEDICINE, OKLAHOMA CITY, OKLAHOMA

At no time perhaps, since the time of Jenner and his discovery of Vaccine for small pox, have the more intelligent investigators within our Medical Fraternity been so intensely aroused since in the early spring of 1910, it was announced from Frankfort Germany, that Paul Ehrlich had discovered a new remedy for Syphilis.

A remedy whereby only one dose or injection was sufficient to cause a complete disappearance of the Spirochete Pallida within the human body, or cause a negative Wasserman Reaction within a period of twenty-four hours to a few days.

This remedy which was soon commonly spoken of as "606" from its laboratory number, was later fully explained to be a sulphur colored powder; about 34 or 35 per cent. arsenic. A modification of one of the main reduction products of atoxyl; known chemically as Dioxydiamidoarsenobenzol, later patented under the name of Salvarsan.

The writer was fortunate in having been in New York City during a part of June, and July, 1910, and after visiting the Rockefeller Institute for Medical Research had more information given him by one of the Laboratory Staff. This institute had been supplied some weeks previous from Professor Ehrlich's Laboratory with enough of "606" for experimental purposes only. Some few days later through the courtesy of Dr. Jno. A. Fordyce, Professor of Dermatology and Syphilogy University and Bellvue Hospital Med. College, we were shown some seven or more cases at the City Hospital, Blackwell's Island, to whom this preparation had been administered previously, ranging in periods from five days to three weeks.

Seeing these patients and noting the change which had taken place in their glandular infections and skin lesions fully convinced us that this preparation was something, which if too many untoward after effects were not observed, the whole of the Profession would be forced to recognize.

I say the whole of the profession, for there is no practitioner of any part of medicine, however limited his specialty, who does not have to deal with this dread disease syphilis in some one of its many phases. Again, however much we may have vaunted our old remedies of mecury and iodides, and spoken of them as "specifics" yet we all, not only appreciate how difficult it has been for us to continue our patients upon these drugs for sufficient length of time, but have also recognized the effects of para-syphilitic conditions in many of those who seemingly have had the best of treatment. No wonder then of the intense interest which is manifested in the much literatute and case reports which are appearing in all our journals, even to the laity through magazines; upon the wonderful "606 treatment for syphilis."

Strange as it may seem we have had practically no chemo-therapy, (or agents which are capable or entering in solution with the blood in sufficient quantity or strength to destroy the desease parasite without doing injury to its host) since the discovery of the effects of quinine upon the plasmodium of malaria. While many have been directing their studies and experiments along the line of serum treatments.

Few it seems. have sought for a spe-

cific human parasiticide.

It was with this in mind that Professor Ehrlich began making experiments upon mice, rates and rabbits which had been previously infected with the spirochete of so called "sleeping sickness." He was using some of the different arsenic dyes which had also been used by Hata and Berthein to destroy the spirillum of recuring fever, when he was led to try the same preparations upon some monkeys in which he had been cultivating the spirochete pallida.

Now that this remedy has been tried upon more than 20,000 human beings of various ages, lesions, and stages of syphilis, we are receiving reports of such marvelous results until it sounds almost too good to believe and we feel more like the "man from Missouri."

On the other hand we have had no great discovery in medicine which was not also followed by many evil or untoward effects, or in many cases untimely deaths. The same is to be expected and is already being reported in the use of "606" or Salvarsan. Quite a number of contra-indications such as: Acute disease, advanced cardiac or cascular deseases, optic neuritis, or advanced lesions and degenerative changes taking place in the nervous system, are already being classified and warned against by Professor Ehrlich and many other careful investigators. A few sudden deaths or cases of temporary or total blindness have been reported.

So not unlike the discovery of anaesthesia, antitoxins, or the X-Ray we shall no doubt have much abuses in the hands of the un-intelligent, the over zealous, or the un-conscientious Charlatan within the next few years.

For this reason, Professor Ehrlich asserts, was his reason for placing the first of this preparation in the hands of only intelligent and cautious experimenters, hence the very limited number of physicians and institutions which were supplied until January 1st, 1911, when it was placed upon the market under the protected name of "Salvarsan."

Although the writer earnestly sought even "a few doses" and registered our order early last fall, we did not receive our first until December 30th, 1910, and then only three ampules or doses. Within a few days we had through the courtesy and assistance of some of our local physicians selected our three cases, each case with such distinct history and lesions as to give no room for doubt of diagnosis.

Sufficient time has not yet elapsed since the administration of "606" to our cases, to determine its full effects, yet such very decided improvement in each of these cases particularly cases Nos. 1 and 2, that we feel justified in predicting that we shall also be an advocate of "606" for immediate treatment for all cases of syphilis whether acquired or hereditary in which no contra-indications are present.

As to the permanency of its effects or the possibility of late manifestations time alone shall prove Already quite a number of reports have been made of the necessity of a second or possibly a third injection before the spirochete were absent or the Wassermann Reaction became negative

Granting a second or third dose may be required in many cases, still it now appears that we have in this remedy the most successful of all methods of treatment for the urgent cases and for those over whom we can have but limited supervision

As to the best methods of preparation and administration, no doubt much improvement shall take place within due time .

Ehrlich first advised the sub-muscular administration of the alkaline solution, but has recently advised the intra-venous. The sub-muscular is given under the fascia and

superficial muscles between the scapula or deep into the gluteals. The solution may be given as either an alkaline or acid in reaction, but is attended with much pain for some hours afterward. Usually it is necessary to administer a hypodermic of morphine to relieve. While if the solution is carefully trituated and drop by drop of 15 per cent. sod. hydrox sol. or Dil. ac. hydrochloric is added until the emulsion becomes neutral to the litmus test, according to Wechselman's method the injection is followed by but little discomfort.

The site of injection in most cases shows more or less tumefaction, inflammation and induration for some days or perhaps two or three weeks following, but rarely needs much treating if done with perfect asepsis.

The above is the method which the writer has been practising to date, though we mean to try the intra-venous later.

The intra-venous is giving directly into the veins, usually the brachial, of a larger quantity of the alkaline solution diluted with normal salt solution. This method appears to be quite frequently followed some minutes later by a chill, rise of temperature, and nervous sensations. The temperature persists however only a few hours or days. It is advised that for the latter method the patient should be placed in hospital in bed for not less than eight days, whereas by former method confinement to bed seems necessary for only three or four days.

For administration either method it is advisable to have a well adapted syringe or a needle and stop cock arrangement. For the sub-muscular, a strong or "record syringe" with platinum needle is advised.

Before we had secured the special syringe we used only a Luers antitoxin syringe, holding about 15 C. C. With this syringe we had some difficulty in forcing the emulsion through the needle, also found it avisable to secure a new needle for each injection.

The following reports were our first three cases treated and represent each a different phase of the disease:

Case reports:

Case No. 1.

Male, age 29, had primary lesion about July 25th, 1910. Several weeks later had the secondary eruption on skin, mucus, patches, etc. During which time he had been taking irregularly mercury. Was referred to us January 7th, 1911, at which time several mucus patches were on peritonsilar muscles, also on mucus membrane of mouth several lesions. Tonsils nearly double normal size, red tender, with distinct ulcer on right. This condition he said had persisted ever since first signs in mouth some months earlier. Cervical, epitrochlear, also glands in each groin quite palpable.

We gave by sub-muscular injection into sub-scapular muscles and according to Weschelman's method, 6 gm. Salvarsan. Pain at time only slight, nor was there any great discomfort at any time thereafter. Put patient to bed for four days· January 8th, temperature 98 5-8, pulse 80, slept well. January 10th, erythema of throat fading, slight tenderness on sight of injection, temperature 99, pulse 80. January 12th, improvement in mouth and throat, quite perceptible, also adenopathy lessened, feels finely. January 15th, throat and tonsils almost clear of lesion, mucus patches healed, some tunufaction and induration site of injection. January 18th, throat and mouth entirely healed, patient never felt better except site of injection showing more inflammation, antiplogistine com. applied to site of injection two days in succession. January 24th, much reduced, lesions in throat and mouth have

entirely disappeared, all glandular enlargement reduced until not palpable, patient has been at work regular since 12th, and is now not suffering any discomfort, at site of injection, but some induration still remains.

Case No. 2:

Male, aged 26, referred to us for diagnosis, first by one of our local eye and throat specialists, about October 15th, 1910, at which time a very pronounced ulcer on right tonsil, skin on forehead, and parts of body, showing very characteristic, secondary eruption. Again referred to us on January 7th, 1911, by another local physician. At this time glandular enlargement was quite perceptible in epi-trochlear and groins. He now had flat elevated, deep red, papular eruptions, scattered over entire body and on forehead. Below the knees being very numerous, and arranged into characteristic annular and crescentic figures. Some scaling of the lesions below the knees appear more like psoriasis at this date January 10th, we injected 6 gm. neutral suspension "606," submuscular. Practically no pain followed. January 8th, temperature 98 3-5, pulse 78, resting nicely· January 9th, temperature and pulse about the same as previous day. No discomfort except slight tenderness at site of injection. January 12th, deep red color of lesions becoming paler. January 16th, fading of color and lessening of elevation of skin lesions, decidedly better. Some tumefaction and induration at point of injection. January 19th, still more improvement in lesions noticeable also adenopathy much reduced. January 23, about one-half of elevated eruptions have disappeared except for reddened macule now level, where formerly elevations were present. Some induration at site but no marked inflammation, adenopathy almost imperceptible, patient eating more, gaining in weight. January 28th, about one-half of lesions have entirely faded.

Case No. 3:

Male, aged 25, referred by local physician, January 10th, had not had the usual secondary eruption but glands in groin now quite palpable. Now has deep erythema of mucus surface of mouth buccal and faucial cavities. Tonsils enlarged, also cervical glands. Has partial anaesthesia of posterior buccal cavity and uvula. External rectus of left eye has recently become paralyzed, both eyes reddened, almost constant headache. Has irregular gait in walking exaggerated patella reflex. Has lost much in strength and weight. January 11th, we prepared submuscular injection. 6 gm. "606" neutral reaction. Choking of needle caused a loss of perhaps one-third, leaving our real dose about .4 gm. instead of .6 gm. as intended. January 12th, temperature 99, pulse 84, resting fairly well. January 13th, temperature and pulse about same, resting better, but headaches still felt at times. January 16th, headache only slight and at periods, sleeps better, adenopathy apparently, partially reduced. January 24th, headache absent and tonsils and other glands much reduced everything of throat fading, eyes clearing, but paralysis same, appetite better. This patient is at this date evidently improved through almost in the contra-indicated class, yet we believe had we given him a sufficient amount we would have

had more improvement, and we shall repeat the injection within a few days.

Although we report only three cases and sufficient time has yet not elapsed for the full effects of the drug, neither has the permanency of its effects yet been proven, it now appears that we shall see an entire disappearance of all symptoms, in cases Nos. 1 and 2, and that our experience shall equal the best of reports which have been made by others who are using this wonderful preparation.

We are using the same preparation upon other cases from our second supply obtained and while too early for reporting indications seem flattering. Each of our patients were confined to their rooms and beds for three days and have as yet suffered no inconvenience or untoward effects.

In conclusion we believe, First, this drug and its administration is attended with but minimum amount of danger in the hands of the intelligent, cautious physician and surgeon. Second, that it shall be the drug of first choice for most cases of syphilis either acquired or heredetary. Third, that if permanency is proven equal to its present indications, it shall be one of the greatest discoveries for unfortunate and suffering humanity that medical science has ever known. Fourth, this discovery may be the step which shall lead to many other remedies with which we may successfully combat diseases of known etiology. January 27th, 1911.

ERGOTIN

BY H. H. REDFIELD, M. D., PROF. OF THERAPEUTICS, ILLINOIS MEDICAL COLLEGE, CHICAGO, ILL., MEDICAL DEPARTMENT, LOYOLA UNIVERSITY

Ergotin is the purified aqueous extract of ergot and represents the full medicinal value of that drug. Standard granule, gr. 1-6.

Physiological action: Ergotin is class-

ed as a motor-excitant, vaso-constrictor, cardiac sedative, and stimulant of involuntary muscle tissue. It is also a hemostatic, ecbolic, anhidrotic and convulsant.

The exhibition of ergotin in large doses

at first produces a temporary fall in blood-pressure; which is due to the depressing action of the drug on the heart; soon however the vaso-constrictor effect of the drug manifests itself, with a resultant general constriction of the blood-vessels throughout the entire body and a consequent rise in blood-pressure, an arterial ischemia being produced owing to the blood-supply being decreased.

Regarding this effect of ergotin considerable controversy has arisen; some physiologists claiming that the action is the result of a combined stimulation of the vaso-constrictor center in the medulla, and the unstriped fibers in the walls of the blood-vessels; while other equally careful and competent observers contend that it is due entirely to an action on the vaso-motor center alone.

In excessive doses ergotin has a depressing effect upon both the heart and the vaso-motor center. The primary fall of blood-pressure which this drug produces is not reversed as it is in the case of moderate doses, but continues, and as a result a paralysis, progressive in nature, of the heart and vaso-motor apparatus is produced.

By its stimulating action on the centers in the cord which govern the uterine muscle-tissue, ergotin produces powerful contractions of the uterus, especially of the parturient uterus. On the impregnated but not parturient uterus this action is not so constant, and though the exhibition of ergotin often produces abortion, yet in many instances it fails utterly to initiate uterine contractions in pregnant females.

Its action as a constrictor of the blood-vessels makes it a valuable agent in controlling post-partum hemorrhage, when it practically seals up the hemorrhagic points in the walls of the uterus, notwithstanding the increased blood-pressure in the vessels.

"The phenomena produced by ergotin are divided into two classes according as the drug is taken in large quantity for a short time, or in small doses for a considerable period of time. In large doses it acts as a gastro-intestinal irritant causing nausea, vomiting, colic, thirst, and purging. It slows the heart, raises arterial tension greatly, dilates the pupils, and produces pallor and vertigo with frontal headache. It stimulates contractions of unstriped muscle-fiber, especially affecting the sphincters and causing contraction of the sphincter of the bladder, making micturition difficult if not impossible. It produces cerebral and spinal anemia, a great fall of the body temperature, coldness of the surface, tetanic spasms and violent convulsions. A very large dose is necessary to produce these results, and as much as three ounces of the fluid extract of ergot have been given daily for a week or more without producing any marked effect."—(Potter.)

Therapeutics: Ergotin is indicated in women who are thin, emaciated, cachectic, of a melancholy turn of mind, and who complain of a constant sensation of bearing-down in the uterus, and who as a rule are more or less sufferers from passive hemorrhages.

In conjunctivitis and general inflammations of the mucous membrane, the local application of ergotin or its exhibition internally is highly benificial.

It should be remembered in headache of a congestive nature, when the pain begins at the back of the neck and extends over the entire occiput and head; the extremities are cold and livid, the patient much distressed and pale, and the face wears an extremely anxious expression.

Incontinence of urine when due to a lax condition of the sphincter of the bladder is quickly corrected by ergotin.

Headaches occurring during the climacteric period, when the hands and feet are cold and clammy, the face pale and drawn; derive marked benefit from the exhibition of ergotin.

It should be studied in diarchea when the skin is shriveled and covered with a cold clammy sweat; the patient although feeling cold objects to being covered up and will throw off the bed-clothing. Sometimes there is an involuntary passage of stools; anuria is present, the abdomen tympanitic, and the patient greatly prostrated.

Ergotin by slowing the rate of the flow in the blood-vessels is of great benefit in hastening or aiding coagulation in aneurism.

It should be kept in mind in cases of spinal meningitis.

According to Da Costa, the internal administration of ergotin will markedly reduce an enlarged spleen.

It is of service in those cases of importance due to an escape of blood from the dorsal vein of the penis, making erection an almost impossible matter.

In mania produced by cerebral anemia, ergotin is very useful.

Compare its action with that of arsenic and colchicine.

STERILIZATION OF THE UNFIT

BY S. M. JENKINS, M. D., ENID, OKLA.

Ever since the beginning of time, it has been a custom of civilized nations to contribute of their earnings to the benevolent cause of charity. It is regarded as a duty by some; while others look upon charitable donations as a special privilege to be enjoyed by the more fortunate ones of God's children. In dividing the products of their labor and shrewd business transactions with their less fortunate or disabled brother. Necessity for such contributions are usually the result of unforseen misfortune, such as floods, fires, repeated crop failures in the rural district, protracted sickness, accident or other misfortune that robs the family of the life or services of the chief bread-winner. Then, it is that these contributions are made most cheerfully and willingly.

To the above disasters are added the ever-increasing burden either by voluntary contribution or by taxation for the suppression of crime, the care of the insane, the feeble-minded, the epileptic and last but not least the "rapist," all of which are increasing at a ratio out of all proportion to the increase in population. The question of dealing with the ever-increasing output of degeneracy is becoming not only national but of international interest. Letters of inquiry now are being received from Europe and other foreign countries with requests for more articles on the operation of vasectomy for the prevention of procreation of the degenerate, from the pen of Dr. G. H. Bogart of Indiana, author of "The Procreation Law" now in operation in that State. Only recently, I resolved to take up the work in Oklahoma and in order to get this paper ready for the printer, I did not have time sufficient to procure data right up to the minute but this is correct of the dates as given: In 1880, there were in the United States 40,492 inmates of the various state institutions; in 1890, 74,028; in 1903, 150,151, an increase of 85 per cent. from 1880 to 1890 and by more than 100 per cent. from 1890 to 1903, as against an increase of less than 30 per cent. in the total population of the United States during the same thirteen years. This applies to the insane asylums alone; other statistics show that the increase of the confirmed criminals, idiots, epileptics and other degenerates are increasing with an equal ratio and out of all proportion to the increase in population.

Many states enact laws for the protection of its animals even to wild birds and the fishes of its small streams; they spend large sums of money and devote much time to meetings, associations, congresses, etc., for the protection and improvement of the quality and breed of their hogs, horses and cattle. Indiana is the first state in the Union to enact a measure for the improvement of the grade of its human beings. A similar bill is now pending before the Texas legislature and I am informed with almost positive assurance of passage at the present session.

Oklahoma (the best state of the entire forty-six) has never been the last in anything, save in getting into the Union. Let us then be up and doing and take third place in the ranks of progress by adopting this safe, sane and rational measure which makes it lawful for our tleemosynary institutions to perform a simple operation for the prevention of procreation by the unfit. Dr. G. H. Bogart, of Brookville, Indiana, says the operation of vasectomy is so simple that it is hardly believeable. He says:

"The seminal cord leading from the testicle to the vesicular seminalis can be found as a rounded cord immediately under the skin on either side of the penis where the cord crosses the pubic bone. To operate, the parts are sterilized, the cord fixed between the thumb and finger and an incision made through the skin; the cord is then exposed on a director. The vas deferens tied and cut between the ligature and the testicle. The cord dropped back and the incision closed with collodion. The operation requires from three to four minutes and is so slight that no anesthetic, either general or local, is used and the patient climbs out of his chair and proceeds to his usual employment with hardly any inconvenience. The testicular end is left open that the orchitic fluid may flow into the scrotal cavity and be re-absorbed and thus prove a benefit to the subject, as this is a wonderful nerve-tonic; in fact is the Brown Sequard 'Elixir. of Life' Tremendous results have been obtained from the operation on confirmed masturbators; the passions are retained as is sexual ability and pleasure. There is ejaculation at orgasm, though the emission is sterile.

The Refromatory of Indiana has a record of over five hundred operations with no untoward cases and universal good results to the individual."

Some states propose a law prohibiting marriage to the viciously diseased or otherwise unfit. In my opinion, such a law would only serve to augment the very conditions that we wish to prevent, the increase of the unfit.

Degenerates, if forbidden to marry, will likely gratify themselves at all hazards; if left to themselves, they will raise babies illigetimately if not permitted to do so legally.

I have observed in many epileptics a mania for large families, some of them harbour an opinion that the more babies they have, the more stars will be added to their 'Crown of Glory' even if the baby is handicapped and unable to ever become an average, useful citizen. It is numbers, and not quality, that they are after; a better quality, even if the number is not so great is the object of this paper. Ex-President Roosevelt's "Race Suicide" has never caused me any uneasiness; from sixty millions to ninety-seven millions of people in twenty years does not indicate that we were lacking in numbers. To improve the quality by selective breeding and castration, as in the lower animals, is neither practical nor desirable in the human being. The simple and humane operation of vasectomy will check the output of the unfit; and improvement of the race when the objectionable are decreased would then only become an operation of one of Nature's laws.

From Dr. Bogart's essay in "The Texas Medical Journal" of September, 1910, allow me to illustrate by referring to the Jukes family:

"Max Jukes, the progenitor, was born in New York, in 1720; he was a drunkard who would not work (two very bad qualities that are sometimes found in citizens of Oklahoma); of his descendents, 1,206 have been identified as inmates of penal and charitable institutions; not one was ever elected to public office; not one ever served in the army or navy or contributed anything to public welfare. They cost society above $1,250,000.00. 310 were inmates of poor-houses on an average of over seven years each; 440 are viciously diseased; 56 were notorious public prostitutes; seven were convicted murderers; 60 were habitual thieves; 134 were habitual criminals."

Now, had Max Jukes' vas deferens been encountered by the little knife of some surgeon, legally authorized to operate, what a saving of misery, sorrow, suffering and crime. A saving, not only to general society but to the wretched offenders who would thus have been left unborn and the above "Box of Pandora" would never have been opened.

An act for the prevention of procreation by the unfit.

PREAMBLE.

Whereas, heredity is a most important element in the transmission to posterity of criminality, insanity, feeble-mindedness, degeneracy and epilepsy,

Be it Enacted by the People of the State of Oklahoma,

Sec. 1. That on and after the passage of this Act, it shall be compulsory for the governing body of each and every institution within the State entrusted with the care of the confirmed criminal, insane, idiot, imbecile, feeble-minded, epileptic and rapist to appoint two surgeons of recognized ability who, with the regular institutional physician shall constitute a Board of Medical Control.

Sec. 2. Such Board of Medical Control shall examine such inmates of the respective institutions for which it has been appointed and who shall be recommended by the regular physician of the institution and, if in the opinion of such Board of Medical Control procreation by such inmate is deemed inadvisable or if the physical or mental condition of any such inmate will be substantially improved thereby, it shall be lawful for any of the members of this Board of Medical Control to perform such operation for the prevention of procreation as shall be decided as safest and most effective.

Sec. 3. For every consultation as to the condition of any inmate under the provisions of this Act, the members of this Board of Medical Control shall receive the fee of not more than $3.00 to each member thereof, to be paid out of the funds appropriated for the maintenace of such institution.

Emergency.

Sec. 4. An emergency is hereby declared, by reason whereof it is necessary for the immediate preservation of the public health and safety that this act shall take effect from and after its passage and approval.

EDITORIAL

PAY YOUR ANNUAL DUES.

It should be remembered that all membership in the State Medical Association has expired and that now is the proper time to pay your annual dues for 1911.

If you know of a neighboring physician

who is not a member induce him to become one of us and help the good work along. The greater fraternalism is made in the medical profession the more satisfactory will the profession be found. Society membership keeps down much bickering and makes the hard path of the physician lighter.

HAVE YOU A PAPER FOR THE ANNUAL MEETING.

If so notify the chairman under whose section it properly belongs of the title and subject and prepare the paper in duplicate in order that a copy may be ready at the annual meeting for the use of the Journal·

Chairman:

Surgery—Ross Grossheart, Tulsa.

Medicince—J. H. Scott, Shawnee.

Mental and Nervous Diseases—F. B. Erwin, Norman.

Pediatrics—W. G. Little, Okmulgee.

Gynecology and Obstetrics—B. W. Freer, Nowata.

Pathology—Elizabeth Melvin, Guthrie.

Eye, Ear, Nose and Throat—Milton K. Thompson, Muskogee·

A GOOD JOURNAL FOR THE PHYSICIAN.

The Physicians Business Journal published in Philadelphia, with Dr. P. B. Thatcher as Editor, is one that should come to the notice of every physician who is deficient in business training and systematic work. It follows necessarily that this class covers a large precentage of the medical profession, who are notoriously lax in business methods and training. This publication is designed for the busy man and a study of its columns will result in great good to the physician in a financial sense. Dr. Andrew Lerskov, of Claremore, is one of the collaborators·

THE ATTITUDE OF THE GOVERNOR ON MEDICAL APPOINTMENTS.

It is stated on good authority that Governor Lee Cruce has decided to follow the wishes of the medical profession of Oklahoma in selecting his Medical Cabinet and has asked that all possible aid be given him by the profession in the selection of proper and competent medical officers. This idea will be most acceptable to the medical profession and follows the principle laid down in many of the newer laws governing such matters. In many of the states where recent medical legislation has been enacted, a clause of the law requires the medical associations concerned to nominate to the governor a list of names from which it is mandatory upon him to select his various Boards and Officers. This is as it should be for no one knows the qualifications of a physician better than his fellow physicians and when the responsibility is with him to select his officers it is reasonable to assume that he will give the matter much consideration and nominate men of the highest fitness.

We trust the Governor will be able to select officers that will reflect credit on the profession and keep the state in the advance column of medical progress.

EXPERT TESTIMONY·

One of the advances much needed in Oklahoma and for that matter in all states is some sane law regulating expert testimony.

Under the present system it is most difficult to get the real condition of a party to a suit before the jury in such a manner as to enable them to decide the truth. If the case be a civil suit the attorneys hunt around to find some physician to testify according to their views and as many conditions are susceptible of a double interpretation it is a rare case where there is not free from any influences that are usually a clash of authority. present when they are called to testify by the attorneys in the case.

It has been suggested in various localities that a law be enacted requiring the appointment of a non-biased board of experts who will make a report to the court of their findings, the experts to have no interest whatever in the issue and to be thus

A law covering the above essentials would prevent many of the present outrageous verdicts and would be especially beneficial to the medical profession in the prevention of bothersome and baseless malpractice suits.

PERSONAL

THE NATIONAL CONFEDERATION OF STATE MEDICAL EXAMINING AND LICENSING BOARDS.

Will hold its Twenty-first Annual Meeting in Chicago, Ills., on Tuesday, February 28th, 1911, at the Congress hotel.

The subjects to be taken up at this meeting will be a consideration of the State Control of Medical Colleges; a report by a special committee on Clinical Instruction; a report on a proposed Materia Medica List by a special committee; the report on a paper presented at the St. Louis meeting by Mr. Abraham Flexner of The Carnegie Foundation for the Advancement of Teaching; and some special papers on such subjects as the Regulation of Medical Colleges, Necessity for Establishing a Rational curriculum for the Medical Degree, and others, by men eminently qualified to prepare papers upon such subjects.

These topics are all of practical and vital interest to medical colleges, medical examining boards, the profession at large and the public. The Symposium will be composed of ten papers and be presented from the view-points of state, law, *medical colleges, state medical examining and licensing boards and the medical profession.* The contributors of papers to the Symposium on State Control of Medical Colleges are men of the highest attainments in matters pertaining to state, law and the medi-

cal profession, and their production will be worthy of the most careful consideration. The chief object of the Symposium is to determine, as far as possible, the feasibility of placing Medical Colleges under State Control. The special committee on Materia Medica made a report at the St. Louis meeting of the Confederation, June 6th, 1910, and it was continued and instructed to report again at the next annual meeting of the Confederation in 1911. The report of this committee made at St. Louis has received very favorable comment by many of the editors of medical journals, and should receive at the Chicago meeting extended and careful consideration. The report on Mr. Flexner's paper is published in the Proceedings of the St. Louis meeting of the Confederation, page 64, and will be open for discussion at the Chicago meeting.

An earnest and cordial invitation to this meeting is extended to all members of State Medical Examining and Licensing Boards, teachers in medical schools, colleges and universities, delegates to the association of American Medical Colleges, to the Council on Medical Education of the A. M. A., and to all others interested in securing the best results in medical education. .

The officers of the Confederation are, Pres. J. C. Guernsey, M. D., 1923 Chestnut St., Philadelphia, Pa.; Secretary-Treasurer George H. Matson, M. D., State House, Columbus, Ohio.

Drs. D. Armstrong, of Mead, and Sydney Hagwood, of Durant, are in New York City, attending clinics and doing post-graduate work.

Dr. O. C. Klass, of Muskogee, has returned from Vienna, after a prolonged stay.

Dr. Robert L. Hull, of Portland, Maine, has located in Oklahoma City. Dr. Hull has just completed an internship in the Hospital for Ruptured and Cripples, New York, and will make a specialty of orthopedic surgery.

Drs. Curt Von Wedel, of New York, and Charles Cross, of Meridan, Mississippi, have located in Oklahoma City.

The Muskogee County Medical Society recently were tendered a reception and smoker at the residence of Dr. H. C. Rogers, the retiring President of the Society.

Dr. C. V. Rice, of Francis, Oklahoma, has located in Muskogee.

Dr. A. K. West, of Oklahoma City, has been appointed delegate to represent the State Medical Association at the Joint Conference on Medical and Medical Legislation, Chicago, March 1-3, 1911.

Dr. E. S. Ferguson, of Oklahoma City, has been appointed to represent the State Association at the meeting of the Association of American Medical Colleges, Chicago, March 27-28, 1911.

COUNTY SOCIETIES

CADDO COUNTY.

The annual election of officers in Caddo County gave the following result:

President—P. H. Sanders, Carnegie.

Vice-President—A. W. Dail, Cement.

Secretary-Treasurer—Chas. R. Hume, Anadarko.

Censors—S. Blair, Apache, three years, Geo. W. Westermeir, two years, M. H. Edens, Verden, one year.

Delegates—P. H. Anderson, Anadarko, W. W. Gill, Gracemont.

POTTAWATOMIE COUNTY.

President—J. B. Ellis, Shawnee.

Vice-President—F. L. Carson, Shawnee.

Second Vice-President—H. G. Campbell, Shawnee.

Secretary-Treasurer—G. S. Baxter, Shawnee.

Censors—Esther Mitchell, J. E. Hughes, J. S. Cannon.

GARVIN COUNTY.

The Garvin County met in Pauls Valley January 19th. The subject for study was Anesthesia and Surgical Shock, the following papers were read:

The Choice of an Anesthetic, Dr. J. R. Calloway.

Indications and Contra-Indications for Chloroform and for Ether, Dr. J. C. Matheny.

Local Anesthesia and General Surgery, Dr. H. P. Wilson.

The Prevention and Treatment of Surgical Shock, Dr. N. H. Lindsay.

PUERPERAL ECLAMPSIA.

F. J. Plondke, St. Paul, Minn. (*Journal A. M. A.*, January 14), describes his method of treating puerperal eclampsia by combined venesection and infusion. Nearly all pathologists, he thinks, agree that the convulsions and concurrent symptoms are the results of irritation of liver and kidney cells, and of the cerebral centers by toxins circulating in and distributed by the blood-current. He follows with modern precautions as to antisepsis and prevention of air in the vein, the usual technic of phlebotomy, using a double ligature, one above and one below the incision into the superficial vein. After withdrawing a certain amount of blood from the distal portion and at the same time infusion into the proximal end of normal salt solution at the proper temperature, in both cases through thin-walled glass cannulas, the ligatures are drawn tight and the vein closed. The amount of blood withdrawn by him ranged from 15 to 32 ounces; the quantity of normal salt solution introduced varied from 1 to 2 quarts and averaged about 40 ounces. · He claims nothing new in the operation except the combination of the two methods, infusion and withdrawal of blood, taking away some of the circulating toxin and diluting the remainder. Three cases are reported in which the method was used with success.

ECLAMPSIA.

J. B. De Lee, Chicago (*Journal A. M. A.*, January 7), says there is no question as to the necessity of prompt delivery in eclampsia. The problem is in the method of accomplishing this. Before the seventh month the fetus always dies and craniotomy may be performed, but after viability an attempt must be made to save it. In a well-equipped hospital the matter is simple, as operative delivery can be brought about, but in a private home and when skilled assistance is lacking, less active surgical measures will have to be employed together with medical treatment. Puncture of the membranes, use of the colpeurynter and, after almost complete dilation, manual dilatation of the balance with episiotomy and forceps delivery or version, and extraction depending on the conditions. The state of the cervix is the all-governing condition so far as rapidity of delivery is concerned· If fully dilated, delivery may be safely effected by forceps if the head is engaged, and version and extraction if the head is movable. If the cervix is effaced but the os not sufficiently dilated, manual or mechanical dilatation is the best, and episiotomy to overcome the resistance of the peritoneum, followed by forceps delivery. The greatest discussion has arisen regarding the condition when the cervix is uneffected and tightly closed, and De Lee gives his experience with each of the methods that have been employed. Manual dilatation is objectionable on account of the bruising and laceration attending it and the time that it requires. Only rarely are the parts so soft and dilatable as to allow safe delivery. Metreurysis is the ideal method if no urgency exists, with soft cervix and large vagina. Its contraindications in eclampsia are, scars on the cervix, abnormal rigidity, complete closure of the cervix in a primipara, edema of the paracervical tissues, local infection, and great urgency. Rigid cervix is a frequent complication of eclampsia as it occurs most often in primiparæ and women of advanced years. He denies the usefulness of instrumental dilation in these cases and considers the cervical incisions as contraindicated. They are also contraindicated if the child is large or presents abnormally. Vaginal Cesarean section has given the best results of any yet obtained, especially when performed immediately after the first convulsion. He refers to Dr. Fry's paper on the subject offered at the same symposium. Abdominal Cesarean section has not obtained the recognition it deserves in eclampsia in De Lee's opinion. It has been used mostly in the worst cases and the maternal mortality has been high, but in some cases the vaginal section is impossible. He does not see the advantages in the extraperitoneal method, or considers them rather overdrawn. The resistance of the perineum is also to be considered and, if episiotomy is employed, he recommends the mediolateral method. Special mention is made of decapsulation of the kidneys proposed by Edebohls. It is made of decapsulation of the kidneys proposed by Edebohls. It is impossible, De Lee says, at the present time, to pass judgment on this procedure and also to advise nephrotomy in addition to decapsulation as recommended by two German authors. It has not had a fair trial since it has been only in cases proving refractory to all other methods. Considering what we know of the causation of eclampsia the operation is not rational but it is perhaps as reasonable as any one of our other "specific" remedies. Early in his practice De Lee learned two facts, one that morphin given to eclamptics killed many of the babies and prolonged the post partum coma, and the other that chloroform is a very dangerous drug in eclampsia. He now restricts his use of anesthetics and narocotics to an irreducible minimum. For the operative delivery he has used ether, but for Cesarean section he uses nitrous oxid and oxygen because the child is delivered so rapidly that the preliminary asphixia is of no moment.

THE MODERN TREATMENT OF SYPHILIS.

J. A. Fordyce, New York (*Journal A. M. A.*, January 1), says that the classical treatment of lues has failed, as is show by the number of cases of late syphilis and parasyphilis that we meet with at the present time. He attributes this in part to the under estimation of the seriousness of the disease in the teaching of our medical schools and the unfamiliarity of the unfamiliarity if the general practitioner with its manifestations, which is a consequence. It is impossible to predict the outcome of the disorder in any case from its early symptoms, and these, moreover, are often inadequately estimated and sometimes altogether overlooked. Fortunately, with the later discoveries we have better means of diagnosis than formerly. The old methods which are still largely in use, of mercurial treatment by ingestion, have been proved to be entirely inadequate, and the best methods for administering mercury are by intramuscular or intravenous injection. It is premature to depose mercury from its rank of first specific and, without discrediting Ehrlich's discovery, we must not ignore the fact that mercury, too, yields clinical results bordering sometimes on the marvelous. Iodid of potassium is too often relied on alone, though it is a valuable adjunct, and arsenic, though long used, has been found to be dangerous in the forms hitherto employed. Fordyce gives a history of the use of the more modern arsenic preparations, leading up to the discovery of the Ehrlich-Hata preparation, salvarsan, or "606." The impression first given by the reports, that it was possible to eradicate the infection entirely by one dose, has been proved erroneous, as has also the opinion that a special susceptibility to the drug could be acquired. The remedy has been used in eighty-four cases so far in the New York City Hospital· The injections are painful, usually requiring morphin, but pain does not last over twelve hours in most cases. In a few cases there appears to be a special susceptibility to the drug and the reaction is very severe. Its effect on primary lesions is very striking, but the most brilliant results altogether have been obtained in mucous membrane lesions and almost as much with gummata. Bone lesions are quickly affected, but these often disappear quickly under mercury. Malignant syphilis with multiple bone lesions, resistant to mercury, were, however, markedly influenced by the arsenical treatment. The treatment in tabes has not been very encouraging, probably on account of the degenerative conditions which have been induced. There is a suspicion, based on certain reports of cases like one here given by Fordyce, that the treatment may have disastrous effects on vision, though no degenerative changes have been found in experimental animals. Two striking cases of hereditary syphilis are briefly reported. Fordyce concludes from the study of his observations that salvarsan has not been found absolutely cura-

tive in a single dose, but that it is a most efficient agent in controlling the early symptoms and limiting the contagious stage. A theapeutic blow in the early stage, when the spirochetes are numerous, must have a marked effect on the later development, and the result of one injection is fully equal to that of a long course of mercury and mercury and iodid, without their unpleasant by-effects. The objections to the use of salvarsan are the pain it produces in its intramuscular injection and the present uncertainty of its effects on the eyes. Administration by the intravenous method, however, obviates the first mentioned difficulty, although it requires more technical skill. He thinks it better for the present not to employ it as routine treatment, but to use it only in cases where it is specially indicated, carefully observing all the precautions laid down by Professor Ehrlich. Every patient should be examined by an ophthalmologist before the drug is administered and patients should have hospital care for four days or a week afterward. It would be better to lengthen the period of hospital observation rather than shorten it.

BOOKS RECEIVED

PRINCIPLES OF THERAPEUTICS.

The Principles of Therapeutics, By A. Manquat, National Correspondent to the Academic De Medicine, Translated By M. Simbad Gabriel, M. D.

Cloth, 298 pages, Price $3.00 net·

D. Appleton and Company, New York and London.

THE PRACTICAL MEDICINE SERIES.

(Nervous and Mental Diseases.)
Nervous and Mental Diseases, Edited

by Hugh T. Patrick, M. D., Professor of Nerology in the Chicago Polyclinic, Clinical Professor of Nervous Diseases in the Northwestern University Medical School; Ex-President Chicago Neurological Society.

And

Peter Bassoe, M. D., Assistant Professor of Nervous and Mental Diseases, Rush Medical College.

Series 1910, Bound in Cloth, $1.25 net.

Chicago, The Year Book Publishers, 40 Dearborn Ave.

BOOK REVIEWS

HYDROTHERAPY.

Hydrotherapy: A Treatise on Hydrotherapy in general. Its application to special affections; the Technic, or Processes Employed; and use of Waters Internally. By Guy Hinsdale, A. M., M. D., Lecturer on Climatology, Medico-Chirurgical College of Philadelphia. Octavo of 466 pages, illustrated. Philadelphia and London, W. B. Saunders Company, 1910. Cloth, $3.50 net.

Hydrotherapy is one branch of treatment that has long been neglected and in this work we have a condensed and practical application of the approved hydrotherapeutic measures.

The work is well illustrated with the necessary appliances used in the treatment of disease and space is given the various mineral water springs and baths as well.

The author disclaims his intention to supplant drugs with physiologic measures, but insists that an intelligent combination is to be desired and that hydrotherapy is one of the great aids of drug treatment. In this view the work will be found very valuable to those who study its principles and the foundation laid down that hydrotherapy is a rational adjunct to a large majority of the affections we have to treat will be approved by all who give the matter thought.

The work is very explicit as to indications for different treatments and their contraindications are closely noted.

This volume should be in the hands of every nurse in the land and the library of the physician will be enriched by it.

THE PRACTICE OF SURGERY.

The Practice of Surgery. By James G. Mumford, M. D., Instructor in Surgery in the Harvard Medical School. Octavo of 1015 pages, with 682 illustrations. Philadelphia and London, W. B. Saunders Company, 1910. Cloth, $7.00 net; Half Morocco, $8.50 net.

This is a clinical surgery, written with remarkable force and clearness.

The author discards much that is to be found in a text-book on surgery and adds a large fund of personal experience and goes into many of the commoner affections with an intimate description of the methods used in his daily work, thus making the book an entertaining one from the start; one that holds the students attention more closely than other styles of writing can possibly do.

The work is divided in such a manner

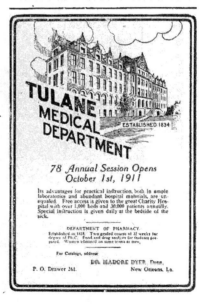

that more space is given those affections most often met, each subject receiving attention in proportion to its importance and its occurence in daily practice.

It is richly illustrated with many original drawings and one of the striking features is the devotion of much space to the minor surgical procedures. In this particular section the cases are taken up and their best treatment is handled in a masterly manner and one can almost see the author delivering his salient points and stressing those that are likely to be overlooked.

It may be assumed that this book will find great favor in the eyes of those doing a general work and to those who are only occasionally called on to do emergency surgery its study will be found invaluable.

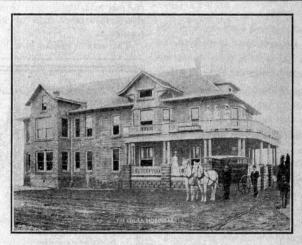

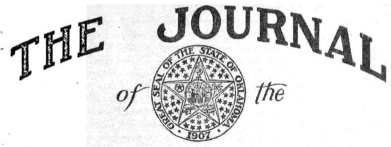

THE JOURNAL
of the
Oklahoma State Medical Association.

VOL. III.	MUSKOGEE, OKLAHOMA, MARCH, 1911.	NO. 10

DR. CLAUDE A. THOMPSON, Editor-in-Chief.

ASSOCIATE EDITORS AND COUNCILLORS.

DR. J. A. WALKER, Shawnee.
DR. CHARLES R. HUME, Anadarko.
DR. F. R. SUTTON, Bartlesville.
DR. I. W. ROBERTSON, Dustin.
DR. J. S. FULTON, Atoka.

DR. JOHN W. DUKE, Guthrie.
DR. A. B. FAIR, Frederick.
DR. W. G. BLAKE, Tahlequah.
DR. H. P. WILSON, Wynnewood.
DR. J. H. BARNES, Enid.

Entered at the Postoffice at Muskogee, Oklahoma, as second class mail matter, July 28, 1910

This is the Official Journal of the Oklahoma State Medical Association All communications should be addressed to the Journal of the Oklahoma State Medical Association, English Block, Muskogee, Oklahoma.

THE OBLITERATED APPENDIX, ITS PATHOLOGICAL AND CLINICAL SIGNIFICANCE. (A Preliminary Report.)

BY A. L. BLESH, M. D., HORACE REED, M. D., C. E. LEE, M.D., OKLAHOMA CITY, OKLA.

Observations extending more than a century have failed to prove an established function for the appendix. Older writers assign it a function such as could be reasonably assumed from its structure. Embryological facts lead us to assume for the appendix a necessary place in the processes of early development and even in early childhood. And the observations of retrogressive changes which take place between childhood and adult life just as forcibly compel us to believe that function ceases as the subject approaches maturity. Nature tries to obliterate those organs or

Read Before the Central Oklahoma Medical Society, at Chickasha, October 4, Nineteen Hundred and Ten.

structures which are no longer needed. In this she does not always succeed. Thus we find a patent foramen ovale in almost fifty per cent. of all subjects (Stoerk), and a Meckel's diverticulum is found in two per cent. of all autopsies (Aschoff.) In four hundred cases in which the appendix was examined by Ribbert, ninety-nine (99) showed partial or total occlusion; twenty-five (25) per cent. (Kelly & Hurden.) The youngest observed case (non typical) was five years of age, and complete obliteration was not observed under the thirtieth year. More than one-half of all cases over sixty years of age show obliteration. In early fetal life the appendix represents not much more than a lengthy, somewhat enlongated, cecum. As the child develops this enlongated portion assumes more and more the worm-like form until, at birth, it has reached that stage in which the demarcation between cecum and appendix is absolute. The lumen, however, remains patent in the child, there being no valvular contrivance to obstruct the free flow of bowel content into its opening. As age advances the lumen gradually narrows and a fold of mucus membrane extends across the appendiceal orifice so that in adult life a valve is quite uniformly to be found. That this valve does not always prevent the leakage of bowel content into the appendix we have all observed. This material is capable of setting up all grades of irritation from the simple so-called catarrhal appendicitis to the most violent and rapidly spreading inflammation and destruction.

From these considerations we are brought face to face with two questions: First, is the obliterated appendix the result of retrogressive changes in a no longer functionating organ, or, second, is a pathological condition, resulting from a prolonged irritation produced by bowell content, acting as a foreign body?

The scientific explanations of these questions cannot be given until the physiology of the appendix is known. In the absence of any known physiology we must content ourselves with the conclusion reached from anatomical and clinical data.

ANATOMY: The histological structure of the appendix is not markedly different from that of the neighboring bowel. It consists of an outer, or serous, coat; two muscular coats; longitudinal and circular sub-mucus and mucus coats. In addition, in the young are to be found large islands of lymphoid tissue resmbling that of the tonsil. This tissue early disappears. Between the different coats are found a network of vessels and nerves. Fibres and branches from these freely perforate the

different coats anastomosing with those beyond. The richest supply of vessels and nerves are to be found in the sub-mucus coat. The blood supply is from the same source as that of the cecum. The nerve supply comes from the superior mesenteric plexus of the sympathetic system. This plexus receives a branch from the right pneumogastric. In the obliterated appendix the various coats become more or less blended. There may remain a column of epithelial cells varying in thickness according to the obliterated channel.

The muscalature is gradually replaced by connective tissue and the blood vessels for the most part are squeezed out and the structure now gives a picture resembling scar tissue.

What becomes of the rich nerve supply —fibres, and terminals? Histolgosists have not, so far as our search in literature extends, answered this question. Do they undergo the same retrograde changes as the other parts and disappear, or do they remain tangled up in the fibrous coat and thus give rise to reflex symptoms such as may be observed when a nerve becomes entangled in a scar in other parts of the body? Clinical experience has strongly impressed us with the probability of the latter theory. Investigations which we now have under way will, we hope, decide this question.

CLINICAL MANIFESTATIONS: Our observations extend back over a period of more than eight years. In our abdominal surgery we have practiced removal of the appendix when it was within reach of the field of operation, provided it showed any abnormality. We have always classified the obliterated appendix as being normal. We have found that a large number of patients have reported a cure of numerous abdominal conditions for which the original operation was not intended but in which the removal of the appendix was incidental. We have never quite believed that an ovariotomy would cure constipation, or that a resection of a tube or a round ligament operation would cure gastric neuroses. These reports, however, became so numerous that we have endeavored to find an explanation for them. A review of our cases has demonstrated that in cases reporting such cures the appendix accidentally removed was either partially or totally obliterated in a large majority of instances. More recently, in the light of these observations, we have advised operation and performed it on a number of patients presenting themselves with numerous abdominal symptoms but which were not directly referred to the appendix.

The operation performed was the removal of the appendix, and in these instances, without an exception, the appendix was partially or totally obliterated. The results of these operations have been marvelous and in a later report we will detail these cases.

CONCLUSION: Laboratory investigation, partially complete, anatomic findings and clinical observations, seem to justify these conclusions.

First: The appendix apparently functionates in fetal life and early childhood.

SECOND: With retrogressive changes there is introduced the pathological element capable of producing various symptoms heretofore classified as neuroses.

THIRD: The intimate nerve supply of the appendix, its close connection with the sympathetic system would justify the belief that the changes which are taking place, or which have taken place in retrogression, are sufficient to exert a reflex, inhibitory action on a part or the whole of the gastrointestinal tract.

FOURTH: In gastric or intestinal neuroses, where there is no other demonstrable cause, the appendix may be assumed as the seat of trouble, and justifies treatment by its removal.

State National Bank Biulding, Oklahoma City.

THE MEDICAL SECRET AND VENEREAL DISEASES.

BY DR M. A. WARHURST, SYLVIAN, OKLA.

What is commonly known as Medical Secret of the physician is really after all the secret of the patient which is intrusted to the physicians keeping this obligation he is supposed to keep inviolate. This secret means much when applied to the relation with the sanitary duties of the profession and health authorities in oberliterating venereal diseases. In taking the physicians liberty of action from him it practically dominates the entire situation. The obligation of this has been prevalent since it was formulated in the precepts laid down in the oath of Hippocrates. The observation of this law of ethics is a professional virtue and is considered so by the wisest and greatest men of the medical profession. Theories and dogmas have their advocates and their opposition but the medical secret or ethical law of the medical fraternity is observed by the entire profession almost to a man. Even the degraded and unethical physician holds to and practices this law as a sacred duty he owes to his patient. Physicians often violate every ethical rule of right toward his brother physician; he may sneer and scoff at his reputation and use his influence to injure his practice, the excuse he puts up for this unprofessional conduct is professional competition, but how does he treat the medical secret? The answer is easy; it is held by this unethical man as a sacred trust and is obeyed to the letter. Observing the medical secret in its relation to venereal diseases considering their private nature and more their shameful character it is the proper estimate of this obligation that it must take on a more rigid and stern application. They are diseases of all others which the patient desires to keep secret even from his dearest friend. It is certain that a knowledge of their existance would not be revealed to the physician if there was any risk of his secret being imparted to others. To this traditional habit our law makers have aided by making the violation of the professional secret a penal offense. In some of the foreign countries physicians, surgeons or health officers imparting the secrets of his profession unless otherwise ordered by the government is punished by imprisonment. In this country it is different as regards punishment while there is a law prohibiting the disclosure of this secret there is no penalty attached to the violation. In another sense the law takes into consideration and throws a protection around the common interest of society by compelling the physician to report all cases of contagious diseases regarded as dangerous to the health of the public, but this compulsion does not extend far enough, it ought to cover venereal diseases also. This compulsion is justifiable since it is a prophylactic measure for the protection of the public health. Perhaps the law of this State is broad enough to cover all diseases which are considred contagious and dangerous to the public welfare. Venereal diseases comply with both of these conditions for they may be considered contagious and surely there is no disease that carries more danger than these diseases do, yet the health board never requires them to be reported. Why are they exempt? Because of the difficult character as a health problem, yet they are a menace to society, cause more sorrow and affliction than any other disease. They give to the surgeon, gynecologist, eye specialist a large proportion of their work yet this is not all, they contribute their share to the insane, the epileptics and other nervous troubles. They are a greater menace to society than tuberculosis; a disease which the intelligent class of people are using their influence and lending every effort to eradicate from society. While never a thought is given to the havoc venereal diseases are causing the human race. If there is a disease that is a curse to mankind it is diseases of this class. Why not include them in disease that are reportable? In Norway and Denmark, reporting of venereal diseases is made obligatory by law; this information is kept secret by the health authorities yet it has proved to be one of the best measures for the prevention of venereal diseases. By this means the authorities are enabled to locate the dangerous sources of contagion and subject them to treatment. It seems to me that the above would be to an advantage if applied to this country. In the usual treatment of venereal diseases the physician can easily adjust his conduct in accordance with his professional duty in cases where the patients interests alone are considered, but when it comes to the question of marriage how different. The interest and welfare of the coming generation must be taken into consideration. Here the physician owes his duty to the wife and her future children and through them to society in general. Often special obligations are imposed upon the physician whereby he is to protect the interests of his patient regardless of the welfare of others, this working a hardship upon the physician. As a rule patients seeking to obtain advice are honest in their intentions and the majority can be prevailed upon to heed the advice and comply with its terms. The principal role of the physician is to point out and make plain the dangers of the disease that he may expect in married life, the necessary treatment to pursue and the period of time to elapse before marriage can safely take place.

There is another class of people to consider and it is very unfortunate to society that this class is not rare. The physician may give them explicit instructions as to the dangers that may be encountered in married life, the sorrow and disease that the future generation would fall heir to through his wilful neglect in carrying out the instruction given. Yet with all the advice and warnings he refuses to heed these. instructions.

He insists, makes excuses that he can not honorably carry out the advice given. Appeals to his honor are ineffective. This conscienceless patient leaves the office of the physician without any intention of carrying out the advice given. But with the full intention of putting his former plans into execution. And in so doing commits a crime; for it is a moral crime, and should be regarded as a legal one. He is a afflicted with venereal disease and knowingly transmits his loathsome disease to a pure innocent woman who has trusted her life and honor to the one whom she has chosen as a husband and father to her future children. Here the hypocratic oath comes up and says my tongue shall be silent as to secrets confided to me I will not use my profession to corrupt maners or aid crime. Here is a contemplated crime, but as yet not committed; but none the less wilful and from a mean ignoble motive. The physi-

cian by his professional relations is the only one that can prevent this crime for he is the only confident, his silence makes of him an accomplice to the crime. One word to the parents or guardian or a hint to some friend of the intended victim would save her from a fate oftimes worse than death. Physicians do not look at this question in its seriousness, but pass it by perhaps without any serious thought as to the future consequences to the human race. He satisfies himself by saying, "I have given the man fair warning and he has not taken heed to it; so, I am not eo blame." So far he is not but he has neglected his duty by not warning the innocent. Why? Because he considers the oath to keep silent. In this case the secret shields a criminal and the physician, without giving it a thought becomes an accessary to the crime. Physicians report tuberculosis, smallpox, measles and all contagious diseases except venereal diseases but these are never hinted. No other disease to which mankind is heir is a greater menace to the race and there is no reasonable excuse why they should not be reported, only custom keeps them back. One of the greatest problems of the age, or should be, is the prevention of venereal diseases. This problem is complex exceedingly so no satisfactory solution has ever been given or proposed to control these diseases. There is always a conflict between the sanitary authorities and other interests involved.

EMPYEMA.

BY D. E. BRODERICK, M. D. KANSAS CITY, MISSOURI.

The very marked difference in the physical findings in children as compared to adults; the neglect or ignorance manifested

Read before the Annual Meeting Oklahoma State Medical Association, Tulsa, May, 1910.

in the recognition of collections of pus in the pleural cavities; and the fact, well known in pediatrics, that many children succumb to undiscovered empyemata, afford the motive in the preparation of this paper. The pneumodynamics of the chests of children, the frequency of the etiological factors in empyema of children and adults must necessarily offer pabulum for fruitful discussion.

ETIOLOGY.

Empyema is more frequently primary than is generally believed. The microbic factor is frequently the pneumococcus. In 109 empyemata investigated by Netter (quoted from Leslie Carr) the pneumococcus was present; in 53.6 per cent. of 28 cases in children; while in 89 cases in adults it was found in 54 of 137 cases or 39.4 per cent. The French authors give 53 per cent. as due to pneumococci and 70 to 75 per cent. of the sero-fibrinous pleurises as tubercular. It is possible that in old empyemata, those showing yellowish-green creamy pus with fibrinous masses the pneumocci have dissappeared, as cultures are frequently sterile. There is a tendency for all pneumococci empyema to tend to spontaneous sterility. The effusion is not always purulent in the pneumococcal form. The classification of the varied forms need not necessarily detain us. One must remember that empyemata is, in all cases, a localized purulent process, therefore a simplified working classification is all that is necessary. Goodhart presents an admirable classification as follows:

1. Pus contained in cavity between outer surface of lung and the costal pleura. (Most common form.)

2. Between diaphragm and the base of lung. (Diaphragmatic form.)

3. Between lobes (inter-lobar) and between lungs and mediastinum. The loculated form may occupy any of these positions and is merely a more localized process.

In Musser's statistics of 12,892 cases of pneumonia, empyema occurred in 2 per cent. there were 5 per cent. of empyema found at autopsy out of 973 cases of pneumonia.

Empyema of the newly born is generally due to strepococci.

SYMPTOMS.

Most frequently empyema in children is secondary to pneumonia, although as previously mentioned it is commonly primary in children. If the pleura be primarily attacked by the pneumococcus the constitutional signs do not materially differ from a primary invasion of the lungs. The onset may be acute or insidious, the latter having a tendency toward chronicity at times exhibiting a septic state which may be difficult of recognition. The onset of a diaphragmatic pleurisy is often mistaken for abdominal disease, due to the referred pain, icterus, etc. The fever in empyema may be high and continuous, intermittent or hectic or absent altogether. All hectic temperatures should excite suspicion of laculated empyema, and most carefully ruled out if the pathological process is confined to the chest. Sweating and diarrhea may be present.

PHYSICAL SIGNS.

The physical signs in diseases of the chest constitute our chief method of diagnosis combined with exploratory thoractomy.

PERCUSSION.

This is our most valuable asset in our examination of the chest of children. The sense of resistance obtained as one is percussing over fluid is marked and when this method of examination is once developed, valuable information is obtained. I am of the opinion that marked sense of resistance obtained while percussing chest is the most valuable physical sign we have. Forcible percussion must be light. The dullness obtained in empyema is stationary and is not affected by position. The upper line is either horizontal or slightly concave, ascending into axilla; in simple cases —flatness over one entire lung in infants is strongly indicative of fluids.

INSPECTION.

The apex beat may afford valuable information in the differential diagnosis. It may be accepted as a general rule that the apex is displaced by all fluid collections in the chest when the amount is sufficient—the displacement is away from the affected side. In fibrotic processes the apex is displaced toward the side affected. One should hesitate to diagnose an empyema when the percussion note shows a marked area of dullness with apex of the heart in its normal position. Bulging of intercostal spaces, etc., are of secondary importance.

GROCCO'S SIGN.

This sign, first elucidated by the Italian physician, is of inestimable value especially in small empyema or it s disappearance after some being present in distinguishing between thickened pleura and persistent effusion. Blumer states that Grocco sign is of distinct value in the recognition of small effusion and of encapsulated effusions provided that these are in contact with the spinal column. When the triangle does occur, as a result of disease below the diaphragm, it is usually symmetrical, differs in shape from the typical triangle of pleural effusion. It is not pathognomonic for Smith reports a case demonstrating Groccos triangle in cyst-adenoma of the ovary. The dullness is probably due to displacement of the mediasterum. In 77 cases in which Grocco sign was noted the dullness was two or three vertebrae lower in about 50 per cent. and in the rest was on the same level. (Rauchfuss), "Perforation of an inter lobar empyema into the pleural cavity was accompanied by the triangular area of dullness."

AUSCULTATION.

This aid to physical diagnosis has been the means of failure of correct interpretation of the findings by many physicians in examining children with pleural effusion—for this information has been gained mostly by study of disease in the adult.

In children bronchial breathing and bronchial voice are heard over fluid. The bronchial breathing is often distant and not harsh or distinctly tubular in type. What is known as baccallis dictum is the phenomena of whispered voice being better transmitted through serous than through purulent exudates. It is rare to find bronchial breathing or bronchopony both absent. Coin sound has not been of any value to me and is corroborative only; vocal resonance may be lost while whispered voice is often present. Auscultation has not the value that percussion has in the recognition of empyemata.

DIAGNOSIS.

The difficulties of diagnosis may be great and often are. The varied group known as Basic diseases are most puzzling methods. One must have resort to exploratory thoracotomy to clear up massive signs in the chest. I have seen an exploratory needle give pus (pneumococci) by perforating a small pocket of pus in a fibrotic lung, and as resection followed to give drainage for a supposed empyema, an entire fibrotic lung was revealed. As obdominal diseases have been studied by exploratory laparotomy, and, as the surgeon has been our chief exponent of pathological conditions of the abdomen, placing our knowledge of the diseases of the abdomen far in advance of those of the chest, so do I anticipate a similar condition for diseases of the chest. The pneumatic cabinets have materially aided in this study since their advent in thoracic surgery. As previously mentioned in this paper, many children and a great many more nurslings succumb to an empyema, which is revealed post-mortem.

The diagnosis of a typical empyema following a lobar pneumonia is, of ocurse, simple; the primary envolvement of the pleura; inter-lobar or diaphragmatic form constitute a different question.

A discussion of non-tubercular basic diseases with reference to differential diagnosis affords much interest. A classification as given by Dr. Goodhart, of London, is as follows:

I. Collapse of lower lobe by effusion, absorption of fluid.

II. Collapse by effusion, absorption, supervening fibrosis and bronchiectasis.

III. Empyema opening into the lung.

IV. Hepatic abscess or hydatid cyst.

V. Collapse by pressure on bronchus, supervening bronchiectasis.

VI. Gangrene of chronic pneumonia of lower lobe of lung.

VII. Bronchiectasis secondary to collapse and catarrhal pneumonia (children.)

To this classification may be advantageously added (a) those rare cases of middle lobe collapse due to progressive obstruction of the bronchial tubes, (b) a haemorrhagic condition of the distal lung substance from emboli, (c) chronic pneumonic condition subsequent to measles, leading to caseous tuberculosis or pure fibrosis, (d) enlarged bronchial glands or mediastinum (I mention this division because of the interscapular dullness which may and often is present in these conditions), (e) a recurring form of pneumonia characterized by a recrudesence of all constitutional signs with physical signs unchanged, later constitutional signs return and run typical course. A detailed discussion is not permissible in the time allowed me, and I must merely state the classification and depend upon your discussion for development. Your ingenuity will often be taxed to say positively the advent of an empyema or a pneumonia. A chronic febrile course may accompany a pneumonia causing death by emaciation. One is necessarily perplexed to decide the question of an empyemata. I am of the opinion that since these cases are in the minority, one is justified in exploring all cases of the lobar form after the usual time has elapsed for a complete recrudesence of constitutional signs and disappearance of physical phenomena. "When tubular breathing is followed by complete absence of respiratory sounds, vocal fremitus and diminished or absent resonance, it must not be hastily concluded that an infusion has taken place into the pleura, for massive pneumonia may have come to pass or mucus may be only temporarily blocking the bronchi." Of course, this condition would be rare in children, but it is a knowledge of the rarities that denotes the diagnostician. In the differential diagnosis of purulent effusion and sero-fibrinous effusion I am giving you the tabulated form quoted from Godlee, of London, with personal addition.

PURULENT EFFUSION —AGE.

Common in children.

SERO-FIBRINOUS EFFUSION:

More common in adults. A tendency become loculated in children. (Case report in appendix.)

MODE OF ORIGIN.

Pneumococcus in children. Streptococci in nurslings.

(Commonly tubercular.)

ONSET.

Severe, may resemble pneumonia. May be primary in pneumococcal form. Insidious form perplexing.

(May be severe, commonly insidious.)

SYMPTOMS.

Dyspnea, rigors, sweats, cough, emaciation, Leucocytosis.

(Usually absent. No leucocytosis.)

TEMPERATURE.

Hectic, continuous or normal.

(Evening elevation. May assume hectic character.)

LOCAL CHANGES.

Fullness of interspaces, pulsation, edeme of chest wall. Rupture of sack. Physical signs same in both.

(Very rare. Physical signs same in both.)

ABSORPTION.

Rare. Occasionally observed in pneumococous cases in children.

(Common. Fibrosis of pleura may remain. Recurrence more common.)

PROGNOSIS.

Good in pneumococcal form.

(To be guarded.)

In regard to the dullness at the left base, described by Cheadle, in pericarditis, with effusion, the only importance is, of course, in the interpretation of the pericardic trouble. This dullness is very apt to be increased from day to day until the whole left base may be dull; no constitutional signs accompany the condition. The real pathology is an atelectasis. The differential diagnosis between an empyenma, pericarditis with effusion or pyo-pericardium, is not often difficult. Unless the apex is displaced I would view with hesitation a diagnosis of empyema. The blood picture in diseases of the chest; the great value of the X-Ray and the more frequent use of exploratory thoracatomy will place our observation of physical signs upon a more rational basis. In empyema and pneumonia we have a pronounced leucocytosis; the X-Ray is of especial value in clearing up a diagnosis of inter-lobar empyema and the finding of pus with the trocar is confirmatory. The latter observation needs reservation. A case to point:—Female, age 2 yrs. 5 months.

Breathing is not labored, is shallow and slow. No dyspnea is apparent while at rest or on assuming the upright position. Temp. slightly irregular, not ascending above 100 degrees F. There is a steady loss of weight. Calamette's reaction is negative. There is an occasional loose cough. No pain. Fingers clubbed. Beneath the left clavicle in front there is a dull, semi-flat percussion note which reaches to the nor-mal cardiac dullness, occupies entire left axilla and all of chest posteriorly on left side. There is distant bronchial breathing as you have patient take a deep breath, accompanied by fine crepitations at the end of inspiration. The breathing assumes the carvernous type over the lower 1-3 of the left lung. Over this cavernous area there is a tubular percussion note. Chest is resistant on percussion. The apex is a little to the left of the nipple line, otherwise the heart is normal. Exploring needle was inserted 6th interspace and 10 m. of pus obtained which showed pneumococci. The diagnosis at this time was empyema. Calamette reaction on second trial proved positive. X-Ray later verified a diagnosis of fibrosis. This case is extremely interesting. The finding of 10 m. of pus, demonstrating pneumococci, was due to puncturing a small packet of pus in a fibrotic lung. More attention should have been given to the apex, as this was drawn to the side of the lesion. The X-Ray proved of inestimable value in this case.

There is perhaps no field of physical diagnosis that the personal equation is of so much value as in diseases of the chest. In the brief discussion of inter-lober empyema, which from the intricacies involved, could easily occupy all our time, I am to be content with the citation of a typical case. Girl, age 4 1-2 years, seen with Dr. Voelkers, of London.

Child was admitted for pneumonia. Illness began with the prodromata of measles followed with some delay by an atypical measles eruption. Ten days later child developed broncho-pneumonia. The course of the pneumonia was of moderate severity until the end of 10 days, when she becomes much worse. Temperature 103, pulse 160, resp. 40-50. *Status Praesens.*

Patient looks ill. Coughs up much purulent material. There is a line of dullness and bronchial breathing extending transversely along the lower border of normal lung, resonance lying over the liver in front. In the back there is a transverse line of dullness, corresponding with breath of interspace. It extends for about 2 inches.

Operation was not deemed advisable at present as further study was necessary. It was Voelker's supposition that the free expectoration of pus was indicative of the rupture of this inter-lobar empyema into a bronchus.

A case illustrating the deceptions encountered in the differential diagnosis between a fibrosis of the lung and empyema is given in order to emphasize the mistakes one makes in his deductive logic.

Girl, age 8 months. Child has been ill for two months. Patient looks ill and anaemic; Mother has tubercular appearance. There has been a gradual loss of weight, but no ascertainable history of an acute illness. Temp. 99.4. Resp. 36. Pulse 120. *Status Praesens.*

From directly below the vlavicle on the left side anteriorly, whole of left axilla and entire left chest posteriorly there is a marked dullness with much increased resistance. Typical bronchial breathing is absent, the inspiratory sound being harsh and bronchial in character. The expiratory sound is not bronchial, nor is it perceptibly prolonged, differing but slightly from the normal. Voice sounds are well transmitted. The apex beat is not displaced nor is there any cardiac hypertrophy. The spleen is palpable. There is no dyspnea, nor does the child's appearance denote a septic process. Physical examination otherwise normal. The needle was inserted and a pus containing pneumococci evacuated. The original diagnosis was empyema. In a more thorough study of the case this diagnosis was changed to fibrosis. The diagnosis of fibrosis was made at operation. Six oz. of pus was also obtained. Anatomical diagnosis, fibrosis of lung.

REMARKS—The diagnosis in this case was partially correct. The pneumococcal empyema was probably engrafted on a tubercular lung. Too much importance was assigned to the absence of expiratory bronchial breathing and likewise the absence of displacement of the apex.

One naturally is placed at a disadvantage in these cases of lung fibrosis. The onset and early history is lost to the consultant. The primary process is often a capillary bronchitis, collapse and subsequent fibrosis.

Diaphragmatic empyema is often difficult of recognition, has a tendency to remain latent and not infrequently associated with sub-phrenic or hepatic abscess. It is impossible to differentiate areas of dullness due to pleural fluid from those due to a subphrenic abscess, if both are present. (Eisendrath.) In paracentesis of a hepatic abscess the pus obtained is chocolate-colored, and without odor.

Space will not allow a discussion of dullness due to enlarged bronchial lymph glands and mediastinal tumors, nor certain areas of pneumonic consolditation which are difficult of recognition.

Among the complication of empyema one must remember a septic state of the body occuring in old undiscovered empyemata. The recovery is doubtful when once this state is fully developed. The development of a pyo-pericardium, complicating an empyema is of hopeless prognosis. The pyo-pericardium may be in partitions as I saw a pathological specimen in the Hospital for Sick Children in London in which pyo-pericardium was diagnosed and operated. The space of the pericardium was normal. Post-mortem it was shown that the pericardium was divided into 4 compartments by adhesions, three of which were filled with puss (pneumococci), the remaining one showing a normal pericardium. Poynton says that 60 per cent. of pyo-cardium are associated with empyema and about 40 per cent. with pneumonia or acute pleurisy. An edema of the lung is not as common in children following withdrawal of much pleuritic effusion as it is in adults.

In explanation of the spinal and vertebral resonance occuring in effusion, giving what is known as the S-shaped dullness Damaiseau, is due to the recession of lung, when laterally compression by fluid into the spinal groove (Ewart). Collapse following exploratory thoracatomy or more radical measures in empyema is reported as 10 per cent. (Sewis & Capps). Traumatic pneumothorax may be alarming. I have a most vivid recollection of witnessing a traumatic pneumo-thorax follow thoracatomy with a marked fall in blood pressure and collapse. Sewis and Capps, in an admirable article, classify the collapse as the cardio-inhibitory and the vaso-motor type. Sewis advises adrenalin chlordie for this collapse.

TREATMENT—Sauerbuch pneumatic cabinet if constructed on a more simplified and economical plan will mark an era of great improvement in operative work in empyemata. The expansion of the lung assisting drainage; the prevention of chest deformity will necessitate its employments by all modern surgeons. The simplification of the pressure apparatus, either negative or positive, will find us resorting frequently to exploratory thoracatomy, fearless of pneumothorax and possessing the knowledge to clasify many choatic physical findings. Pathology will be elucidated thereby, and the future may find us as thankful to the thoracic surgeon as internists have been to the abdominal surgeons in the development of our knowledge of intra-abdominal conditions. I am of the opinion that many cases of frank empyemata in children are allowed to die without even a suspicion of the true pathological condition being known. In a recent experience this statement is well exemplified.

Briefly, a girl, age 8 years, was sick for 8 weeks with a condition simulating typhoid fever. I was asked to post her.

The right chest contained fully a quart of pus, and the left chest 1 pint.

Exploratory thoracatomy over all areas of consolidation, not clear in their pathology, would save many lives.

There seems to be a tendency toward irrigation in pleural exudates. I think this is to be deprecated. Murphy, Wyeth and others inject 1 dram of a 10 per cent. solution of formaldehyde following evacuation of pus, or a 2 per cent. solution of formalin in glycerin. Auto-serum injections are advocated by Gilbert, Morcan, Dehis, "The technique consists in injecting 1 to 5 c. c. without withdrawing needle, plunging it into the subcutaneous substance. They repeat injections at intervals of 2 or 3 days." In thoracic paracentesis the indications for stopping the fluid flow are:

(a) Signs of cardio-inhibitory or vaso-motor collapse.

(b) Persistent pain and coughing.

(c) Bloody fluid.

The seats of election for paracentesis are 5 or 6 interspace or 9th outside of angle of scapula.

There is some differences of opinion among equally competent surgeons whether to operate on a double empyema at one time or defer operation on the other side until later. My opinion is that the sooner both sides can be drained the better the patients will do. In the treatment of old fistulous tracts, Beck's paste has been of advantage. Beck gives his formula for this work as 33 per cent. Bismuth Subnitrate with 67 per cent. vaselin—5 to 8 drams as a dose. Suction hyperaemia combined with inflation of lungs and the injection of sodium citrate chlorid) 4 pts. Nacl., 1 part of Sodium Ciratre, 100 pts. of boiling H_2O)

is advised for the treatment of these fistulae by a prominent English surgeon. Towel breathing may be of value in deformity of the chest, following atelectasis. The child is supported by a towel supporting the sound side and the child suspended.

THERMOGENESIS.

BY G. H. THRAILKILL, CHICKASHA, OKLA.

Animal heat may be defined as the thermic energy stored up in an animal body under both normal and pathologic conditions, as measured by the thermometer. These units may be similar but not identical, for the same animal species; since each individual of the same species may, technically speaking, have its own standard; so that in studying this complex physiologic mechanism, we must needs compromise science on some general average for the warm-blooded animals; also for the so-called cold-blooded animals; while we are compelled to reverse the position in this classification, under certain external surroundings of the so-called cold-blooded animals, since their range of temperature may be very much lower or very much higher than the warm-blooded animals.

Cold-blooded animals have been frozen by the surrounding media, and have been resuscitated after this suspended animation, and their temperature raised, surrounded by a liquid media, to a temperature beyond the possibilities of the warm-blooded animal; thus, it may be readily seen, that no general average can be fixed even for the same species of the cold-blooded animal; while, for any species of the warm-blooded animal a general average temperature can be approximately determined. The youth of warm-blooded animals sustains a higher general average than the aged of the same species; while the general average of the different species would each have its own general standard; this general average also differs in the sex of the same species; females being higher than males. Studying all species of warm-blood-

ed animals, the general average of each species gives us a wide difference of general averages; so, also, the temperature in any warm-blooded animal for any given time differs for the different parts of the animal anatomy from which the temperature is taken; the liver being hottest, the cutaneous surface the coldest. The lowest average general temperature among warm-blooded animals is that of the Duck-bill Plohbus, which is seventy-six degrees F., while the highest is that of the Sparrow, which is 110 degrees F.; while we note averages raging between these for the different species, we also note that there is a daily remission and exacerbation, varying from a half degree to a degree and a half, in the same animal, in a comparatively quiet state. Physical exertion, increased respiration, accelerated heart action, the ingestion of a hearty meal, excitement, mental exertion, physical trauma, toxic reaction, metabolism, and so on, increases body temperature. In the human species man has an average normal temperature varying from 98 to 99 1-2 degrees F., with a daily excursion of 1 1-2 degrees F.; this general average normal temperature is subject to minimum variations constantly.

Hyperthermacy is any temperature of the body above normal; hypothermacy is any temperature of the body below normal. These points, as we can readily see, must be determined in a general way to be practical; yet, they must necessarily differ by 1 1-2 degrees F. between the low temperature and high temperature. They must necessarily, at times, occupy common positions.

Thermogenesis is today a speculative field for the physiologist. Yet many facts have been proved, demonstrating that in the base of the brain, we have thermogenic centers which control the heat mechanism of the body, through the reflex of sympathetic system; that we have afferent and efferent nerve centers and nerve fiber which to their possessor unkonwingly control heat production, and heat dissipation. Thermogenesis, or heat production, being excited by all pathogenic toxins, physical violence, as an electric current producing a spasm of the skeletal musculature of the body, or a chemical violence, as the increased muscular tone resulting from physiological action of drugs, as strychnine, digitalis, curara, or any drug, increasing decreasing physiologic function of an organ; the venom of any serpent, insect, cold or heat, increases oxidation and stores heat energy in the animal body; nature's method of resisting extrensic intrusion, thus, waging a battle for the survival of the fittest.

The factors of heat and cold first manifest themselves on the sensory nervous system; the following being a good example—About twelve years since, while passing over the mountains at an altitute of about 11,000 feet above sea level, one cold winter night, your humble essayest was caught in a mountain blizzard; found it impossible to urge the team against the cold wind, or get his breath while facing it, stopped and turned around to breathe, and in a short time experienced the pains of severe cold, which were replaced in a short time by a comforting glow of warmth and a self-satisfied physical condition, which forced itself upon him; and, except for the mental agony of the knowledge that he was freezing, could have lain down and gone to sleep; however, my destination was finally reached, due to calming of what had been a severe but short blizzard; for four or five weeks after this the nerves of sensation were so injured that tactile sensation was lost in the fingers of both hands. The thermogenic centers had saved my life.

The thermogenic centers may be classified as acceleratory and inhibitory centers. Thermolysis employs the inhibitory centers and efferent nerves and diminishes body heat, as follows: By radiation, perspiration, and respiration; while the extrinsic factors of absorption by surrounding media aids nature's battle; shock and syncope assist at times in diminishing temperature by temporarily suspending animation. Thermotaxis is that nervous control that regulates hyperthermacy and hypothermacy, and does so by either increasing, excretion, or diminishing excretion, by exciting inactivity of the skin, kidney, or alimentary canal; thus storing up heat in the animal economy. The appearance of so-called goose flesh is a guard against loss of heat, and stores up, temporarily, heat energy in the animal body; while flushing hastens elimination temporarily; both is a kind of momentary reflex and produces a hysterical action of very short duration.

Heat stroke (insolation) is followed by high temperature; due to internal congestion, and may involve vital organs—as the stomach, heart, liver, spleen, kidney, or may be followed by evidences of central nerve exhaustion, as evidenced by mania, meloncholy, neurasthenia, neuritis, and often insanity; due to high temperature affecting nerve tracks, and impoverishment of blood corpuscles; when the person so affected survives the stroke; while persons dying of insolation usually die in collapse, and a low temperature maintains throughout; a moderately high temperature in heatstroke, prognosticates recovery, while a low temperature is eminent of collapse.

Fever may in some infectious diseases as Typhoid, Erysipelas, and Diphtheria for example, increase the activity of anti-bodies and thus lessen malignancy, however, for the safety of our patient this beneficial fever should be maintained within medium limits, ever bearing in mind that a long standard is only comparative; that all patients should not receive a routine management; that individual temperaments depend on individual physiologies as well as generalities as to sex and age.

Sub-normal temperatures are more frequently observed than might at first seem possible; peritoneal injury; surgical shock and brain trauma furnish many examples; alcoholism and various neuroses furinsh examples. In these cases we usually find a diminished oxidation and faulty elmination.

In collapse there is always present a depressed condition of the nervous system, volition is abolished or much diminished; while dermal elmination is increased; however, this will not account for the loss of body heat; thermolysis in these cases is active, while thermotaxis is paralyzed; since this activity in normal physiological processes would tend to a normal equillibrium; hence in shock only, that medication which restores normal physological processes is indicated; strichnae, normal saline solutions by enema or transfusion, external heat dry, rest in a recument position, while in the secondary shock cold packs locally are most efficient.

Fever and hysteria is seldom observed, however emotional energy may cause it; the fever being transient in most cases; and best controlled with sedatives. Personally. I have never seen what I considered a fever in hysteria.

If hyperthermacy remains reasonably low even though it be continuous, the degenerative changes to the organs effected by physological heat whether it be toxobicrobic, toxochemic or physic is comparatively slight, the less so when the diurnal excursion is not excessive as in Malaria, Typhoid and clinically speaking should not cause

great anxiety for the patient. well fare, nor require active medication; much harm has been and may be done by medicating fevers; happy was the introduction of hydrotherapy in the treatment of fevers; we are glad to note the tendency at present to give but little medicine in efforts to reduce fever; the bath and cold pack have displaced medicine much to the comfort and safety of the patient.

Fever is a result of a pathological change going on in the animal economy, and is pathognomonic of a diseased condition. When called to the bedside of a patient with a thermometric record above or below normal, we should decide at once that there is a diseased condition, and search for the same; the disease may be toxochemic or toxomicrobic or physical in origin, thus requiring diagnostic acuteness, which may require several visits to determine and locate. We may never locate the pathologic condition; however, we may be always assured there is one. A sub-normal temperature is just as positively a pathognomonic index as a super-normal temperature, and should demand as careful examination; it may mean impending brain or circulatory lesions; it may be the result of pathogenic toxines recently thrown into the circulation, by a very recent fission of pathogenic germs, as in the early rigor of a pernicous malaria or a very malignant diphtheria or eresypalis. The experience of all bacteriologist confirms the lowering of body temperature when a pathogenic toxine or vaccine is first injected into the circulation, followed soon. however, by a rise of temperature. The rigor being nature's method of resisting the invasion, and the beginning of nature's battle for the survival of the fittest.

In conclusion on this point, when we have a patient with a temperature above or below normal, we must at once look for a pathological condition, for such surely ex-

ists. Theremometers do not lie. The temperature may be ephemeral or may be hysterical, but a pathologic condition has called it forth; and, it is our duty to so acquit
ourselves as to be able to intelligently
search out the etiology. Let us hope that
the day of symtomatic treatment is nearing an end. Whatever good symptomatic
medication may have served us in the past,
it is but an acknowledgment of a condition not yet thoroughly investigated. An
open admission of ignorance, a frank ac-
knowledgement of indolence and mental
turpitude, a poor apology for a frank I
don't know.

I hope the day shall soon come when
we shall cease to hear such misnomers as
lung fever, bilious fever, brain fever, typhoid fever, hay fever, puerperal fever,
remittant fever, as ordinarily used, scarlet
fever, splenic fever, and yeilow fever, et al.
They mean nothing within themselves, and
have no patholigical significance. The sooner we drop them, the sooner shall we begin to know something of the pathology of
fevers and the morbid anatomy of disease.
Let us consider all fevers as having a pathologic origin, and soon these meaningless
terms will be absolete, and we will be directing pyrexias by other means than coal
tar derivatives; that are fraught with many
dangers and must only reduce temperature
at the expense of an already weakened physiological body; as a result of a pathogenesis.

Clenically, fevers may be classified as
remittent, intermittent, and continuous, as
they relate to the normal average temperature, and with this meaning only; remembering that their excursions on the fever
chart will show variations between the
youthful and the aged.

Last but not least, let us endeavor to
assist the thermogenic mechanism in the
control of body heat, in accord with physiological processes, namely, by keeping in
mind the metabolisms of the normal physiologic, animal body.

SUMMARY.

1. Fevers in most cases depend directly upon infectious toxaemia and are of
bacterial origin; having a definite pathology.

2. Fever may be toxochemic having an
indefinite pathology.

3. Fever may be due to physical exer-
tions the pathology of the same coming late
and of a definite character.

4. That fever has nothing to do with
the organ or organs diseasesd and is only a
symptom of a condition and should have
nothing to do with the naming of disease.

5. That hypothermacy is a pathological symptom as well as hyperthermcay.

6. That hydrotherapy either cold or
warm is more efficient in controlling body
temperature and more safe than internal
medication, except in emotional fevers.

April 30, 1910.

PHYSICAL CHARACTERISTICS OF THE NEGRO.

BY DR. ALBERT C. HIRSHFIELD, NORMAN, OKLA.

When I began the preparation of this
paper, I asked a friend, casually, "What do
you know about the physical characteristics
of the Negro?" His reply was, "Well, he

*Read before the Oklahoma Academy of
Science, at the First Annual Meeting, Nov.
26, 1910.*

has a black skin, kinky hair, and thick
lips." But in my investigation of this subject, I find that these are really but very
incidental differences between the black and
white race. Beyond being of passing scientific interest, I hope to show that the negro's physical characteristics are of vast

sociologic and economic importance. In fact, these characteristics explain the social, moral and industrial inferiority of the blacks, the fact of which inferiority is acknowledged by all except a few prejudiced sentimentalists.

With the leading sociologists of the day, I have come to believe that within the facts of primary racial characteristics, physical and psychological, lies the solution of the often discussed and apparently troublesome American Race Problem. But more of this anon.

Before going into discussion of this question, I wish to disclaim any originality for this work. The inspiration and much of the material for this paper emanate from the work of Dr. Dowd, Professor of Sociology in Oklahoma University, and the writings of other students of this question, constitute the balance of the basis of this paper, together with some clinical observations of my own.

In studying the American negro, it is important to take a peep at him in his natural surroundings and original home in Africa. Here must we study the conditions that have moulded the race, for not in a century or two is a race formed, but through ages.

First, let us bear in mind that one negro is not a representative of a single type or tribe of the native African, but a mixture of the five great distinct negro races of Africa. 1. It is a mistake that many missionaries and some writers have made that the American negro is a descendant of any particular race of negro; usually the lowest types having been considered the ancestors of our ex-slaves. No more is this true than that the American of today is the descendant of the Puritan Fathers. But to five different and largely dissimilar negro races, must we trace the ancestry of the American negro. Briefly these are: 1.

The Negritos, including the dwarf races of the equatorial regions, the Bushmen and the Hottentots. 2. The Nigritians, all the natives with dark skin and wooly hair, occupying the great Soudan territory. 3. The Fellatahs a race supposed to have sprung from crossing of the Berbers of the dessert with the Nigritians of the Soudan. 4. The Bantus, of somewhat lighter colored and less negroid features. 5. The Gallas, a light colored and very superior race. 2. The great differences between these people are largely due to the difference in the surrounding climate and economic conditions. 3. We find four distinct zones in negro Africa, each of which possesses special conditions, which in turn contribute toward the formation of different types of negro.

First we have the banana zone which, as the name signifies, is a tropical country, abundant in fruit and other natural resources. Here the native scarcely has to turn his hand for a livlihood. In this zone we find the lowest type of the physical negro. He has a small head, with a very receding forehead and an extreme prognathism, and a relatively larger occipital development. This configuration gives him a long, sloping, egg-shaped head. The centres of thought, reason and intellect being housed in the fore brain, it is seen at once that these have scarcely developed. The large occipital development signifies a predominance of growth of the objective centers, or centers of animal instinct. 4

As is to be expected, knowing that there is a well defined connection between mental and physical energy, these negroes show a very conspicuous lack of physical energy.

Leaving the Banana Zone, we find to the Northward the Millett Zone. Here the conditions of life demand more mental effort, hence the brains of these people are somewhat larger and better developed. Going West from the Slave coast, the heads of the natives become less dolichocephalic and foreheads less receding. 5.

Another step Northward and we are in the cattle zone, the natives of which lead a nomadic, pastoral life. Here the heads are larger and better formed. The Kanuris of this region have larger heads, and high foreheads.

Lastly we have the Camel Zone, the natives of which bear no greatly dissimilar physical characteristics to those of the cattle zone. 6.

To return to the American negro and his physical make up.

Beginning with his head, we find it dolichocephalic, prognathus and with a somewhat receding forehead, indicative of a low development of the intellectual centers. We of course find brachycephalic heads upon some black shoulders, but this is more common among the Mulatoes, or those having more or less white blood.

As to the anthropometry of the negro, Mr. F. L. Hoffman, Statistician of the Prudential Insurance Co. has published some very comprehensive statistics in his "Race Traits" and "Tendencies of the American Negro." From these I shall quote frequently.

First, relation of weight and height,— the negro is on the average of greater weight in proportion to both age and height than the white. The best statistics on this point are taken from the reports of the Sanitary Commission and of the Provost Marshal General of the U. S. Government. The former work deals with recruits at the time of the application for enlistment, while the latter deals with the soldier in the field. 7. These statistics show an excess of weight, from five to ten pounds, for the negro, with an average of about seven pounds for all statures. Also these statistics show that for the same chest measurements the negro is from eight to ten pounds heavier than the white man. From a medical view-

point, I would rather present this statistical fact turned around—that is to say, for the same weights, the negro's chest circumference is from one to one half inches less than that of the white man. For example, white men averaging one hundred and forty-three pounds in weight will possess an average chest circumference of thirty-six inches, while a negro of the same weight will have a circumference of thirty-four and five-tenths inches. For the greater weights, the difference is only about an inch, but these facts are interesting, in view of the negro's great susceptibility to respiratory diseases, of which I shall speak later. Negro children, as well as adults, show an excess of weight over white children of the same height and age.

The average weight of the negro lung is four ounces less than that of the white. 8.

The average mobility, e. g. expansion of the negro chest, is less than that of the white.

Also in lung capacity the white lung exceeds that of the black by from 8 cu. inches at 5 ft. of height to 14.5 cu. inches at 6 ft. of height, and from 2 cu. inches at 40 inch chest girth to 25.5 cu. inches at 30 inch chest girth. 9.

Also in frequency of respiration the negro exceeds the white by one and three-tenths, or eight per cent. This in a condition of health. In disease, the comparison is still more unfavorable to the negro, for here his rate is nearly four respirations greater, or about 25 per cent. This shows a much higher degree of susceptibility of the negro lung to disease. The same favorable condition is to be noted in the rate of the pulse. 10.

In mean lifting strength, the negro averages 8 3-4 pounds less than that of the white man for all ages, this disproving the common belief that the negro is of superior strength. 11.

The power of vision of the negro is inferior to that of the white, 12 but he is less liable to diseases of the eye, especially color blindness. 13. It is interesting in passing to note that, in the power of vision, the Indian surpasses all others. 14.

It is noteworthy that in all the conditions noted, where a comparison was made, the negro falls short of the white man in physical strength and development. This comparison shows a marked physical deterioration of the blacks in the last half century, as in 1861 the male negro was considered the equal, if not the superior, of the white man. While the scope of this paper does not permit comprehensive quotations in support of this view, let me offer one or two quotations from army examining surgeons, who had a wonderful opportunity of comparing white and black males at the time of the Civil war. The Kentucky negro of war time was described thus, by Dr. James Foster of London, Ky., "For symmetry, muscular strength and endurance, I do not think the Ky. negro can be surpassed by any people on earth. The stoutest and most muscular men I ever examined were the negroes I examined at this office—he is certainly more muscular than the white man. He is in addition generally better developed in the chest than the white man." 15. Dr. John C. Maxwell, of Lebanon, Ky., wrote as follows: "I think I may state without fear of contradiction that the colored man in this locality, if bone and sinew, chest measurements and general physique are the criteria, presents the greatest physical aptitude for military service." 16.

So much for the anthropometry of the negro. Now let us consider the practical results of such a make-up, that is his susceptibility and resistance to the various diseases to which the human flesh is heir.

The first diseases to which the negro shows an alraming susceptibility and which are his prevalent ones are respiratory and venereal diseases. In my service in a large free dispensary, in a city with a large negro population, I was continually struck with the fact that of the great number of negroes who presented themselves for treatment, the vast majority were afflicted with consumption or venereal diseases. The great prevalence among the negroes of venereal diseases is a result not so much of any special susceptibility to the same, but to his extremely licentious and almost uncontrolled sexual life. While this statement may not be contradicted by any who know the negro, in support of this statement I offer the following quotation from the "American Negro," by William Hannibal Thomas, himself a negro: "My study and questioning of the average negro as he exists in the U. S. today has convinced me that he is bestial by nature, that he holds in regard whatever such virtues as may be present in the mothers, daughters, wives and sisters among them. They revel in lewd conversation, erotic practices, and unlimited sexual pursuits. Especially do they delight in encouraging the approaches of the whites among the woman of their kind." That such licentiousness is prevalent, is not surprising when we reflect that animal impulse is the sole master to which both sexes yield unquestioning obedience. 17.

While it is horrible to think of the almost universal prevalence of these diseases among them, what is it when I say, without fear of contradiction, that once contracted, probably 90 per cent of the cases of these diseases among the negroes are never cured. As a physician, I know that tuberculosis, gonorrhea and syphilis, are practically incurable unless taken in hand early and given long and skillful treatment. How many negroes could and would give up their surroundings and spend two or more years in some favorable climate for the cure of tuberculosis, or what negro will take five years regular treatment for a case of syphilis? It is my experience, and that of all physicians, that as soon as the distressing acute symptoms of venereal disease are over, the negro ceases treatment. It is almost axiomatic that a negro once infected is always infected. In the case of tuberculosis, the disease progresses until it claims its victim, and has infected those about him. I know of one case of tuberculosis which was followed by 13 others in the same dwelling, all fatal. In the case of venereal diseases, the acute symptoms shortly subside, but the infection remains dormant, infecting all his partners in licentiousness and resulting in blind and degenerate offspring, most of which die before reaching the age of productiveness and reproductiveness.

Not only are these diseases terribly prevalent, but they are increasing in prevalence. Prior to emancipation it was an undisputed statistical fact that tuberculosis had a greater mortality rate among the whites than among the blacks, but the reverse is now true, for among whites the mortality from this disease has been steadily decreasing, while it is increasing within the black race. 18.

Pneumonia is also very prevalent among the blacks, especially in the North, and the mortality rate from the same is very high. In explanation of this, you will remember that the negro has a small or tropical lung, that his lung has a proportionate smaller capacity, and that both his chest circumference and expansion are smaller than that of the white

While the above are the diseases having the greatest effect on the increasing mortality rate of the blacks, I shall not close without considering briefly some of the other common diseases.

Malaria and typhoid fevers. While it is the belief of many that the negro is relatively immune from these diseases, statistics show just the opposite to be the case, at least during the Civil war, and ever since emancipation. During the Civil war, the average rate of admission to hospitals for malarial diseases was 522 per 1,000 for the white troops and 829 for the colored troops, a difference of 307 per 1,000. The average death rate for the same was 3.36 per 1,000 for the whites and 10.03 for the colored troops. 19. For more modern statistics, I read the following tables of mortality from malaria and typhoid per 100,000 population in three large cities. 20.

MALARIAL FEVER.

		White	Colored
Charleston,	1865-94	42.45	66.63
Washington,	1890	25.21	77.94
Baltimore,	1890	27.78	29.72

TYPHOID FEVER.

		White	Colored
Charleston,	1865-94	67.34	100.73
Washington,	1890	74.34	112.29
Baltimore,	1890	42.49	8.35

The greater susceptibility of the negro is interesting in view of the fallacious belief that the negro is adapted for swampy and alluvial districts. The U. S. census of 1890 shows that the white race in these districts has a greater rate of increase than the blacks. 21.

It is also claimed that the negro enjoys an immunity against yellow fever. This is not true, but the negro is not as susceptible to this disease as the white. With smallpox the reverse is the case, the negro being very much more susceptible than the white. However, I believe I can attribute this difference to two causes; the very much worse average sanitary surroundings, and second, the smaller rate of vaccination among the negroes.

For measles, scarlet fever, diphtheria and croup, the mortality is undoubtedly less among the colored than among the whites, but by no means does the negro enjoy an absolute immunity against any of these diseases. 22.

There is also a trio of pathologic conditions, not mentioned, to which the colored man is much less susceptible than the white. These are alcoholism, insanity and suicide. These are encouraging conditions, but are probably due to the less highly organized structure of the negro brain.

While I have been reading of the high death rate among the negroes, did I hear some one say, "Well they are prolific enough to balance the excessive mortality." This brings me to the statement, that in the South the excess of births over deaths is less for the colored race than that of the white, and that in the North, deaths among the colored race exceed the births, which means that the race is not holding its own. The increases in the negro population of the Northern cities is due to migration.

I think I have succeeded in demonstrating that the negro has a higher mortality at all ages, but especially at the earlier age periods, and this mortality is increasing, already exceeding the birth rate in the North. What then is the answer, or what is the solution of the negro problem? It is ultimate extinction, resulting from intrinsic ra-racial characteristics.

In closing, I quote from Dr. Dowd, that after the negro has ceased to be, the most remarkable fact in his history will be the rapidity with which he vanishes from the earth.

BIBLIOGRAPHY.

1. Dowd, J. Lecture, Okla. U. Sept. 18, 1910.
2. Dowd, J. The Negro Races, N. Y. 1907.
3. Dowd, J. Lecture. Okla. U. Sept. 26, 1910.
4. Dowd, J. The Negro Races I, N. Y. 1907.
5. Dowd, J. The Negro Races I, N. Y. 1907.
6. Dowd, J. The Negro Races I, N. Y. 1907.
7. Hoffman, Race Traits and Tendencies, N. Y. 1896.
8. Flint, Sanitary Memoirs of the War of the Rebellion, p. 333, N. Y. 1867.
9. Gould, Military Statistics, p. 22.
10. Gould, Military Statistics, p. 523.
11. Gould, Military Statistics, pp. 461 and 465.
12. Gould, Military Statistics, p. 530.
13. Annual Reports of the Surgeon General U. S. A. 1888-1895.
14. Hoffman, p. 168.
15. Provost Marshal General's Report, Vol. I, p. 384.
16. Hoffman, p. 174.
17. Folk, The Negro as a Health Problem, Journal A. M. A. Oct. 8, 1910.
18. Hoffman, Ch. 2.
19. Hoffman, p. 97.
20. Hoffman, p. 100.
21. Census of U. S. Population Vol. I, p. 48 et seq.
22. Hoffman, p. 114.

CARDIAC MURMURS AND THEIR CLINICAL SIGNIFICANCE.

BY LEWIS J. MOORMAN, M. D., PROFESSOR OF PHYSICAL DIAGNOSIS, OKLAHOMA STATE UNIVERSITY MEDICAL SCHOOL, OKLAHOMA CITY, OKLA.

Auscultation of the heart sounds was first practiced by Harvey, but to Laenec (1819) belongs the credit of developing clinical auscultation. He attributed the first sound of the heart to the contraction of the ventricles and the second sound to the contraction of the auricles. Not many years later it was demonstrated that the contraction of the auricles preceded that of the ventricles and thus Laenec's theory as to the cause of the second sound was exploded. Since then many theories have been proposed to explain the cause of the heart sounds and though certain general views have been accepted, the subject is not yet closed.

With the investigation which has lead to our present understanding of the normal heart sounds, we have also acquired a certain knowledge of abnormal heart sounds, or heart murmurs. For a time heart murmurs were looked upon as almost synonymous with heart lesions, and those who laughed at Laenec's exploded theory working under a more dangerous fallacy, and even today, notwithstanding the progress of the past thirty years in the pathology and diagnosis of cardiac lesions, we are still attributing to heart murmurs much more importance than they merit. We seem inclined to forget that heart lesions of the gravest character may exist without heart murmurs, and that pronounced heart murmurs may occur independent of heart lesions.

FREQUENCY OF CARDIAC MURMURS.

Statistics from the combined hospitals of Vienna show that lesions of the heart and vessels rank third as a cause of death (Stoerk.)

In 1901 and 1902 there were 9,227 deaths. Of this number 1,152 were due to lesions of the heart and vessels, and 459, or 40 per cent. of the latter were due directly to valvular lesions. This means that about five per cent. of the total number of deaths resulted from valvular lesions. This, it must be understood, does not represent the frequency of valvular disease, but merely the number of deaths attributed directly to this cause. Records compiled by Gillespie show that of two thousand, three hundred sixty-eight cases (2,368) of cardiac lesions 80.8 per cent. showed valvular disease.

I believe the majority of cases that come to autopsy show either active valvular endocarditis, or the results of old endocarditis. Perhaps many of these do not give rise to murmurs.

In addition to the murmurs caused by valvular changes, we have a large percentage of functional murmurs which must be considered in the examination of the heart.

ORGANIC MURMURS.

Organic murmurs have their origin in valvular deformities which result, as a rule, from valvular endocarditis. Rheumatisim is the most frequent cause of endocarditis, giving rise to over eighty per cent. (Strumpel) of organic murmurs. This includes the heart lesions from rheumatism and chorea in children. In those cases in which there is no history of rheumatism, not even growing pains, chorea, or frequent attacks of tonsilitis during childhood, we are to think of scarlet fever, diphtheria, erysipelas, or other infectious processes.

We may have, in a limited number of cases, valvular deformities arising without a history of acute endocarditis. In these there is a gradual thickening with subsequent contraction. We have also the valvular changes accompanying general arterio-sclerosis. These are usually aortic. Aortic lesions, especially before middle life, carry with them the suspicion of syphilis.

Valvular lesions are of two types: (1) Those which cause partial obstruction of a valve orifice and give rise to stenosis; (2) Those which produce leakage or prevent perfect apposition of valves, thus giving rise to regurgitation or insufficiency. Stenosis results from adhesions between the free borders of the valves and from thickening and stiffening. Stenosis probably never exists without some degree of regurgitation. The same lesions which give rise to stenosis render perfect closure of the valves impossible. Regurgitation is caused by deformity of the valves or by weakening of the heart musculature.

The competency of the mitral and tricuspid valves is dependent partly upon the papillary muscles and the auriculo-ventricular rings. This accounts for the regurgitation occurring in connection with lesions of the myocardium. This is termed relative insufficiency and usually is classed with functional murmurs, as such murmurs may disappear with improvement in the condition of the cardiac muscle.

Murmurs are classified as systolic and diastolic. Those occurring synchronously with systole, and those occurring during diastole. The murmurs occurring in the latter part of diastole and leading up to the beginning of systole are called presystolic.

The quality or character of a murmur has little diagnostic worth. As a rule, the rough, rasping murmur indicates stenosis, and the soft, blowing murmur attends regurgitation. A musical quality has no special significance. The intensity or loudness of a murmur may have some prognostic value. As a rule, a loud murmur indicates a fair degree of compensation. If

Murmurs produced at the mitral valve have their point of maximum intensity in the region of the apex beat.

Murmurs heard most distinctly in the second left interspace are produced at the pulmonic orifice.

Murmurs heard with maximum intensity in the region of the ensiform cartilage are usually produced at the tricuspid orifice.

Murmurs produced at the aortic orifice may be heard best in the aortic area, but have their point of maximum intensity in the fourth left costal cartilage.

It is not within the scope of this paper to discuss in detail individual valvular lesions and their possible combinations, however, the accompanying table is useful in that it presents some physical signs of the most frequent organic murmurs and also serves to emphasize the importance of inspection, palpation and percussion.

FUNCTIONAL MURMURS.

Functional murmurs, according to some authorities, constitute not less than fifty per

AUSCULTATION	PERCUSSION	PALPATION	INSPECTION	LESION
1—A loud systolic murmur at the apex and accentuation of the 2nd pulmonic.	Hypertrophy of the left ventricle, and later also the right ventricle.	Strong radial pulse. Systolic thrill at the apex.	Strong heaving apex beat, displaced downward and to the left.	Mitral Insufficiency.
2—A diastolic or pre-systolic murmur at the apex; the first sound often loud; 2nd pulmonic accentuated.	Hypertrophy and dilatation of right ventricle.	Diastolic thrill at apex. Small pulse often irregular.	Increased cardiac action; epigastric pulsation.	Mitral stenosis.
3—A loud diastolic aortic murmur over the 4th costal cartilage or upper sternum. Short systolic sound in the peripheral arteries (brachial and femoral.)	Great hypertrophy and dilatation of left ventricle.	Strong heaving apex; often heaving precordia.	Apex beat increased in strength and area. Displaced to left and downward. Sometimes bulging of precordia. Visible pulsation of peripheral arteries.	Aortic Insufficiency.
4—A loud systolic aortic murmur. Absence or enfeeblement of aortic 2nd sound.	Hypertrophy of left ventricle.	Hearts action not very strong. Pulse small, lazy and usually slow. Aortic thrill.	Apex dislocated to left and downward.	Aortic stenosis.

a murmur entirely replaces the valvular sound it is safe to infer that there is considerable deformity of the valve.

cent. of all cardiac murmurs. They are practically always systolic and are usually heard best over the pulmonic valve. However, they may have their maximum intensity over the mitral or aortic area. They are usually soft and blowing, but may be loud. They are not transmitted to axilla or back. They are not accompanied by evidence of organic lesions, as hypertrophy, dilatation, cyanosis, dyspnea, hepatic or other visceral engorgement. They are more readily influenced by position and exercise than are the organic murmurs, often disappearing when the patient is in the upright position, and becoming more pronounced after exercise. They are more common in children than in adults, and often occur in febrile conditions. They are to be found especially in the anemic, poorly nourished and over-taxed. Butler found that in one hundred children from six to fourteen years of age, supposed to be free from vascular or blood diseases, sixty-four presented cardiac murmurs. Of these all but eighteen disappeared when in the upright position. The absence in the history of rheumatism or other infections which might have caused endocarditis suggest functional murmurs. Some cases may have to be kept under observation a few weeks or months before a differential diagnosis can be made.

THE NEED OF SYSTEMATIC EXAMINATION OF THE HEART AND A MORE RATIONAL INTERPRETATION OF CARDIAC MURMURS.

The large percentage of unrecognized cardiac murmurs is due principally to want of examination rather than to want of knowledge or skill. It is our duty to examine the heart of every case coming under our observation before we presume to give an opinion or a prescription. This duty is multiplied by anything in the history suggesting the possibility of a cardiac lesion. In connection with this we must remember that growing pains and chorea mean rheumatism; and that rheumatism in the child may be manifested by fever and endocarditis without joint symptoms. Also, that tonsilar and pharyngeal affections may give rise to endocarditis. No doubt many of the valvular lesions first discovered in the adult have their origin in childhood. They are overlooked because the heart is not carefully and frequently examined. If these lesions were anticipated and recognized early, much damage might be averted. The same is true of valvular endocarditis originating in the adult. The condition is often overlooked at the time of origin and discovered accidentally when the individual applies for life insurance, or when, on account of some particular symptom or condition, his physician deems it necessary to make a careful physical examination, or refers him to some one for diagnosis.

I have chosen to speak of cardiac murmurs rather than of valvular lesions, because of the prevailing tendency to depend too much upon auscultation in the diagnosis and estimation of cardiac conditions. Heart murmurs must be interpreted in the light of inspection, palpation and percussion. With the intelligent employment of these methods, which must constitute a part of every systematic examination of the heart, many of our errors in diagnosis and prognosis might be eliminated. The individual possessing a functional murmur might be spared the anxiety and worry, and, in some cases, the material loss, attending the announcement of a heart lesion; and the unfortunate victim of an organic murmur might have his strength conserved and his life prolonged by the well-directed management which naturally follows a definite determination of the lesion and a correct estimate of the degree of compensation.

LEWIS J. MOORMAN, M. D.
Oklahoma City, Okla.
September, 1910.

EDITORIAL

THE FEE SPLITTING QUESTION.

The following editorial is copied complete from the February number of COLORADO MEDICINE, the official Journal of the Colorado State Medical Association, for the reason that no words can be more applicable to the same question which is confronting the profession of Oklahoma at this time and has been one of a vexatious nature for some time in the past:

A deliberate division of a fee, prearranged or not, by the surgeon and family attendant, without the knowledge of the patient is a crime and should be so regarded by the profession.

"EVERY MAN WHO DOES GOOD WORK SHOULD BE PAID FOR WHAT HE DOES, AND NO MAN SHOULD BE PAID FOR WHAT HE DOES NOT DO."

(1) *A surgeon who leis it be understood that he will give to every doctor sending him a case, a certain proportion of the fee, whether he earns it or not—say half as its frequently done—really makes every one who agrees to this his hired agent, just as much as if he sent him out to canvass the incoming railroad trains with the promise of a fat commission for every patient he might steer in.*

These agents are sometimes beginners in practice or else more or less unsuccessful and unscrupulous practitioners. They soon discover that they can make more money and make it easier by furnishing cases on commission than they can through legitimate practice, and their hunt for subjects for operation becomes a frantic one. With a poorly paying practice on the one hand and a rich bait of 50 per cent of the fee dangling within easy reach on the other, they soon begin to strain a point and urge operations where operations are unnecessary. It becomes easy to say; "If you are not operated upon you will die." Under the circumstances excuses for this questionable conduct are easily found.

Now, the surgeon who employs these agents is a more or less unscrupulous man, who is wildly grasping for work and does not care how he gets it. He is not willing to earn it by proving to others that he can do things well, thus establishing a legitimate reputation—the recognized and approved method—but he is anxious to buy his work and let the proof of ability come afterwards, if it ever does come.

It may be said that such a man may soon become an expert operator, owing to the amount of work which he will do. True; but an expert operator does not constitute a good surgeon—this requires, in addition, judgment, learning, conscience, and an undeviating purpose to do that which is best in every respect for the patient, irrespective of fees and operative statistics. In this sense, he who buys his cases can seldom become a good surgeon.

When an agent sends a case to such a commission-paying employer, the necessity for an operation has often been exaggerated so as to make sure of bagging the game. Hence, in order to protect the interests of his agent, as well as the interests of his pocket, the surgeon *MUST* operate; but it can readily be conceived that his already elastic conscience is usually equal to the emergency; and I venture to say that few such cases are ever turned down even when an operation is not really called for.

(2) Hence, *the commission business leads to indiscriminate, reckless and useless operating;* and in these days, when the tendency in this direction is already too great, owing to the comparative ease with which many operations can be done, this

is unfortunate, to say the least.

(3) *Individual ability in different lines of work should be encouraged and not hampered.* In every community there are surgeons who are noted for certain things, —one is particularly skilful in hysterectomy, another in operating upon the brain, a third in the surgery of the appendix, a fourth in stomach and gall-bladder work. The general practitioner is supposed to find out in the course of time who these men are and his patients have a right to expect that he will use this knowledge for their benefit. But how can a fine, or even a course, discrimination be exercised with 50 per cent of the fee obscuring the vision, and with nothing to do but reach out and take it? The doctor's employer, the commission-paying surgeon, inevitably gets the case, whether he is the best man to handle it or not.

Suppose your wife were very sick and required the services of a surgeon, and you trusted your family physician to pick out the one best suited to operate on this particular case; and you found out afterwards that the surgeon had really been selected not because of fitness, but because he paid your doctor half the fee for selecting him. How would you feel about this? Would you not feel that you had been buncoed? Would you not call it on unjustifiable traffic in human misfortune? Would you not feel like shooting your family physician, especially if disaster resulted to your wife?

(4) *Publicity is what is needed:*—If but two doctors resided in a small town and one was known to be a "commission-doctor" while the other carried on a legitimate business of his own, being in the employ of no one and choosing his surgeons according to their merits alone—if this state of affairs existed, other things being equal, how long would it take the populace to make a selection between these two men?

And this suggests the easiest, best, and quickest manner of doing away with the commission evil—*publicity.* Such things flourish in darkness. Turn on the light and they run for cover. Is there any doubt that if the public *knew* a surgeon obtained his work by paying commissions rather than by proving his skill it would express its disapproval by avoiding him?

(5) *Every man should be paid for what he does, and no man should be paid for what he does not do:* Simply referring a case to a surgeon without further action should usually mean a consultation fee only, which the patient will generally pay without question. It is true, however, that in surgical cases the responsibility is often increased by advising operation; but if the case is one which *should* go to the surgeon, is not the responsibility even greater if he is not so advised? In fact, the responsibility can not be escaped either way. It would be right, however, for medical men to demand a larger fee for the added responsibility, and trouble accompanying the diagnosis of many surgical cases, the selection of a surgeon, and other matters incidental to the necessary arrangements for an operation. When this matter is presented in a proper light to the public it is always quick to see its justice.

When a case is sent to a surgeon, especially to a strange surgeon in a strange city, the patient often desires his physician to accompany him. Even when this is not actually necessary it contributes a feeling of security and backing which would otherwise be absent. In addition, most individuals wish their physician to be present at an operation, and it gives them confidence to know that he is there and watching over their interests. They also want him to see them during their convalescence, to cheer them up and to make such suggestions as his knowledge of their peculiarities may prompt. .

There can be no question that these attentions should be paid for according to their value; but this is not yet sufficiently recognized. Physicians too often give their time and skill and receive no pay in return. Undoubtedly the proper method would be for the patient to meet these obligations directly. At present, however, he often does not see it in this light, and in order to educate the people up to this point (6) *it is permissible for the surgeon and the physician to present a joint bill*— for services rendered by Dr. A. and Dr. B. This can be itemized if desired or at least it should be if the patient request it. Understand, what makes such a joint bill legitimate is that it is clearly indicated that it is for services rendered by both the attendants, and not by the surgeon alone. In this way it not only assists the physician in collecting his just dues, but also helps to educate the public to understand that the physician's time and services in connection with an operation are worth something—a point well worth driving home at every opportunity, because services for which nothing is charged are usually estimated as being worth nothing.

The other day a Denver surgeon remarked. "It is nobody's business what I do with a fee, as long as I do not overcharge—if I want to give half of it away, that is my affair, and does not concern the patient or anyone else." But it *does* concern some one else. It concerns the patient, the public and the whole medical profession.

If we wish to retain the confidence of the public, and our own honesty and self-esteem, no transaction should be entered into that we cannot openly lay before the patients and his friends.

This is a precept which we cannot afford to neglect. The tendency is already too great to distrust the actions and motives of doctors, and we should do all in our power to combat it rather than to encourage it. We should in every way endeavor to convince people that we are honest men with right motives, who are trying, within our limitations, to cure the sick without taking undue advantage of them. This is really what separates us from the charlatan and the quack. It is the standard raised by our forefathers, and we should endeavor to maintain it.

(7) *When an agent receives part of a fee without earning it, somebody suffers— either the surgeon gets too little or the patient pays too much.* In the former instance, the rights and dignities of the profession are trampled upon and in the latter the individual is buncoed.

For the surgeon's agent to receive from the patient something for nothing without the patient's knowledge, is as culpable as if he engaged in a get-rich-quick scheme, or robbed a bank, or held up a citizen on the highway. Because surgeons are popularly believed to make more money than the general practitioner, which in the long run is questionable, is no reason why the latter should graft either upon the surgeon or upon the public. If there is a real grievance it should be rectified in some more legitimate manner, in accord with the high ideals and moral responsibilities which physicians are supposed to possess —for instance, by educating the public to understand that with the growth of surgery increased responsibilities and duties have been thrust upon the general practitioner, which should receive increased remuneration. It goes without saying, that every surgeon will be glad to assist in such a campaign of education so far as lies within his power. For instance, a few words to the patient in explanation of the situation are usually sufficient to bring about a proper understanding of the value of the services rendered by the physician before the operation, during or after it; assuming, of course, that the physician is not a grafter and desirous of obtaining renumeration for something he does not do. It is usually easy enough to convince a patient that a good diagnosis, involving the responsibilities and trouble of an operation, is worth more than ordinary medical services, and should be paid for accordingly but this can never be done by the medical man pretending to work for nothing and then getting half the fee from the surgeon.

(8) *Buying cases is worse in some ways than advertising in the daily press, because the public has no way of protecting itself against this form of graft.* All members of the profession recognize that advertising in the newspapers or upon bill-boards is a serious breach of ethics. This is one thing upon which we fully agree and are extermely "touchy." The reason for this is not so much because it lowers our dignity and cheapens us, although this is of importance, but because advertising enables men to make false and wonderful claims to deceive the public, the extent of which is limited only by their ability to write and pay for advertisements. From time immemorial it has been recognized that the only decent and honorable course for the doctor to pursue is to let his work speak for itself, and not cry his accomplishments from the house-tops, this being left to the quacks and to the charlatans. If we acknowledge this to be true, how do we reconcile with it the actions of the commission-paying surgeon? Instead of letting his work speak for itself, he *pays* for his cases—he does not make his reputation, he buys it like any other charlatan. He introduces into the profession a form of advertising much more pernicious than that which employs the newspapers, because against its secret practice the public can not defend itself. People may be too intelligent to be misled by the allurements of an ordinary advertisement; but when they are steered against a commission-paying surgeon by his paid agent they are helpless, because the game of graft and bunco is a hidden game and not an open one, like that of the ordinary quack.

PERSONAL

Dr. A. T. Blaylock, of Madill, is in Chicago, for Post-graduate work.

Dr. J. O. Callahan, of Muskogee, has been extremely ill for several weeks.

Dr. J. H. Barnes, of Enid, Councillor for the 5th district, is spending a few weeks in New Orleans.

Dr. M. D. Belt, of Woodville, is spending the month of February in New Orleans, taking in the clinics.

Dr. C. T. Scott, formerly of New York City, has located in Oklahoma City. He will specialize in Genito-Urinary work.

Dr. James C. Johnston, formerly of Waurika, has moved to McAlester, and has been elected Superintendent of All Saints Hospital.

Dr. J. H. Sanford, formerly of Baton Rouge, La., has located in Muskogee. Dr. Sanford will make Genito-Urinary work a specialty.

Dr. Charles Blickenderfer, of Shawnee, has been appointed surgeon for the Rock Island Railway System. This is a deserved compliment to a worthy member of the medical profession and will be appreciated by the doctor's friends.

DR. WALKER MARRIED.

Dr. J. A. Walker, of Shawnee, one of the Councillors of the State Association and Miss Minnie May Kirst, were married December 31st.

The doctor's many personal and professional friends wish for him and his wife a happy and prosperous life.

The Thirty-fifth Annual Session of the Arkansas Medical Society will be held under the auspices of the Sebastian County Medical Society, at Ft. Smith, on the 2nd, 3rd, 4th and 5th of May, 1911.

COUNTY SOCIETIES

KAY COUNTY.
Elected officers at their annual election in Ponca City, as follows:
President—A. S. Risser, Blackwell.
Vice-Pres.—W. S. Lemmon, Nardin.
Secretary—R. E. Waggoner, Ponca City.
Treasurer—H. H. Bishop, Tonkawa.
Delegates—A. P. Gearhart, Blackwell; W. A. T. Robertson, Ponca City.
Censors—H. H. Panton, Ponca City; Allen Lowery, Blackwell; W. A. Lockwood, Ponca City.

GARFIELD COUNTY.
President—M. A. Kelso, Enid.
Vice-President—John N. Shaunty, Carrier.
Secretary—Walter M. Jones, Enid.
Censors—W. A. Aitken; C. J. Lukens and G. W. Boyle, Enid.
Delegate—E. J. Woolf, Waukomis.

CLEVELAND COUNTY.
President—J. A. Davis, Norman.
Vice-President—H. C. Childs.
Secretary-Treasurer—C. D. Blackley.
Censor—F. B. Erwin, Norman.
Delegate—C. S. Bobo, Norman.
Alternate—Walter Capshaw, Norman.

COMANCHE COUNTY.
President—Jackson Brashear, Lawton.
Vice-President—T. J. Gipson, Taupa.

Secretary-Treasurer—D. A. Myers, Lawton.
Delegates—E. B. Mitchell, L. T. Gooch.
Alternates—Brashear and Mead, Lawton.
Board of Censors—Drs. Angus, Dunlap and Knee.
Social Committee—Young and Meradith.
Committee on Public Safety and Health—Milne, and Webb, Temple, Okla., and Myers, Lawton.
Program Committee—Gooch, Angus and Meeker.
This society has inaugurated a plan by which two lecturers are appointed to hold their positions for one month. These lecturers prepare their work and deliver it verbally.

ALFALFA COUNTY.
President—Z. J. Clark, Cherokee.
Vice-President—J. H. Medaris, Helena.
Secretary-Treasurer—F. K. Slaton, Goltry.
Censors—A. J. Decker, Jett.
Delegate—F. K. Slaton, Goltry.
Alternate—J. H. Medaris, Helena.

LATIMER COUNTY.
President—J. F. McArthur, Wilburton.
Vice-President—Geo. A. Kilpatrick, Wilburton.
Secretary-Treasurer—H. L. Dalby,

Wilburton.

Censor—R. L. Rich, Red Oak.

Delegate—J. F. McArthur, Wilburton.

Alternate—Geo. A. Kilpatrick.

JACKSON COUNTY.

President—S. H. Landrum, Altus.

Vice-President—S. P. Rawls, Altus.

Secy.-Treasurer—Raymond H. Fox, Altus.

Delegate—W. E. Sanderson, Altus.

LINCOLN COUNTY.

President—F. H. Norwood, Prague.

Secy.-Treasurer—E. F. Hurlburt, Chandler.

Delegate—H. M. Williams, Wellston.

OKMULGEE COUNTY.

President—J. A. Oliphant, Okmulgee.

Vice-President—W. O. Weiskotten, Morris.

Secretary-Treasurer—J. E. Bircaw, Okmulgee.

Censors—W. M. Cott, V. Berry, Okmulgee; H. E. Breese, Henryetta.

Delegate—A. H. Culp, Beggs.

Alternate—W. M. Cott, Okmulgee.

WOODS COUNTY.

President—A. J. Sands, Capron.

Secretary-Treasurer—E. P. Clapper, Waynoka.

ELLIS COUNTY.

President—H. W. Hubbell, Arnett.

Secretary—J. F. Sturdivant, Arnett.

CANADIAN COUNTY.

President—R. F. Koons, El Reno.

Vice-President—S. S. Sanger, Yukon.

Secretary-Treasurer—James T. Riley, El Reno.

Delegate—A. D. Aderhold, El Reno.

Alternate—Dr. H. C. Brown, Okarche.

Censor—R. E. Runkle, El Reno.

MARSHALL COUNTY.

President—J. I. Gaston, Kingston.

Vice-President—T. A. Blaylock, Madill.

Secretary-Treasurer—John A. Haynie, Aylesworth.

Censor—A. H. Bray, Madill.

Delegate—John A. Haynie.

Alternate—J. S. Welch, Madill.

CARTER COUNTY.

President—W. T. Bogie, Ardmore.

Vice-President—Walter Hardey, Ardmore.

Secretary-Treasurer—Robt. H. Henry, Ardmore.

Delegate—F. P. VonKeller, Ardmore.

Alternate—J. C. McNees.

Censor—F. W. Boadway.

CHOCTAW COUNTY.

President—H. H. White, Hugo.

Vice-President—J. B. Allen, Grant.

Secy.-Treasurer—J. D. Moore, Sawyer.

Delegate—E. R. Askew, Hugo; H. L. Wright, Hugo.

GARVIN COUNTY,

This society held its meeting February 16th, and the following program was carried out.

The Value of Blood Examinations in Surgical Infection—S. W. Wilson, M. D.

The Clinical Diagnosis of Septicaemia and Pyemia—M. M. Webster.

Prophylaxis of the Surgical Infections —G. L. Johnson.

GRADY COUNTY.

President—G. H. Thrailkill—Chickasha.

Vice-Presidents—J. E. Baid, Pocassett; R. R. Hume, Minco; P. D. Vann, Chickasha.

Secy.-Treasurer—W. H. Cook, Chickasha.

Censors—J. E. Stinson. Chickasha; R.

J. Gordon, Ninnekah; A. B. Leeds, Chickasha.

Delegates—Walter Penquite; J. C. Ambrister, Chickasha.

BOOK REVIEWS

DIFFERENTIAL DIAGNOSIS.

Differential Diagnosis. Presented
through an Analysis of 383 cases. By
Richard C. Cabot, M. D., Assistant Professor of Clinical Medicine, Harvard Medical School. Octavo of 753 pages, illustrated. Philadelphia and London. W. B.
Saunders Company, 1911. Cloth, $5.50 net.

This work differs from the usual diagnostic works in its very unusual text arrangement. It may be said to be a very
practical history of 383 cases of illness with
the means of diagnosis and the conclusions
resting on the various tests made for diagnosing the conditions. Hardly in any instance is the typical case given, but the
cases were selected from a large number
with a view of throwing light on the authors means of determining the trouble. He
very candidly admits that in some instances
exception may be taken to his conclusions,
especially in those cases where no operative
procedure was had, which usually clears the
diagnosis in obscure acses. The book is of
immense practical value and one that a student reads straight through from cover to
cover with avidity. A perhaps just criticism may be made of the arrangement of
the text; there is no grouping of the subject matter, which places under one head all
that may be found o nthat subject, but the
cases are intermingled in such a manner
that the reader must jump from page to
page for the substance of one subject. However, this is all that may be said against it;
the writer feels impelled to, say that it is
one of the most entertaining books lately in
his notice and that the style is of that intimate character which causes the reader to
feel that he is at the bedside making his
diagnosis.

COLLECTED PAPERS BY THE STAFF OF ST. MARY'S HOSPIT-AL, MAYO CLINIC, 1905-1909.

Collected Papers by the Staff of St.
Mary's Hospital, Mayo Clinic, Rochester,
Minnesota, 1905-1909, Octavo of 668 pages,
illustrated. Philadelphia and London: W.
B. Saunders Company, 1911. Cloth, $5.50
net.

This volume may be said to be an accurate compilation of the means of diagnosis,
treatment and conclusions of the various
members of St. Mary's staff during the
past five years. Naturally it is almost wholly surgical, but a great deal of attention is
devoted to the findings by all the late means
of diagnosis and the conclusions following
the various steps taken are clear and pointed. While the work is a reprint of articles which have formerly appeared in medical publications of the country and of papers read before medical meetings at different times its reduction to book form renders it convenient and accessible to the profession.

The papers, as would be expected, go
largely into differential diagnosis and for
this reason the work is extremely valuable.

It will be found of great service to the
surgeon and to the physician who is called to attend the borderland cases of surgery and medicine.

The popularity and recognized standing
of its authors, the Mayo Brothers, Plummer, Judd and others of the Staff and the
splendid illustrations accompanying the
text should command it to every student
of medicine.

MISCELLANEOUS

READING NOTICE.

DOCTOR.

LOOK YOU.

UPON THIS PICTURE!

A poisonous agent should not be used for antiseptic douches and dressigns.

According to a report of the Council on Pharmacy and Chemistry of the American Medical Association, a 1 to 5,000 solution of bichloride of mercury does not kill the staphylicoccus phogenes aureus in five minutes contact. That is, it is not germicidal in that strength in that length of time yet it is highly poisonous to the individual, if kept in contact with an absorbing surface for that length of time.

"Bichloride of mercury even in this dilute lotion (1:10000) has, when used, in the peritoneal cavity, given rise to toxic symptoms." Hare's Therapeutics.

Koch states that where albumen is present, bichloride is decomposed and rendered inert.

AND THEN UPON THIS.

Containing, as it does, those agents which are antiseptic in action, as well as inflammation allaying, and repair inducing, Tyree's Antiseptic Powder is indubitably the most effective preparation thus far evolved for employment in the treatment of either acute or chronic inflammation of the muccus surfaces, or other soft structures. It is especially efficacious in leucorrhea, gonorrhoea, vaginitis, pruritus, and chronic catarrhal affections of the female genital tract.

Dr. Jacob Geiger, Professor of Surgery, at the Ensworth Medical College, St. Joseph, Mo., in speaking of Tyree's Antiseptic Powder, says that it has been used in the above hospital with very satisfactory results. He considers it a good dressing powder, non-irritating in its effects.

Dr. T. E. Potter, Secretary of the Ensworth Medical College, St. Joseph, Mo., says that it has been used at St. Joseph's Hospital, St. Joseph, Mo., with very satisfactory results.

A liberal supply is furnished doctors free, upon request.

J. S. TYREE, Chemist.

WASHINGTON, D. C.

ELIXIRS DE LUXE.

Parke, Davis & Co. announce some important improvements in their line of medicinal elixirs, a line numbering more than one hundred and twenty-five preparations and highly esteemed by physicians on the score of therapeutic excellence. The improvements cited are in manufacturing processes, in the interest of palatability, permanence and physical appearance. They are set forth at some length in the current issue if Modern Pharmacy, from which these interesting extracts are taken:

"Three or four years ago, in the gradual development of our scientific staff, we secured the services of Professor Wilbur L. Scoville, a pharmacist well known to the country and a man pre-eminent in the field of what has been termed pharmaceutical elegance. Professor Scoville may well be considered, an artist in questions concerning odor, flavor and appearance of galenicals. The first task assigned to Professor Scoville was to go systematically and patiently through our entire line of elixirs—regardless of what other workers had done before him, and regardless of what changes were under consideration at the time. He was given carte blanche to go ahead and suggest any modifications and improvements which seemed to him necessary.

"Professor Scoville at once began an exhaustive series of experiments which took him nearly three years to complete. He went over the entire line, improving here the flavor, there the color, elsewhere the odor, and in other instances the permanence of our products. How well he succeeded may be seen by comparing any one of our elixirs with others on the market. It is our honest opinion that there is no other line of elixirs in the United States to-day possessing an equal degree of therapeutic efficiency which will stand up on the druggist's shelves and retain their physical properties and clearness so long as Parke, Davis & Co.'s.

"During this three years of work we have made hundreds of experimental lots which have been kept under observation for a period of from six to eighteen months. The experiments have included such things as increasing and decreasing the percentage of alcohol, noting the effects of different solvents upon the stability of the elixirs, the increase and decrease in the proportion of the sugar present, and the effects of acids. We have studied the effect upon permanence of the elixirs of using fluid extracts or percolating the mixed drugs direct. The matter of aging and also the use of refining agents such as egg albumen and similar proteid matters have been tested out. The essential oils and perfumes employed have been subjected to careful criticism; many of these have been changed with the idea of getting a better blend or a more agreeable flavor.

"We might sum it up by saying that we have attempted first to make our line more stable; secondly, to improve the physical properties which appeal to the eye; and thirdly, to improve the flavors which appeal to the palate. But we want it understood that in making these improve-

ments we have not in a single instance sacrificed the medicinal activity of the preparation."

CORRINNA BORDEN KEEN RESEARCH FELLOWSHIP OF JEFFERSON MEDICAL COLLEGE.

The accumulated income of this fund now amounts to $1,000,00. The fellowship will be awarded by the Trustees upon recommendation of the Faculty to a graduate of the Jefferson Medical College of not less than one, nor more than ten years standing, upon condition that he shall spend at least one year in Europe, America, or elsewhere, wherever he can obtain the best facilities for research in the line of work he shall select, after consultation with the Faculty; and that he shall publish at least one paper embodying the results of his work as the "Corinna Borden Keen Research Fellow of the Jefferson Medical College."

Address J. W. HOLLAND,

Dean.

AMERICAN MEDICAL ASSOCIATION NATIONAL CONVENTION.

Los Angeles, Calif., June, — 1911

A rate of $50.00 for the round trip has been granted for our convention. Tickets will be on sale June 10th and 22nd, with final limit of September 15th. and are good on the California Limited trains, to Los Angeles, thence to San Francisco, and return via same route or via the northern route, through Salt Lake and Denver and Colorado Springs, with stopovers in either direction.

We could go via the Santa Fe from Kansas City and other junction points convenient from Oklahoma and use the California Limited, with a special through sleeper from Oklahoma, which would make the trip much more pleasant and convenient and retain our through sleeper while visiting the Grand Canon, petrified forests, Indian villages, etc. Tickets may be routed returning from San Francisco via Portland, via Northern Pacific Ry. via Seattle and Spokane, Livingston via Mont., for a slight additional amount and a side trip can be made from Livingston, Mont., through Yellowstone Park and return to Livingston at a very reasonable rate.

Please notify the undersigned at your earliest convenience if you would like to make up a party of this kind to be composed of the Oklahoma delegation and their families.

C. A. THOMPSON, Secy

FOR SALE.

Wanted to sell—A Genito-Urinary Practice in one of the best towns in Oklahoma. A choice practice amounting to about Five Thousand Dollars cash per year. Write "Genito-Urinary," care of the Journal.

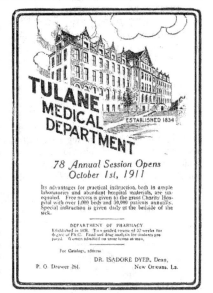

BEWARE OF ITINERANT MORPHINE AND COCAINE TABLET PEDDLERS.

Manufacturers, jobbers, dispensers and others obliged to keep considerable stocks of morphine, coacine and various forms of tablets of the same; suffer considerable loss from theft owing to an illegitimate demand and the ease with which the drugs are concealed about the person.

A man described as about 5 feet 10 inches, light brown hair, wearing a light gray overcoat, well dressed, nice looking, with a nice way, seeming to know the price of morphine and cocaine, etc., called on the Hort-Schaeffer Drug Co., Omaha, Neb., about January 23rd, and tried to sell 5,000 H. T. 26 P. D. & Co. at $5 per M; said he had sold 30,000 already and had 5,000 more to sell. Refused to call again to see Mr. Hort. When the clerk tried to get finishing number he took package away from him with the remark: "If you don't want them o. k., I can sell them without any trouble." He claimed to be from the East—either New York or Philadelphia— saying he sold different things at different times, and now was the time to get in easy as morphine, etc., was going up all the time.

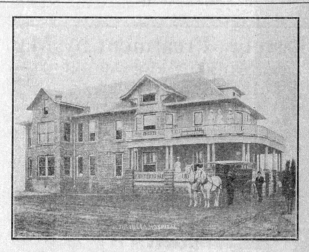

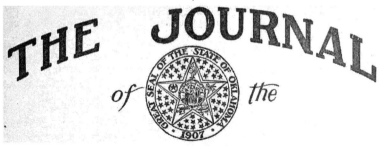

THE JOURNAL of the
Oklahoma State Medical Association.

VOL. III.   MUSKOGEE, OKLAHOMA, APRIL, 1911.   NO 11

DR. CLAUDE A. THOMPSON, Editor-in-Chief.

ASSOCIATE EDITORS AND COUNCILLORS.

DR. J. A. WALKER, Shawnee.
DR. CHARLES R. HUME, Anadarko.
DR. F. R. SUTTON, Bartlesville.
DR. I. W. ROBERTSON, Dustin.
DR. J. S. FULTON, Atoka.

DR. JOHN W. DUKE, Guthrie.
DR. A. B. FAIR, Frederick.
DR. W. G. BLAKE, Tahlequah.
DR. H. P. WILSON, Wynnewood.
DR. J. H. BARNES, Enid.

Entered at the Postoffice at Muskogee, Oklahoma, as second class mail matter, July 28, 1910

This is the Official Journal of the Oklahoma State Medical Association All communications should be addressed to the Journal of the Oklahoma State Medical Association, English Block, Muskogee, Oklahoma.

THE REPAIR OF FRACTURE.

BY J. H. SCOTT, M. D., SHAWNEE, OKLA.

The diagnosis of fracture having been made we will first consider what repair is likely to be necessary. After a limb has been broken, in a little while it swells and feels sore and in a few hours or a day or two echymoses appear on the surface of the limb at the seat of and at various distances from the seat of the fracture. We first have shock and excitement and then some, fever for a day or two. Within the first few hours after a fracture has occurred the con- tusion and laceration produces a haema- toma and oedema. This oedema increases for about two days then gradually subsides. In this stage the periosteum and all the tissues are cloggy and thickened, and the bone ends lie in a cavity full of semi-coagu- lated blood. In the gross superficial appear- ance and signs we have the pain swelling echymosis, and abnormal mobility with more or less of an inflammatory process. The echymosis persists for a variable length of time. It may clear up in a week or ten days or it may persist for weeks; some- times until after firm bony union. It first gives place to a yellowish discoloration of the skin and finally assumes a normal color. After complete union and removal of the splints the limb is found to be shrunken and its surface dry and rough. The joints be- come stiffened from disuse and the limb swells when allowed to hang down. After the inflammatory swelling and oedema have subsided a firm ovoid mass can be felt about the bone at the seat of the fracture and gradually becomes smaller and harder until finally nothing is left but the callus which unites the fracture. The process of repair in the long bones might be said to proceed by three stages.

When a fracture takes place the bone marrow is crushed the periosteum torn though and the adjoining mucles, connective tissue and blood vessels lacerated to an extent that varies with the degree of displacement. Blood is poured out from the torn ends of the blood vessels and partially coagulates between the fragments and in the muscular spaces. The continuity of the periosteum covering the fragment is probably preserved in part, forming what has been called the perio-teal bridge, but this membrane is torn and stripped from the bone of one or both fragments. All of the parts the bone, the bone marrow, the periosteum and the adjoining connective tissue take part in the process of repair. This is done by the gradual formation of simple granulations of all the lacerated structure filling the gap between the fragments, and become structurally united with, and completely surrounding them. This is called the provisional callus and varies in amount according to how well the bones are coapted. This may be said to complete the first stage.

The granulations usually spring from the periosteal bridge but are also produced from the bone marrow also by thickening of the perosteum and granulation from the soft parts and the bone end.

Stimson: "The first effect of fracture is traumatic irritation and injury of the soft parts adjoining the fracture, and this is the explanation of the large ovoid swelling which can be distinctly felt after the first day or two. After displacement has been reduced and the limb immobilized the irritation and with it the swelling diminishes. The periosteum thickens and pours out a viscid gelatinous substance between itself and the bone for a short distance beyond the edge of the fracture or beyond the point to which it has been stripped up. Then be-gins the process of granulation. Those furnished by the soft parts and the marrow are first to appear those from the periosteum next and those from the broken edge of the cylindrical shaft last as they can only appear after rarefication of the bone by enlargement of the haversian canals has opened a way for them. These granulations which are termed provisional callus are at first large and spongy." The callus arising from the periosteum being the greater part of all the callus first change to cartaliginous and then to bone. The callus coming from the bone marrow goes through no cartaliginous farmation but becomes bone directly. This osseus formation begins at the inner surface of the bony shell and persists inward until the entire medullary canal if full and outward until it meets periosteal callus and the medullary plug of the opposite fragment. After this process is completed the soft parts have thoroughly healed the echymoses are disappearing and the cartilage and bone without, make everything firm except over the broken edges of the fragments, the slow solidification at the ends of the fragments is due to the slow process of bone granulation. The bone granulation is slow at this point partly because of the deficient circulation and partly because of the bone absorption that must take place before the bone repair can be completed. The splinters of the bone that are usually present at the seat of the fracture must be absorbed as well as a thin shell along the surface of the bone which is cut off from the circulation. This about completes the second stage of repair and consumes three or four weeks of time.

At the beginning of the third stage the fragments are reasonably firm and immovable but no bony union exists between the bone ends. While held in this position the osseus callus unites the bone ends in about the same manner as a mass of solder unites the two ends of a pipe except that in the bone union the lumen of the pipe is filled solid with the bone solder and extends beyond the circumference.

Druing the remainder of the third stage the superabundance of callus is gradually absorbed. The lumen of the bone is cleared, the callus between the bone ends become more firm and the more compact approaching in structure very nearly to that of the bone which it conects. The external callus is absorbed until in some cases when the bone is perfectly set there remains no trace of the fracture.

The process of osification in fracture repairs is much the same as original osification.

In case of completely detached fragments of the bone the process is different varied and interesting. They are either absorbed, revived by a newly established circulation or permenantly encopsulated by the callus. For the most part the small splinters are absorbed. The larger fragments are surrounded by the granulation callus, and if the fragment takes kindly to the overtures of the granulation circulation, the fragment renitaliyed and takes an important part in the reconstructive process. But if the new criculation communication between the fragment and granulation callus is not established, then the fragment remains dormant and encapsulated in the callus for years and their presence be first known when on account of debility or inflammation elsewhere in the organism they become centers of suppuration which go on to abscess and fistula, and removal of the fragment by nature or by the surgeon.

In fracture of the skull the repair is effected chiefly from the diploe which is not capable of producing large callus or of closing large defects.

The fracture of spongy ends of long bones is repaired chiefly by the bones themselves.

Fracture of cartilage is slow to heal and the repair is chiefly fiberinous if there be repair is chiefly fiberinous if there be repair at all, except in isolated cases when there is an exuberant callus.

In compound fracture the process of repair differs in several ways from that of simple fracture. The primary oedema and haematoma are less or absent on account of the free escape of the blood and serum through the opening. In case of infection there is a more important difference if suppuration occurs, healing is delayed by the casting off of all fragments by the death of a layer of some thickness along the broken edge, and especially by the destruction of the periosteum. The union between the bone ends is first fibrous and is slowly replaced by the bone formation from the medullarly plug. The bone is formed entirely by the medullary plug and grows slowly. Thus making final union and solidfication tedious and discouraging. Fragments of dead bone may prolong suppuration indefinitely, and likewise markedly prolong final union.

In case of non-infected compound fracture, the soft parts heal enough in a few days to close the external communication and the compound fracture is thus converted by nature into a simple fracture and the repair is the same as that heretofore described under simple fracture except that the quantity of blood and oedema is not present.

There is sometimes a fibrous union of bone especially in elderly people who have an intra-capsular fracture of the neck of the femur. Also in cases of defective immobilization of the fragments of the long bones in cases where the natural process of repair is defective from any cause.

ANTI-TYPHOID VACCINATION.

BY JOHN W. RILEY, COMMISSIONER OF HEALTH, OKLAHOMA CITY

In 1883 Metchnikoff attributed recovery from infectious diseases, decreased susceptibilty to any infectious disease from which an individual has recently recovered and in certain cases natural immunity, to the ability of the leucocytes to ingest and destroy bacteria.

He did not recognize the role that the serum played in preparing the bacteria for phagocytosis, but believed that it acted solely in the manner of stimulating the leucocytes to greater phagocytic activity.

Wright and Douglas demonstrated that in response to actual infection with or inocculation with killed bacteria typhoid, cholera and some others, the blood serum is found to have acquired the power of agglutinating, killing and dissolving the organisms when brought in contact with them in vitro, although the serum was highly diluted.

These substances were named according to their effect agglutinous, bactericidains and bacteriolysins.

In the bodily reaction against typhoid those substances play a most important role.

However besides these anti-bacterial substances, known as bacteriotropins there is a fourth factor the opsonin, which accomplishes the destruction of bacteria by combining with the leucocytes and other phagocytic cells in the following manner, by combining with the cell protoplasm of the bacteria and rendering them palatable to the leucocytes and that in the absence of this opsonin, the leucocytes have very little effect on bacteria.

The opsonin and other bacteriotropins probably originate from the connective tissue cells as a result of the stimulation of the specific poison which cause these connective tissue cells to produce these protective substances.

Thus much for the theory, as to the cause of recovery from typhoid, to date.

There is much evidence to prove that these same substances can be artifically produced by inocculation with killed bacteria.

opsonized bacteria................................

.................................vaccine injected.

.................................connective tissue cells.

serum

.................................bacteriotropins.

.................................opsonin.

It was along this line that Wright in his experiments found, that as a result of a single injection of killed typhoid cultures, into man, the bactericidal power of the blood was increased, sometimes a thousand fold after a single injection, and that there was also a high agglutinating power and a high opsonic power.

That there followed as a result of the injection of these killed bacteria an elaboration of the same specific anti-bacterial and typhotrophic substances as were found in the individual infected with and recovering from typhoid fever.

Wright reported his first two cases of anti-typhoid inocculation in 1896. These two cases showed after a single dose, a considerable increase in agglutinins found, and in the bacteriolytic power of the blood.

In January, 1897, he reports the results of anti-typhoid to limit the spread of epidemics and in the time of war.

Wright's work was the means of placing prophylactic vaccination against typhoid on a working basis, and it is now used extensively in the various armies of the world.

In 1898 he vaccnated 4,000 men of the British Indian Army, and the following year he vaccinated many of the troops of the Boer War.

In the 19,000 men immunized, the morbidity was only half and the mortality was reduced two thirds, as compared to the non vaccinated men.

Colonel Leishman furnishes the following accurate and reliable statistics:

	Innocculated.	Non Innocculated.
Number	5473	6610
Cases of typhoid	21	187
Deaths	2	26
Comparative sick per cent per 1000	3.7	32.8
Comparative death per cent per 1000	.36	3.93

Only four of the 21 cases had had two doses, all recovered.

17 had received but one dose.

The observation of these 12 000 men extended over a period of three years and no more perfect or convincing statistics are needed to show the value of this method of prophylaxis.

The duration of protection.

Too short a time has elapsed and there are too few facts to base an opinion on the duration of immunity.

We do know however that it will last three years and this is quite long enough from the army point of view, and for the protection of hospital internes and nurses during their training period.

And right here I wish to say is where this method of prophylaxis can accomplish an unusual amount of good, for you all know of many internes and nurses who have contracted typhoid during their hospital life and many have died as a result of this infection.

It therefore behooves every training school, hospital and institution to see that all conected with it are protected by prophylactic vaccination.

One can readily see that it means a great deal to the nation when it can marshal raw recruits, and in thirty days time have a practically typhoid proof troop.

The necessity for anti-typhoid vaccina-

tion and the inadequacy of other treatment is shown by the great prevalence of typhoid in modern war.

In the civil war there were 80,000 cases in the northern army, in the Franco Prussian war there were 73,396 cases, and 8,789 deaths among the Germans. In fact 60 per cent. of their total mortality was due to typhoid. In the Boer war there were 31,000 cases and 5,877 deaths. In the Spanish war there were 20,730 cases and 1,580 deaths among 120,000 men or one case to every 5.6 men, 86 per cent. of all deaths were due to typhoid.

These figures mean much, it shows the crying need of some method of prophylaxis to obviate this terrible mortality.

And I believe that the time is fast approaching when anti-typhoid vaccination will be as common as anti-small pox vaccination.

I will not enter into a discussion of the preparation of the vaccine for it can be obtained in a syringe package from several of the labratories.

I have used the H. K. Mulford and Co. vaccine.

If this method of prophylaxis is to become popular, its results must not be too unpleasant, painful, or disagreeable.

I have vaccinated 37 patients with 3 doses of anti-typhoid, 5 patients with 2 doses, 10 patients with 1 dose.

The dose of the anti-typhoid is 500,000,-000 for the first injection and not sooner than 10 days nor longer than 14 days a second injection of one billion, and again in an equal length of time a third injection of one billion. The technic of giving these injections is the same as for giving any aseptic hypodermic, the hpodermic should be sterile and the skin should be washed with a 70 per cent. alcohol and painted with tincture of iodine.

I have never seen an infection following the injection.

I have never seen an infection following the injection.

The reactions are described as none or mild; second, moderate, the temperature 101 to 103; third, severe, temperature 103 and above.

After each injection there is usually a reaction, this as a rule is a red and tender spot, ranging in size from a dollar to the palm of the hand, around the point of the inocculation, and sometimes the axillary glands are enlarged, it usually makes it appearance in 6 to 8 hours after the injection and reaches its full development in about 12 hours, and then gradually subsides, usually in 48 to 72 hours. Some patients show no reaction.

The reaction in my own case was quite marked after the first injection, I had chills, severe headache, and my arm was swollen from acromion process to elbow and quite painful, temperature ranged from 101 to 103. Appetite was perfectly normal during this 48 hours and after 48 hours I felt perfectly normal. The other two injections I did not notice at all.

Dr. Raver, the City Bacteriologist, was quite sick after the first and second and refused to take the third.

Quite a number complained of sore throat, and said they felt as though they had taken cold or were coming down with the grippe.

In the 52 patients treated, 49 had mild or no reaction, three moderate reaction after the first injection; 39 had mild or no reaction, and three moderate reaction after the second injection. 37 had mild or no reaction after the third injection. I had two moderate reaction after first and second injection. 10 took only first dose, but I ascertained that the reaction was mild, and that they forgot to come for the other injection, 5 took only first two injections, none of these patients had a severe reaction.

The dose of anti-typhoid for a child is reckoned on the percentage weight of a child to an adult 150 pound man. If the child weighed 30 pounds then he would take 1-5 of the amount of the anti-typhoid.

If given about 4 p. m., reaction will have disappeared by next day.

According to Major Russell, in his report of 120 cases of vaccination in patients known to have had typhoid previously, the reaction was much more severe than in those who had never had typhoid. The percentage of severe reactions in these cases must be more than a mere coincidence and is probably coupled with the immunity to typhoid. He advises against giving it to patients who have had typhoid or are more than 50 years of age.

The reaction, both local and systemic, in children is exceedingly mild, and they stand the injections well.

I have vaccinated several families, where one of the family had typhoid and none of the vaccinated developed typhoid. In Wright's negative phase is a positive thing, than this would not be the proper thing to do. But Leishman claims that the negative phase is a neglible factor.

Conclusion:

1. That innoculation treatment is effectual and harmless.

2. That it is the most valuable means of preventing the disease, and probably the most valuable of combating it.

3. All nurses, physicians, hospital attendants and medical students should be protected by inoculation.

4. Inoculation should be done in families where one or more cases exist and early.

5. In as much as typhoid is always with us, no matter how careful we may be with sanitation, water, milk, flies, and the possibility of typhoid carriers, we can only keep more or less free from the disease by inoculation.

6. And last, I believe that it is without

a peer in preventive medicine since Jenner immortalized vaccination.

No.	Before Innoculation.	After Innoculation.	1-40 N M	1-80 N M	Time Hr.
" 2		First		G P	"
		Third			"
" 3				M	"
" 4		Second		M M	"
" 5		Third		M M	"
" 6				M	"
" 7		First		M M	"
		Second	N		"
" 8			P	- P	"
		Third	M	M 1-2	"
" 9			M	M	"
" 10		Second	L	L	"
" 11			M	M	"

Reaction strong and positive and marked clumping in three cases, ten days after second and third injection.

Moderate reaction, moderate clumping with plenty of motility in five cases after second and third injection.

Poor reaction very little clumping and plenty of motility in two cases ten days aftter third injection.

In two cases of typhoid where temperature continued after six weeks a lvidal was practically negative, and after first injectior temperature dropped to normal in 48 hours, patients began to improve, lvidal positive in ten days. I believe that the vaccine will do good work in these long drawn out typhoids, and infected gall-bladders, for it is apparent that the cells are not sufficiently active to produce an opsonin.

TUBERCULOSIS OF THE FALLOPIAN TUBE.

BY DR. CHARLES NELSON BALLARD, OKLAHOMA CITY, OKLA.

Those diseases which are of common occurrence are thought of and studied most. They are brought to our attention often, and are not forgotten. It is the disease that is more obscure, occurring in the part of the body where it is not easily noticed, or examined. More likely are these diseases to be overlooked, and not properly diagnosed. We are often careless and neglectful in our efforts to differentiate difficult complications. The organs in question are not easy of access and hence their pathology is frequently unnoticed.

We know of no other disease that destroys more human lives, and occurs in a greater variety of tissue, isolated or complicated, than does tuberculosis, it being the cause of one death in every seven occurring among our people. It is found coexistent with many other diseases, fact other diseases seem to increase its severity.

The history of tuberculosis of the female genitalia dates back to 1744, when Morgagni, making a necropsy on a young woman who had died from tuberculous peritonitis, found the uterus and both fallopian tubes filled with caseous material The tubes and ovaries were firmly adherent, so that it was impossible to separate them and he considered the lesions as being the primary focus of the disease. Similar observations were reported by Louis and by Senn of Geneva later on.

In 1831 Reynaud gave a description of two cases of uterine tuberculosis found in tuberculosis patients. Lesions of the tubes were figured by Cruveilhier, and tuberculosis of the uterus describe by Kiwish and Paulsen. Up to this time genital tuberculosis had been considered merely as a pathologic curiosity, and of no clinical interest.

Bouardel in 1865, in a thesis corrected the early information on the subject, and gave a good account of the gross pathology.

Koch's discovery of the specific germ of tuberculosis aroused fresh interest in the subject, which was increased by Babes finding the tubercle bacilli in the vaginal secretions, and by the publication in 1886, of Hagar's exhaustive and classic contribution of the pathogenesis, diagnosis and surgical treatment of the condition. We owe to Conheim and Verneuil (1883) the suggestion that coition might be the starting point of the tubercular localization.

The order of frequency with which the organs of the genitalia are involved is, the tubes, uterus, ovaries, vagina, and vulva.

Tuberculosis of the uterus is almost invariably a descending infection originating in the Fallopian tubes.

Hematogenic infection is met with in the disseminated milliary form. The affection has been found at all ages, from infancy to old age, but is most common during the period of greatest vitality. This last statement seems contradictory to the general rule, and needs some explanation. This tissue, during the time of greatest activity, is most exposed to infection and tracma and hence more susceptable to infection at those points where trauma and irritation is greatest. As examples, the epithelium lining the tube, following a gonorrheal infection, has lost much of its power of resistance, and becomes fruitful soil for the development of the tubercular bacilli; after the puerperium, when the parts are exposed to more or less trauma; after a miscarriage, when the parts have been unnaturally disturbed. The vaginal secretions being acid and the cervical alkaline, they act as a protection against infection, by continuity of surface. A microorganism that thrives in one of these secretions is usually destroyed in the other, hence the time of greatest danger from infection is when these secretions are diluted or rendered neutral by fluids foreign to the normal secretions; as after the puerperium; after a miscarriage or during a profuse leucorrhoea. Greatest care is required at these times on account of these protecting agencies being rendered neutral and allowing the microorganisms to pass undisturbed. The body of the uterus at the ostium tubea is the sight of election for the origin of the disease. It is a disputed point, however, whether the acutal origin is in the tubal tissue or uterine tissue. It extends throughout the tube without interference, while it usually stops short, in the descending type, at the internal os.

The sources of infection by the bacilli in the production of genital tuberculosis may be classified as hematogenous, lymphatic, contiguity of tissue and continuity of surface.

Kleinhaus mentions three arguments in favor of infection by means of the blood current.

(1)   The existence of tuberculosis in the genitals following tuberculosis of the lungs, with no intervening foci.

(2)   The localization of tuberculosis on the sight of the placental attachment.

(3)   The transmissibillity of the bacilli from the mother to the foetus Any disease which confines its secretions long enough within the tissue to produce an exfoliation of a portion of the lining epithelium, greatly enhances the extension of the infection.

So frequently do we find postpartum tuberculosis that we are satisfied that the puerperal state, with its attendant traumatism, is a common source of primary infection.

Merletti reports five cases out of a total of sixteen milliary tuberculosis, in which caseous foci were found at the end of the tube.

Duherssen cites a case in which catheterization of the uterus for sterility led to acute tuberculosis of the tube and peritoneum. General tubercular infection has followed operative procedures on tubercular ovarian cysts and tubal complications.

Strassman reports two incidences: Adhesions between tubercular loops of the bowel and the tube may cause infection of the tube.

One a butchers wife who contracted genital tuberculosis—the meat handled by the butcher being infected. The other, a domestic who attended the cows on a farm. She developed genital tuberculosis, and investigation proved that the cows were infected with tuberculosis.

Voight states two facts which he considers is in opposition to so frequent occurrence of genital tuberculosis during the period of sexual activity. He is a supporter of direct ascending infection, however in the experience of many authors it is found just as often before puberty as afterward, but on account of the age of the patient opportunities are not so frequently offered to detect its existence.

Direct infection may be caused by unclean instruments, clothing, bed linen, the accouchers, or patients fingers, and especially by coitus. The tubercle bacillus may be deposited on the external genitals by the dust of the street put in motion by the skirts of the female. Genital tuberculosis may be either primary or secondary. By primary, we understand that the focus in the genital apartus is the only one in the body.

The following facts establish without a doubt, the existence of primary genital tuberculosis.

(.1) People who are otherwise strong and healthy have primary manifestations in the genitalia.

(2.) If this primary focus is removed while local only, the patient remains free from the disease for years or possibly permanently.

(3.) Children, otherwise apparently healthy, are found to have tubercular infection of the external genitalia.

Cases of primary tuberculosis contracted from the husband during coition are reported by Murphy, Amann, Merletti, and others.

Primary infection of these organs is much more rare than secondary.

In genital tuberculosis, Schram finds one primary in 34 cases: Spaeth finds 27 in 119 cases; Mosler finds 9 in 46 cases: Frerichs finds 1 in 15 cases. The second-

ary form is frequent in pnthisis. Turner found 5 out of 27 with 7 more suffering with suspicious catarrhal salpingitis. Stolper finds an average of about 20 per cent.

Remarks:

To produce primary tuberculosis, two possibilities must be considered:

(1.) Penetration of germs from the outside directly to the mucosa of the vagina, uterus and tubes.

(2.) Penetration of germs through minute breaches of continuity in the genital canal into the lymphatics.

We speak of the two forms of tubal tuberculosis as acute secondary and chronic primary. In the first we find few giant cells, but an abundant of bacteria. Necrosis of the mucosa occurs rapidly. It is agreed by most authors that primary tuberculosis of the tubes occurs in about 18 per cent. of all cases of genital tuberculosis in the female. This form is more chronic in all its phases. Though the swelling may be marked, the mucosa may remain unaltered for a long time.

The infection is usually hematogenic, although it has been proven that it has been transmitted by sperm containing tubercle bacilli. It has been carried through the mendium of the spittle used for lubrication during coitus from a man suffering with pulmonary tuberculosis to an otherwise healthy woman.

The abdominal end of the tube is more likely to be sealed by adhesions. The tube is enlarged, the walls thickened and its caliber enlarged at the abdominal end.

If the abdominal end is patent, a discharge is seen at the opening, caseous in nature, if non-mixed infection exists. Should it be closed pyosalpinx usually forms, often of considerable size. Adhesions may attach the diseased tube to hollow organs and evacuation take place through a sinus.

Nodules may often be detected while examination is being made, which practically establishes our diagnosis. We must not lose sight of the fact however that a similar nodular salpingitis of the insthmus of the tube is found in chronic gonorrhoea. These nodules are due, it is thought, in both conditions, to a swollen, thickened mucus membrane encroaching upon the muscularis and thus producing the characteristic nodular feeling.

Early the mucosa of the tube may become infiltrated with round cells, vascular, and thickened, containing many giant cells. At this stage, in these cases, the muscularis is unchanged. Later the epithelium degenerates and disappears. Necrotic changes follow, affecting the tubercle first and then the muscle tissue is encroached upon. If the necrosis affects all the coats or coverings of the tube, rupture and escape of the contents occur. This is rather rare unless it be mixed infection.

Secondary tuberculosis of the tubes may occur by extension from the peritoneum, ovaries and uterus. The disease is usually bilateral, yet both tubes may not be affected to the same degree. In our observation of many cases, we are convinced that the tube presents fertile soil for the production of the tubercle bacillus. We can assign no definite reason for this unles it be due to the previously existing inflammatory or circulatory disturbance, and disorders arising during menstruation and the puerperium.

If the infection is of the descending type it generally begins in the mucus membrane of the ampeulla. The affected tube is thickened, more or less tortuous. The musculat coat is hypertrophied and the fimbria are thick, firm and shortened. Many adhesions are found about it, binding it firmly to adjacent tissue. On incising the tube in the earlier stages the mucosa is found swollen and reddened and the folds are adherent. It has the appearance of chronic productive salpingitis. As it becomes more advanced, greyish points show themselves in the mucosa, or caseous nodules or streaks are seen.

Microscopically in the secondary form, the mucus membrane is swollen and infiltrated with round and epithelioid cells. Tubercles are to be seen near the lumen, with central caseation. As the disease advances the mucosa becomes largely caseous, with the progress noticeable in the muscular and serous coats. In the earlier stages the lesions produced are not unlike those of lesions produced are not unlike those of chronic salpingitis from any other cause. Microscopically the resemblance is close in both forms there being added, in the primary form, giant cells in the neighborhood of the cellular infiltration. Caseation soon sets in and the tubercles are recognized as greyish elevations. The epithlium of the crypts show evidence of cloudiness and degeneration. The crypts disappear in the course of the coalesence of the caseous masses and the formation of tuberculous granulation tissue. The lumen of the tube becomes filled and distended with a caseopurulent detritus. The process of destruction extends into the muscularis. The walls become greatly thickened, adhesions form and the tube becomes tortuous. Small caseous foci may be formed or simply areas of cellular infiltration with giant cells.

The caseous detritus retained in the lumen may undergo degeneration, becoming liquified and puriform. This often results in sacculation causing tuberculous pyosalpinx.

Ulceration and perforation in purely tubercular cases are rare, as the abscess is usually walled off by adhesions, attaching it to the uterus, appendix or other adjacent tissue.

Pus infection may occur in tubercular disease, or it may be a mixed inftction from the beginning, both forms taking place from the one foci. When the primary focus is a mixed infection, its extension is by ulceration, coagulation necrosis and other than extension by continuity of surface, or through the lymphatics.

If the primary focus of mixed infection is the tube, the end of the tube becomes sealed, and a pyo-tubercular salpingitis is established. The extension may be by ulceration through the fimbriated end, and the formation of an abscess in the Cul-de-sac, ovary or anywhere the end of the tube may become attached. Extension from a mixed infection salpingitis is by ulceration through its walls to the adjacent tissue. If it becomes attached to the ovary, the result is a tubercular abscess in one of the graffian follicles.

If it become adherent to the intestines, perforation most likely will take place and a tubo-intestinal sinus result.

This is one of the conditions to be apprehended in operating for tuberculosis of the tube or peritoneum, and is one of the most serious conditions with which we have to contend. Fistulas of the bowel, of tubercular origin, are difficult to suture on account of the infiltrations of the wall of the intestine and the adjacent tissue.

Resection is difficult and should seldom be undertaken on account of the extensive adhesions.

The rapid healing tendency of the peritoneum, which is so all important, has been destroyed by the tuberculous process, and therefore it is difficult to get primary peritoneal union sufficient to support the walls. If repair is inevetable, several rows of sutures must be inserted to approximate enough surface that apposition may be insured during the process of tissue regeneration.

The fundus of the uterus has been utilized, by suturing it to the opening in the bowel, so as to secure enough normal peritoneal surface to repair the opening.

Many cases might be mentioned where the fimbriated end of the tube is united to the bowel and the disease transmitted to the bowel in this way, the disease being primary in the tube.

There being no pathognomic symptom of genital tuberculosis, we find it necessary to make a systematic microscopic examination of the scrapings, and discharges for the bacilli.

We must remember, however, that the bacilli may not be found on every slide, for as an average, it exists only in one out of every 47 slides examined. Hence it requires a careful examination of many specimens to make a positive diagnosis. The smegma bacillus is so very similar to that of tuberculosis that much pains is required to differentiate them. The inoculation method is sometimes a useful adjunct to the microscope. In doubtful cases, a general systemic examination is necessary. The thermometer is of great help in tubal tuberculosis. A constant slight rise in the evening temperature, and a normal or slightly subnormal morning temperature, are very suggestive of the tubercular nature of the tubal affection. Our attention is often directed to the frequent coincident of tubal pregnancy and tubal tuberculosis. This is of much interest from a diagnostic standpoint. When we are confronted with a tubal pregnancy we are to take into consideration the possibility of tubal tuberculosis.

Sterility is the rule in tubal tuberculosis. Early, the menstrual disturbance is slight. Later, there may be either amenorrhoea or menorrhagia. Menorrhagia in young girls should arouse our suspicion, as to there being tuberculosis. Many times will our efforts be rewarded by finding the bacilli, while it would have otherwise remained undetected. Caseous mases may be found in the discharge and yet not especially significant unless the bacilli be found. Pain is not common unless it be confined principally to the tube and salpingitis exists.

The tubes are predisposed to tuberculosis because of their spiral form and the irregular mucosa which tends to stagnate the secretions. The delay of the passing of the secretions produces an irritation of the mucosa, congestion follows, and this existing catarrhal condition favors infection.

The source of the infection may be through the peritoneum, the blood stream, the lymph vessels, or from outside the body. The constriction of the tube near the uterine body favors the accumulation of the bacilli at this point, seemingly the point of selection for infection in the tube. This point of constriction favors infection from any bacteria, and this is the most prominent etiological factor of gonorrhoeal pyosalpinx.

McCallum, gives as his experience, that all foreign material placed in the peritoneal cavity moved in the direction of the diaphragm, but Murphy states that tubercular material deposited in the peritoneal cavity of the female would invariably gravitate to the pelvis. Seldom has he seen nodules above the line of the umbilicus. Material thus deposited and moving downward would most likely infect the tube if the abdominal end were not closed.

In simple tuberculosis of the tube, where the fimbriated end is free, there are manifested periodical attacks, acute in character as soreness, pain, nausea, and rise of temperature.

The attacks pass in a few days, only to recur in 4 to 6 weeks. They are due to the irritation of the retained secretions, and their expulsion periodically. These cases may easily be mistaken for recurrent appendical pelvic infection.

One very important point for us to consider most carefully, is that the soreness in tubercular tubal trouble preceeded the pains while in acute appendicitis the pain comes on suddenly, followed by the soreness. While symbiosis between the gonococcus and the ordinary microbes, is rare it is not exceptional to see this occur between Neissers coccus and the tubercle bacillus. Should the entrance of the infecting microorgan-

isms occur simultaneously, the increase of the tubercle bacilli would be masked by the much more rapid growth of the gonococcus During the time of the greatest activity of the Neisser coccus, the progress of the tubercle bacillus is decreased, but after this activity has ceased then the bacilli become more active than ever on account of the destruction of portions of the epithelium lining the tube, and the lowering of the vitality of the underlying tissue.

The puerperal state plays as important a role in tuberculosis of the tubes as it does in general genital tuberculosis.

It may be asked why we speak of the tubes being the most frequent location of the tubercular infection from without, or the ascending type, while the intermediate tissue escapes. It is for the same reason that the upper air passages are practically immune in pulmonary tuberculosis; the resisting power of these intervening structures is greater.

The symptoms of uterine tuberculosis are similar to those of endometritis, so the symptoms of tuberculosis of the tube are not unlike those of salpingitis.

From the conditions determined by the foregoing investigation we can not consider anything but extirpation of the organs, provided the patient's general condition will permit. As in malignant disease of these organs my preference is the abdominal route.

The uterus and ovaries if not diseased, may be left.

Seelingman reports a case of lupus on the face and scalp which healed after extirpation of a tubercular tubo-ovarian tumor. This slow progressive disease of the tubes needs more careful consideration than is usually given it. Its chronicity is characteristic and is one of our best guides to the nature of the disease.

The infection from the Neisser coccus simulates it more than any other disease, yet its more rapid progress distinguishes its presence. Pain exists in both cases, but more acute and severe in the latter. Soreness is present in both but more severe and sudden in the gonorrhoeal infection.

A carefully taken history will reveal a possible exposure to specific infection.

A careful microscopical examination of the vaginal secretions of the young girls will surprise us as to how often we will find the tubercle bacilli.

A constant profuse leucorrhoeal discharge, in these young girls, should be warning enough, to cause us to make more careful search for a positive diagnosis.

Should we make an exhaustive search and find neither the tubercular bacilli nor the Neisser coccus, well and good, we have done our duty, but should we neglect to do so, and wait for developments sufficient to diagnose the case without such careful examination, until the disease has progressed beyond our control, then we certainly have been, to say the least, neglectful of our duty as diagnosticians.

The disease is transmissible from one school girl or playmate to another and should be included in the examinations made by the physician selected to watch over our school children, to precvent the spread of disease. This is a point wholly neglected and unthought of by the parent and laity and should be made a part of the duty of our school examining physicians who alone can realize its importance.

In conclusion:

1st. Remember, that surgical interference must only be considered a *means* to an *end*, for without it be followed by rigid *dietetic* and *hygienic* treatment it can not accomplish the desired results.

2nd. Remember the importance of an early diagnosis in these cases; that this disease, like malignant disease of these parts, if localized and diagnosed early is positively curable, but if neglected until the disease has invaded the more vital tissue showing pronounced cachexia, our patient is beyond medical and surgical skill, and we must consider ourselves resposible for the final result.

"A DUTY OF THE PHYSICIAN TO HIMSELF."

BY L. H. HUFFMAN, M. D., HOBART, OKLA.

The duties of a physician may well be classed under four different heads: The duty to his patient—to the medical profession—to the community at large, and to himself. In this paper I wish to speak briefly on the last one mentioned.

The duty of the physician to his patient is as old and well defined as sickness itself. Endowed with intelligence, courage, tact and tenderness the physician finds constant exercise of these qualities in his administration to the sick.

A thorough understanding of the obliga-

tions to the members of the profession is an attribute which will figure largely in the successful work of a physician. The acts and works of each physician reflect upon every other physician. An incompetent or irregular physician can do much to discredit the profession among the people, many of whom it is true are prone to suspicion an injustice. On the other hand receiving as he does the full confidence of the patient, the physician is in duty bound to so act as to justfy this confidence and trust, to render to his patient the care and medical skill that will result in the fulfillment of every obligation imposed upon him.

Having fulfilled his duty to his patient and to his co-workers and to the commun-

Read before a joint meeting of the Washita, and Custer County Medical Societies, September 17, 1910, Clinton Okla.

ity at large, there remains a duty, which if neglected must soon destroy his efficiency, his march with modern progress, a duty to himself and that is—*a more careful interest in his own financial welfare.*

Within the last ten years, it is conceded that living expenses have increased 40 per cent. The wages of the skilled mechanic has increased, the salaries of office clerks, teachers, etc., have also advanced. The fees of professional men have not advanced more than 10 per cent., leaving us 30 per cent behind the game.

On every side there have been changes of policies, methods, and adjustments made because of the changed times in which we live. Does the public prefer a cheap doctor to a good one? Is it possible that a good doctor can exist today without a high fee as an accompaniment? The world demands a practical, sensible worker in the twentieth century sick-room. One who is energetic and up with the times. The demand is for the higher ideal. The public clamor for a high degree of skill. We can infuse a different spirit in our profession. Does the public demand a short course medical school, an inferior education and a less expensive physician? No—but on the other hand it is our duty to carry out high practical ideas, train men in the profession in an expensive manner.

The general advance in the science of medicine makes it necessary to change our method of treatment and we must bring to our patients the very best treatment derived from careful investigation of the later and improved ways for the prevention and cure of disease. In other words we should have the best information and cure of disease. In other words we should have the best information that can be had along our line of work. To do this we, as general practitioners are required to get away from our regular work, and get among our superiors that make a specialty of one line of work

at the post-graduate schools and clinics. This takes time and money. The duty which I wish to emphasize is—"A duty to ourselves to charge a fee proportianate to the requirements, efficiency and time required in preparing for the practice." All of which are greater than in the past.

No class of people work so dilligently against their own financial interests as the physician. The education of the public in a general way on the prevention of diseases means what? It is this—ultimately a smaller quantity and better qualify of physicians than we have at the present time.

It is evident that the cabinet of the president at Washington will soon have an addition made to it. Steps are being taken to create a general commissioner of health for the entire United States. This will mean much to the public health inasmuch as this will place much profitable literature into the hands of the public to read on the prevention and spread of diseases and at the expense of the government.

I am glad of the opportunity to be able to present to you an outline of the very practical method by which we have organized and established in Kiowa County a Physicians' Protective Association. There is no question that such a practical method, so complete and efficient fills a long felt want and its universal adoption must be regarded as an important advance step for physicians. By the adoption of this business association we are able to collect our fees and keep up with delinquent patrons who are able to pay, thus making our work more pleasant and profitable and by these methods will be better able financially to keep in touch with the constant dangers and improvements in the practice of medicine.

It is true we have the deserving poor to attend and care for, a service that will nevel be paid for in the coin of the realm. Let us not be afraid to look after these poor unfortunates and that our dignity may not be lowered by stepping into a house of the poor to stop the cry of pain. These patients deserve the same care and skilled work that the people get who are able to pay for it.

It is the purpose of this organization to have a complete association in at least the western part of the state. The secretaries will be able to keep all the member-familiar with facts that will be of mutua benefit.

We will be more appreciated as we become more progressive.

Times have changed somewhat, since we do not now attempt to establish the fact with our patient that taking a certain number of powders or pills at a certain time or intervals will save his life, but use the powder or pill and watch for physiological effects.

The great public health meetings in which the physicians work so diligently and earnestly are for the purpose of getting the public interested in the prevention and spread of disease is another example of an unrewarded service. In days gone by we had ideals that were different from the present, we had invested a small amount of time, money and energy in the preparation for the practice. With four years in college and the required preparatory education for matriculation of a higher degree at present is more evidence of the necessity for a uniform advance in fees.

In addition to all these requirements it is but a question of a short time until graduates will have hospital bedside experience added to their course to become licensed practitioners among the laity.

Therefore it becomes a duty to ourselves to keep our fees proportionate with these conditions for higher ideals and general advancement of the profession.

A REPORT OF CASES FROM THE CLINIC OF ALLEN B. KANAVAL, M. D.
(Professor of Surgery, Post Graduate Hospital, Chicago, Illinois.)

BY T. S. WILLIAMS, M. D., STILLWELL, OKLA.

Among the various clinics given at the Post Graduate Hospital is that of Dr. Kanavel. He ordinarily holds a clinic on Thursday morning, which students of the Post Graduate Hospital as well as some from the Northwestern University Medical (School attend. He usually shows the cases first, then operates on what material he has and intersperses this with a talk from one of his assistants upon some phase of experimental work which they are carrying on, since he makes it a rule that each one of his assistants shall have some work of that kind on hand.

The following is a report of one of the clinics. The first case reported, I have had occasion to observe after operation and the amount of function is almost complete at the present time.

Case 1. Fracture of lower end of humerus with dislocation of fore-arm. Male; age 39; occupation carpenter.

Present trouble: Fell from building about twenty feet, landing on elbow; accident occurred three months ago.

Examination: Shows elbow joint fixed at angle of about 120 degrees, marked distortion of relation of tip of olecranon to condyles of humerus.

X-Ray examination shows fracture of internal condyle of humerus and dislocation of ulna backward; also 8 fractures of coronoid process and head of radius through articular surface, with displacement of radius outward.

Treatment: Ether anesthesia, preceded by nitrous oxide. An attempt was made at reduction but failed, and patient having been prepared surgically, open operation was resorted to.

Operation: Incision was made over radial side of olecranon down to the bone, and finding reduction still impossible, a part of triceps tendon and ligaments attached to head of radius were incised. It was now found that a fragment of the coronoid process acted as a wedge in the olecranon fossa preventing the ulna being returned to its normal position. After removal of this fragment and small fragments of the humerus, reduction was easily accomplished. All divided structures were now brought together with catgut sutures and wound closed in usual manner. The forearm was brought into acute flexion and retained in this position by plaster splint.

After Treatment: Careful manipulation under anesthesia at intervals of ten days to two weeks, continued for several months.

Of special interest in connection with this case we might note the value of the landmarks at the elbow joint, in diagnosis; especially the relation between the condyles and tip of olecranon and Hueters line, also the value of a raidograph taken in two places at right angles, this showing the position of the parts. It might also be well to mention the value of the acute flexion position in retaining the fragments in fracture of the condyles, the position affecting reduction of itself in many cases.

Case II. Fracture of lower end of radius or Colles' fracture complicated with fracture of the carpal schaphoid.

Male: Age 35; Laborer

The occurrence of fracture of the scaphoid alone or complicating Colles' fracture is more frequent than we formerly thought. We have seen a number of cases in this clinic in the past year and it is important to recognize this condition as we frequently have to resort to operative measures to remove a fragment in order to restore function to the carpus. The diagnosis can be established clinically, and there is one characteristic sign, viz: that pressure over the depression back of the base of the metacarpal, commonly known as the snuff box, causes exquisite pain. The X-Ray makes the diagnosis a certainty.

Treatment: Immobilization if no dislocation of fragments. Open incision if dislocation of fragments interferes with function.

IMPORTANCE OF THE ROENTGEN RAY AS AN AID TO SURGICAL DIAGNOSIS.

Dr. B. C. Cushway who is first assistant and has charge of the X-Ray work in the clinic was then introduced and he said in part:

"The value of the radiograph in diagnosis of fractures and dislocations is so well known that little need be said in regard to its use in this class of cases, except to emphasize its value and urge its use in every case, not only to establish a diagnosis, but to study the pathology present in a given case. Three points are worth hearing in mind: I always have two views at right angles if possible; 2. Take symmetrical parts for comparison; 3. Get a picture after reduction in every case to be sure you have obtained the proper result.

"*Cranial Surgery.* Here the X-Ray findings are of value as for instance: Tumor of the pituitary gland; pus in the antrum of Highmore; mastoid and frontal sinus.

"*Malignant and Benign Tumors of Bone.* Here the X-Ray diagnosis is positive and will serve to differentiate, bone cysts, osteoma, etc., from sarcoma.

"*Inflammatory Conditions in Bone.* In the chronic inflammatory diseases of the toe, the X-Ray is especially valuable, and diagnosis can be made as follows:

1. *Bone Syphilis.*

Recognized by deposits of new bone,

thickening of periotteum and density of radiograph.

2. *Tuberculosis.*

Atrophy of the structure, hazy radaiograph.

3. *Osteomyelitis.*

Destruction of bone without production of new bone. No atrophy; fairly clear radiograph.

4. *Diseases of Joints.*

Here the X-Ray serves to differentiate between simple synovitis, arthritis, tuberculosis, and the more infrequent lesions as tabetic joints and arthritis deformans. In conclusion, we might mention the value of the radiograph in diseases of the renal system, diseases of the thoracic organs and digestive viscera and while in some of these instances, the results are not as yet perfect, the field is a comparatively new one and much can be expected for the future.

Dr. J. J. Cole was introduced and gave a short resume of the use of Bacterial Vaccines and Tuberculin in the Clinic.

Definition. A vaccine is a killed bacterial culture, suspended in normal salt solution, to which has been added lysol or carbolic acid to the strength of 1-4 per cent. of the former or 1-2 per cent. of the latter.

Classes. There are two main classes, the autogenous and the stock vaccines. The former is prepared directly from the local lesion, the discharge or the blood of the patient, the latter from a known specie of bacterial culture.

Standardization. Blood from a normal individual is taken and the corpuscular content determined. Definite quantities of this blood and vaccine are mixed thoroughly. Smears are then made, dried and stained.

The slide is placed under the microscope and the numbers of red cells and microbes in many separate fields are counted.

In this way the number of bacteria in each c. c. of the mixture is estimated. Af-

ter testing for sterility, the vaccine is put up in glass bulbs containing approximately one c. c. and sealed.

Varieties. At the present time the vaccines most commonly in use are the staphyloccic, streptococcic, gonococcic, typhoid and dysenteric vaccines. Some of the forms of tuberculin are essentially vaccines.

Dilution. Since the different stock vaccines as we receive them from the pharmacentical houses are put up in more or less concentrated form, it is necessary to dilute them before beginning the treatment of a selected case. Sterile normal salt solution to which has been added about one drop of 95 per cent. carbolic acid to each ounce of the solution, has been found the most suitable diluting agent.

ARTICLES NECESSARY TO MAKE THE DILUTION.

1. An ordinary sterile hypodermic syringe and needle, with a capacity of one c. c.

2. Two or three sterile medicine glasses.

3. Sterile normal saline solution preserved with 1-4 per cent. lysol or 1-2 per cent. carbolic acid.

4. Bulb of vaccine to be used.

The bulb of vaccine is taken and placed in a sterile piece of gauze or cotton and the neck of the bulb broken between the fingers, after which the contents of the bulb is drawn up into the syringe and then deposited in one of the sterile medicine glasses. Into another of the medicine glasses is poured the normal salt solution. Next, as many syringefuls of the normal salt solution is mixed with the vaccine as is required to make the necessary dilution and the whole mixed thoroughly.

To explain: Supposing we have a c. c. bulb of stock vaccine which contains 500,-000,000 dead bacteria and we desire to give 100,000,0000 of these bacteria as a single dose. We would then dilute the contents of this bulb with 4 c. c.'s (or 4 ordinary syringefuls) of the salt solution and then draw up one syringeful of the mixture which would contain approximately 100,-000,000 bacteria. We should bear in mind that the dilution for children and babies should be 5 to 10 times greater than for adults.

Methods of using vaccine. There are two methods in use at the present time, the laboratory and the clinical.

The former is practically Wright's method and treatment is guided by the opsonic index determinations. Owing to the fact that a well equipped laboratory is necessary to carry out Wright's plan of treatment, that a good technical knowledge is essential and that considerable time is required to make opsonic index determinatione, it is obvious that for the general practitioner, not familiar with Wright's technique, the clinical method is the one most generally selected.

Theory of action of vaccine. In the blood serum there are various agents concerned in the protection of the organism against infection. The most important of these are the white blood corpuscles, the agglutinins, the bacteriolysins, the bacterio-trophins and the opsonins, the latter term being given by Wright, of London, to those agents which act on the infecting bacteria and prepare them for digestion by the white blood corpuscles.

A minimal dose of vaccine inoculated into an individual suffering from a local or general infection produces a slight rise in these protective substances of the body which is usually of short duration and is followed by a return to the normal.

When a larger dose is given it at first produces a fall in these protective substances, designated by Wright as the negative phase. This is soon followed by a general rise in the opsonins to or above normal and is known as the positive phase. This rise may be of long or short duration, depending on the dose of vaccine employed. Following this rise there will then occur a gradual fall of these protective agents to the normal level or below.

Preparation of Patient. Having selected a case suitable for vaccine therapy, we prepare the skin area to be inoculated by sterilizing the same with a piece of sterile gauze or cotton saturated with alcohol. No other cleansing is necessary.

The injection is made directly under the skin or may be given intramuscularly.

Selection of Cases. As a general statement it may be said that the local infections are the most adaptable to treatment by vaccine injections. These include boils, carbuncles, acne, adenitis, arthritis, etc. The general infections do not seem to be so favorably influenced by vaccines as the local, although some clinicians have reported good results in this class of cases. However, general infections do not contraindicate the employment of vaccines which should be carefully given.

Dose and Interval of Dosage. After determining the kind of bacteria with which we have to deal, with either by direct smear or culture or both, we begin the treatment with the corresponding vaccine. And I may say here that we have used the stock vaccines exclusively in our work at the Post Graduate Hospital.

The determination of the proper dose and the interval between doses are the most essential factors in vaccine therapy.

Our success or failure in the employment of these agents will depend very largely on these two factors.

Since at present there is no fixed standard by which we may ascertain the initial dose to be given, we will have to depend greatly on our experience in this line of work and by carefully studying the nature and degree of the infection to be treated.

Having in mind the theory of action of vaccines as previously stated we have a working basis as a guide in selecting the proper dose and the interval that should elapse between each successive dose.

In general we may say that the beginning dose should be small enough to cause a slight rise in the protective agents of the body and this is indicated by a slight improvement in the local and general symptoms of our patient. When this improvement subsides it is time to give a second injection of vaccine and here the dose is a little larger than the initial one. In this way we continue the injections, gradually increasing the dose according to the signs and symptoms until we arrive at the maximum dose which may be repeated as though necessary. The maximum dose is regarded as the contents of one of our vaccine bulbs undiluted.

It is plain that we do not wish to cause a lowering of the protective agents which would be the case if too large a dose of vaccine were given and in a general infection such a result would be productive of serious consequence. As our experience in vaccine therapy at the Post Graduate Hospital has had most to do with localized infections, the staphyloccic and gonococcic vaccines are the ones with which we are best acquainted.

In the ordinary local infections occurring in adults we have found that an initial dose of 50,000,000 of the dead staphylocci and 5,000,000 of the gonococci to be a safe initial dose. Children and babies, of course, receive correspondingly smaller doses. At times we may feel that a still smaller dose would be indicated in order that we may work within the limits of safety.

The interval between the first and second injection will depend on the effect produced by the first and varies in the average case from three to six days.

As the dose is increased the interval is likewise increased and when the maximum dose is reached it would usually not be safe to repeat it inside of a week or ten days.

The gonococcus vaccine in cases of acute gonorrhoeal urethritis does not seem to have given the results hoped for, although it has proven of value in complications of this disease particularly the arthritic cases. Why it does not act more favorably in the urethral cases is hard to say but its failure may be ascribed to the fact that there, are various strains of the gonococci organism making it difficult to select the appropriate vaccine.

In conjunction with vaccine therapy the medical and surgical treatment is not to be neglected as is evidenced by the following case:

Mrs. D., age 26 years, entered the dispensary February 25th, '09, suffering from a right axillary adenitis, due to an infection of the right index finger one month previous. No evidence of the finger infection was to be found on her entrance. She complained of considerable pain in the right axilla, especially on pressure made there. A probable diagnosis of straphyloccic infection was made and the patient was given treatment for two weeks with the combined staphyloccic vaccine at the end of which time little or no improvement was noticed.

The right axilla was then opened and almost a quart of pus evacuated.

Evidently, if surgical procedure was neglected in this case serious results would have followed.

It is possible that when this patient entered the dispensary suppuration may have been present, which owing to the fact that the woman was corpulent, pus could not be detected on examination which would explain the failure of the vaccine treatment to effect cure.

Two typical cases are reported here, showing the beneficial effect of vaccine therapy.

Mr. B., age 25, entered the dispensary December 17, '08, suffering from a carbuncle located between the scapulae and about two inches in diameter. Seven or eight smaller carbuncles in the process of formation were scattered over different parts of the body. The large carbuncle was immediately opened by a crucial incision, the pus evacuated and the wound packed with a moist boric acid dressing.

Smear and culture from the wound showed the presence of a staphyloccus albus infection and he was accordingly given treatment with the corresponding vaccine. The operative wound healed rapidly and it was noticed that under the vaccine therapy the other local infections on his body began to heal so that at the end of two weeks, during which time he was given four injections, these smaller lesions had all disappeared without further suppuration.

Mr. W., colored, age 28, entered the dispensary August 12, '09, giving a history of acute gonorrhoeal urethritis which was subsiding and a painful, swollen, left wrist joint, a diagnosis of gonorrhoeal arthritis was made and treatment instituted with gonococcic vaccine, together with immobilization of this wrist with a plaster splint.

Altogether four injections within two weeks were given and at the end of the first week all pain had left this wrist joint and the swelling was perceptibly diminished. at the third week all the swelling disappeared and the patient received a perfect result. The immobilization of the wrist joint was very likely a valuable aid to the vaccine in the cure of this patient.

Other favorable results could be stated but space will not permit.

To conclude, we may say that while vaccine therapy is more or less in it's infancy, it is a scientific and practical aid to our treatment of various infections and when properly employed is usually productive of beneficial results. Improperly used the results will be nothing but failures and often disastrous.

That it fails in some cases we cannot deny but with an improved knowledge concerning the mechanism of immunity and a more perfect technique in applying this form of treatment we may hope that the future will throw more light on this important and interesting subject, producing a less per cent. of failures and a greater degree of success.

TUBERCULIN AS A DIAGNOSTIC AND THERAPEUTIC AGENT.

Nothing more than a brief discussion of some of the principles involved in the use of tuberculin will be attemtped here.

AS A DIAGNOSTIC AGENT.

Tuberculin at present is used in four different ways diagnostically, namely, by vaccination, known as the Von Pirquet test, by inunctions (the Morro teet) by instillation into the eye, (the Calmette test) and by subcutaneous injection.

That there is a certain element of danger connected with the use of tuberculin dropped into the eye or injected subcutaneously for diagnostic purposes most clinicians will admit. Used properly by vaccination or inunction no serious results should follow.

Since our experiments with tuberculin as a diagnostic agent have had most to do with the Von Pirquet test, the method is here briefly described:

Articles required for this test:

1. Bulb of Koch's Old Tuberculin.

2. Two sterile needles or two scarifiers of the Von Pirquet type.

3. Two sterile medicine droppers.

4. A solution of normal salt and glycerine equal parts, to which is added carbolic acid to the strength of 1-10 of 1 per cent. This is known as the control solution.

5. Sterile cotton and gauze and adhesive plaster.

The skin area to be vaccinated is sterilized with ether for a distance of about five by three inches. The arm is usually selected.

One drop of Koch's Old Tuberculin, undiluted or diluted with normal saline solution to the strength of 25 or 50 per cent. is dropped on the upper part of the sterilized area and a second drop is placed about four inches below the first.

Midway between these two drops is placed one drop of the control solution, the other sterile medicine dropper being used for this.

One of the needles or scarifiers is then taken and the skin scarified through the upper and lower drops of tuberculin just enough to allow the serum to exlude. .

The center drop is likewise scarified with the other sterile needle or scarifies.

After five or ten minutes a piece of sterile gauze is placed over the vaccinated area and held there by adhesive straps or a bandage.

The Reaction. From three to seventy-two hours usually twenty-four hours after vaccination a red indurated papule at least an eighth of an inch should be seen.

THE USE OF TUBERCULIN FOR TREATMENT.

This subject is such an extensive one that it will be only briefly considered here, the reader being referred to the various articles and works on the tuberculin theapeutics for a more detailed on the tubercupeutics for a more detailed discussion of the subject.

The treatment of tuberculosis by tuberculin aims at the establishment of an artificial immunity. Our success or failure by attempts at immunizatioon depends to a great extent on the method employed in producing this immunity.

Undoubtedly in tuberculin we have an agent capable of rendering most satisfactory results when correctly employed but when our method is faulty unfavorable or serious consequences will ensue.

It is well then to use extreme care in the use of this therapeutic agent, to understand that it has its's limitations and that a good knowledge of the subject is neces-

sary, especially for the beginner in this line of work.

Selection of Cases. All cases of tuberculosis are not suitable to tuberculin treatment. As a general statement it may be said that the more quiescent and chronic the tubercular process, the more adaptable it will be to this form of treatment.

Those cases showing evidences of marked toxemia in which the process is active had better vaccination with Koch's Old Tuberculin gave a very positive reaction in each of the three cases. Here we see the importance of making a correct diagnosis and the great aid the Von Pirquet test rendered.

It should be borne in mind however, that in the very active forms of tuberculosis, indicating a marked toxemia, we will now and then find the vaccination giving a negative result which may be explained by the fact that such a patient is so saturated with tuberculin toxin that the amount of tuber-, culin introduced into the skin is not sufficient to cause a reaction. In these cases the diagnosis is usually plain so that we could dispense with the tuberculin test anyway.

The beginning and chronic forms of tuberculosis are the ones giving the most typical reactions.

Sometimes we find a case of tuberculosis not reacting to the first vaccination but giving a positive result on the second test two or three weeks afterward so that it is well to vaccinate a patient the second time if the first vaccination was negative, before we exclude tuberculosis.

A positive reaction indicates that the patient has or has had tuberculosis. Cases showing tuberculin reaction, we will observe the following:

A varying degree of redness is noticed around the upper and lower marks and these areas are slightly swollen. In the center of each of these scarifications will be noticed a papule forming.

. The amount of redness will vary from a slight congestion o fthe capillaries around the areas inoculated with tuberculin, to a marked redness the size of a dime or quarter. It lasts from one to fourteen days, depending on the degre of reaction, gradually fading until the vaccinated areas assume their normal appearance. No scar remains and the arm is but slightly sore at most. Constitutional reaction is absent or slight in the great majority of cases.

[VALUE OF THE VON PIRQUET TEST.

The more experience we have with this test the more we are impressed with its value as a diagnostic agent.

By the Von Pirquet est we can frequently make a diagnosis of tuberculosis when the physical examination and sputum findings are negative.

I have in mind three cases, in which the physical examination did not reveal the presence of a local lesion and all three patients giving practically neuresthenic symptoms, first placed on general medical or surgical treatment as indicted in each particular case, until such a time as the active symptoms and signs of the disease have subsided before instituting tuberculin treatment.

Having made our diagnosis and selected a suitable case, we next consider the kind of tuberculin to be used and the method to be followed. It matters not so much as to the form of tuberculin employed as it does the method used.

The varieties at present used most clinically are Old Tuberculin, (Koch), Tuberculin, (R), Bacillen Emulsion, (B. E.), (Koch), Broth Filtrate, (B. F.), (Deny's) and Dɔranecks Tuberculin. Since our experience at the Post Graduate Hospital has had most to do with the B. E. product (Parke, Davis & Co.) a brief account of the method employed in its use is here given:

Parke, Davis & Co. supplies this Tuber-culin B. E. in bulbs of one c. c. which contain one milligram of tuberculin solids. Since this is a concentrated solution, before commencing its use it is necessary to dilute this product.

Tuberculin B. E. is made from the germ bodies pulverized and suspended in glycerine solution. A dilution of 1 to 500 I have found very convenient in beginning the use of this product and is prepared thus:

Sterile normal salt solution, to which has been added carbolic acid 1·2 per cent is used as the diluting agent.

499 c. c.'s of this solution is accurately measured out in a sterile bottle or graduate and to this the contents of the bulb (1 c. c.) of tuberculin B. E. is added. A dark brown bottle which has been sealed with collodion is preferable for keeping this mixture.

This we call our stock solution.

For convenience of using, a sterile wide mouth, brown bottle, with a capacity of two to four ounces is selected and over the top of this is stretched a sterile rubber cover such as a piece of rubber glove which can be secured around the neck of the bottle with a stout rubber band. This bottle contains a portion of the stock solution.

In drawing out the solution from this smaller bottle all one has to do is to first sterilize the rubber cap with 95 per cent. carbolic acid, insert the needle attached to a sterile hypodermic syringe and withdraw the required amount of tuberculin. The punctured rubber is then sealed with collodion.

Dose and Interval of Dosage. As in the case of vaccines previously described, here we come to the most important phase of tuberculin treatment. And since we have no set standard by which we may judge the initial dose, our experience and careful study of the case will have to be our guides.

The principles of the theory of action of tuberculin correspond in general with what has been discussed in regard to vaccines and should be kept in mind in the selection of the proper dose and interval.

The most important rule to be remembered is to begin with very small doses, to avoid constitutional disturbance and violent reactions and to increase the dose very gradually.

Since the formation of antibodies is slow, the treatment will have to extend over from eight months to one or two years depending on the case. Nothing is to be gained by haste in giving this treatment and it is well to have our patients understand beforehand that the completion of a course of treatments requires time.

Patients running a temperature above 100 degrees fahrenheit or showing marked constitutional or local symptoms should not be put on tuberculin treatment until the temperature is below this mark and the symptoms in abeyance.

I have found that for surgical tubercular cases, occurring in adults an initial dose of 1-1,000 of a mg. of the B. E. product is a safe dose as a rule and in medical cases 1-10,000 mg.

To obtain this dose of 1-1,000 mg. we draw up one c. c. or an ordinary syringeful of our 1 to 500 dilution and dilute this with 4 c. c.'s of normal salt solution. By drawing up one syringeful of this mixture we have approximately 1-1,000 mg. in our syringe. For the second dose we use about two minims less of the first diluting agent and the same amount of the tuberculin, so that our increase in dosage would be by about 2 minimums of tuberculin. This same amount of increase is followed until we give one c. c. of four tuberculin mixture undiluted or 1-500 mg. We will then have to make up a fresh solution whose strength is 1-200 mg. and in this way continue until we have finally gradually worked up the dose to the strength of 1 mg., when we discontinue the treatment and observe our patients for one or two months. If signs of the tubercular process return,

a second course of injections would be indicated but here we may use larger doses of the tuberculin since our patient has become accustomed to large doses. The second series of treatments then would not require so much time as the first.

Other methods of making the dilutions may be used but the plan here given seems to me to be simple and easily carried out.

All treatments are given hypodermically, either by the subcutaneous method or intra muscularly, the sites selected being where the tissue is loose.

On an average of two injections a week are given and as we arrive at the larger doses it is well to gradually increase these intervals. After we have given an injection of this tuberculin we instruct our patient to keep a careful record of the temperature and symptoms until the time for the next treatment.

Since we use the clinical method, we judge the time for giving the next dose by the temperature and constitutional and local symptoms. When the temperature is above 100 degrees we do not repeat an injection until the fever goes below this mark.

The constitutional and local symptoms are of more importance than the temperature record, since we may have marked symptoms and no rise in the temperature.

We omit the next dose when these symptoms are marked and wait until they disappear before continuing our treatment.

It is difficult to complete a course of injections without observing some reactions which usually are noted when the larger doses are given.

Our work in tuberculin immunization at the Post Graduate Hospital has convinced us that tuberculin used properly in the chronic forms of tuberculosis is really productive of beneficial results in the majority of cases. We have learned to be exceedingly careful in its use, knowing the dangers liable to follow its injudicious employment.

Space will not permit a citation of the various cases treated.

That the medical and surgical treatment is to be used in conjunction with tuberculin therapy is understood.

After the conclusion of Dr. Cole's paper, Dr. Kanavel demonstrated a case of Von Volkman's Contracture, which he had operated upon at a previous clinic. The operation was a dislocation of the ulnar and median nerves from their bed of scar tissue, placing muscle flaps beneath them. At the operation, the median nerve was found inbedded in scar tissue, and lying upon a fragment of the humerus, separated at time of injury, the ulnar nerve seemed free but lacked the luster of a healthy nerve. This case followed a fracture at the elbow joint where anterior and posterior splints had been used and were probably a little too tight. Dr. Kanavel hoped to get some improvement but could promise very little in the way of perfect function.

The next case was one of great interest, that in which the diagnosis of tumor of the pituitary body had been made. Dr. Kanavel drew attention to the infrequency of these tumors and the fact that about fifteen or eighteen cases had been operated upon, some by the cranial route after the method of Horsley but for the most part the operation now used is by the trans-sphenoidal route by which method the nose is turned down or sideways and the structures of the nose removed, by removal of the tumor through the sphenoid cells. Dr. Kanavel operated by a new method, that of turning the nose up from below and the technique of the operation was in general as follows:

TECHNIQUE OF OPERATION. INFRANASAL ROUTE.

Incision around lower half of nose, close to crease at alae, close under nares, turning the nose back and cutting through the septum along its inferior parts. and attachment to perpendicular plate of ethmoid. It will be seen that this is essentially an entrance into the infranasal cavity. Now after removal of inferior turbinates and deflecting to one side, a perfect view of the sphenoid is obtained. The sphenoidal foramen was next located, the anterior wall of sphenoid cells broken in and entrance to the tumor obtained.

The tumor was now removed in pieces, partly by aid of a curette, care being taken to prevent removal of all of pituitary body; in this case hemorrhage was severe from the tumor substance and a clinical diagnosis of sarcoma was made, which was proven to be correct by microscopic section later. The operation was completed by packing the sphenoidal opening down to site of tumor, the nose being sutured into its normal location, the packing brought through the nostrils, and the septum held in place by packing the inferior meatus on both sides. After the completion of this operation it was remarkable what a perfect cosmetic result was obtained.

"The anesthetic given was ether, given by the rectal route and proved a very satisfactory anesthetic in this case as has been found to be the case in other operations about the face in this clinic. The patient showed no signs of shock at any time and forty-eight hours after operation was taking nourishment frely, and able to carry on rational conversation with his friends and attendants.

"A more detailed account of this operation will be found in the article by Allen B. Kanavel in the Journal of the American Medical Association of November 20th, 1909: Volume LIII, Number 21. The Removal of Tumors of the Pituitary Body by an Infranasal Route."

(Note. This case had a primary recovery and an examination of the tumor removed showed it to be a sarcoma, at the present writing he is still alive.)

Dr. Frederick A. Berry, another assistant who has had charge of the cancer investigations, was now introduced and spoke as follows:

"Certain European investigators, Jacobs and Geets of Brussels, have made studies in which they have arrived at the conclusion that in concerous cachexia there is present a specific micro-organism, the microroccos neoformans of Doyen, and that it is practicable to immunize a patient by the use of a micrococcus neoformans vaccine when it is controlled by deformation of the opsonic power of the blood. They have cultivated the organism from 90 per cent. of tumors examined and have succeeded in producing neoplasic lesions in 30 per cent. of the cases by inoculating cultures of the organism into mice and white rats.

We are using in the clinic in our in-operable cancer cases a microrocci neoforms vacine. It is too early as yet to make even a preliminary report as to the efficacy of the vaccine and at present we neither recommend its use nor can we discredit it but reserve our opinion and conclusions as to its value until some later date.

Jacobs and Geets report (The Lancet, April 7, 1906) on forty-six cases in which inoculation of micrococcus neoformans vaccine have been used.

"Cure" maintained after several weeks, 7.

Lasting improvement 12.

Transient result, 7.

No result, 11.

Under treatment, 9.

ELECTRICITY AND THE NERVOUS SYSTEM.

BY TOM A. WILLIAMS, M. B., C. M., (EDIN.) WASHINGTON, D. C.

Member Corresp. Soc. de Neural, de Paris; Member Corresp. Soc. de Paychol. de Paris; Member Assoc. Soc. Clin. Med., Mant., France. Neurologist to Epiphany Free Dispensary.

This had been the agent of more bunkum and charlatanry than all other physical agents combined. Even now, one hears apologies for the psychic efect of imposing appartatus. That it has a psychic effect is true; but it is the payable effect of the quack. It is not an effect aimed at the origin of the disease, but to impress the patient with the power of the remedy, and to delude him into the idea that he must be receiving benefit from so wonderful an agent. When his intelligence is thus obfuscated, he can be made to believe anything. A parallel is found in the procedure of a christian scientist, who by the mysterious agency of immortal mind wipes out of the patient the consciousness of every inconvenience which conflicts with that conception.

Electricity, like other remedies, should be used only with a clear object conformable with its physical properties. One of the most useful of these objects is the maintaining of life in muscles which would otherwise degenerate on account of injury or disease of peripheral motor neurones which supply them. Such are cases of poliomyelitis and of trauma of peripheral nervces. In each of these, the life of the muscles should be maintained by galvanism (Poliomyelitis, Virginia Semi-Monthly, Aug. 25, 1910; Monthly Cyclopedia, Nov., 1910,) for perhaps a year, until it is ascertained what cells or fibres are definitely destroyed, and which of them can be restored to function. I can not speak from experience of the ability of galvanism to promote nutrition other than by the excitation of contractility; but many authorities believe that its intelligent application fosters regeneration of the tissues.

LACERATED CERVIX.

BY J. H. HANSEN, GRANDFIELD, OKLA.

I desire to discuss some of its symptoms and treatment and to call attention to some errors that are frequently committed in treating women who suffer from this complaint.

It has been known for many years that diseases of the uterus may cause many reflex symptoms, notably: headache, nervousness, pains in the back, bladder, urethra, etc.

When a woman presents herself with a history of pain or other symptoms of disease it becomes our duty to find the cause and remove it if removable; until this is done our researches should not stop. We should labor on the case until a pathological condition is found that explains the symptoms.

It may be desirable to give some symptomatic treatment in the meantime and frequently it becomes necessary to do so. If the symptoms disappear and there is no further trouble, we may stop our investigations, but if there are recurring attacks we must not fall into the habit of giving some opiate and let a habit be established.

To illustrate: In the year 1900, Mrs. R.—, called on me and asked if I could cure "gall stones." She stated that she had suffered from that disease for several years and named several doctors who had treated her for the same for some months she had been taking phos. soda, and olive oil.

On examination, I found no typical signs of gall stones. She had repeated attacks of pain in the region of the liver. These were somewhat like the intermittent attacks of pain on passing gall stones; but there was no jaundice, no tenderness over the gall bladder, no enlargement of the liver, in fact nothing to mark the liver as the cause of trouble except its anatomical location and with a nervous woman suggestion would be a sufficient cause.

Suggestion! Unconscious hypnotism. how often has it misled doctor or patient:

None of the doctors who had treated her had examined her feces for gall stones, after an attack.

She was at this time intending to go to Mineral Wells, Texas.

On further examination I found a greatly enlarged uterus. There was a bilateral laceration. The cervix was as large as a silver dollar greatly eroded and covered with a mucopurulent discharge.

I did a Schroeder operation on the cervix and replaced the uterus. She made a prompt recovery and remained in good health for about five years when she had an abortion. The pains returned. Her doctor declared she had gall stones. I was again sent for and corrected the diagnosis and curretted the uterus. Her doctor gave her a few local treatments and she was well.

Some time in the year 1898, Mrs. W., called on me. She had been treated 18 months for ovarian enlargement. I found a lacerated cervix and repaired it. She made a good recovery. Her ovarian enlargement disappeared, also the pains in her pelvis.

Mrs. E.—, had been in poor health for years. She was very nervous, had frequent attacks of palpitation of the heart and fainting spells, was hardly able to be up. Had been under the care of doctors off and on for years. On examination I found a very deep laceration, the deepest I ever saw. I operated restoring the cervix. All her old chronic ailments disappeared and she was able to do her own work and to take in sewing.

Mrs. B.—, suffered a laceration 18 years

before I saw her. From that time until I operated she had suffered from leucorrhea and extreme tenderness of the vagina to such an extent that maritial relations had been entirely suspended during all these years. The operation removed all her troubles and restored her to perfect health.

These cases illustrate the importance of making a careful examination in every case, especially if after a reasonable length of treatment your patient does not recover.

Dudley in his work on gynecology, reports one case where a cervical operation cured an optic neuralgia and also a case where it cured a persistent headache.

Laceration of the cervix is perhaps the most frequent pathological condition to be treated in pelvic diseases.

The zeal of the doctor to deliver a woman quickly. The giving of ergot and the using of forceps needlessly cause many unnecesary lacerations.

A large child, a rigid os or an inflmmatory condition of the cervix account for many more lacerations.

Whatever the cause, the effect is subinvolution with its train of evils such as endometritis, erosion of cervix and displacement.

The displacement and enlargement of the uterus in turn produce displacement and disease of the ovaries, bladder and urethra.

A common complaint is pain in the right side any place from the lower border of the rigs to pouparts ligament. This pain has led to many operations on the ovarian and the vermiform appendix and in one of the cases reported above would have led to an operation for gall stones. In another one

it would have led to an ovarian operation if the case had not fallen into my hands. This pain in the right side is often reflex. We should be sure that there is a direct cause before we consent to operate for its relief.

Dysuria is another common effect of pelvic disease. It has given me more trouble than any other single symptom in the diseases of women. Often it is purely nervous, and resists all kinds of general or local treatment. In most cases, curing the pelvic disease will cause its disappearance.

Constipation is a frequent result, nervous prostration is very frequent.

Local treatment in these cases is a waste of time and brings the doctor into ill repute. True in some cases they give temporary relief and in the case of light lacerations or when a woman is near the menopause it may become permanent.

The proper treatment is to repair the laceration and among the different operations for its repair I believe that in most cases "Schroders" is the best.

The Emmett operation removes some of the tissues in the line of the tear making the cervix narrower than it was before and hence more liable to laceration in the next labor. It also predisposes to dysmenorrhea by making the cervical canal smaller and flatter.

Most of these cases are complicated by a displacement of the uterus. The cervical operation and the rest that follows it will cure the risplacement in most cases but it is best to let your woman wear a pessary for a month or two after she gets up.

PYLORIC OBSTRUCTION DUE TO EXTRINSIC CAUSES.

BY DR. GORDON A. BEEDLE, KANSAS CITY, MO.

In reporting the following cases em-

(Read before Medical Association of the Southwest, Wichita, Kansas, October, 1910.)

braced in this article, the chief purpose is to bring before you for consideration the demonstrated importance offered by adhesions towards the productions of pyloric obstruction. Considering the anatomical intimacy of the pylorus with that compact area in the right hypochondrium composed of the gall bladder, ducts, pancreatic head and duct receiving portion of the duodenum, associated involvments resulting from inflammatory lesions of this frequently invaded field are clearly conceivable. When we consider the varied and extensive symtomatology of stomach trouble, generally termed indigestion, and appreciating the facts that this indigestion is so often a sequence or adjunct to various other lesions, such as Appendicitis, Gall Stones, Ect., obscurity in diagnosis is often made possible.

The increased realization of the frequent occurring chronic stomach trouble dependent for its relief upon some surgical intervention or organs directly or indirectly associated, is essential evidence that we can mate and close association of the surgeon and stomach internist, thus broadening the view of the internist to the advantage of exploratory incision, giving the surgeon an opporunity at the operable stage of dawning malignancy, gall bladder invaluement ad adherent appendices, adhesions, cecal involvement, etc.; on the other hand importance of surgical recognition of the valuable assistance bestowed by the internist through laboratory and chemical findings of stomach, stool and urinary contents, aided by various additional procedures of diagnosis; with finally the clinical judgment of both united in conference. However, an exhaustive treatise could but sparingly cover the importance of close intimacy between the surgeon and internist in cases of obscure stomach conditions. The following is the history of case of Mr. W. Farmer, referred by Dr. Ninestead of Le Loup, Kans., age 36, weighed 135 lbs., regular weight 146, height 5 ft. 10 in., parents both living, father troubled with slight stomach trouble; ten children in family, all

living and healthy, but one brother, who complains with similar trouble of stomach, but not constant or severe; patient's history of ill-health commenced about twelve years ago, or at the age of 24, attacks beginning with pain in stomach, belching large quantities of gas; attacks occurring two or three hours after eating; relief afforded by the taking of food, or by free emesis; constipated at time of attacks; constant attacks recurring for two or three days, when, through elimination and dieting, condition would gradually subside into normal state and continue so for several months. Blood never observed in emesis or stool, no appearance of jaundice; early history of attacks continued the same over a period of years. Pain always localized and tenderness limited to the epigastrium; about three years ago obtained complete relief, after receiving medical treatments by his home doctor; the period of freedom lasted about two years, when similar attacks commenced again, continuing until the time of his operation, during past two months distress almost constant. Saw patient June 14th, 1910. General history as presented above; had been under series of medical observers for past six months. Patient in almost constant pain; tenderness over the epigastrium and right hypochondriac regions; stomach dialated, peristaltic contraction of stomach wall on stimulation; pain increased on traction upward of left thorax during inspiration; rigidity of th e upper right rectus; referred to Dr. Roberts for stomach analysis, which was as follows: Test meal, total quantitty, 45 C. Cn. total acid 66 free H. C. L. 40 _____; _____; 14 deg.; finely divided fluids in great excess; small amount of mucus; starch digestion good; no sarcinaoppler boas; yeast fermentation profuse. Duration test, positive, 2 quarts; diagnosis, obstruction at pylorus of benign type.

Operation—Stomach exposed cardiac

half of the stomach free, plyoric half of the stomach appeared congested, the pylorus pulled high up under the liver and held firmly in a cramped position by extensive adhesions; a slightly thickened area in stomach wall of the pyloric half of greater curvature about one inch long and one-half inch wide, but did not extend to the pylorus; gall bladder seemed free of adhesions and normal in appearance; the apiplaic vessels greatly enlarged and hard; the omentum was involved in the mass of adhesions; no glandular enlargement detected. The abdomen was opened in this case for the purpose of performing a gastro-jejunostomy for obstruction of the pylorus, evidently resulting from healed pyloric ulcer, after thorough intra-abdominal examination, the kinked position of the pyloris, the same being bound down by adhesions; and the evident freedom of scar tissue in the pyloric lumen made conservatism seem the proper procedure. After careful freeing of all adhesions, we decided to postpone the anastomosis, doing the same later, if present efforts were not sufficiently successful. Post operative convalescence was all that could be desired one lavave following the operation; liquid diet for three days, followed by light diet ,and general diet at the end of first week; no pain after third following operation; general post operative attention was accompanied by rapid improvements; left hospital at the end of two weeks, with every appearance of complete relief from his trouble, it being four months since operation. I was pleased to receive a recent report from this patient, stating that there had been no return of his previous trouble, increasing in weight and enjoying good health in general.

In my opinion, this case represents a much larger class of stomach sufferers than we have been inclined to recognize. When we may consider the large percentage of stomach ulcers properly treated medicinally and healed, never having developed a sur-

gical stage, such as extravagant hemorhages, perforation, ect., proceeding for a varying length of time with apparent freedom, later gradually developing symptoms similar to the former trouble, possibly varying slightly in symptomatology, with distress of less severity; obtaining temporary relief, but discouraged from the repeated recurrence, he begins shopping from one doctor to another, confidence fluctuating in a comparative degree to the medical relief obtained. So may a case of this character, bounded in obscurity of its actual etiology, travel on for years under the head of gastric neurosis, gastric catarrh, etc. Fortunate is this man should he fall in the hands of the thorough up-to-date internist of today who isolate and differentiate through repeated findings, and if the case be deemed necessary, will promptly recommend surgical interference, or, in obscurity, will advise exploratory incision.

M. B., of Marian, Kans., recommended by Dr. Sanders of Rosedale, Kans.—History taken by Dr. Sanders, April, 1908. Male, age 38; single; 5 ft., 11 inches; weighed 130 lbs.; family history good; past history good, with exception of an attack of indigestion several years previous, occurring periodically once a month, apparently free from same, however, for the last year or two, or until about October, 1907, when similar symptoms returned; attacks would begin by headache, vertigo, belching of gas, vomiting large quantities of sour fluids, no blood, pain in epigastrium extending around to the upper lumbar region on right side; distress and acid eructations coming on frequently in the early morning hours; some relief after emesis stubborn constipation always constant at time of attacks; stool matter lumpy and light in color during attacks, but no blood apparent; patient treated medicinally for these attacks during the past six months, with but temporary benefits; attacks becoming more frequent and severe in character. Patient developed severe attacks February 9 th, 1910. When first seen by Dr.Sanders,temperature 103, pulse 110; severe pain of epigastrium, extending over right side sligthly jaundiced; constipated; vomiting large quantities of sour fluid; urine containg bile; leucocytotis 18000; muscular rigidity over upper right abdomen; had been unable to retain anything in stomach for several days jaundice increased markedly during the next twelve hours, patient growing apparently weaker; stomach analysis normal, but showing increased quantity. Gall bladder pouted into the wound when abdomen was opened, dilated and thin walled; adhesions extensive; bladder drawn up on top of liver about one and one-half inch, and plastered there with adhesion; the colon adherent to the inferior surface of gall bladder. After freeing same, we found adhesions more dense as we neared the duct. The pyloric end of the stomach was drawn over towards the gall bladder and extensively involved in adhesions; no abnormal appearance in stomach wall except general congestion of vessels, with general enlargement of the organ; adhesions were freed and gall bladder opened and explored for stones; none were found. The bladder contained large quantities of extremely thick black bile; gall bladder drained and incision closed; patient improved rapidly, with no recurrence of pain or vomiting; digestive functions apparently normal on leaving the hospital. A recent communication from Dr. Sanders states that patient has had no reurn of his gastric sympstoms, and is in excellent health. This, in my opinion, was an operable gall bladder case, but adhesions impinging the pylorus as result of his long standing cholecystitis was the chief cause of the man's gastric discomfort for years. The anatomical distortion discovered on intra-abdominal exploration in this case, demontrasted clearly the extensive scope that adhesions secondary to gall bladder infections can play towards the production of obstruction at or near the pylorus, bringing before us for consideration the frequency of such a complication associated with gall bladder lesions; or, more important, the possibility of the frequent obstructive influence of such adhesions resulting from mild inflammatory attacks of the gall bladder. It appears to me a safe conjecture that a great many chronic obscure gastric disturbances can be traced to this latter conclusion. The tendency of some individuals towards the rapid formation of abdominal adhesions, the close anatomical association of the organs in question and the frequent recuperation of acutely infected gall bladders, regaining and maintaining a normal condition, all bear witness to the plausability of the conjecture above, at least placing the same before as (worthy of thought in formulating a diagnosis) the possibility of adhesions being a prime factor in all cases bearing the symptomatology associated with the gastric obstruction.

The following case of Dr. Wise, operated on at Carthage about a year and a half ago, seen but once before operation, history meager: Widow, between 50 and 60 years old; family history good; no tuberculosis; no cancer; had enjoyed good health all her life, with exception of last few years; had been troubled with dyspepsia; attacks of same coming about ten years ago, at that time being mild in character. consisting chiefly of distress after eating, with belching of gas and slight distention; attacks would last a few days, then pass away for a month or two; attacks gradually becoming more frequent, accompanied with nausea, and vomiting about three hours after eating; extreme constipation, with apparent bloating of abdomen; diffuse tenderness over entire epigastrium; coated tongue, with foul taste in the mouth; as attacks become more frequent symptoms incresed with severity; nausea and vomiting became an early factor; no blood in emesis, but quantities of acid fluid frequently containing particles of food eaten the day before were noticed; slight chills with fever occurred at times; jaundice developed during later attacks; stools light and constipatedffi urine normal.

Physical Examination—Patient extremely fat and slightly jaundiced; temperature 102; complained of cutting pains throughout dypochondrium and epigastrium; extending through to back on right side, opposite lower thoracic vetrebra; tongue coated; nausea and vomiting; stomach distended; elicited no peristaltic wave on massage; extension upward and backward of left arm caused material increase of pain; tenderness diffuse over epigastrium, diagsossd gall stones complication, with adhesion involving the stomach, and advised operation. Incision revealed a mass at site of the gall bladder, which porved to be a reflected portion of omentum containing hard tallous mass of tubercular deposit, wedged down on the gall bladder, and adherent in every direction. Careful exsection revealed the pyloric half of the stomach drawn down and firmly anchored, tumor pressure and malposition caused by adhesion, clearly defining the cause of the obstructive symptoms; there was a slight amount of fluid in the cavity, and a few scattered tubercules could be felt on the peritoneum; the gall bladder, although slightly dilated and full, and appeared normal, and was not cpened. This patient recovered with complete freedom of her previous symptoms, in good health, six months after operation. In this case, had a stomach analysis been made, the findings, no doubt, would have strongly indicated obstructon, with dilation and motor insufficiency, but arrival at the actual cause could be made positive only through incision. The tuberculous invasion of long standing, with adhesion development from early perigastric irritation, most probably accountable for early disturbance

of gastric function. Differential diagnosis of obstructive adhesions of this character, their responsibility as a complete or partial factor in the production of symptoms, may present a picture of comparative clearness or dense obscurity. Valuable as a chemical analysis is, there are times that they fail to bear out or confirm a diagnosis based upon physical examination and clinical history. The stomach may develop an atonic stage early under obstructive influence, and not devolp the beginning muscular hypertrophy which is frequently an early compensation associated with dilatation. In such a case the customary findings of the increase amount of gastric secretion would be absent, in connection with the same H. C. L. finding taken alone point towards malignancy. Again, as the various degrees of involvement exist, may we expect complicating variations which may or may not coincide with a clinical and physical aspect. The plyorus, in normal position under the crest of the liver, is inaccessible to palpatation, while with dilation the pylorus, with movable portion of duodenum, is drawn downward, permitting more successful palpatation, which may reveal the bubbling sensation to the palpatating fingers at the constricted pyloric passage. In this position may be dstinctly evident the peristaltic wave of contracting stomach muscles, brought on by stimulating massage over the shurface of the epigastrium. This sign is present in many cases of obstruction, but may be absent, or not apparent. If obstruction is due to adhesions, a diagnostic sign which I have found of frequent existence, is a drawing pain radiating through the right hypochondrium during extension upward and backward of left arm, thus drawing up the left shoulder and thorax. In cases of obstruction unaccompanied by ulcer or cancer, sharp pain may occur after the intake of food, or associated spasmodically with a peristaltic contraction of the stomach wall, especially in cases where the involvement has reached an extreme gastritis. This symptom, however, is rare, and is more commonly associated with stenosis, accompanied with ulcer or carcimona. Failure at obtaining relief after free emesis, or continued and frequent vomiting, with pain after the stomach is emptied, is strongly indicative of advanced gastritis with accompanying lesion. In such cases, important aid in differenciation should be acknowledged through chemical analyss and microscopical findings.

DISCUSSION ON THE PAPER OF DR. BEEDLE.

Dr. Horace Reed, Oklahoma City, Oklahoma.—This paper is very clear and thorough, and I have enjoyed it very much. The question which came up to my mind was, the site of the adhesion which bound down the pylorus.. Pylorus is normally fixed. There are two fixed points to the stomach—the lesser curvature and the pylorus. It is true, the pylorus is not firmly fixed, but it is impossible to move it by adresions which for mwithout disturbing its lumen. It strikes me, that the good results which the doctor reports were due not so much to the breaking up of the adhesions, as to the pathology which existed at the same time.

In the matter of gall bladder cases, in my experience I have not been able to satisfy myself whether or not the adhesions which existed there had anything to do with the reflex symptoms, such as vomiting and stomach trouble, or whether the trouble was due to adhesion or to involvment of the gall bladder itself. We know that gall bladder infections are most always referred first to the stomach. A patient may insist that the only trouble he has exists in the stomach, and after that stomach trouble is relieved he is alright. Personally, I have not paid so much attention to the adhesions which I find in these cases, but content myself with draining the gall bladder n cases of nfecton or stones whch indicate a previous or existing infection, and I have found the results have been satisfactory.

Dr. Howard Hill, Kansas City, Missouri.—The question of pyloric obstruction from extragastric causes is an extremely important one. We should not confuse the symptoms which exist with anything else, because we. have usually a history of dilatation of the stomach, so that whatever was found in the neighborhood of the pylorus must have been responsible for the dilation. Of course, patients often vomit and have much pain and disturbance, but gastric retention is a sign of obstruction. We may not be able to locate the seat of the obstruction definitely. The obstruction may be at or near the ileo-cecal valve. In given cases, often gas will produce dilatation. I recall the case of a patient who had a dilated stomach, as was shown by tubage and a test meal. This woman had pronounced symptoms of dilatation of the stomach, and I made an incision over the stomach, and there was absolutely nothing the matter with it. I looked around and found that the omentum was attached down in the pelvis, and I could not reach the point where it was attached. I sewed up the incision in the upper abdomen, and then found that the omentum was adherent to both tubes. I resected the tubes, separated the omentum, and it floated up out of the way. Following this operation, the symptoms of the patient disappeared. In another case, in which there was an adherent gall bladder, there was an acute angle in the duodenum. I removed the gall bladder in this case on the theory that if I separated the gall bladder the chances were, at least, that the adhesions might reform. Dr. Andrews of Chicago has suggested in these cases where we find adhesions, to take the lesser evil and sew the colon to the surface of the liver to prevent these adhesions. I wish to draw attention to one fact—that in the separation of adhesions between the duodenum and other structures, the duodenum is thin, so that if a blood vessel is oozing, I would ligate it. In the presence of dense adhesion around the pylorus and dilation of the stomach, it is better to do a gastro-enterostomy. That would suggest itself, based largely on the effect of the extreme danger attending the dissection or separation of adhesions around the duodenum. This case would not fall in that category, but I would suggest it in case such an oportunity should develop, because if you have stasis you get excellent results from gastro-enterostomy.

Dr. John F. Kuhn, Oklahoma City, Oklahoma.—I would like to ask as to whether the early history of this case did not point to acute cholecystitis? I saw this particularly, because I have been treating a case of acute cholecystitis, non-operative. The patient refused operation. When I suggested that drainage of the gall bladder was the only proper method, she would not have it done. I treated her the best I could, but what is going to be the after history of that case I do not know.

Dr. Jabez Jackson, Kansas City Missouri.—I would differ with Dr. Beedle as to the first case he reported, as there is nothing in the clinical history before the operation, nor in the description of the pathological findings at operation to show that it was a case other than that of typical duodenal ulcer. The question arose in my mind as to whether the adhesions which he found were subsequent to the duodenal ulcer, and were Nature's efforts to prevent leakage of the duodenal ulcer into the cavity or not. The question, therefore, arose whether the simple separation of the adhesions will completely cure the ulcer of its own accord. It may be that these protective adhesions would not do any damage, and it is a question whether the patient may not have what he had before. He had had several intervals of comparative quiet, and

then exacerbations or recurrence of the trouble, and while he has been free from pain for three or four months, he may still have duodenal ulcer, which has healed or unhealed, with the gatric contents pasing over that area. I would have been better satisfied to have done a gastro-jejunostomy as a protective recourse anyhow, because it is an alternative operation. I believe gastro-jejunostomy in the hands of an experienced surgeon is not a difficult operation, and one would feel more secure by giving an extra vent to that stomach.

Relative to the case of cholecystitis with adhesions, I must confess that my experience has rather led me to the method suggested by Dr. Hill, which he carried out in one of his cases, namely, that simple drainage of the gall bladder which is sufficiently infected to be attended by a considerable amount of adhesions, has not been followed by brilliant results, so far as permanent cure is concerned. I have had a few patients of my own on whom I have done a conservative operation, but have had to do a more radical one later on, particularly in the general service of the City Hospital, I have had a number of patients come to me for a secondary operation who had been operated on by someone else outside of the hospital or in the hospital. I recall one case I had about a month ago. A man had been operated on twice. A diagnosis of chronic cholecystitis was made, and drainage was resorted to, and in the second operation an attempt was made to break up the adhesions. A third attempt was made, with no relief, and then the gall bladder was here taken out. As a rule, the infection has been sufficiently severe in the gall bladder in these cases to produce extensive peritonitis, with extensive adhesions, and then the patient is better with the gall bladder out of the body than in it, as well as the fact that, after removing it, you can apply cosmetic stitches, close the raw surfaces, so that tracted exerted on the duodenum will disappear. To sum up: It has been my observation that in these cases of pyloric adhesions, with infected gall bladder, the results are better by removing the gall bladder rather than resorting to drainage, because the symptoms have recurred later on in patients whose gall bladders have been simply drained.

Dh. S. N. Mayberry, Enid, Oklahoma. —Dr. Jackson's remarks on this paper were very interesting to me, from the fact that I had a case a year and a half ago which gave me considerable trouble. From the history of the case, I was led to make a diagnosis of infection of the gall bladder. I operated, and when I got in there I found adhesions of the gall bladder and duodenum. Under the circumstances, the only thing left for me to do was to break up the adhesions and let the case go. I did that, and sent the patient home at the end of two weeks. The patient has had no further trouble. She did have a few recurrent attacks the first month, but she has been well of her gastric disturbance since the operation. I have wondered if I did enough in this case, and a short itme ago I had a conversation with Dr. Charles Mayo and presented this case to him and he said, "If you will look over our record in 1898, you will find sixteen of these operations were undertaken, in which nothing more was done than to break up the adhesions. The gall bladder was normal." He said th y had done nothing in these cases, except separate the adhesions and drain the gall bladder.

DR. BEEDLE (closing the discussion) I wish to thank the gentlemen for their remarks on my paper. There are a few points I would like to take up in closing the discussion. In the first place, in reply to the remarks made by Dr. Reed, I believe the pylorus is more movable than he thinks it is. The motility of the pylorus was not the point in question, but it was the compression caused by the adhesions around

that region I had reference to in my paper.

With reference to the first case being one of ulcer of the stomach, there is no doubt that there had been an ulcer of the stomach and it had healed. The indurated point seems typical to me of such a condition. The appearance of the condition in there, and the presence of adhesions high up all bore out that conclusion. An analysis of the stomach contents showed that a quantity of the contents was not passing out of the stomach at all, and this bore out the diagnosis of dilatation of the stomach.

As to the question of draining the gall bladder, mentioned by Dr. Jackson, who also spoke of removing the gall bladder where there are extensive adhesions, it is a question in my mind whether we should remove the gall bladder in these cases. Of course, a perigastric condition or a gall bladder condition may in one case result in a great many more adhesions than another, resulting in more perigastric disturbance or disturbance about the gall bladder. Some or prone to form adhesions that are more dense than others, but when a gall bladder appears infected and involved in dense adhesions, it is proper to remove it in every case, but before doing so we should thoroughly inspect and see the appearance of the gall bladder.. The gall bladder is undoubtedly put in the human economy for a purpose, as a reservoir with a contracting bulb to force the bile on into the ducts. I believe if the conditions do not point to a pathological lesion advanced and infected, it is a question whether it should be removed or whether prolonged drainage would not be of a great deal of good. By opening the gall bladder and draining it a little longer than necessary, we will get more thorough rejuvenation of the gall bladder in a great many cases.

Dr. Hill spoke with reference to the adhesions being dense about the duodenum. I agree with him in that regard. In such a case as that, the operation of gastro-jeju-nostomy would be preferable rather than attempteing to break up the adhesions which might do so much damage to the walls of the bowels.

With reference to conservatism, I think anything is conservative in surgery when we do what is necessary inside the abdomen. While gastro-jejunostomy is an operation that is accompanied by a comparatively low mortality, still it is an operation that jeopardizes the life of the potient more or less. If in this case I had any suspicion that there was a duodenal ulcer, I certainly would have done a gastro-jejunostomy. However, time will reveal the story in that case.

EDITORIAL

CONTRIBUTORS TO THE ANNUAL MEETING.

Contrbutors to the annual meeting will confer great favor on the Secretay by preparing their papers and fully correcting them before presentation to the meeting.

Heretofore, many men have gone on the program and never been present at the meeting, and all efforts to secure their papers for publication has been futile. We believe that there is some responsibility attached to the promise to present a paper, and that the advertsing men receive by reason of being on the annual program should prompt them to reciprocate by presenting the paper promised.

If it is possible to prepare the program in time, it wlil appear in full in the May Journal, whch should be out of press by the first of May.

THE COUNTY MEDICAL SOCIETY AND THE PUBLIC HEALTH.

The Public Health Education Committee of the American Medical Association, through ts Secretary for Oklahoma, Dr. Leila E. Andrews of Oklahoma City, is calling attention of the various county secretaries of the State Medical Association to the work she is commissioned to undertake.

The plan adopted by this committee, and which seems to be most feasible, is to call on the qualified physicans in different localities to deliver to the laity o nstated occasions an address on some interesting public health matter.

That this is the only possible way in which the great mass of the people can be brought to realize the importance of prevention, rather than treatment of disease, has long been evident to observers; until the matter of prevention of disease is made a part of our educatoinal efforts, no great succes can be attained. The propaganda set forth by this committee should have the hearty support of physicians of all clases, and the County Medical Society should endeavor to call the attention of the people to this movement and enlist their co-operation; to do this requires years of patient and persistent education.

COUNTY SOCIETIES

COUNTY SOCIETIES.
TEXAS COUNTY.

President—James McMillan, Goodwell.

Vice President—W. H. Langston, Guymon.

Secretary—R. B. Hayes, Guymon.

CARTER COUNTY.

President—W. T. Bogie, Ardmore.

Vice President—Walter Hardy, Ardmore.

Secretary-Treasurer—Robrt H. Henry, Ardmore.

Delegates—F. P. con Keller, Ardmore; J. C. McNeees, Ardmore.

Censor—F. W. Boardway, Ardmore.

GARVIN COUNTY.

The election of officers in Garvin County for 1911 was as follows:

President—R. L. Baker, Wynnewood.

Vice President—T. C. Branum, Pauls Valley.

Secretary-Treasurer—N. H. Lindsay, Pauls Valley.

Censors—J. C. Matheney and S. W. Wilson of Lindsay and A. W. Gray of Pauls Valley.

Delegates—G. L. Johnson, Pauls Valley; J. C. Matheney, Lindsay.

CUSTER COUNTY.

President—J. M. Gordon.

Secretary—O. H. Parker.

KAY COUNTY.

The February meeting of this society elected:

President—A. S. Risser, Blackwell.

Vice President— .WG. Lemmon, Nardin.

Secretary—R. E. Waggoner, Ponca City.

Treasurer—H. H. Bishop, Tonkawa.

Delegates—A. P. Gearhart, Blackwell; W. A. T. Robertson, Ponca City.

LEFLORE COUNTY.

President—M. O. Moore, Braden.

Vice President—J. N. Sommerville, Howe.

Secretary—R. L. Morrison, Poteau.

Delegate—E. L. Collins. Panama.

Alternate—W. O. Hartshorne, Spiro.

BOOK REVIEWS

INEBRIETY.

A Clinical Treatise on the Etiology, Symptomatology, Neurosis, Psychosis and Treatment, and the MedicoLegal Relations, by T. D. Crothers, M. D., Superintendent Walnut Lodge Hospital, Hartford, Conn., editor of the Journal of Inebriety, author of Morphinism and Narcomania, Drug Habits and Their Treatment, Etc,; Recording Secretary of the American Medical Society for the Study of Alcohol and Other Narcotics, member of the American Medical Association, honorable member of the British Society for the Study of Inebriety, Etc., Etc.; 1911; Harvey Publishing Company, Cincinnati, Ohio.

This is a cloth bound volume of 365 pages devoted exclusively to the consideration of inebriety and allied diseases due to drug addictions. The history of inebriety is carefully considered and no form of the condition is untouched. The chapters devoted to the Medico-Legal phases are valuable to all classes of physicians, and those chapters devoted to the cause of inebriety enter largely into the question of the use of many of our so-called harmless drugs as a factor in producing the condition. The question of heredity as a cause is also considered in many parts of the work. Every phase of the different treatments used in the treatment of the disease is considered, and there is a great deal of valuable information as to the home treatments; this will especially appeal to those physicians who are so often called on to treat their clientele at home, who, for one reason or other, refuse to enter an institution exclusively operated for attention to such cases as they present.

The well known standing of the author, Dr. Crothers, warrants this work a most kindly reception from the profession.

INTERNATIONAL CLINICS, VOLUME I, TWENTY-FIRST SERIES.

Edited by Henry W. Cattell, A. M., M. D., Philadelphia, Pa., with the colaboration of other men of note. Bound in cloth; price $2.00 net; Philadelphia and London. J. P. Lippincott Company.

This volume is the first of a series of four to be issued in the year 1911, following a system now in operation by the authors and publishers for many years. A description of the work is not necessary, as it is well and favorably known to the profession.

The wor kcomprises a large variety of subjects, all of which are interesting to the general practitioner and are brought up to date by the contributors.

MALARIA AND ITS MANIFESTATIONS.

A Careful Study of Malaria and Its Manifestations, with the most thorough and exhaustive methods of treatment of any work of its kind on the subject. By J. H. McCurry, M. D., Grubbs, Ark.; cloth $1.50.

ABSTRACTS AND EXCHANGES

SODIUM CACODYLATE.

H. J. Nichols, Washington, D. C. (Journal A. M. A., February 18), gives the results of the aplication to sodium cacodylate of the experiments which demonstarted the wonderful destructive action of salvarsan on the spiro chete of syphilis. They consist briefly, first, of the determination of t hetolerated dose of a given substance in a normal rabbit, and, second, of the determination of the curative dose for rabbits infected with *Spirochaeta pallida*. The results are expressed in the form of a ratio, C:T. The interest excited in this country by Murphey's observations with sodium cacodylate have caused others to employ it, and the results have not been uniform. The experiments are reported and the results show that sodium cacodylate has no spirillicidal action on infected rabbits in hoses short of seriously injuring or killing the animals. Of course, facts gained by experiments on animals cannot be transferred directly to human medicine, but much of our knowledge of salvarsan has been obtained in that way. Dawes and Jackson have shown that the therapeutic effect of sodium cacodylate is really due to decomposition and reduction products, such as cacodyle, arsenious an darsenic acids. The amount of reduction depends largely on personal idiosyncrasy, and this introduces a very uncertain element. For all practice purposes salvarsan should be regarded, not as an arsenical compound, but as a new substance not specifically related to ordinary arsenic. While there is no indication from experimental evidence for the use of sodium cacodylate in syphilis, it does not interfere, as has been suspected, wit hthe action of salvarsan usde subsequently. This is shown by a case here reported by Dr. M. O'Arcy Magee of Washington. At present, Nicholas says, it may be taken for granted that salvarsan is a specific against syphlis, and the important question now is what is the best dose and what is the best method of its administration in a given stage of the disease. There Is considerable evidence to show that the size of the dose should vary invedsely with the duration of the disease. Alt's original method of injecting intramuscularly seems to hold its own for certainty of results. The Wechselamnn method has been somewhat discredited by the slow absorption and liability to necrosis of tisue. A single intravenous injection in some cases seems to be too brief in action, but further experience is needed on all these points.

RETROVERSION OF THE UTERUS.

R. C. Coffey, Portland, Ore. (*Journal A. M. A.*, February 18), points out the importance of the peritoneum in the formation of the ligamental supports of the uterus which requires peculiar mechanism for its support. Ligaments are formed by the uniting of peritoneal surfaces and the so-called round ligaments being muscular tissue have properly a motor function and do not take up the work of a ligament proper. Their function is that of automatically poising the uterus during the various positions assumed by the individual and preventing its becoming a dead weight on the broad ligaments. The ideal operation for retrodisplacement, therefore, is to shorten the broad ligaments and at the same time avoid permanently fixing and hampering the movements of the round ligaments. The operation recommended by him is described as follows: "Before beginning the operation proper, break up adhesions and treat adnexae, lifting the uterus and packing a sponge back of it. Then seize the round ligament about an inch and a half from the uterus, and with No. 2 or No. 3 chromicized catgut, stitch to the anterloatal border of the uterus at the beginning of the vesico-uterine fold. Place 3 or 4 similar sutures between this point and the uterine end of the ligament. Thus a double fold of the broad ligament is brought over to the side of the uterus.

'Seize the ligament an inch and a half further on and bring it up to a point just above and internal to the uterine end of the round ligament and fasten with a cromicized catgut suture. Place 3 or 4 more suures between this and the first suture at the vescio-uterine fold. Thus 2 more peritoneal or broad ligament layers are brought over to the side and front of the uterus. Wit ha No. 1 or 2 chromicized catgut continuous suture bring a fold of peritoneum from each side over the line of interrupted chromicized sutures. This continuous suture may include as much of the peritoneum as necessary to bring it taut; care must be made to avoid pulling in the bladder. Be careful not to include the entire thickness of the round ligament in any part of the rows of sutures." The operation is illustrated. Coxey has personally performed 272 operations for retrodisplacement by using this method and gives the results. He has heard of only 2 cases of recurrence and considers that teh results show that all the anatomic and surgical requirements have been filled. He mentions 2 other physicians who have also used the method with satisfaction. One of them has deliberately performed the operation in 2 cases in the second month of preganncy to prevent theatened abortion and in both instances the child was delivered without difficulty at full term.

COMPLEMENTAL FEEDING OF THE INFANT.

T. S. Southworth, New York (*Journal A. M. A.*, February 4), advocates supplemnting the more or less deficient secretion of mother's milk instead of abandoning the latter entir, as is too often done, he thinks. Much that has been accepted as to the occurrence of poor or injurious breast milk must be givn up in the light of later researches. We must recognize the fact that mucoid and somewhat frequent stools, ranging in color from dark green to golden brown, and containing but little fecal residue of milk, are the stools of relative starvation and not of digestive disturbance caused by abnormal mother's milk. The breasts function poorly often because of defective nutrition of the mother and her nutrition should be attended to and the natural breast milk should be utilized as much as possible in the important early weeks of life. After the first postnatal loss of weight the infant's growth should be progressive, and when this does not happen, or, having happened, ceases, experience tells us that the matter is more serious than mere stationary weight. There may be loss of assimilative power. If, after waiting ten days or two weeks, attention being given to the diet and nutrition of the mother, the breast milk is still in sufficient, small supplemental feedings are advisable instead of discarding the breast milk altogether. It is better, Southworth thinks, to give small bottle feedings each time the baby finishes nursing. For these he prefers the term "complemental feedings," as distinguished from the supplemental feedings given occasionally to nursing infants, instead of the breast. These complemental feedings must first furnish food in simple and assimiable form, not dissmall in quantity as not to exceed, together with the previous nursing, the normal capacity of the stomach of the infant at this age. One-half ounce at first and later 1 ounce are usually sufficent for a recently born infant. This increase may be made when the age and growth of the child indicate a larger stomach capacity, or earlier if the residue in the stools or the weight of the infant before and after nursing show a larger deficiency of breast milk. The materials used have been barley water, whey, or one of the proprietary combinations of maltose, dextrose and dry condensed milk; o fthe latter a fairly level teaspoonful is used to half ounce of boiled water. Barley water has small food value and cannot be used alone for long at a time, but it is an aid to the proper digestion of over-rich breast milks and an excellent medium for the addition of cow's milk. If the subsequent progress of the case shows that, with further failure of the breast milk, more food is needed, an infant so fed makes the transition to bottle feeding very easy. Whey and the maltose-dextrose-milk combinations have proved useful in Southworth's hands, and may be continued for considerable periods if the breast milks holds its own. If it increases they may often be discontinued, but if the nursing gradually fails they should be remilk, since neither is suitable to maintain well-rounded development when given exclusvely. Artificial feeding of the very young child requires close and long-continued supervision, and this for many reasons is not possible in the majority of cases. The safer progress of the infant receiving breast milk needs no argument.

PICRIC ACID AND BURNS.

A. Ehrenfried, Boston (*Journal A. M. A.*, February 11), after a brief historical review of the uses of picric acid in surgery and a statement o fits chemical and antiseptic qualities, so far as stated in the literature, reports experiments as regards the latter. Fresh virulent culture of *Staphylococcus aureus and Bacillus pyocyaneus* were used, the former being selected as a resistant, and the latter as a milder pus-producing agent. The rod method was employed, the bacilli having dried in air, and thec ultures were passed through guinea pigs to increase their virulence. The results are shown in tabulated form, and indicate that a saturated aqueous solution of picric acid (1.2 per cent) kills bacteria from a fresh virulent culture of B. pyocyaneus which have been exposed to the air for one hour, in half a minute, and basteria from a fresh virulent culture of *S. pyogenes aureus* in about two minutes, as compared with 1 per cent solutions of phenol under the same conditions, which takes twenty minutes and ninety or a hundred minutes respectively, to do the same. Picric acid solution, therefore, is fifty times as strong as the phenol solution. Within five years he has employed the phenol in practice on about three hundred patients, practically using throughout a saturated aqueous solution of the C. P. crystalized picric acid. Stronger solutions in alcohol and water sometimes recommended are momentarily very painful on large raw surfaces and it is of course more liable to cause symptoms of absorption. The surgical use in the for mof ointment is illogical and also dangerous. By his method and strength of solution he has never seen sufficient absorption to show in coloration of skin or urine. He describes the method of preparing sterile saturated solutions which should be applied on gauze. In case of a superficial burn of hand or foot, the part may be completly immersed in the solution for some minutes before aplying the gauze dressing.. In fresh burns of the first and second degree, or superficial lacerated wounds, no preparation is necessary if the parts are tolerably clean, but if the skin is dirty it should be gently washed clean; blebs should be opened antiseptically at their dependant points, and the contents expressed. One dressing usually suffices in these cases, unless the lesion is extenive. In burns of mixed degree, the same principles are to be followed, but more care should be exercised to render teh lesion aseptic. Extensive third degree burns should not be treated by picric acid. He recommends this saturated aqueous solution as superior to any other method in first and second degree burns, as being cheap and simple in application and inducing rapid regeneration of the skin without pain or irritation. Deeper lesons may be made to heal by the formation of a smooth, level non-secreting, granulating surface over which dermatization will proceed rapidly, or whch will serve as an ideal base for the recepton of Reverdin or Thiersch grafts. The mild toxic symptoms which have been occasionally reported as occurring will never be seen if reasonable care is exercised.

MISCELLANEOUS

SODIUM CACODYLATE IN SYPHILIS.

Few articles apptaring in the medical press in recent months have attracted more attention and comment than that by Dr. John B. Murphy of Chicago, published in he *Journal of the American Medical Association* of September 24, 1910, in which the writer detaled the striking results obtained by him through the hypodermic administration of Sodium Cacodydate in the treatment of syphils. Uhysicians who have not seen the article in question will be interested in the following abstract, as publshed in Therepeutic Notes:

"Administered in doses of 1-2 to 2 grans hypodermically, its action was prompt and efficacious. Chancres became clean ulcers without induration in forty-eight hours; mucous patches cleared up in twenty-four to forty-eight hours; ulcers of the palate and pharynix healed in three to six days. In a child 9 months old 1-4 gran injected into the pectoral muscle caused a papillary syphilide to disappear in forty-eight hours. Two 2-grain doses, twenty-four hours apart, completely relieved the pain of a patient who suffered fro mactive gasthic crises (luetic) which usually lasted three weeks. An advancing perforating ulcer of the palate, which had resisted injections of 1-4 grain of mercuric bichloride daily, promptly yielded to Sodium Cacodylate. tow injections of 3-4 grain each. The ulcer was healed in six days.

"Dr. Murphy suggests that Sodium Cacodylate be employed in primary odses of 2 to 4 grains, depending on the size and strength of the patient, and not repeated within three or four days unless there are special indications for it."

Sodium Cacadylate, in sterile solution, is marketed by Parke, Davis & Co., in sealed glass compoules containing 3-4 grain and 3 grains, respectively, of the arsenic salt. In this conection it s proper to emphasize the importance of specifying a preparation that is known to be pure. Parke, Davis & Co. lay especial stress upon the prity of their product.

THE NEW LOCAL ANESTHETIC IN AMPOULE FORM.

In consideration of the growing demand for Quinine and Urea Hydrocloride for local anesthesia, Parke, Davis & Co. are now marketing this valuable combination in convenient ampoule form, and the physician can procure it in. 1 per cent solution, absolutely sterile an dready for use. The ampoules contain 5 Cc. of the solution each and are suplied to the trade in boxes of six.

Quinine and Urea Hydrochloride is being used in a great variety of operative procedures with pronounced success. As a local anesthetic it is held by many physicians to be superior to cocaine, a contention which would seem to have warrant in view of the fact that the preparation is not toxic in large doses, that it tends to restrain or prevent hemorrhage, and that the anesthesia produced by it is persistent. The latter point is worthy of especial emphasis. The anesthetic effect lasts for hours, sometimes for days, an important factor in connection with rectal and other operations that may be classed as painful.

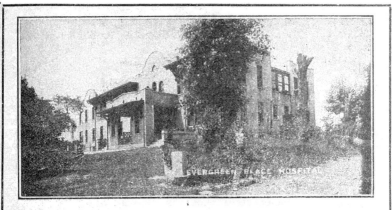

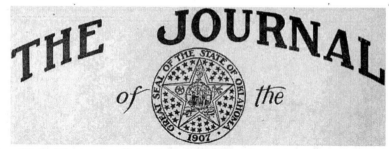

Oklahoma State Medical Association.

VOL, III.	MUSKOGEE, OKLAHOMA, MAY, 1911.	NO: 12

· DR. CLAUDE A. THOMPSON, Editor-in-Chief.

ASSOCIATE EDITORS AND COUNCILLORS.

DR. J. A. WALKER, Shawnee.   DR. JOHN W. DUKE, Guthrie.
DR. CHARLES R. HUME, Anadarko.   DR. A. B. FAIR, Frederick.
DR. F. R. SUTTON, Bartlesville.   DR. W. G. BLAKE, Tahlequah.
DR. I. W. ROBERTSON, Dustin.   DR. H. P. WILSON, Wynnewood.
DR. J. S. FULTON, Atoka.   DR. J. H. BARNES, Enid.

Entered at the Postoffice at Muskogee, Oklahoma, as second class mail matter, July 28, 1910

This is the Official Journal of the Oklahoma State Medical Association All communications should be addressed to the Journal of the Oklahoma State Medical Association, English Block, Muskogee, Oklahoma.

FRACTURES OF THE ELBOW.

BY CHARLES BLICKENSDERFER, M. D., SHAWNEE, OKLA.

Fractures of the elbow are comprised in fractures involving the lower end of the humerus, of the external and internal condyle of the epi-condyles, supra-condyloid fracture and that known as the "T" fracture. Elbow fractures in which the lesion lies in the bones of the forearm are those of the olecranon, coronoid process, fractures of the radial head and epiphyscal separations in and about the join.

Age. is the predisposing factor of greatest importance, since a large majority of these injuries occur in childhood and early youth.

In older subjects, the state of physical being and occupation operate more or less as predisposing to these accidents. Determining causes are injury more or less great, operating directly upon the structures comprising the elbow joint, as a blow or a fall upon the elbow or indirectly, as a fall upon the hand or a wrench of the forearm and is expended upon the joint structures causing the fracture. In this discussion, the diagnosis and treatment of injuries involving the lower end of the humerus will alone be considered.

Diagnosis and treatment can be successful only by the exercise of a knowledge of the normal relationship of the several anatomical landmarks concerned.

The most prominent of these are the external and internal condyles of the humerus and the olecranon process of the ulna. With the forearm in extension, these three points are in a line transverse to the long axis of the humerus, the condyles at either side of the lower extremity and the olecranon in a medium line posteriorly. They can be easily located both by palpation and inspection.

With the forearm flexed at a right angle with the arm, the tip of the olecranon is lowered but lies in the same plane with the posterior surface of the condyles and the posterior surface of the arm.

In the event of a fracture or dislocation involving any or all of these parts, these anatomical relations are to this extent disturbed.

DIAGNOSIS.

The classical signs of fracture, crepitation, loss of function, and preternatural mobility, serve in a general way to distinguish such injury from a dislocation, the characteristics of which are in great measure the opposite, i e., absence of crepitation, preternatural immobility and consequent functional loss. But there are other features that are equally distinctive of the several lesions to be mentioned. Supracondyloid fracture is usually more or less transverse to the condyles and the line of fracture is more commonly above the epiphysical line. This fracture may be complicated by a line of fracture, perpendicular to the joint lying between the condyles, an example of the "T" fracture. These may also be compound, comminuted or both. Supracondyloid fractures may be oblique from side to side, but are most usually oblique from behind downward and forward, or from before downward and backward.. As a result of a fall upon the palm with the arm in extension, the line of fracture is usually oblique from behind downward and forward and the inferior end of the superior fragment is displaced forward, the force of the blow or fall and the contraction of the muscular tissue serving to push and pull the tissues below, upward and backward, a not infrequent complication being the penetration of the soft tissues in front by the sharp edge of the lower end of the superior fragment. The brachial artery may be torn and the radial median and ulnar nerves may also be torn or compressed by the same agency. This is known as the "extension fracture." Following a blow or fall upon the flexed elbow or forearm, a supra-condyloid fracture may be produced, and in this the line of fracture is oblique from before downward and backward......

In this variety the inferior end of the superior fragment is directed downward and backward, while the superior end of the inferior fragment is displaced and directed upward and forward. The superior sharp extremity of the inferior fragment may produce similar injuries of the soft structures in front as the lower end of the upper extremity in the preceding form of fracture, i. e., laceration or compression of vessels, nerves, muscle and skin.

In both these fractures, there is likely to be inward displacement of the lower fragment and the other portion of the lower fragment is tilted downward or lowered, giving us as a result the deformity known as "gun-stock" deformity.

In rare instances we may have a splitting of the condyles with more or less impaction of the inferior end of the superior fragment between, a result of great violence.

Fractures of the internal epicondyle is an accident of youth occurring most frequently between the ages of ten and twenty, frequently occurring with luxation of the elbow. The displacement is usually downward and forward.

Fracture of the internal condyle is rare in children, more common in adults.

"The most frequent form of displacement is upward and inward and somewhat backward." "The ulna remains attached to the fragment and pulls the radius with it, causing it to be partially or

completely   dislocated." — (1
Keen.)

Fractures of the external condyle are of
fairly common occurrence in children, and
are also more common in adults than is
fracture of the internal condyle.

The fragment is usually displaced
downward and tilted forward, or it may be
rotated inward with the fractured surface
looking outward, backward and upward.
It would appear that the displacement of
the fragments in the two fractures under
consideration must depend somewhat upon
the length of the vertical axis of the fragment in question, and the degree of muscular development of the patient. Thus,
in fracture of the internal condyles, the
fragment remains attached to the ulna and
unless the line of fracture extends sufficiently high to include parts of the muscular attachments of the brachialis and triceps, the fragment should be tilted downward, forward and outward, by the action
of the pronator radii teres, palmaris olngsu
and the flexors of the forearm. In this instance the ulnar attachment acts as a ful-
crum. In the event of the fragments extending farther up and into the triceps
and brachialic attachments, it could then be
elevated, these muscles serving to pull it up
and the flexors rotating it as before. As
a rule, the displacement in this injury is not
great.

The fragment in external condyloid
fractures remains attached to the radius
and the ulna and the traction exerted by the
attached supinator brevis and the extensor
muscles tend to tilt it forward and downward, while the traction of the attached
portion of triceps serves to raise the fragment in the direction of the long axis of
the humerus. In fracture of the condyles
lateral motion of the elbow can be elicited
but is more marked in fracture of the internal condyle than of the external.

In these injuries, swelling is at first over
the injured condyle, but later becomes more
uniform around the joint.

DIFFERENTIAL DIAGNOSIS.

In the supracondyloid fractures, there
are crepitus, preternatural mobility, pain,
swelling and a bulging in front of the elbow joint due to the projection of the superior end of the inferior fragment or the
inferior end of the superior fragment. The
traction of the triceps upon the olecranon
pulls the elbow backward and upward. The
three points of anatomical interest, the condyles and the tip of the olecranon sustain
their normal relations to each other, but lie
behind the plane of the back of the arm.
A line let fall from the tip of the acromion
to the condyle will show shortening of the
humerus as compared to that of the uninjured arm.

Comparative measurement and inspection will show an increase of the distance
between the epicondyles in a "T" fracture,
especially marked where there is impaction of the superior fragment between them.
In a dislocation of the bones of the forearm
backward, there is immobility marked unless complicated by accompanying fracture; the olecranon now assumes an abnormal position in relation to the condyles,
is out of line and posterior to the place
both the condyles and back of the arm.
There is no shortening as shown from the
acromion to the condyle, but there is shortening of the distance from the condyles to
the styloid processes of both radius and
ulna.

In fracture of either condyle, there is
crepitus, increased mobility and a disturbed relation of this point when compared to the olecranon and uninjured condyle.

In all injuries of this joint, swelling
first appears at the seat of injury, and
is immediate, soon becoming marked, involving the entire elbow. The diagnosis,
reduction and treatment of these and other fractures of the larger bones should

never be attempted without general anesthsia. This is of first importance, since the pain attendant upon manipulation of such injuries is intolerable, besides the anatomical displacement of the fragments are often masked by muscular rigidity incident to an involuntary effort to maintain the parts at rest. The patient anesthetized, the surgeon, by placing the tips of the thumb and second finger upon the epicondyles and the tip of the first finger upon the olecranon, should first determine their relations.

In supracondyloid fractures, reduction is effected by flexing the elbow at right angles, and making traction downward from the condyles, while an assistant makes countertraction above the point of injury. Gentle manipulation of the parts will aid materially in the adjustment and reposition of the fragments. Primary swelling may render necessary an extemporaneous or temporary dressing for forty-eight or seventy-two hours, after which the swelling subsides and a permanent dressing may be applied. The treatment instituted in this injury may be one of two kinds, rectangular or the acutely flexed position. Those in which the line of fracture is low and transverse, not oblique, may be treated in the acutely flexed position, while those higher up on the shaft of the bone may require the right angular position with a corresponding internal splint. In a general way, it may be said that the position in which the fragments are most easily maintained in reduction, is that in which the permanent dressing should be applied. Before applying any dressing, the skin should be thoroughly washed in soap and water, dried and a dry dusting powder freely applied. This may be of talcum or starch. The splints may be of metal, cardboard or plaster of Paris, accurately molded to the parts. With the internal rectangular splint, care must be taken that the angular portion of the splint fits snugly into the elbow in order to maintain the parts in reduction. Metal and cardboard splints should be covered with sheet wadding before being applied, and may be held in position by adhesion strips, bandages, or both. In addition to this, there may be applied an external right-angular splint and the arm, midway between supination and pronation, supported in a broad sling from around the neck.

Where the line of fracture is oblique, and the subject muscular, it may be necessary to attach a weight in addition to the dressings mentioned, in oder to prevent the displacement incident to slipping upward of the lower fragment due to muscular contraction. The weight must of course be proportioned to the amount of muscular development. Fractures of the condyles and some supracondyloid fractures are best treated in the acutly flexed position. This in our experience is particularly applicable to the treatment of these injuries in children. The skin should be washed and dried as before mentioned. The condyles should be grasped by one hand and by traction in the bend of the elbow with the other, the arm should be slowly and gently flexed to an acute angle. Lateral pressure and manipulation of the condyles will materially aid in their reduction. The amount of swelling present will govern the degree of flexion to be used necessitating a readjustment of the dressings as the swelling subsides. Fractures of the condyle and transverse fractures of the supra-condyloid type, which are low down toward the extremity of the bone, should always be treated in the acutely flexed position, for the reason that the fragments are held in reduction by the coronoid process in front and the ligamentous and musculotendinous structures behind. Besides, the relaxation of the attached muscles allow of the maintenance of the fragments in reduction more readily than if these muscles were put upon the stretch as in extension. A small gauze pad should be placed in the elbow and a thin gauze pad may be placed in the axilla to prevent chafing. A gauze pad should be placed beneath the arm and forearm where they come in contact with the skin of the body, and an adhesive strip —a wide one—around the arm just below the axiliary fold and around the forearm just above the wrist joint. The whole may now be supported by a swathe sling encircling the body or by broad gauze bandages encircling the body and supporting the extremity, securing perfect immobility.

AFTER TREATMENT.

Fractures are more productive of legal difficulty to the surgeon than all the rest of his practice combined. For this reason, the daily inspection of the injured member, either within or without the dressing, is imperative. In cases of much swelling at the first dressing, these may be changed and the position readjusted to suit the conditions. Inspection and rebandaging where the internal angular splint is used, should be done daily to insure against malposition. A gentle stroking of the skin from the wrist to the elbow stimulates the circulation and promotes absorption of excessive exudate.

In supracondyloid fractures, attempts at passive motion should not be made until union is fairly firm, the fourth or fifth week. In children passive motion may be used earlier.

These injuries should all be diagnosed, reduced and dressed without the use of the X ray, but should, where possible, be confirmed by this means of diagnosis. The X ray is an exceedingly valuable aid in many injuries of this character, but when used as the chief means to diagnosis and reposition of fragments, the tendency is toward the prostitution of the surgeon's skill, both in diagnosis and treatment, causing him to overlook many essential features in both diagnosis and the treatment. A knowledge of the mechanics of the func- in question is of far greater importance in the treatment of injury than that that may be gotten by use of the X ray. Again, it is to be remembered that the X ray often magnifies and distorts the extent of the injury, and excellent functional results are quite common even where reduction is far from complete.

GERMI-PHOBIA.

DR. ARCHA K. WEST, OKLAHOMA CITY, OKLA.

When Hippocrates divorced medicine and superstition and taught the world that disease was not of supernatural origin, but in obedience to natural law, the most important epoch in medicine was marked. Of scarcely less importance, a discovery made 2500 years later, namely, that microscopical plants and animals may be and are the cause of disease.

To Lewis Pasteur first, John Tyndall second, and Jos. Lister third, con-jointly belong the honor of marking this second epoch-making period in the history of medical science. I know of no single discovery of our delving for truth of more momentous importance to the whole human race. When we contemplate the hundreds of thou-

sands of lives that have been saved within the few short years since this truth was demonstrated, and try to compute upon this basis the beneficent influence upon all future people in all future time, it fairly staggers the imagination. It is no wonder, then, that we, as medical men, are at times intoxicated with exultant zeal to open wider the window of light and make further applications of this discovery. To become almost fanatical in our effort; to spread faster the glad tidings of great joy, "The cause of disease has been found."

Over-stimulated by a most praiseworthy motive, to be of service to humanity we are prone to allow imagination to run away with reason to allow plausible theories and clever hypotheses to take the place of demonstrated facts. To attempt to run, before our feet are accustomed to walking.

A word of warning against this danger is the prime object of my contribution today. Let us survey the field for a moment, and see how many tares have already sprung up amidst our wheat. I can see a close psychological analogy .between the medical profession of today and the theological profession of yesterday. Both show a penchant for playing the imaginatoin, and talking most about what they know least. The preacher of my boyhood painted in lurid colors the unspeakable sufferings of the lost soul writhing in the bottomless pit of fire and brimstone, and this to the end that man might be made better and happier, that the sum total of good in the world might be augmented. The result was, instead of making man happy, the impressionable and imaginative who really believed, were burdened through life with a distressing fear that they might accidentally stumble, and at last be lost, world without end. The more hard-headed, and, as the preacher said, hard-hearted, in rejecting the unbelievable hell of fire, rejected also, to their great loss, the important and beautiful truths, the real value of the Christian religion.

Some of our modern doctors, likewise overzealous to save the population from death by infection, tell horrible stories of more horrible germs; how they inhabit the heaven above and the earth beneath; are lying in wait for us at ever turn, until the nervous and over-sensitive are continually in anxious distress, lest they be contaminated by these unseen harbingers of death. Their whole environment is peopled with microscopical foes who, like "goblins, will get you if you don't watch out.'" Food and drink, even the air we breathe, raiment, room and bed, is a possible means of contagion from which escape seems well nigh impossible. Our fruit and vegetables, ice and water,

milk and butter—in fact, nearly our every article of necessity or luxury is under the ban. "Touch not, taste not, handle not," until it is sterilized is the dictum. About the only thing left that is now free from the odium of b. ing a possible germ carrier, is "Good old Bourbon," taken straight out of of the bottle. The laity, in my opinon, are being imposed upon by this crusade of imaginative exaggeration and overstatement. not intentionally, perhaps, but again analogous to the preacher—some of our doctors, no doubt, really believe what they preach.

During the past year more especially, the public print of whatever sort—newspapers, periodicals, monographs, both professional and lay—have been filled with glaring headines: "Don't Kiss the Baby;" "Wash Your Fruit and Vegetables;" "Boil Your Drinking Water;" "The Deadly Oyster;" "Baccillus Carriers;" "Swat the Fly," while the demon drinking cup and the old oaken bucket is labeled with a skull and crossbones. The objectionable feature of this sort of crusade is that it is based upon certain scientific truths, concerning which the public should be enlightened, not frightened. For instance, the anxious mother asks: "Doctor, is it not possible for my baby to be infected by tubercle baccilli as a result of kissing?" I am obliged to answer that it seems to be theoretically possible under certain peculiarly favorable circumstances, so likewise is it possible to be maimed or killed in a railway accident, but that is not a sufficient reason why the comfort, not to say the necessity of railway travel should be abolished.

Is it not possible for infectious germs to settle from the circulating dust of the street on our fruit and vegetables? Yes, no doubt, but pathogenic bacteria have been demonstrated on those commodities, but are we not forced to continue to brathe this same dust-laden air dawn into the innermost recesses of our lungs? How absurd, then, to think we are protecting ourselves by reason of rinsing a bunch of grapes in a little cold water. It reminds me of a son of Ham carrying an umbrella to protect his complexion.

"Boil your water." Quite certain it is if this be done, sealed in sterilized receptacles and served in sterilized cups, we would not be infected from this source, but when we consider the unpalatable drink, the constant annoyance and anxiety, the fact that people who drink only sterilized water. do develop typhoid, that the conclusions reached by one of the most scientificaly conducted investigations of water supply in recent times, were "that at least in the city of Washington, water had little if anything to do with the dissemination of the typhoid epidemic." Is the game worth the candle? "Baccillis carriers," "Swat the Fly." Here, an open-minded agnosticism only can be maintained. The character of evidence in favor of these as imminent dangers was duplicated in quality and far exceeded in quantity only a few years ago, in support of the doctrine of the contagiousness of yellow fever.

The cup, with the skull and cross bones. Here, I am persuaded our zealous pseudoscientists, have indeed builded a mountain out of the veriest mole hill. Within a year, two editorials have appeared in one of the leading—I may say, the leading—ladies' magazine in this country, detailing the pitiable case of a young, beautiful and innocent girl who contracted the initial lesion of a loathsome disease while visiting away from home, presumably by contact with an infected drinking cup, the presumption being based upon the fact that this particular young woman, considering her station in life, education and invironment. etc, was like Caesar's wife—above suspicion, and by no stretch of the imagination, could it be conceived that she could have b.en kissed and fondled by a syphilitic man. With regard to such evidence, I can only say that a physician of fifteen or twenty years' of city practice behind him, can hardly be expected to be deeply impressed by such a story.

Editorial No. 2 gravely advised mothers to deny their children water entirely while on board cars, unless an unquestioned supply had been taken along, because forsooth he had actually seen a railway employee put ice in the cooler without first taking the trouble to boil his hands.,

Now, again, I do not deny the possible infinitesmal danger from this source, nor do I affirm. I simply, have as yet no conclusive evidence upon which a dogmatic statement is justifiable. To make my attitude clear, I do not wear lightning proof coat of conducting mail and ground myself carefully when there is a cloud overhead, I prefer to take the chance of being struck by lightning, in preference to enduring a lifetime of anoying inconvenience. For the same reason, I do not pester myself by carrying around eternally an individual drinking cup. This analogy I believe to be entirely reasonable. It certainly can be shown from experience and statistics that death by lightning is far commoner indeed than initial syphilitical lesions which can be accounted for *only* by cup infection. With those who advocate the use of the individual cup from an aesthetic viewpoint, I have no argument; but as a member of a reputed scientific profession, I protest against the lurid exaggeration of danger of infection. This over-statement and mistatement of the known facts in bacteriology. The laboratory nature faker which has for his object not so much the uncovering of a new truth, as the promulgating of a new and bizare theory to catch the itching ears of the morbid public, has no place in the catalog of true men of science. I protest against our profession taking up and teaching as truth these iridescent possibilities merely because they appear in the leading medical journal, or have the stamp of authority.

If medicine is to be indeed a science, we must distinguish clearly between demonstration and opinion. Harvey did not opine that 'the blood circulated—he proved it. The great Koch did not merely believe that a certain baccillis was the cause of tubercule—he produced indisputable evidence. Walter Reed did not surmise that yellow fever might be desseminated by the stegomia, but by painsaking experiment, eradicating every source of error—he established the fact.

In the presence of these, and others of the type, I uncover my head. This is real authority. I plead for a healthy, openminded skepticism, for conservative statement, for dogmatizing only within the bounds of demonstarted truth any other method, instead of furthering the ends of scientific medicine, can only result in humiliating reaction to the discredit of our profession. Even now, much of the time of the student in our medical colleges is consumed in unlearning the learning of our predecessors. Shall we, in turn, load our progeny with the same burden? We ridicule or pity the ignorance of our fathers when we review some of the sanitary laws of but recent years, for instance, the fumigation of mail matter to prevent the spread of yellow fever. Will our children ridicule us for some of our present legislative activity?

I do not know, but this I assert, that the evidence upon which our fathers based their belief in the contagious nature of that dread scourge, was the same in character as that upon which we, for instance, base our belief in the water-borne character of typhoid infection. Both voluminous in mass of medical observation and expert opinion—both lacking experimental verification.

Aside from the abstract love and truth,

allow me to call your attention to some of the results which must follow in the wake of such loose, unscientific generalizations. First, the anxiety and mental distress, amounting in the susceptibie almost to an obession. This, within itself, is no small consideration.

Second: The loss of prestige and power for good adherent in the medical profession, for directing sanitation and health legislation. Even now one of the serious obstacles in the way of establishing a national department of health, is lack of confidence in medical men as cool, clear-headed scientists.

We have left in our wake too many fads, too many hobbies ridden to death. Too much rainbow chasing. The hard-headed taxpayer has not yet forgotten the squandered money and paralysis of business incident to the enforcement ot our late quarantine regulations. Nor do they fail to point to such recent illumination upon the subject as the expediture of 1 1-2 millions of dollars on the water supply of the nation's capital, with the promise of checking the yearly epidemic of typhoid fever, whereas the death rate next year was slighter than ever before.

The great difficulty of getting municipal, state or national appropriations for sanitary purposes is proverbial. This is now fashionably alluded to as merely the selfish pneuriousness of our substantial business men, the placing of dollars above human life. With this view, I have no patience. I have a far better opinion of the character and humanity of my fellow citizens. The reason we are not now trusted, is simply because we have not always been trustworthy in the past.

"The truth itself, is not believed by one who often has been deceived." The sins of the father are now being visited upon the children. Will we profit by past experience? I do not know. Candidly, I see little hope until the rank and file of our profession cease being the mouthpiece, the parrot of the faddist—cease the blind following of so-called authority—cease fathering laws and ordinances based upon hypothetical conclusions, and insufficient evidence, until the rank and file think for themselves, develop the backbone to say to the laity, "I don't know;" develop independence to say to authority, "show me."

In the words of the Lime Kiln Philosopher, "It is better not to know so much, than to know so much that ain't so."

Gentlemen, for fear of being misunderstood, allow me this reiteration in closing: I am not here to deny the possibility of danger lurking in the kissing of the baby, eating raw fruits and vegetables, drinking unsterilized milk and water, using the public drinking cup. I am here to protest that these dangers have not as yet been demonstarted with that mathematical certainty necessary to classify them as matters of true scientific knowledge. I am here to assert that in the light of such knowledge of biological laws as I possess, the observations and experience of a lifetime, I cannot but feel that whatever modicum of truth there may be underlying some of our later hypotheses, has been so exaggerated and luridly overstated as to have reached an importance in the minds of the people in sanitary laws and regulations little short of the absurd and rediculous.

THE HUMAN TONGUE.

BY W. C. CUMMINGS, M. D., OKLAHOMA CITY, OKLA.

The diagnostic condition of the tongue, which, in many instances, are the only guide in selecting the proper therapeutic agent, and the only point in giving us a definite knowledge of the finer or more intricate pathological conditions, and without which information we put ourselves upon a level with some Old Granny with her recipe book. In the first place, we must arrive at a knowledge of the pathological tongue by comparison with the physiological organ, and which can be done only by having the image of the normal tongue constantly in our mind, so it will be seen that a close study of this normal tongue is of the same importance to the practitioner as the study of the organ in disease conditions.

Diagnostic:—The color, shape, coating and manner of protruding the tongue all carry the most valuable diagnostic information to those who are learned in its silent language. To the average physician, the inspection of the tongue is a sort of habit or to "buncombize" his patient to a certain extent, by trying to appear learned to an extent greater than he really is. He says: "The tongue is white; he has had a fever." Now what do we care what he has had? We want to know what he has now, and we want these pathological conditions that are shadowed out as symptoms to point us directly to the right medicinal agents that will rectify these wrongs. As an old physician told me: "I can't tell anything about the looks of the tongue any more than I could by looking at a slice of calf liver.' And he was honest in his assertion and spoke the sentiments of no doubt great many of physicians who are practicing medicine today.

The study of the tongue enables us to treat diseases of the digestive tract with a degree of certainty that is astonishing to the average practitioner. The same can be said of rheumatic troubles; and, in fact, the whole line of pathological conditions are so closely interwoven that certainties in therapeutics make it an absolute necessity.

The shape of the tongue tells us of the condition of the sympathetic nervous supply. With the narrow tongue we note the irritation of over stimulation of the important function. The nerves seem to pull upon the musclar fibers of the tongue and narrows it, and with the opposite condition, that is a condition ot broadness, the the nerves have let go of these fibers and the tongue spreads out like a duck's foot in the mud, and indicates a prostration of these nerves, and the greater the degree of this broadnss and "pin cushion" puffness, the greater the degree of prostration will be noted. So in the narrow tongues we find use for nerve sedatives, such as bromids, aconite, etc., while remedies that are stimulating in their effect are always strictly contra-indicated, and with the broad tongue the opposite are called for, such as quinine, nux vomica, strychnia and general restoratives, and remedies that cause nerve prostration or are depressing in their ef-effects are contra-indicated. So it will be seen that much thought must be given to these matters, and those who have no capacity for sound thinking must content themselves with the old method of guessing at conditions.

When we add to this narrow tongue a red tip, we have, plus the irritation of these nerves, and irritation of the stomach, which may be from the extent of a slight uneasiness of this organ to serve nausea and vomiting, which can be determined by the degree of redness shown; and here we find use of calomel, nux, etc., or, in fact any agent that is stimulating should be avoided, unless in some instances where we find the tongue coated at its base with a coating slightly a yellowing, when we have in addition to the other conditions a torpor and loaded condition of the liver. But these conditions will seldom be found together, but should they be then it may be necessary to even cause more cirritation of the stomach by remedies to get the liver in working order, then turn your attention entirely to the stomach. In making this plain, I draw a horizontal line upon the

blackboard, which is to represent the normal man, or any part, we may designate, and measure the deviation from this normal as excess (above this line), or defect (as being below this line), and with this excess we always want sedatives, and with effect always prescribe those agents that are stimulating or tonic in their action, and thus this method of comparison will always keep the physician upon the right track, or mistakes will be less liable to take place.

Now this broad tongue with red edges tells us of the irritation of the bowels; the extent of this irritation is in proportion to the degree that these red edges extend inward toward the center line of the tongue, tinued fevers, the red edges increase until nearly the whole tongue is invaded, when, if the trouble (blood deprivation) is not stayed, they change to a dusky red and then to a brown or black, when we note severe typhoid conditions and we look out for hemorrhages of the bowels. Here we want a liquid diet.

With the broad tongue without any coating, but a white fur, we note a complete atonic condition, and "boasters" are in demand to call more blood into the lining of the stomach, such as nux, quinine, with or without, bitter tonics, alcoholic stimulants, strychnia. We hardly need cathartics, because this white fur does not indicate any accumulations in the digestive tract. This white tongue tells us of still another condition, that is of a hyper-acidity of the fluids of the body, and which demand alkalies, and in rheumatic cases it guides us in the administration of the salicylates between the salicylic acid and the soda salicylate; or it may show us a case of rheumatism that plain bicarb. soda will cure, or if the tongue is very red we may cure with lemon juice or hard cider alone.

Should we have an abnormal red tongue, we note a desire for acids; the patient wants lemonade or anything that is sour, and it will be noted that after a fever has run for a time, that these natural acids seem to have been burned out, and when these acids are indicated and supplied that the fever will decline and every part function better, because the demand has been supplied. Still, we have an exception to this red tongue that I designate as calling for acids in the one that is made red by irritation of the boewls, which can generally be differentiated by the tenderness and other evidences of this irritation.

We are all familiar with the strawberry tongue characteristic of a scarlet fever, so we will say little about that.

Another tongue is the one that is spotted, patches of the epithelium being off from the size of a kernal of corn to as large as a diet. Here we note a poor nutrition. In such cases always look for worms, and in the large majority of cases you will find them. In these cases tonics do not seem to do good until the cause is first removed.

Another tongue is the fissured tongue; it is mentioned as the mapped tongue. The patient complains that whenever he eats cheese or tomatoes, the tongue smarts and burns. Many writers tell us that with these tongues we always have a condition of renal inflammation or congestion, and point to a coming morbus-brightii, etc.

When a man is hunrgy and his stomach is empty, the tongue is much lighter in color than at the end of a meal. Why? Because when this stomach is empty the blood vessels are contracted and depleted and very little blood is sent to the walls of the stomach, but when the food is introduced the blood is called in and the stomach gets red, the gastric follicles begin to throw out the digestive juices and the tongue being the index of the stomach, turns red also.

In the great majority of ladies that are not very strong, or, I may say, all of them, we note at the time of menstruation that they have a puffy tongue, indicating a torpor or prostration of these sympathetics.

Now I ask my physician friends to read this carefully and re-read it; try it at the bedside, get these indications straightened out in your mind so you can use them at will, and you will be astonished at the help it will be to you in your every day practice, as the many perplexing diagnostic conglomerations that will lead you out of the field of uncertain therepeutics into a line of certain results.

THE TREATMENT OF CERTAIN INFECTIONS OF THE SKIN WITH VACCINES.

BY WILLIAM H. MOOK, M. D., SAINT LOUIS, MISSOURI

The introduction of vaccine, by Wright. as a method of therapy, has produced a new clissification of certain varieties of skin diseases, serving to identify them quickly, and to cure many of them with wonderful rapidity. It has long been known that certain irritating discharges flowing from the various cavities of the body over the adjacent skin, produces a dermatitis of that particular area, and that relief is only obtained by treating the source of the infection, after which time nature, in many instances, cures the dermatitis. Some years ago, Engman, of St. Louis, called attention to the fact that once started, this infection may be spread to other parts of the body, far removed from the original lesion, by scratching, rubbing of clothing, etc., at the same time producing lesions of quite diffeent characters than the original ones.

The staphylococci are ever present organuisms on the entire surface of our body, but only under certain conditions do

Read before the Medical Association of the Southwest, Wichita, Kansas, October, 1910.

they give evidence of their presence. Whenever the organism is introduced into, or under the skin, a new condition obtains. Anti-bodies are immediately manufactured in the blood, and leucocytes are rushed to the affected area to overcome the invading enemy. If the organisms are overcome, at once the lesions disappear, and we say that an individual's resistance power towards the organism are perfect. If, however, the lesion persists, or spreads, we asume that his resistence powers are below par. In other words, the blood is not able to produce anti-bodies of such strength or number as to overcome the infection.

This may possibly be shown by the opsonic index, but is not necessary for treatment with vaccines. Once established, this lowered opsonic index, or resistance to the organism, may persist for an almost indefinite period of time.

Skin diseases are peculiar, in that any one, or all of them, may, under certain conditions, be complicated by a secondary infection. This infection may be caused by staphylococci, streptococci, diphtheria bacilli, and probably most of the organisms that invade the system. The staphylococci, however, are many times the variety encountered. The loss of the physiological equilibrium of the skin, by the development of any kind of skin affection, immediately favors the development of the usually present secondary organism, and thus we have a complication of the original affection. The most common example probbly being furuncles developing an eczema.

Engman called attention to the fact that there existed an eczema consisting of erythematous, crusted patches: from small to unlimited areas of development, symmetrical or asymmetrical, due entirely to a staphylococci in cultures, (as they are also found in dermatitis from other causes) for when we inoculated another individual, an abscess or perhaps furuncles, impetigo, or entirely different lesions resulted. Personal equation or individual reaction is difficult of explanation. Why, for instance, does one individual develop furuncles and another an abscess, or impetigo, while a third may only have a mild crusted dermatitis form the same strain of organisms?

The treatment and rapid cure of this variety of eczematoid dermatitis with vaccine alone proves the etiological factor, and establishes a new entitty in dermatology. The lesions usually begin as minute, papulae follicular, inflammations, which soon coalesce to form a cohfluent patch. This patch in then red, slightly elevated, and covered with crusts and scales of varying degree. It spreads peripherally, the follicles usually being the focus of primary involvement. There is, in nearly all cases, marked pruritus, and with the inevitable scratching, the infection may be spread over the entire body. The source of the infection can usually, though not always, be traced to some localized infection. I will illustrate by a case recently treated. Mrs. M. consulted me for a skin affection, which had begun on the abdomen, and had been present for a month, involving most of the trunk, the external genitals, the inner surfaces of the thighs, the legs and the ankles. She remarked that her condition was intolerable from the pruiritus. Examination revealed large and small intensely red patches, covered with crusts and scales, over the entrie abdomen and thighs. On the back and on the legs and ankles were seen the typical small follicular inflammations. The confluent patches on the abdomen, thighs and hips consisted of a diffuse crusted dermatitis. Further examination revealed that she had a small sinus in the left iliac region, from which a small amount of pus could be pressed. Investigation showed staphylococci. She was given an injection of 100 million, stock staphylococcic vaccine. Her improvement began within 24 hours. The injections were given at 5 to 7 days' intervals until now, five weeks later, the skin is entirely well. Her sinus was the result of an operation three years ago for peritonitis, and has persisted ever since. Her resistance to staphylococci, for some unknown reason, suddenly dropped below par, and the eczematoid dermatitis resulted. She will, of course, be liable to suffer a relapse, until her sinus is cured by operation.

Another case reported by Egman in a paper read before the last meeting of the American Dermatological Association, was that of a man, G., treated in the St. Louis Skin and Cancer Hospital. His lesions were exactly the same, and had persisted for months, though they were much more extensive, and many of them were bullous. He entered the hospital under the service of Dr. Engman. He was put to bed; 100 m. staphylococcic vaccine was injected at five and six-day intervals. His improvement was very rapid. About the time he was nearly well, he was allowed to get up, when he suffered an immediate relapse. He was allowed to remain up, but very little impovement resulted from the vaccines until he was kept in bed. A cure was invariably followed by a relapse when he was allowed to remain up. After long observation it was noticed that the relapse always began around the waist line, especially over an old inguinal hernia. Inquiry developed the fact that he had worn the one truss for twelve years. It was destroyed and a new one purchased, which he was not allowed to wear until perfectly well, and he has had no relapse for the past eight months. Leg ulcers, syphilitic ulcers, abcesses, sinuses, etc., may all be mentioned as possible source of infection from these extensive skin affection. These cases will suffice to illustrate this class of eczematoid dermatitis.

Fordyce, of New York, read a paper on this subject before the Section on Dermatology of the American Medical Associa-

tion at the last meeting in June. His paper will shortly be published.

Another variety of affections very amenable to vaccine treatment are those occuring on individuals who perspire freely in summer, usually as a complication to prickly heat. The latter affection is pruritic, and the individual soon infects himself by scratching himself. In a short time small vesicopustules appear at the sites of the follicles, and the puritus, with the consequent scratching, soon produce large areas of involvement. Soothing antiseptic lotions and salves will give some relief, but a few injections of vaccines usually rapidly cures the staphylococcic involvement.

Recently I treated a woman for a typical dermatitis of the external genitals and genito crural region. Soothing salves and lotions, and proper diet gave only temporary relief from the intolerable itching. Microscopical examination of the urine showed great numbers of staphylococci. She was cured within a few weeks by injections of staphylococcic vaccine, and most of the bacteria disappeared from the urine. Undoubtedly the condition was a staphylococcic infection of the skin, engrafted on a diabetic dermatitis, which could not be benefitted by sugar free diet alone.

The experience of Dr. Engman and myself, in our private practices, and at the St. Louis Skin and Cancer Hospital, in the treatment of furuncles with vaccine, has been so uniformly good that we use it as a routine method.

Ance necrotica, a persistent necrotic, follicular infection of the forehead, temples and scalp, by some thought to be luetic, and by others tuberculous, has always yielded in a very short time to staphylococcic vaccine.

The treatment of various kinds of eczema, when complicated by secondary infactions, will be greatly enhanced by the use of vaccines, even in those due to other disturbances.

Usually the stock vaccines as prepared

by the commercial houses, and put up in convenient forms in small bottles, suffice for treatment of a majority of the cases. The usual course and method is to give small doses, after which improvement is rapid and progressive for three days; then a slight relapse occurs. The succeeding injections should be given about the time of the beginning of the relapse. Care must be exercised not to give too large doses or a

negative phase will be established, and a relapse occurs at once, after which, little or no improvement will be obtained.

Great care must be used in sterilizing the instruments. Only an all-glass or metal syringe, which can be sterilized by boiling, should be used. The injection is given in the arm or thigh, celansing the area thoroughly with sterile cotton and alcohol.

THE METRIC SYSTEM SIMPLIFIED FOR PHYSICIANS USE.

BY C. T. SCOTT, M. D., OKLAHOMA CITY, OKLA.

The metric system has as its unit the meter 39.37 inches, which is the ten millionth part of the distance from the pole to the equator. From this as a basis, all other measures and weights are formed. The system is arranged on a decimal scale—that is, all the divisions are connected by the multiple ten, in exactly the same way as the coins in the United States monetary system. The names given to the different divisions and multiples of the unit are formed in Greek, which is placed before the name of the unit. It is the custom in all countries where the metric system is used, in writing prescriptions, to express all quantities by weight, fluids as well as solids being expressed in this way. We have only to do then, with the gram and its decimal divisions, that being the name given to the unit of weight. A gram is the weight of one cubic centimeter of water at 39° Fahr. The subdivisions of the gram are as follows:

1 gram—weight of 1 C. C. water at 39° F. written ....1.
1 decigram—1-10 of a gram, written . .1
1 centigram—1-100 of a gram. .01
1 milligram—1-1000 gram .001

The United States Pharmacopela Eighth Revision, limits its use to the metric system to grams, milligrams and cubic centimeters.

1 gram is equal to 15.432 grains.

1 cubic centimeter is equal to 16,23 minims.

1 milligram is equal to .015432 grains.

EQUIVALENTS OF APOTHECARIES' IN METRIC WEIGHTS.

Grain.	Gram.
1	.0648
15	1.9720
30	1.9440
60	3.888

EQUIVALENTS OF APOTHECARIES' IN METRIC MEASURES

Minims.	Cubic Centimeters.
1	0.0616
15	0.924
20	1.23
30	1.84
60	3.7
480	29.57

RULES FOR THE CONVERSION OF ORDINARY WEIGHTS AND MEASURES INTO THE METRIC SYSTEM AND THE CONVERSION OF METRIC WEIGHTS AND MEASURES INTO THOSE IN ORDINARY USE.

First Method.

1 Cubic Centimeter=1 millilitre or 16.23 minims, or better expressed in fractions as

1000....61.6 or 61.6=.0616 C. C. in each

    16.23   1000

minim.

The gram equals 15.43 grains. 10 deci-
1000=64.8=grams in each grain.

15.43 1000

1. To convert 20 grains into grams,
multiply 20×.0648=1.296 grains.

2. To convert 4 grams into grains, divide 4×.0648=61.72 grains.

3. To convert 20 minims into C. C.,
multiply 20× .0616=1.232 C. C.

4. To convert 4 C. C. into minims, divide 4×.0616=64.92 minims

Second Method.

To Convert

Grams into grains, multiply....................15.432
Cubic centimeters into fluid ounces
  multiply by.................................. 0.338
Cubic centimeters into minims, multi
  ply by.......................... ....16.23

To Convert

Grains into grams, multiply by.......... 0.648
Fluid ounces into cubic centime-
  ters, multiply by........................29.572
Minims into cubic centimeters, mul-
  tiply by.................. .... 0.0616
Troy ounces into grams, multiply
  by 31.1035

A QUICK, ACCURATE METHOD FOR EXPRESS-
ING QUANTITY BY WEIGHT OF THE
APOTHECARIES' SYSTEM IN

METRIC TERMS.

RULE—Reduce the quantity to grains
and multiply by .66, then convert the number of grains used to drams and multiply
the corresponding number of drams used
by 2 and add to the first figure to the right
of the decimal point.

1. *Conversion of Grains into Grams—
Examples:*

Drams 1 or 60 grains, multiplied by
.0648=3.88 grams exactly. Accordng to
the rule, after first multiplying the
number of grains by .06, then
convert the number of grams to drams,
multiply by 2 and add to the figure to the
right of the decimal point, as; 60 grains
multiplied by .06=3.60 grams, then drams
1 multiplied by 2=2, then, 5.60 plus 2
equals 3.80 grams.

Drams 2 or 120 grains, multiplied by
.0648=7.77 grams exactly. 120 grains multiplied by .06=7.20 grains.

Drams 2 multiplied by 2=4, then, 7.20
×4=7.60 grams.

Drams 3, or 180 grains, multiplied by
.0648=11.66 grams exactly. 180 grains
multiplied by .06=10.80 grams.

Drams 3 multiplied by 2 equals 6, then
10.80×6 equals 11.40 grams.

Drams 4, or 240 grains, multiplied by
.0648=15.55 grams exactly. 240 grains
multiplied by .06=14.40 grams.

Drams 4 multiplied by 2=8, then, 14.40
×8=15,20 grams.

From 5 on, add 2 to the left of the decimal paint, as, drams 50, or 300 grains, multiplied by .0648=19.44 grams.

300 grains multiplied by .06=18. Grams
18×2, to the left of the decimal point=
20 grams.

Drams 6, or 360 grains, multiplied by
.0648=23.32 grams, exactly. 360 grains
multiplied by .06=21.60×2=23.60 grams.

Drams 7, or 420 grains, multiplied by
.0648=27.21 grams.

420 grains multiplied by .06=25.20×2
=27.20.

Drams 8, or 480 grains, multiplied by
.0648 equals 31.104 exactly.

480 multiplied by .06=28.80×2=30.8 grams.

In applying this. rule to liquids, reduce to minims, multiply by .066 and add the figure corresponding to the number of fluid drams used to the first figure to the. right of the decimal point.

Examples.

Fluid drams 1, or 60 minims, multiplied by .0616=3.696 C. C., exact. 60 minims. multipliede by .06=3.60×1=3.70 C. C.

Fluid drams 2, or minims, multiplied by .0616=7.392 C. C., exactly. 120 minims multiplied b yo6=7.20×2=7.40 C. C., or grams.

Fluid drams 3, or 180 minims, multiplied by .0616=11.088 C. C., exactly. 180 minims multiplied by .06=10.80×3=11.10 C. C., or grams.

Fluid drams 4, or 240 minms, multipli d by .0616=14.784 C. C., exactly. 240 minims multiplied by 60.=14.40×4=14.80 C. C.

Fluid drams 5, or 300 minims, multiplied by .0616=18.48 C. C., exactly. 300 minims multiplied by .06=18.×5=18.5 C. C.

Fluid drams 6, or 360 minims, multiplied by .0616=22.17 C. C., exactly. 360 minims multiplied by .06=21.60×6=22.20 C. C.

Fluid drams 7, or 420 minims, multiplied by .0616=25.872 C. C., exactly. 420 minims multiplied by .06=25.20×7=25.90 C. C.

Ounces 1, or 480 minims, multiplied hy ,0616=28.57 C. C., exactly. 480 multiplied by .06=28.80×8=29.60 C. C.

This is the only comparatively accurate, mental method that I am familiar with for converting the ordinary weights and measures of the apothecaries' system into those of the metric system.

THE SYMPTOMATOLOGY AND DIAGNOSIS OF INFANTILE PARALYSIS.

BY LOUIS J. MOORMAN, M. D., OKLAHOMA CITY. OKLA.

The frequent occurence, the wide distribution and the disastrous consequences of infantile paralyisis during the last few years, have stimulated the study of its clinical manifestations, and have also led to much experimental work with a view of determining the exciting cause, the mode of infection, and, if possible, a specific remedy. Its infectious nature has been definitely determined by animal experiment. That it is also contagious seems very probable from the results of recent clinical observations. These two facts serve to emphasize the importance of an early diagnosis.

Infantile paralysis predominates in late summer and early autumn. Eighty to ninety per cent of the cases occur in children under six years of age. It is more common in adults.than formerly supposed, as shown by recent reports. Perhaps many adult cases have passed as Landry's paralysis, typhoid, or other infectious processes with a complicating neuritis.

It is believed that teething, overheating, sudden chilling, over exertion and errors in diet predispose to infection. The cases have been divided by different observers into clinical types varying in number from three to eight. Holt classifies them as mild, severe and those with bulbar symptoms. The bulbar cases seem to be more frequent in empidemics than in th sporadic forms. The incubation period varies from three to thirty days. The average being about nine days.

The onset is sudden, usually with fever and constitutional symptoms. Muller, observing fifty cases, evolved three cardinal symptoms: (1) Profuse perspiration; (2) Cutaneous hyperesthesia, and (3) Leukopenia. There are usually some gastro-intestinal symptoms, diarrhea, or constipation, and sometimes vomiting. Constipation is found more often than diarrhea. There is prostration and muscular weakness. The paralysis follows in from a few hours to three or four days.

In the mild cases the constitutional symptoms are slight, or, perhaps, absent. The paralysis may appear without warning, or there may be mild constitutional symptoms, followed in a day or two by paralysis of certain groups of muscles in one extremity, or recovery may take place without paralysis—abortive cases. In such cases the diagnosis is impossible, except during an epidemic, and where there are other cases in the family. Holt reports two cases in which the paralysis apparently came on while the child was playing in the street, there having been no previous symptoms observed.

The severe type, which embraces the majority of all cases, is characterized by sudden onset with vomiting, prostration, fever from 103 to 104, diarrhea or constipation, restlessness, with pain in neck and back; also pain in the extremities where paralysis supervenes. There may be retention of urine. There is general hyperesthesia and often profuse perspiration and muscular rigidity. Unconsciousness and delirium are rare, except in fatal cases. After two or three days, loss of power in one or more of the extremities is noticed, and a flaccid paralysis follows, usually reaching its maximum about the sixth day, coincident with the constitutional symptoms.

In the bulbar cases the onset may be similar to that just described, or there may

be convulsions followed by delirium and stupor. However, the symptoms may be less pronounced, and the paralysis may first appear in the extremities, extending to trunk and neck, finally, with paralysis of the face and disturbances of respiration and of the heart's action. Death usually takes place in a short time, due to failure of respiration. The primary paralysis may be limited to groups of muscles in one lower extremity, this being the most frequent finding. However, it may vary in extent and distribution from the involvement of one extremity to the general paralysis of all the extremities, with extension to portions of the trunk.

The sphincters usually escape. Atrophy of the paralyzed muscles soon appears and the affected limb is distinctly smaller than its mate. Sensory disturbances are absent except early in the course of the disease. The tendon reflexes are absent for the muscles involed.

Within a week or ten days reaction of degeneration is present in the muscles in which permanent paralysis develops. The muscles in which recovery is to take place may respond to the faradic current, but the degree of contractility is less than normal.

Infantile paralysis is to be differentiated from cerebro-spinal meningitis, multiple neuritis, cerebral palsies, rheumatism, rickets, scurvy and other infectious processes.

Those cases with general hyperesthesia, severe pains in the back and extremities, with rigidity and high fever, cannot be differentiated from cerebro-spinal meningitis without an examination of the spinal fluid for the purpose of determining the presence or absence of specific micro-organisms. Until Fexner's most recent reports, we thought that the spinal fluid in infantile paralysis, in direct contrast to that of cerebro-spinal meningitis, remained clear thoughout the coarse of the disease. Flexner has shown that in monkeys, where a daily puncture is made, there seems to be a period covering one or two days, coincident with the onset of paralysis, when the spinal fluid becomes turbid. This, of course, discounts the diagnostic value of the micrscopic examination.

Multiple neuritis is rare in children, except after diphtheria. Here the history of the case is essential in making a diagnosis. The conditions presented may correspond exactly to those found in some cases of infantile paralysis.

In cerebral palsies there is usually rigidity. There is no reaction of degeneration, and there is a history of cerebral symptoms. The intense muscular pains and prostration, in rare cases, may mask the developing paralysis and lead to a diagnosis of rheumatism. One must also bear in mind the pseudo-paralysis of rickets and scurvy. A thorough examination, together with the history of the case, usually suffices to make the diagnosis clear. If doubt remains, the presence of the reaction of degeneration will eliminate these affections.

Some of the inital cases of recent epidemics were diagnosed as grippe. The acute eruptive diseases and gastro-intestinal disturbances must be eliminated.

MYOPIA OF THE MEDICAL PROFESSION.

DR. W. R. ALLISON, PEORIA, ILL., IN THE ILLINOIS MEDICAL JOURNAL

The relation of medicine to social and business life is constantly changing, necessitating readjustment from time to time. Labor has organized for protection while capital has combined for protection, and each of them receives medical and surgical care for a fee much less than the customary charges.

The labor unions reduce the number of working hours at increased wages. They elect a physician who contracts to give medical and surgical aid for so much per head. The fee is often a dollar or less per year for each member, with no objection if the women and children are thrown in for good measure. The doctor must make calls night or day, and as often as desired, for $1.00 per year. Many of the fraternal orders have, as their chief attraction, a free doctor any time you want him. Some of these orders are finding medical men willing to do this work for practically nothing. Organized labor will expel its members for working less than contract price, or outside of working hours.

This does not apply to the doctor's fee or hours. If organized labor is not paid as per contract, there is a strike and tie-up. If a unionist does not pay his physician there is no tie-up in the profession. The laborer is so much ahead and a score of doctors ready to take the place of the unpaid doctor. You can not point to an instance of organized labor breaking their scale because the contractor is poor. If you can not pay the scale there is no work.

The employer has sought protection by insuring the employee against accident, in a company which has a doctor under contract for one-third to one-half the fee customarily charged for such work. The doctor is paid for his first aid only. The employer has now dumped the injured into the care of the surgeon for the price of first aid charged at half the customary price, and is repaid by the insurance company, while the doctor cannot legally decline further treatment, and must continue to give his services which are gratuitous.

If the patient could pay he would decline because he would say he was insured and let the company pay. So it is safe to say that this class of work is now done for one-third to one-half what it was done for before beef and cabbage were cornered.

I have used these comparisons to show what can be done by organization and to negative the common expression that it would be impossible to get the medical profession together. It has always been a conundrum just why men who boast of intelligence, who pose as leaders of men in society, who are keen students, can not govern themselves as well as the mechanic or common laborer. Suppose I violate the adopted fee table of this society; what is the result? Nothing more than that I have labored for less than I might have received, hurt myself, lowered the profession, and robbed my professional brother.

Suppose a provisional wholesale house of this city would cut the price for a poor widow, with a sick child. What would happen? There is no danger of anything happening. That is fixed, that is all arranged. If the widow gets provisions she must pay for them or be blacklisted. Suppose the truckster should retail? Do you suppose he could find a market for his produce?

Not so with us. A few days ago a doctor made arrangements to operate for a $45 fee and was underbid by a member of this society, who charged $25. Another member of this society contracted to perform a herniotomy for $100 and deferred the operation until the money was ready, when another member of this society did the work for $50. Have we not the same ability, as much brain and sense as

commercial men, for our own interests and protection? .

This argument may be met by the claim of charity and refuted by asking who is suffering most, the hungry, the unclothed, or the sick? If to doctors belong the charge of caring for the sick, can you point to an individual so poor as not to have a doctor? What a wail of complaint should we refuse?

Is there any noise made against those who refuse food and clothing and are they censured for not supplying the needy? The daily papers have for weeks been notifying us to pay our coal bills, or we will not get more coal. That's business. Suppose doctors would take a similar stand, would that be business? Is it not true that we have made provision for the needy poor by delegating two of our profession for such emergencies?

Do not for a moment doubt that there is a business understanding between the retail stores, and there should be. It is essential to a continuous and profitable business. Have you not noted the uniformity of prices? Have you not also noted the steady advance and promptness of collections? Do you realize that doctors are working for less than they were receiving twenty years ago?

Some may deny this; but look it up. Those of us who have seen twenty years of service, know that house rent, office rent, expense of conducting practice, has doubled in twenty years.

If business so intricate as commercial with all its lines can be brought under control and be regulated so as to increase profit in cost of production and sale, what then do you think of the medical business under present conditions? Do you know that we are the only class of business men on the face of the earth which is cutting fees?

What do you think of the liveryman charging more than the doctor for making a call? What do you think of the plumbers of this city who are receiving nine dollars a day and one half-holiday every week? $263 each month, over $3,000 per year. No night work, no office, no irregular hours. Do you realize that many of us are not making wages as good as this and work seven days a week, subject to call any time day or night. The charity of our profession is abused and misdirected. It is too often of the kind reacting on us, to our harm. You can find no other trade or calling that is trying to lessen its output or destroying its livelihood. I have looked in vain for a nurse from any of our manufacturers telling me how to escape buying their wares. There is no nurse from the grocery organization going about telling the housewife that vegetables are so cheap outside of this city that it does not pay to send them to market, and if there was such an attempt how long would the grocerymen let such a thing exist?

Now, why should this not be, for if it is right for one class it should be right for all. Let the missionary spirit prevail everywhere, not only a tubercular nurse but a pneumonic nurse, a surgical nurse, a genitourinary nurse and an obstetrical nurse. Let each of these carry some business cards directing the sick to their favorite physician. Now, when we apply this in its broad sense, it sounds ridiculous; and yet am I not right?

How many mechanics are there in this city out of employment? Try to employ one and they are all busy. This is a great age, a prosperous year. None were more productive than 1910. During this year of great activity in commerce and industry every workman was busy, increasing wages, better clothes, prosperity unbounded. Compared with this how many idle hours, waiting for patients; how many days have you had this fall when you did not make expenses? If it does not come now when will it come? When may you hope for a change? You are deceiving yourself by thinking a better day will come under the present circumstances. You have been deluded into thinking medicine a great lucrative field. You have been deceived, and yet you tell us you are doing well, busy all the time—getting rich, and yet since the history of this city began, not one doctor has been able to retire as the result of the practice of medicine.

When the prophets first foretold the benefits of united labor, of happy homes and blessings of higher wages, people hung their heads in doubt, but such is the change that the plumber gets better wages by stopping a leak than we do. The weekly wages of the hod carrier for this week is more coin in his pockets than some of us received. We are twenty years behind in our business methods.

The mechanic has for years been limiting the number of graduates in his school, by limiting the number of apprentices and increasing the period of time of the apprenticeship, and yet they have received more praise than censure, for doing this. Do we not say the life of the mechanician has vastly improved? Is this not a lesson from which we can learn something?

On the other hand we are increasing the number of graduates, lessening the amount of sickness, and are now reaping our folly. This may seem pessimistic but it's truth. I am dealing with the business side of life. Suppose it was within our power to foster free dispensaries, free clinics, charity everywhere, until disease became so rare that doctors would have nothing to do. Suppose we killed the goose that laid the golden egg. In other words, who pays us for such laudable charity, who pays us for prophylactic measures? Only the good of knowing you killed your business and mine. That's not the moving spirit, nor the intention of this mode of advertising. It is one method of increasing business and belongs in the same class with bankrupt stocks and selling out at cost. It's a sale of fire goods at wholesale prices, with the middlemen cut out. What's the difference between such methods of conducting business and the quack who treats free? Why does the advertiser give free examination? You know why, and what's the difference between them?

Peddlers, street hawkers, and fire sales interfere with the retail merchants. Free medicine shows interfere with the retail druggist, so that our City Code contains a stiff license fee, meant to be prohibitive and also to help the retailer.

Dispensaries and free clinics only hurt the business of doctors not connected with the show. So dub it with charity, with a chunk of religion, and nobody will see the point until they become a public nuisance, a curse to the profession, which, like an obnoxious weed, can not be killed out, so long as we have such advertisers in our profession.

The press is now giving a friendly ear to our profession. Mystery and ignorance of medicine are giving way to fundamental facts written by able men for the dailies and magazines.

Jealousy and backbiting will change to a united profession. Soon we will be represented in the cabinet of national affairs. United we can teach the people the wisdom of obeying our teachings and granting to us better protection. Then all together we can legislate for our common good. Then we can say to our representatives, when voting on medical subjects (just as organized labor demands anti-election pledges) to vote intelligently and right to represent the doctor squarely on medical subjects. Then will it be possible to go to our representatives and say: "you voted for obnoxious bills"—just as Gorman and Butts did at the last General Assembly—and are now asking that your and my vote return them, to slap us in the face again. Gentlemen, remember these facts when voting. We have a vote and influence.

The whole trouble in medicine is in our own ranks. From time to time the subject of increased fees have been before us and here it is up again. Some of you are increasing your charges. Some say you are, but are not. Suppose you adopt the fee table as endorsed by this society, and attempt to follow it, and I talk for and urge you to stick to it, and then I quietly take your business by giving cut rates. That very thing is going on in this society. It looks like a scheme whereby those of you who are honorable, wait and hope for a square deal, while I am playing traitor to my own organization. Show me one case of this kind in organized commercial or industrial life. Why should we be the only exception and how can we succeed when the universal verdict of labor and capital is emphatic that it is by combination that hope of success may be had.

When a patient calls a doctor he does not consider who is the cheapest but who is best. The charge is an after consideration for the courts to settle six months or a year after recovery of the sick.

Each of us owes to his brother doctor, if not to himself, the duty of maintaining the dignity of the profession, which can be lowered no more quickly than by being cheap.

If you charge $2 for making an ordinary call, and I take your patient by charging $1.50, you can only get your patient back by charging $1. Then I begin to talk about you and you about me, until we have hurt each other, taught the patient that we are both cheap, spiteful, jealous creatures and they become disgusted with both of us and employ another physician. It is not our charity the sick are calling for. It is our ability to cure.

I have always believed the cheap doctor a conscientious man, and when he underbids me I say each doctor surely knows what his services are worth and if one charges more than the other it is because he thinks the job is worth it.

I believe in advertising and so do you. Some of us advertise one way and some another. We must blow our own horn. I will not blow yours, you will not blow mine but let's tune up, blow together in unison and make a band with more than a local renown. Stop this discord, blow your part and I mine, blow so that people will applaud, and blow so well that competition will not be in it. Blow so perfectly that the sick will find that medicine has charms to soothe, etc.

Free dispensaries and free treatment sound good to the layman, but no doctor will encourage such unless the advertisement brings some gain. Free treatment is a feeler for reaching the sick. It's the place to increase ac quaintance with the afflicted.

In every city where free treatment has been introduced, they are now

trying to stop it. The universal desire is for its abolishment. It is to be hoped that the members of this society will see the error of introducing this kind of practice in this city and stop it. It is certainly one of the advertising features that must be discouraged.

Why not introduce free plumbing for the needy poor. Free carpentry where we could get help for the asking. Are not these ludicrous questions? No more so than that we should give time for nothing. No more demanded than other necessities. Our course is such that our income is gradually lessening. Sanitation and hygiene have greatly lessened disease. Epidemics are a thing of the past. As time goes on the doctor will be in less demand. The sick are made to recover in shorter periods of time than formerly. With progress of time we prescribe less medicine. The layman asks and receives our advice until he can many times dispense with our services; all brought about by ourselves, our free clinics, sanitation and hygiene; and what is there to take the place of this loss, which has come to stay. We are today applying old ideas to new conditions. Twenty years ago not onehalf was expected that is now demanded to make a proper diagnosis. There was more sickness than there is today, fewer doctors and better fees than there are now.

Here is a patient who has taken to idolatry, to the She God who gave life to the book called "Science and Health." There are those who have displaced bones and nerves and get cured without reduction, all of whom pay larger fees to these prophets of deception than one charged by doctors who endeavor to practice sane medicine.

It is amusing to see the idolatrous teacher charging $2 per call, without training, without knowledge of the normal, much less any knowledge of disease, treating matter which does not exist, and we professors of the true faith asking $1.50. Do you think any of our patients have gone over to these cults because of our charges? Not at all. It's because of our own bickering, because of our lack of attention to small details, because of lack of unity. It's our looseness that leaves a place, when the fickle needs tickling, when the neurasthenic wants coddling. There are three classes: the well, the sick and the intermediate who thinks he is sick. We must recognize this division and we have here to awaken to the new condition.

Medicine is largely a one man power. You must represent yourself. We can not increase our output, for there never yet has been a day and night of more than 24 hours. But we can be made to understand that what is good for you is good for me. If you use treachery to get my patient and I get him back by using your methods of getting business, we surely can realize that neither of us can hold this patient so long as either of us has enough baseness to get business. If I am blinded to my own good, help me to see myself, and when enlightened it is reasonable that I will no longer be in error.

I am not advocating a fixed fee table at so much per hour or call. I am trying to see further than organized labor. Let every man have just recompense. Some of us excel others. Your time may be worth more than mine is to me. A calico doctor should be cheaper than a silk doctor. Let each know his worth and let each go beyond the demand of union labor by none being so dishonest as to charge more

than he is worth. If I choose to make night calls at day rates, convince me of my error. Help me to reason that I could have had more for my services, and still hold the gratitude of my patient. For my persistent blindness, let me have as my reward, a life of hard labor, known as a man poorly paid with a dejected family.

I believe in strikes, but not in tying up the profession because my brother was not paid for his labor, but strike in defense of his honor and ability. I will strike for a part of his burden when called by him to do so. I admire the doctor who can take my patient from me because of his wisdom, because of his able diagnosis and skill. It is then I realize I have more to learn, more ability to acquire. It makes me see myself. But should a doctor with such ability make a fee not in comparison with his ability. I would reason that I had overestimated his worth, and the patient would naturally arrive at the same conclusion. I would think the consultant was bidding for my patient and the patient would wonder why was the doctor so cheap.

Why does the medical profession boast of being overworked no time to eat or sleep; horses are too slow; compelled to use an auto? Why do we deceive by telling each other of making twenty calls a day and three confinements during the night? What delusion is this that pictures an office with a long row of waiting patients? Is this not the exception? If it were true and you were making what you told me, you would have some evidence of it; some property to show, lift mortgages and be free of debt.

The down-trodden farmer, the retired capitalist, all ask our reduction for labor bestowed upon them for we have educated the people to believe we have a mecca, a real bonanza for making money, that money is a secondary consideration, that we do not need it, for we are making money so fast that it is a pleasure to make a reduction for cash, while in truth you need the cash so badly that you are forced to do something to get it quick.

It is this kind of hot air that is crowding the profession. The baker has heard it and is saving enough money to join our ranks. Men in all callings of life look at us with a desire to some day be able to be a doctor, live in ease and luxury, to have an easy time, and make money.

Our profession has done noble work in looking to the needs and ills of fellow man, but has taken little heed of self. Now, let's be considerate of ourselves. Learn a lesson from organized labor which teaches that to labor belong the spoils.

There is no charity in this, we must look further than such teaching and organize for the good of those who may become our charges. Do not fret away our substance in pretence of greatness, but remember that the well paid doctor has money for books, aids to diagnosis and an incentive to aid the afflicted. We would not say as does the labor union: "To us belong the proceeds of labor"; but, "give us proper recompense, that we may be prepared to minister to the sick." Can you do this under present conditions; can you equip your office modernly? Why have you not so much as a reasonably equipped office? Because you cannot afford it. Why are you using strict economy? It is because you are apeing a professional brother. He wears good clothes, looks progressive, and you try to look like him. He is apeing you and wears good clothes because you do. Neither can afford it.

If I have a poor business, and you are busy, run nearly to death doing laparotomies and cutting to beat thunder and every doctor I talk to is busy, I get blue, I cannot understand it but trust a change will come and I keep on spending the little my wife inherited. I know it's a lie, but I tell my brother I am doing all right, better than I expected. I delude him and he lied to me and we become confidential and in a moment of confidence he said he was not making a cent and then I took new courage and realized that I was not alone.

Why should members of this society set themselves on a high pedestal and tell the laity that there are only two or three doctors in this city who are sufficiently qualified for them to consult with? What is wrong with the doctor when he ignores the meetings of this society because he says there is nothing here he can learn? What's wrong when he sneers at us, and shakes his head when our name is mentioned. The same thing exists in the mind of the fractious colt when hitched up with the old mare from which the colt is expected to learn the duties of a well broken horse. The colt is excited, champing its bit, sweating, and thinks the old mare ignorant of her duty because she don't get out of place.

When I need help, let me turn to my brother, speak for him words of confidence to my patient. Teach the people that this society membership can give them good service. Tell them that we have here good surgeons, good specialists and talk as if you had good sense. If I can not get a good fee, why should it not be better to help you get it than to give it to Chicago. If I am behind the times and don't know much, then come to our meeting and teach me. If then I am convinced you

know it all, I surely shall call you, when needed.

Here, in this society, is the place for discussing our deportment in the practice of medicine. Just as long as medicine is progressive, so long will there be a difference of opinion between the progressives and those who stand still. This organization should be and is our post-graduate school. Prepare for and fix right here those things that lessen our personal loss in practice. You and I are integral parts of the medical decorum of this city. I can not destroy your medical career without blacking my own.

Why should not your fellowship in this society be as dear and revered as the unionist card. If the unionist card was ignored and members treated as we do each other, it would be despised and rejected. This want of harmony, too much jealousy, still the ambition

and blasts the hope of a McDowell, Gross or Sims rising up among us. If you doubt it let this society endorse and praise the work of the earnest doctor and see how quick the news is spread, while honor and prestige would make for us one whom it would be our pleasure to say had sat among us.

To be such you must merit our confidence. Not by egotism and self conceit, but as a teacher imparting wisdom, a leader; be a progressive and an independent thinker. When you find it is impossible to know it all and learn that some can even learn sermons from running brooks, or be confounded by the simplest atom; that your spurned doctor might be your guide; then why not ask him, thank him, give him credit for possibly the one talent that was needed. That's brotherly. That's professional ethics, pure and simple.

Nineteenth Annual Meeting Oklahoma State Medical Ass'n, Muskogee, May 9-10-11, '11

All meetings will be held in the Leighton Building, on South Fourth Street near Okmulgee, unless otherwise announced. The first meeting will be called to order at 2 P. M., May 9th, and at that time the House of Delegates and Council will be organized for work and the addresses of welcome will be delivered. There will be a smoker on the evening of May 10th, preceded by an automobile ride over the city which will be tendered the Association at 5:30 P. M.

SECTION ON SURGERY.

Wednesday, May 10th, 1:30 P. M.
Ross Grosshart, Chairman, Tulsa.
Address of the Chairman.

1 "Treatment of Compound Fractures and Lacerated Wounds,"
..............Virgil Berry, Okmulgee.

2 "Indigestion From a Surgical Point of View,"
..............LeRoy Long, McAlester

3 "Joint Manifestations of Hemophilia,"
..............C. S. Neer, Vinita

4 "Prevention and Treatment of Superficial Infections,"
..............E. H. Troy, McAlester

5 Subject unannounced.
..............Jackson Brashear, Lawton

6 "Chloroform,"
..............Wm. Fowler, Alderson

7 "Cancer of the Uterus,"
..............F. H. Clark, El Reno

8 "The Importance of Early Recognition of Peritonitis,"
..............G. H. Butler, Tulsa

9 "Surgery of the Tonsil,"
..............I. B. Oldham, Muskogee

10 "Remarks on the Diagnostis of Surgical Diseases of the Kidney,"
..............J. Hutchings White, Muskogee

11 "Bone Tuberculosis, Including Pathology, Symptomatology and Treatment,"
Millington Smith, Oklahoma City

12 "Surgery of the Urachus,"
..............R. V. Smith, Guthrie

SECTION ON MENTAL AND NERVOUS DISEASES.

Wednesday, May 10, 9:00 A. M.
F. B. Erwin, Chairman, Norman, Okla.
Chairman's Address.

        F. B. Erwin, Norman, Okla

1 "Brain Tumors,"
        John S. Turner, Dallas, Texas

2 "Chronic Alcoholism,"
        Jhn W. Duke, Guthrie, Okla

3 "Chloroform Delirium and Its Causes, a Clinical Illustration,"
S. Grover Burnett, Kansas City, Mo

4 "Better and More Humane Laws Governing the Admission of Patients to Our State Hospitals for the Insane,"
        D. W. Griffin, Norman, Okla

5 "Nervous Phenomena Due to Pathologic and Physiologic Changes in the Female Pelvis,"
Charles Nelson Ballard, Oklahoma City, Okla.

SECTION ON OBSTETRICS AND GYNECOLOGY.

Tuesday, May 9, 1911, 8:00 P. M., and
Wednesday, May 10, 1911, 9 A. M.
B. W. Freer, Chairman, Nowata, Okla.
Chairman's Adrress.

1 "Uterine Prolapse,"
Horace Reed, Oklahoma City, Okla

2 "Pelvic Abscess,"
        W. E. Dicken, Oklahoma City

3 "The Pitfalls for a General Parctitioner in Eclampsia, Etc,"
        Walter A. Howard, Chelsea

4 "Practical Obstetrics in Country Practice,"
        F. R. Wheeler, Manford

5 "The Treatment of Gonorrhoea by the General Practioner as a Pre-Preliminary to Operation,"
        John F. Kuhn, Oklahma City

6 "Puerperal Sepis,"
        F. L. Hughson, Vinita

7 "Puerperal Sepsis a Preventable Disease,"
        J. C. Mahr, Oklahoma City

8 "The Puerperium,"
        Andrew J. Lerskov, Claremore

9 "Extra Uterine Pregnancy,"
        W. C. Graves, McAlester

10 "Sigmoido-Colporrhaphy, With Report of Two Cases,"
Frank D. Smythe, Memphis, Tenn

11 "An Obstertrical Recor dof Forty Years,"
        Wm. Nairn, Alluwee

12 "Some Peculiar Cases of Obstetrics, and How I Would Handle Them, Etc,"
        L. T. Strother, Nowata

13 "Failure or Success in Obstetrics, With Case Reports,"
        G. R. Gordon, Wagoner

SECTION OF GENERAL MEDICINE.

Tuesday, May 9, 1911, 8:00 P. M., and
Wednesday, May 10, 9:00 A. M.
J. H. Scott, Chairman, Shawnee, Okla.
Chairman's Address,

1 "Influenza,"
        M. A. Warhurst, Sylvian, Okla

2 "The Various Forms of Icterus,"
        H. M. Williams, Wellston, Okla

3 "Pernicious Malaria,"
        G. A. Reber, Okemah, Okla

4 "Practical Helps on Malaria,"
        G. S. Barger, Wayne, Okla

5 "Drugs and Their Administration,"
        R. I. Bond, Hartshorne, Okla

6 "A Plea for More Rational Therapeutics,"
        A. B. Leeds, Chickasha, Okla

7 "Auto-Intoxication,"
Wm. R. Bevan, Oklahoma City, Okla.

8 "Elephantiasis, With Presentation of a Clinic,"
        C. A Peterson, Tahlequah, Okla

9 "My Experience With Typhoid Fever,"
Walter L. Capshaw, Norman, Okla
10 "The Value of Uterine Hemorrhage as a Symptom,"
..........J. A. Hatchett, El Reno, Okla
11 "Looking Ahead,"
..........A. K. West, Oklahoma City
12 "Preventive Medicine,"
..........................H. L. Wright, Hugo
13 "Rabies, With Report of a Case,"
..........G. A. Morrison, Poteau
14 "The Cure of Morphine and Opium Addicts,"
..........W. E. Rammel, Bartlesville
15 "Chronic Alcoholism, What Can and What Cannot Be Done by Treatment,"
..........Geo. F. Petty, Memphis, Tenn
16 "The General Practitioner as a Surgeon,"
..........................A. S. Risser, Blackwell
17 "Cretinism, With Report of a Case,"
..........................J. C. Watkins, Hallett
18 "The Early Diagnosis of Tuberculosis and Its Importance,"
..........P. H. Anderson, Anadarko
19 "Scarlet Fever,"
..........................Jas. L. Shuler, Durant
20 Subject not announced,
..........................L. T. Gooch, Lawton

SECTION ON PEDIATRICS.

Thurdsay, May 11th, 9:00 A. M.

W. G. Little, Chairman, Okmulgee, Okla.

Chairman's Address,
"The Conservation of Child Life an Economic Factor to the State."

1 "Nasal Obstructions,"
..........................J. H. Barnes, Enid
2 "Some of the Preventable Causes

of Infant Mortality During the First Months of Life,"
..........Effia V. Davis, Oklahoma City
3 "Infantile Paralysis, Etiology, Pathology and Treatment,"
Leila B. Andrews, Oklahoma City
4 "Open Parliament,"
Five-Minute Talks by Various Physicians on Topics of their Own Selection.
5 "Clinic."
6 "Varicella,"
..........J. F. Duckworth, Tahlequah

SECTION ON DISEASES OF EYE, EAR, NOSE AND THROAT.

Wednesday, May 10th, 1:30 P. M.

M. K. Thompson, Chairman, Muskogee, Oklahoma.

Chairman's Address.

1 "Trachoma,"
Daniel W. White, Eye and Ear Expert, United States Indian Service.
2 "The Eye as Seen by the General Practioner,"
.....Graham Street, McAlester, Okla
3 "Choroiditis,"
..........S. M. Jenkins, Enid Oklahoma
4 "Paper,"
..........W. Albert Cook, Tulsa, Okla
5 "Otitis Media Suppurative,"
..........D. W. Miller, Blackwell, Okla
6 "Vestibular Nystagmus,"
Edward F. Davis, Oklahoma City
7 "Case Reports,"
.....D. D. McHenry, Oklahoma City

Meeting of House of Delegates, Council, etc., for the election of officers. After this election is held such Section programs as are unfinished will be concluded.

EDITORIAL

REDUCED RATES FOR ANNUAL CONVENTION OKLAHOMA MEDICAL SOCIETY.

Muskogee Traffic Bureau.

Muskogee, Okla., April 13, 1911.

Dr. W. T. Tilley, Chairman,

Local Committee on Trans. & Accommodations, Oklahoma Medical Society Annual Convention, Muskogee,

Oklahoma.

Dear Sir:

I take pleasure in advising you that Chairman Hannegan of the Southwestern Passenger Association has announced that Oklahoma railroads have individually authorized a rate of fare and one-third for the round trip, with a minimum of 4 cents per mile, subject to a minimum selling rate of 50 cents, from all points in Oklahoma to Muskogee, on account of the Annual Convention of the Oklahoma Medical Society, which convenes in Muskogee May 8-10 inclusive, 1911. Tickets on sale May 7, 8, and 9, with final return limit to reach original starting points prior to midnight of May 12th.

Yours very truly,

R. D. SANGSTER,
Secretary.

THE WORK OF THE LAST LEGISLATURE.

A study of the measures proposed at the last session of the legislature shows us that the irregulars and under standard gentlemen are still active and able, by unity and concert of action to block necessary legislation improving the standard of medical requirement though they are not strong enough to do anything really harmful to the existing regulations.

A bill creating a separate board of examiners for Chiropractors never saw the light of day, while to offset this a bill increasing the educational requirement and strengthening the definition of the practice of medicine was killed by their efforts.

The Optometry Bill became a law and so long as the Governor uses discretion in selecting a Board it is believed no one will be hurt by the measure, yet the attention of the profession should be called to the fact that both in Ohio and Illinois Optometry bills failed of passage by reason of the veto of the Governors, who gave as a reason in both cases that it was their understanding that in order to properly refract and correct defective vision a knowledge of medicine was necessary and that such knowledge was not in the possession of an optician per se.

It was noticeable in our legislature that many members considered all measures looking to the raising of the standard as a move in some way beneficial to the medical profession rather than a benefit to the State. So long as this idea is prevalent and until our legislative body understands that the medical profession is doing more work today along the lines of prevetive medicine than any other kind and that hardly a year passes that a great deal of work and study is not added to the requirements creating a finished physician, just so long will the advance be delayed. It seems almost criminal to have the advances of medicine and the raising of the standard of medical education and requirement held up on the demand of some small ism represented by men who have no scientific standing, and who at the mose devote a few months of so-called study to a so-called and unproved and untried science—pardon the word—and then impertinently and ignorantly demand to be legalized and turned loose on the general public.

Where would we be today if our Army and Navy, the Marine Hospital service, the great and protective quarantine stations and our public works were turned over to these so-called scientists to handle. We pause here to ask what lasting benefit, yes even what temporary and fleeting benefit have any of these obstructionists conferred on humanity. It is scarcely a decade when this southwestern country was flooded with a laughable set of alleged physicians called magnetic healers, their ignorance was of that character that nothing was sacred from their manipulations and folderol; in each town marvelous things were heard of performed at the hands of this wonderful body of men, who like the negro exhorter had "received the call of the Lord," dropped the handle of the plow, the razor and the dishcloth entered the "Institute" for sixty days, graduated after a strenuous laying on of hands and then entered the house of sickness as physicians. These men were as much entitled to legal protection as the farcical set of men called Chiropractors who importuned our legislature for an act creating them a separate board of examiners, yet they are no more with us, after a brief and destructive career their science like other sciences untried and without foundation other than fraud and ignorance faded away under the strong glare of public scrutiny and common sense and so will go the Chiropractor, for that matter any other ism proposing to make a finished healer without preparation and study.

However, a law absolutely prohibiting them from even existing would hardly protect the people for tomorrow they show up under a different guise and name, and commence their same old practices. This is well illustrated in the manner of advertisers who are exposed or prohibited the use of the mails on account of fraud; the order is hardly issued until they have simply turned their hat around, called themselves Smythe instead of Smith and are at the public pocket book again. From this it will be seen that a law specifying them is inadequate; the law should be broad enough to require every man entering the sick room to be a diagnostician and to

prove it to the satisfaction of educated men and then we have a basis from which we may hope to do some good.

SUBSCRIPTION TO THE JOURNAL

It seems necessary to again call attention to County Secretaries and members that membership in the State Medical Association no longer carries with it subscription to the Journal.

This rule, put in force on account of a ruling of the Postoffice Department has now been in force a year, yet members are still writing letters complaining that they do not receive the Journal and investigation discloses they are simply members by reason of having paid $1.50 for dues and neglecting to pay the additional fifty cents for subscription. There is no doubt that this is often due to the neglect of the County Secretary in his failing to call attention that the membership and subscription lists have long been separate matters and the member goes along under the assumption that the Secretary's office is neglectful of the matter.

It might be worth while to note in this connection that membership costs $1.50, subscription fifty cents additional and that the members' $1.50 is largely expended in the publication of the Journal from which he receives no benefit unless he pays an additional fifty cents in addition to his annual dues.

We believe that every man should give the Journal his moral as well as financial support and the sum asked is a mere pittance compared to the benefit received. A subscriber to the Journal is kept fairly well informed of the happenings to his fellow practitioner and has an opportunity which he should not neglect for keeping in touch with the standards of the Oklahoma Medical Profession. A perusal of the columns of the Journal and comparison with the offerings from other States leads one to the conclusion that our State profession is well up and abreast of the profession in other States. Another phase not occurring to many men is this: Our profession is changing and growing daily and only through the columns of the Journal can even a small acquaintance with the men and their attainments be secured and for this reason alone the Journal should be in the hands of every member.

After this issue those members who have not subscribed through their county secretaries will have their names taken from the rolls.

This notice is given for the information of all concerned, so that the responsibility may be removed from the office of the secretary.

THE PROGRAM FOR THE ANNUAL MEETING.

Following the custom inaugurated last year the program of the annual meeting appears in this Journal and no other program will be mailed to the members. A program for the use of those attending the meeting will be issued and placed in the hands of the attending members as they arrive.

This plan saves the expense, which is not small, of mailing a program to each member separately, a large percentage of whom do not attend the meetings and therefore are saved the trouble of receiving and digesting a second program if it were mailed in the small and compact form used at the meeting.

卍 COUNTY SOCIETIES 卍

LOGAN COUNTY.
President, E. O. Barker.
Vice-Pres., E. L. Underwood.
Secy.-Treas., R. V. Smith, Guthrie.
Censors, L. A. Hahn, C. F. Cotteral, C. B. Hill, Guthrie.
Delegate, R. V. Smith, Guthrie.

WASHINGTON COUNTY.
President, G. F. Woodring, Bartlesville.
Vice-Pres., A. P. Owens, Bartlesville
Secretary, W. E. Rammel, Bartlesville.
Treasurer, J. V. Athey, Bartlesville.
Censor, H. C. Weber, Bartlesville.

KIOWA COUNTY.
Elected the following officers for 1911:
President, A. Barkley, Hobart.
Vice-President, A. H. Hathaway, Mt. View.

Alternate, J. F. Duckworth, Tahlequah.
Secy.-Treas., J. M. Bonham, Hobart.
Delegate, G. W. Stewart, Hobart.

OKFUSKEE COUNTY.
President, B. J. Vance, Checotah.
Vice-Pres., A. H. Barton, Onapa.
Secy-Treas., W. A. Tolleson, Eufaula.
Delegate, Geo. W. West, Eufaula.

SEQUOYAH COUNTY.
President, A. A. Hicks, Sallisaw.
Vice-Pres., T. F. Wood, Sallisaw.
Treas., S. B. Jones, Sallisaw.
Secretary, M. D. Carnell, Sallisaw.
Delegate, Sam A. McKeel.

CHEROKEE COUNTY.
President, W. G. Blake, Tahlequah.
Vice-Pres., Israel Hill, Tahlequah.
Secy.-Treas., C. A. Peterson, Tahlequah.

Censors, Jos. M. Thompson, L. E. McCurry, J. L. Dement, Tahlequah.

Delegate, J. D. Bewley, Peggs.

Seminole County

President, W. L. Knight, Seminole.

Vice-Pres., W. R. Black, Little.

Secy-Treas., M. M. Turlington, Seminole.

Delegate, J. N. Harber, Seminole.

THE NEW BOARD OF MEDICAL EXAMINERS.

Regulars, F. B. Fite, Muskogee; John W. Duke, Guthrie; LeRoy Long, McAlester; Philip E. Herod, Alva.

Electics—M. Gray, Mountain View; R. E. Sawyer, Bochito.

Homeopaths—Dr. W. L. Bonnell, Chickasha; C. F. Stilwell, Piedmont.

Osteopaths—J. A. Price, Oklahoma City; alternate, H. J. Shackelford, Ardmore.

Garvin County.

The Garvin County Medical Association meets in Paul's Valley April 20, 1911, at 8 p. m.

Program:

"The Diagnosis and Treatment of Congenital Heart Disease,"

......................................W. E. Settles

"The Treatment of Convulsions in Infants and Children,"

......................................J. R. Callaway

"The Early Diagnosis of Tuberculous Meningitis,"

......................................S. W. Wilson

"The Diagnosis and Treatment of Cerebro-Spinal Meningitis,"

......................................N. H. Lindsey

WOMAN'S AUXILIARY

The fourth annual convention of the Women's Auxiliary to the State Medical Association will be held in Muskogee, May 10 and 11, 1911.

The first day's program, commencing at ten a. m., will be given at Miss Alice Robertson's home, "Sawokla," at Agency Hill.

Following is a partial list of the good things to be enjoyed by those who attend this convention:

Wednesday, May 10, 10 A. M.

Call to order by the President,

......................Mrs. W. G. Little, Okmulgee

Invocation,

......................Rev. Hugh J. Llwyd, Muskigee

Welcoming Address,

......................Miss Alice Robertson

Response,

......................Mrs. F. H. Morton, Okmulgee

Vocal Solo,

......................Mrs. C. L. McCallum, Sapulpa

President's Address.

Song—"A Garden Coronation,"

......................Galela Peterson, Tahlequah

Piano Solo,

......................Miss Marsh, Muskogee

Paper—"Our Proposed Law on Medical Inspection in the Public Schools,"

......................Mrs. W. C. Bradford, Shawnee

Discussion,

......................Led by Mrs. H. L. Wright, Hugo

Vocal Solo,

......................Mrs. J. O. Callahan, Muskogee

Paper—"Methods and Results of Medical Inspection in Our City Schools,"

......................Mrs. R. E. Looney, Oklahoma City

Reading—"Rewarding Our Heroes,"

......................Mrs. H. L. Wright, Hugo

Talk on Medical Inspection in the Muskogee Schools,

......................Dr. A. B. Montgomery

Vocal Solo,

......................Mrs. Edmund S. Ferguson, Oklahoma City. Mrs. Wayman Jackson, Accompanist.

Symposium—"The Physician's Wife as a Social Factor,"

Five-minute Talks by Mesdames O. E. Howell, Oktaha; R. M. Sweeney, Sapulpa; W. C. Mitchner, Okmulgee; T. C. Sanders, Shawnee.

Vocal Solo,

Mrs. Wayman C. Jackson, Muskogee. Mr. Gamble, Accompanist.

Adjournment.

Luncheon will be served those in attendance at Miss Robertson's home, after which a drive over the city will be enjoyed.

Thursday, 9:30 A. M.

Place of meeting to be announced.

Call to Order.

Reading of Minutes.

Reports of Co. Auxiliaries.

Reports of Officers.

Open Parliament—"General Hygiene."

Recitation,

...............................Dryl Butler, Tulsa

Paper—"Public Sanitation,"

...............Mrs. H. E. Breese, Henryetta

Reading—Selected,

Mrs. Wm. L. Kendall, Oklahoma City

Song,

...............................Maurienne Butler, Tulsa

BOOKS RECEIVED

MODERN OTOLOGY. Second edition revised. The Principles and Practice of Modern Otology By John F. Barnhill, M. D., Professor of Otology, Laryngology, and Rhinology, Indiana University School of Medicine; and Ernest de W. Wales, B. S., M. D., Clinical Professor of Otology, Laryngology and Rhinology, Indiana University School of Medicine. Second edition, revised. Octavo of 598 pages, with 305 original illustrations, many in colors; 1911. Cloth, $5.50; half Morocco, $7.00 net. W. B. Saunders Company, Philadelphia and London.

GOEPP'S STATE BOARD QUESTIONS AND ANSWERS. Second edition, revised. State Board Question and Answers by R. Max Goepp, M. D., Professor of Clinical Medicine at the Philadelphia Polyclinic. Second edition revised. Octavo volume of 715 pages; 1911. Cloth, $4.00 net; half Morocco, $5.50 net. W. B. Saunders Company, Philadelphia, London.

DIAGNOSTIC METHODS. Second edition revised. A treatise on Diagnostic Methods of Examination. By Prof. Dr. Hermann Sahli, Director of the Medical Clinic, University of Bern. Edited, with additions, by Nathaniel Bowditch Potter, M. D., Assistant Professor of Clinical Medicine, College of Physicians and Surgeons, New York. Octavo of 1229 pages, containing 472 illustration; 1911. Cloth $6.50 net, half Morocco $8.00 net. W. B. Saunders Company, Philadelphia and London.

DIAGNOSTIC AND THERAPEUTIC TECHNIC. Diagnostic and Therapeutic Technic. By Albert S. Morrow, M. D., Adjunct Professor of Surgery, New York Polyclinic. Octavo of 850 pages, with 815 original line drawings; 1911. Cloth, $5.00 net. W. B Saundes Company, Philadelphia and London.

The Practical Medicine Series, Volume 1, General Medicine.

Edited by Frank Billings, M. S., M. D., Head of the Medical Deartment and Dean of the Faculty of Rush Medical College, Chicago, and J. H. Salisbury, A. M., M. D., Professor of Medicine, Chicago Clinical School. Series 1911. Cloth $1.50, entire set of ten volumes, $10.00. Chicago: The Year Book Publishers, 40 Dearborn Street.

New and Nonofficial Remedies, 1911: Containing descriptions of articles which have been accepted by the Council on Pharmacy and Chemistry of the American Medical Association, prior to Jan. 1, 1911. Price, paper, 25 cents; Cloth, 50 cents. Pp. 282.

This is the 1911 edition of the annual New and Nonofficial Remedies, issued by the Council on pharmacy andChemistry of the American Medical Association, and contains descriptions of all articles approved by the Council, up to Dec. 31, 1910. There are also descriptions of a number of unofficial non-proprietary articles which the Council deemed of value. The action, dosage, uses and tests of identity, purity and strength of articles are given.

In the arrangement and the scope of individual descriptions, the present edition does not differ widely from the 1910 edition, but it contians about twenty-five additional pages, these being required to describe the articles accepted by the Council during 1910.

Besides indicating to physicians the proprietary articles which the Council's examination has found to be honestly marketed, and contaming accurate descriptions of these articles, all similar articles are arranged under group headings; thus the physician at a glance can learn that atoxyl and soamin are practically identical articles, and that arsacetin is a closely related body. Again, the several proprietary solutions of the blood-pressure-raising principle of the suprarenal gland are listed under a general title "epinephrin," and the manner in which the solutions differ from each other can be learned at a glance. In the same way, the medicinal foods are brought together and their relative value compared.

ABSTRACTS AND EXCHANGES

INNOCENT GALL STONES.

W. J. Mayo, Rochester, Minn., (Journal A. M. A., April 8), says that symptoms must now be acknowledged to be incorrect. We have become better informed by operative experience with the disease. He questions the high percentage of gall-stones in the general population as estimated by some good authorities and thinks that it is more probable that not over 0.5 per cent. would be a fair estimate of the frequency of gall-stones in individuals of all ages, although evidence at hand shows that from 5 to 8 per cent. of women and from 2 to 4 per cent. of men have gall-stones after the age of 50. The symptoms may not be recognized as regards their source though appreciable to the individual and to the observer. He has been impressed with this fact on finding undiagnosed gall-stones in operating on women for pelvic trouble. After the recovery of the patient he has nearly always been able to elicit a satisfactory history. The hypothesis of Lartigau as to the bacterial causation of gall-stones is probably correct, though it is difficult to demonstrate it experimentally. Their place of formation is in the gall-bladder, and Mayo describes and discusses the anatomy and functions of this viscus. It cannot be considered merely a storage house for bile, he says, and it is most reasonable to suppose that its function is to relieve temporarily the pressure on the common and hepatic ducts and also, if necessary, the ducts of the pancrease. Another function is the production of mucus which, mixed with the bile, protects in· a· measure the pancreas from injury if the mixture is forced into the pancreatic duct. That the gall-bladder is important as a means of protection, especially to the pancreas, is evident, and this is an argument against its unnecessary removal. The greater frequency of gall-stone disease in women than in men must depend on some sexual difference; 90 per cent. of the cases in women are in those who have borne children, and 90 per cent. of these identify the beginning of the symptoms with some particular pregnancy. Every patient with chronic gastric distress should be questioned intelligently to obtain any former history of gall-stone colic, since this may have escaped the patient's attention. Gallstone disease sometimes causes serious circulatory distrubances, such as endocarditis, which, though rare, is of a specific type and in its origin is coincident with the gall-stone attack. Subsequent attacks aggravate the heart action. While stones are the most common cause of cholecystitis, this is not always the case, but the patient still requires operative relief. It is usually in these cases accompanied by habitual tenderness in the region of the gall-bladder and colic is not so prominent. Complications were found in more than two-thirds of the patients found in the common duct in 531 cases with an operative mortality of 6.5 per cent., while serious complications involving the liver, duodenum, transverse colon, etc., were the rule. Carcinoma was found in eighty-five cases (2.25 per cent.) In a number of the cases slightly advanced cases of carcinoma were accidentally encountered before they had advanced sufficiently for diagnosis in removing thick-walled functionless gall-bladders, and five of these patients are still alive and well from two to six years after operation. Gall-stones are foreign bodies bodies and Mayo asks why delay operation until complications ensue. In their experience at Rochester simple operation for uncomplicated gallstones has had a mortality of less than 0.5 per cent., and this was due more to the condition of the patient than to the operation. While temporary paliation may be obtained with non-operative measures, the patient can only be thoroughly cured through surgery.

ANTITYPHOID VACCINE.

The method of administering prophylactic antityphoid vacciinations in the United States Army is described by J. P. Fletcher, Fort D. A. Russell, Wyo. (Jorunal A. M. A., April 8.) In brief, the method used consists in making three subcutaneous injections at ten-day intervals of a killed culture of B. typhosus prepared in the laboratory of the Army Medical School at Washington, D. C., sent out in sealed ampoules and containing 1,000,000,000 dead bacilli per cubic centimeter. The injections are made in the posterolateral aspect of the arm with a syringe with a plane ground nipple on the barrel fitting the base of the needle so that it can be easily attached and detached and also give a tight joint even after repeated boilings. A freshly sterlized needle is used in every case. The men are rapidly placed, after scrubbing up and the application of antiseptic and alcohol, and when the soldier reaches the medical officer the arm is grasped between the thumb and forefinger of the left hand to steady it, the skin is pinched taut, the needle plunged downward and slightly forward into the subcutaneous fat; the needle is then quickly withdrawn. The needle puncture is touched with a glass rod moistened with pure trikresol, which dries rapidly, and the man leaves by another door. The cleaning-up process is then managed quickly and orderly and the slight burn made by the tribresol prevents any man receiving two doses the same day, as some may try to do. The needles are boiled and sterilized and placed in a special needle-holder so that sixteen needles can be used for the work of two surgeons constantly at work in the vaccination. With four assistants to do the scrubbing, etc., and a non-commissioned officer to keep the notes, an average of four or five doses can be given every minute for an hour or more, and the vaccination of from 100 to 200 men, which is not infrequent, becomes merely an incident in the day's work. The vaccine ampoules used are kept in a 1 to 500 mercuric chlorid solution and are removed and dried as needed and scattered with a file and broken at the neck, the sterile needle inserted and the syringe filled. A little practice is required to hit the opening every time, but infection is pretty well barred by the method of taking the vaccine at once from the original container and avoiding dust contamination by the use of the small opening. Dr. Fletcher thinks that the time will soon come when civil practitioners will be confronted with the problem of wholesale vaccination against typhoid in schools, etc., and an acquaintance with the army experience will then be of advantage.

SALVARSAN TECHNIC.

A long list of "don'ts" in the use of salvarsan are given by J. F. Schamberg and N. Ginsburg, Philadelphia (Journal A. M. A., February 4.) These, slightly abbreviated, are as follows: 1. Don't use salvarsan in mild carditis, advanced tabes and paresis, syphilis of nervous centers, in grave kidney disease, in cachexia or marked debility, unless due to syphilis, in aneurism, optic neuritis or in persons with lesions (such as gastric ulcer) where increased blood pressure may produce hemorrhage. 2. Don't use intravenous injections of salvarsan until you have fully qualified yourself to do so. 3. In the preparation for the intravenous injections do not use common salt solution or undistilled water, but have all materials chemically pure and sterile; otherwise you may not have a clear solution. 4. Don't under any circumstances inject a solution which is not perfectly clear. 5. Don't use a solution any more alkaline than is absolutely necessary to secure a clear solution. 6. Don't inject the salvarsan into the vein without previously running in physiologic salt solution. If the needle is not in the vein you will infiltrate the surrounding tissues and cause unnecessary pain and inflammation. 7. Don't infuse the solution into the vein too rapidly. It is best to have a needle of such capacity as will take eight minutes to introduce 200 c. e. of fluid. With the gravity apparatus the rapidity of inflow can be readily governed. 8. Don't infuse a cold solution, but use one about blood-heat. 9. Don't use glass pearls in the mixing jar, as small parts may chip off and cause embolism. 10. Don't use a routine dosage of the drug, but gauge it according to the weight of the patient and the condition to be treated. 11. Don't employ intravenous injection in your office or in dispensary. The patient should be in bed in the hospital and be carefully observed for not less than three days. 12. Don't persist in intravenous injection if the patient shows signs o collapse during administration, but stop at once.

INDEX VOL. III, OKLAHOMA STATE MEDICAL ASSOCIATION.

Abstracts and Exchanges. 135, 171, 205, 278, 316, 393.
Address of the President .... 1.
Allison, W. R., ...413
Anesthesia, local, ... 92
Annual Meeting Program, 1910, ... 24
Appendix, the obliterated 323
Appendicitis 221
Appendicitis, observations in connection with 46
Armstrong, D. 232
Autointoxication 58
Barnes, J. H. 59
Ballard, C. N., 195, 363.
Berry, V., 22, 292.
Beedles, Gordon A., 382,
Blickensderfer, Charles, 5, 398,
Blesh, A. L. 323
Block, J. 301
Bone Tuberculosis 146
Book Notices, 74, 106, 140, 207, 208, 239, 281, 320, 321, 352, 392.
Bradford, W. C. 1
Breese, Harry E. 111
Broderick, D. E. 327
Broncho-Pneumonia 270
Byrum, Mrs. J. M., ...132

Cardiac Murmurs 342
Carcinoma of Skin, ...177
Cervix, Lacerated 382
Cerebral Meningitis 218
Children, Dependent 258
Childhood, hygiene of, ...141
Clubs, the Womens and Tuberculosis,..132
Concussion, ...162
Constipation, Chronic 107
County, the Medical Society 232
County Societies, 30, 42, 73, 236, 276, 317, 350, 425.
Cretinism, ...184
Cummings, W. C. 406

Davis, W. L. 296
Diabetes, Diagnosis and Treatment of, ...111
Diagnosis, Typhoid Perforation 88
Diagnosis, and Treatment of Diabetes 111
Diagnosis, and Treatment Extra Uterine Pregnancy 156
Diagnostic Relationship, between Medicine and Surgery 301
Dicken, William 52
Diphtheria, Laryngeal 49
Disorders of Sleep 289
Donohoo, J. 232
Duke, John W., ... 43
Duty of Physician, ...369

Eclampsia 159

Edtorial, 29, 69, 105, 134, 166, 202, 234, 273, 314, 346, 391, 422.
Electricity and the Nervous System 381
Empyema 327
Erwin, F. B. 218
Ergotin 310
Ethics, Medical, 61, 193.
Etiology, etc., of Hernia 124
Exudates, Prevention of, ... 52

Fallopian Tubes, Tuberculosis of, ...363
Fee Bills, ...129
Fisk, Chas. W. 213
Foltz, J. A. 228
Fortner, B. F. 162
Fractures of Extremeties 228
Fractures of Elbow 398
Fractures, Repair of, ...357
Fractures, Internal Splint in, ...168
Frick, W. J. 124

General Practitioner, The 213
Germi-Phobia 401

Hansen, J. H. 382
Harper, R. H. 13
Hernia, Etiology and Tr. of, ...124
Herniotomy and Lipectomy 195
Hirschfield, A. C., ...337
Huffman, L. H., 146, 369.
Hughes, J. E. 186
Hygiene of Infancy and Childhood 141

Infancy and Childhood 141
Infantile Paralysis 413
Infections, Septic 245
Insanity of Puerperium 43
Intestinal Obstruction 224
Irland, R. D. 124

Jenkins, S. M., ...312

Kanavel, Allen B., Clinic, ...371
Kidney, Infected Cystic 293

Lain, E. S., 177, 306.
Laryngeal Diphtheria 49
Lee, C. E., ...323
Leeds, A. B. 262
Lerskov, Andrew 61
Lipectomy 195
Little, W. G. 141
Local Anesthesia 92
Long, LeRoy 46

Mahr, J. C. 153
Malaria, Atypical Forms, ... 82
Medical Ethics, 61, 143.
Medical Society, the County 232
Medicine, Internal and Special Surgery ..301
Meeting, 18th Annual 24
Melvin, Elizabeth 11

Meningitis, Cerebral 218
McAlester, J. S. 167
...cCormack's Dr., Itinerary 138
Modern Research 78
Montgomery, A. B., ...49
Mook, William H., ...408
Moorman, L. J., 342, 413.
Murmurs, Cardiac 342

Negro, the Physical Characteristics of, ...337
Nephritis, Chronic 63
New Orleans Clinics 22
Noble, F. W. 16

Obstetrics, Modern Trend of 262
Obstetrical Surgery 252
Ochsner, E. H. 245
Officers of County Societies, ...42
Oklahoma, Dependent Children of, ...258
Oldham, I. B., 88, 156.
Ophthalmia Neonotorum 256

Pathology, General 11
Pearse, Herman E., ...188
Pediatrics 8
Perforation, Typhoid 88
Personal Notes, 29, 75, 109, 137, 168,
    209, 275, 316, 349.
Pemberton, R. K., ...82
Physicians Duty to Self 369
Pneumonia, Broncho 270
Pneumococcus in the Eye 59
Poliomyelitis, 153, 201.
Practice of Medicine 13

Practitioner, the General 213
Pregnancy, Extra Uterine 156
Program 19th Annual Meeting 420
Prostatectomy, Suprapubic 16
Puerperum, Insanity of, ...43
Puckett, Carl 258
Pyloric Obstruction 383

Reed, Horace 323
Redfield, H. H. 310
Renfrow, T. F. 120
Repair of Perineum 252
Respiratory Tract, Diseases of 116
Research, Modern 78
Riley, John W. 360

Sanberg, Eric 129
Scott, C. T., ...411
Scott, J. H, ...357
Sectional Lines, Elimination of 67
Secret, the Medical and Venereal Di-
    seases 129
Septic Infections 245
Skin Affections and Vaccines 408
Skin, Carcinoma of, ...177
Sleep, Disorders of, ...289
Splint, Internal in Fractures 188
Sterilization of the Unfit 312
Suprapubic Prostatectomy 16
Surgery, Special, etc., ...301
Surgery, Obstetrical 252
Surgical, Difficult Cases, ...292
Surgical Section, Address of Chairman....5

Surgical Treatment 146
Syphilis, "606" in, ...306

Thermogenesis 334
Thompson, M. K., ...256
Thrailkill, G. H. 334
Thrush 296
Tilly, W. T., ...221
Tongue, the Human 406
Trigg, J. M. 252
Treatment of Diabetes 111
Treatment of Hernia 124
Treatment of Fracture 188
Treatment of Bone Tuberculosis 146
Treatment of Extra Uterine Pregnancy 156
Treatment of Syphilis 306
Tuberculosis of Fallopian Tubes 360
Tuberculosis, Women's Clubs, and 132

Typhoid and Modern Research 78
Typhoid, Diagnosis and Treatment of
    Perforation 88
Typhoid, Vaccination In, ...360

Vaccines and Certain Skin Affections 408
Vaccines in Typhoid 360

Watkins, J. C. 224
Watson, L. F. 92
West, A. K., 78, 401.
White, J. H., 88, 156, 299.
White, A. C., ... 63
Williams, H. M. 8
Williams, T. S. 371
Williams, Tom A., ...381
Willour, L. S., 58, 193, 270.

Young, A. D. 289

This Space For Sale

DR. RALPH V. SMITH
SURGEON

PHONE NO. 237   GUTHRIE, OKLAHOMA
OFFICE PHONE 8   RESIDENCE PHONE 3

W. ALBERT COOK, M. D.
PRACTICE LIMITED TO
EYE, EAR, NOSE AND THROAT—GLASSES FITTED
308 AND 309 FIRST NATIONAL BLDG.

HOURS: 9 TO 12—1:30 TO 5.   TULSA, OKLA.

E. S. LAIN, M. D.   M. M. ROLAND, M. D.
OFFICE PHONE 619
DRS. LAIN & ROLAND
PRACTICE LIMITED TO DISEASES OF
SKIN, X-RAY AND ELECTRO-THERAPY
SUITE 707 STATE NATIONAL BANK BUILDING
OKLAHOMA CITY, OKLA.

DR. S. R. CUNNINGHAM
PRACTICE LIMITED TO
SURGERY AND DISEASES OF WOMEN
PHONE 158

MAIN AND HARVEY   OKLAHOMA CITY, OKLA.

OKLAHOMA PASTEUR INSTITUTE
OKLAHOMA CITY, OKLA.
FOR THE
PREVENTATIVE TREATMENT OF HYDROPHOBIA
S. L. MORGAN, M. D., DIRECTOR.

411 WEST RENO AVENUE.   L. D. 'PHONE 3311

OFFICE HOURS: 10 TO 12 A. M., AND 2 TO 4 P. M.

SUNDAY HOURS: 10 TO 11 A. M., AND 3 TO 4 P. M.

W. E. DICKEN, M. D.
SURGEON AND GYNECOLOGIST
OFFICE 312, 313, 314 AMERICAN NATIONAL BANK BUILDING.   PHONE 483.
OKLAHOMA CITY, OKLA.
RESIDENCE, 410 W. 10TH STREET, PHONE 484.

L. HAYNES BUXTON   H. COULTER TODD
DRS. BUXTON & TODD
PRACTICE LIMITED TO DISEASES OF
EYE, EAR, NOSE, THROAT
OKLAHOMA CITY, OKLA.

DR. ANTONIO D. YOUNG
DISEASES OF THE MIND AND NERVOUS SYSTEM
SECURITY BUILDING   OKLAHOMA CITY, OKLA.
LONG DISTANCE 'PHONE 384-X

DR. F. H. CLARK
(FORMERLY OF DRS. HATCHETT AND CLARK)
GENERAL SURGEON
FIRST NATIONAL BANK BLDG.   EL RENO, OKLA.

PRACTICE LIMITED TO DISEASES OF
EYE, EAR, NOSE AND THROAT.
DR. R. D. McHENRY
COLCORD BUILDING   OKLAHOMA CITY, OKLAHOMA
OFFICE PHONES: MAIN 194-X—RESIDENCE 6684.

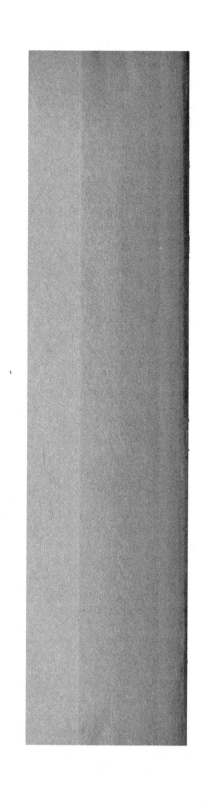

www.ingramcontent.com/pod-product-compliance
Lightning Source LLC
Chambersburg PA
CBHW071356050326
40689CB00010B/1671